a LANGE clinical manual

D0460279

Neonatology.

Management, Procedures, On-Call Problems, Diseases, and Drugs

fifth edition

Editor

Tricia Lacy Gomella, MD
Part-Time Assistant Professor of Pediatrics
The Johns Hopkins University School of Medicine
Baltimore, Maryland

Associate Editors

M. Douglas Cunningham, MD
Clinical Professor, Division of Neonatology
Department of Pediatrics
College of Medicine
University of California, Irvine
Vice President for Special Projects
Pediatrix Medical Group
Orange, California

Fabien G. Eyal, MD
Professor of Pediatrics
Chief and Louise Lenoir Locke Professor of Neonatology
Medical Director, Intensive Care Nurseries
University of South Alabama Children's and Women's Hospital
Mobile, Alabama

Karin E. Zenk, PharmD, FASHP
Practice Consultant and Associate Clinical Professor of Pediatrics
College of Medicine
University of California, Irvine,
Irvine, California

Lange Medical Books/McGraw-Hill
Medical Publishing Division

New York Chicago San Francisco Lisbon London Madrid Mexico City
New Delhi San Juan Seoul Singapore Sydney Toronto

Notice

Medicine is an ever-changing science. As new research and clinical experience broaden our knowledge, changes in treatment and drug therapy are required. The authors and the publisher of this work have checked with sources believed to be reliable in their efforts to provide information that is complete and generally in accord with the standards accepted at the time of publication. However, in view of the possibility of human error or changes in medical sciences, neither the authors nor the publisher nor any other party who has been involved in the preparation or publication of this work warrants that the information contained herein is in every respect accurate or complete, and they disclaim all responsibility for any errors or omissions or for the results obtained from use of the information contained in this work. Readers are encouraged to confirm the information contained herein with other sources. For example and in particular, readers are advised to check the product information sheet included in the package of each drug they plan to administer to be certain that the information contained in this work is accurate and that changes have not been made in the recommended dose or in the contra-indications for administration. This recommendation is of particular importance in connection with new or infrequently used drugs.

This book was set by PineTree Composition
The editors were Janet Foltin, Harriet Lebowitz, and Barbara Holton
The production supervisor was Richard Ruzycka
The cover designer was Mary Scudlarek
The index was prepared by Benjamin Tedoff
R. R. Donnelley, Inc. was the printer and binder.

This book is printed on acid-free paper.

To my twin sons, Leonard and Patrick, and singletons, Andrew and Michael

Contents

Contributors

Marilee C. Allen, MD
Professor of Pediatrics, Associate Director of Neonatology
The Johns Hopkins University School of Medicine
Co-Director of NICU Clinic, Konnedy–Kreiger Institute
Baltimore, Maryland
Follow-up of High-Risk Infants; Counseling Parents Before High Risk Delivery

Gad Alpan, MD
Professor, Department of Pediatrics
New York Medical College
The Regional Neonatal Center
Westchester Medical Center
Valhalla, New York
Patent Ductus Arteriosus, Persistent Pulmonary Hypertension of the Newborn, Infant of a Drug Abusing Mother

Hubert Ballard, MD
Fellow, Division of Neonatology
University of Kentucky Medical Center and Children's Hospital
Lexington, Kentucky
Apnea and Periodic Breathing

Fayez Bany-Mohammed, MD
Assistant Clinical Professor
Division of Neonatology
Department of Pediatrics, College of Medicine
University of California, Irvine
Irvine, California
Hyaline Membrane Disease

Daniel A. Beals, MD
Associate Professor
Division of Pediatric Surgery
University of Kentucky College of Medicine
Lexington, Kentucky
Neonatal Bioethics

Pasquale Casale, MD
Chief Resident, Department of Urology,
Thomas Jefferson University
Philadelphia, Pennsylvania
Renal Diseases

Carol M. Cottrill, MD
Pediatric Cardiologist
Professor Emeritus- University of Kentucky
Lexington, Kentucky
Central Baptist Hospital
Lexington, Kentucky
Arrhythmia; Congenital Heart Disease

M. Douglas Cunningham, MD
Clinical Professor, Division of Neonatology, Department of Pediatrics
College of Medicine, University of California, Irvine
Vice President for Special Projects, Pediatrix Medical Group, Inc.
Orange, California
Exchange Transfusion, Hydrocephalus, Intraventricular Hemorrhage

Nirmala S. Desai, MD
Professor of Pediatrics
Division of Neonatology
University of Kentucky Medical Center and Children's Hospital
Lexington, Kentucky
Intrauterine Growth Retardation (Small for Gestational Age Infant)
Nutritional Management, Management of the Extremely Low Birth Weight Infant
During the First Week of Life

Fabien G. Eyal, MD
Professor of Pediatrics, Division of Neonatology
Chief and Louis Lenoir Locke Professor of Neonatology
Medical Director, Intensive Care Nurseries
USA Children's and Women's Hospital
Mobile, Alabama
Temperature Regulation, Sedation and Analgesia in a Neonate, Anemia

T. Ernesto Figueroa, MD
Chief, Pediatric Urology
Alfred I. duPont Hospital for Children
Wilmington, Delaware
Associate Professor of Urology
Jefferson Medical College
Thomas Jefferson University
Philadelphia, Pennsylvania
Renal Diseases

Catherine A. Finnegan MS, CRNP
Neonatal Nurse Practitioner
Department of Neonatology
Johns Hopkins Bayview Medical Center
Baltimore, Maryland
Percutaneous Central Venous Catheterization

Maureen M. Gilmore, MD
Assistant Professor of Pediatrics
Johns Hopkins University
Director of Neonatology and Medical Director of NICU
The Johns Hopkins Bayview Medical Center,
Baltimore, Maryland.
Death of an Infant; Hyperbilirubinemia, Direct (Conjugated Hyperbilirubinemia);
Hyperbilirubinemia, Indirect (Unconjugated Hyperbilirubinemia); Hyperglycemia;
Hypoglycemia; Is the Baby Ready for Discharge? No Stool in 48 Hours; No Urine
Output in 48 Hours; Pulmonary Hemorrhage; Traumatic Delivery

W. Christopher Golden, MD
Instructor, Department of Pediatrics
The Johns Hopkins University School of Medicine
Baltimore, Maryland
Eye Discharge (Conjunctivitis), Hypertension, Seizure Activity

Tricia Lacy Gomella, MD
Part-time Assistant Professor of Pediatrics
The Johns Hopkins University School of Medicine
Baltimore, Maryland
Assessment of Gestational Age, Newborn Physical Examination, Procedures, On Call Problems, Transient Tachypnea of the Newborn

Janet E. Graeber, M. D.
Associate Professor of Pediatrics
Chief, Section of Neonatology
West Virginia University School of Medicine
Robert C. Byrd Health Science Center
Department of Pediatrics, Morgantown WV
Retinopathy of Prematurity

Deborah Grider, RN
Nurse Clinician, Neonatal Intensive Care Unit
University of Kentucky Medical Center and Children's Hospital
Lexington, Kentucky
Management of the Extremely Low Birth Weight Infant During the First Week of Life

George Gross, MD
Professor of Radiology
Director, Division of Pediatric Radiology
University of Maryland Medical System
Department of Diagnostic Radiology
Baltimore, Maryland
Neonatal Radiology

Wayne Hachey, DO, LTC, USA
Assistant Chief of Pediatrics
Chief, Newborn Medicine
Tripler Army Medical Center
Program Director, Neonatal-Perinatal Medicine
Tripler Army Medical Center/Kapiolani Medical Center
for Women and Children
Assistant Clinical Professor, Department of Pediatrics
John A. Burns Assistant Professor of Pediatrics
Trippler Army Medical Center
Uniformed Services
University of the Health Sciences
F. Edward Herbert School of Medicine
Trippler Army Medical Center
Honolulu, Hawaii
Meconium Aspiration

Bryan D. Hall, MD
Professor Emeritus
Division of Genetics and Dysmorphology
Department of Pediatrics
College of Medicine
University of Kentucky
Lexington, Kentucky
Common Multiple Congenital Anomaly Syndromes

Charles R. Hamm, Jr., MD
Associate Professor of Pediatrics, Division of Neonatology
University of South Alabama Children's and Women's Hospital
Mobile, Alabama
Respiratory Management

C. Kirby Heritage, MD
Pediatrix Medical Group
Miami Valley Hospital
Dayton, Ohio
Infant of a Diabetic Mother

H. Jane Huffnagle, DO
Associate Professor of Anesthesiology
Thomas Jefferson University
Philadelphia, Pennsylvania
Obstetric Anesthesia and the Neonate

Beverly Johnson, RN, BSN, CIC
Infection Control Practitioner, Kaiser Permanente Hospital
Fontana, California
Isolation Guidelines

William G. Keyes, MD, PhD
Medical Staff Vice-President
Children's Health Care of Atlanta
Atlanta, Georgia
Multiple Gestation

Janine Kruger, MD
Clinical Assistant Professor
Department of Obstetrics and Gynecology
University of Wisconsin
Madison, Wisconsin
Prenatal Testing

Christoph U. Lehmann, MD
Assistant Professor
Eudowood Neonatal Pulmonary Division and Division of Health Information Sciences
Department of Pediatrics
The Johns Hopkins University School of Medicine
Baltimore, Maryland
Studies for Neurologic Evaluation

Drew Litzenberger, MD
Co-Director, NICU
Mission and St. Joseph's Health System
Asheville, North Carolina
Infant Transport

Janet Murphy, MD
Associate Professor of Pediatrics
Division of Neonatology
Department of Pediatrics
University of Washington
Seattle, Washington
Resuscitation of the Newborn

Ronald Naglie, MD
Attending Neonatologist , Pediatrix Medical Group, Inc.
Medical Director, Neonatal Intensive Care Unit
Saddleback Memorial Medical Center
Laguna Hills, California
Infectious Diseases

Jeanne S. Nunez, MD
Attending Neonatologist
The Johns Hopkins University Bayview Medical Center
Clinical Associate, The Johns Hopkins University School of Medicine
Baltimore, Maryland
Abnormal Blood Gas, Apnea and Bradycardia, Bloody Stool, Cyanosis, Gastric Aspirate, Gastrointestinal Bleeding from the Upper Tract, Hyperkalemia, Hypokalemia, Hyponatremia, Hypotension and Shock, Pneumoperitoneum, Pneumothorax, Poor Perfusion, PostDelivery Antibiotics, Vasospasms, Polycythemia

Ambadas Pathak, MD
Assistant Professor, Emeritus of Pediatrics
The Johns Hopkins University School of Medicine
Clinical Associate Professor of Pediatrics
University of Maryland School of Medicine
Baltimore, Maryland
Neonatal Seizures

Keith J. Peevy, JD, MD
Professor of Pediatrics
Division of Neonatology
USA Children's and Women's Hospital
Mobile, Alabama
Polycythemia and Hyperviscosity

Andrew R. Pulito, MD
Professor and Chief, Division of Pediatric Surgery
University of Kentucky College of Medicine
Lexington, Kentucky
Surgical Diseases of the Newborn

Rakesh Rao, MD
Fellow, Division of Neonatology
University of Kentucky Medical Center and Children's Hospital
Lexington, Kentucky
Nutritional Management

Tracey Robinson, RN
ECMO Coordinator
Neonatal Intensive Care Unit
University of Kentucky Medical Center and Children's Hospital
Lexington, Kentucky
Management of the Extremely Low Birth Weight Infant During the First Week of Life

Jack H. Sills, MD
Clinical Professor, Division of Neonatology
Department of Pediatrics, College of Medicine
University of California, Irvine
Irvine, California
Perinatal Asphyxia

Galdino Silva-Neto, MD
Assistant Professor of Clinical Pediatrics, Division of Neonatology
Department of Pediatrics, University of Miami
Miami, Florida
Attending Neonatologist, Pediatrix Medical Group, Inc.,
Broward General Medical Center
Fort Lauderdale, Florida
*Fluids and Electrolytes, Rickets and Disorders of Calcium
and Magnesium Metabolism*

Lizette Sistoza, MD
Fellow, Division of Neonatology
University of Kentucky Medical Center and Children's Hospital,
Lexington, Kentucky
Air Leak Syndromes

Kendra Smith, MD
Assistant Professor
Division of Neonatology
Department of Pediatrics
University of Washington
Seattle, Washington
ECMO

Ganesh Srinivasan, MD
Fellow, Division of Neonatology, University of Kentucky
Medical Center and Children's Hospital
Lexington, Kentucky
Thyroid Disorders

Christiane Theda, MD
Assistant Professor, Department of Pediatrics,
The Johns Hopkins University School of Medicine,
Baltimore, Maryland
Neonatologist and Medical Geneticist
Johns Hopkins Hospital
Baltimore, Maryland
Frederick Memorial Hospital
Frederick, Maryland
*Ambiguous Genitalia, Inborn Errors of Metabolism with Acute Neonatal Onset,
Neural Tube Defects*

Jorge E. Tolosa MD, MS
Assistant Professor, Obstetrics and Gynecology
Director, Division of Research in Reproductive Health
Department of Obstetrics and Gynecology
Thomas Jefferson University
Philadelphia, Pennsylvania
Prenatal Testing

Cherry C. Uy, MD
Assistant Clinical Professor, Division of Neonatology
Department of Pediatrics, College of Medicine
University of California, Irvine
Irvine, California
Hyperbilirubinemia

Feizal Waffarn, MD
Professor and Chairman
Department of Pediatrics and Chief, Division of Neonatology
College of Medicine, University of California, Irvine
Irvine, California
Necrotizing Enterocolitis

Richard Whitehurst, Jr., MD
Associate Professor of Pediatrics, Division of Neonatology
Assistant Professor of Pharmacology
USA Children's and Women's Hospital
Division of Neonatology
Mobile, Alabama
ABO Incompatibility, Rh Incompatibility

Jacki Williamson, RNC, CPNP, MSN
Clinical Nurse Specialist, Neonatal Services,
Kaiser Permanente Hospital
Fontana, California
Isolation Guidelines

Karin E. Zenk, PharmD, FASHP
Practice Consultant and Associate Clinical Professor of Pediatrics
College of Medicine
University of California, Irvine
Irvine, California
*Commonly Used Medications, Effects of Drugs and Substance on Lactation and
Breastfeeding, Effects of Drugs and Substances Taken during Pregnancy,
Emergency Medications and Therapy for Neonates*

Michael M. Zayek, MD
Associate Professor of Pediatrics, Division of Neonatology
USA Children's and Women's Hospital
Mobile, Alabama
Bronchopulmonary Dysplasia, Thrombocytopenia and Platelet Dysfunction

Preface

I am pleased to present the fifth edition of *Neonatology*. The manual continues to be widely accepted both in the United States and internationally. It has been translated into many languages including Russian, Spanish, Portuguese, and Polish, to name a few. This wide acceptance is only made possible because of the contributions of our outstanding group of associate editors and contributors.

As the specialty of Neonatology continues to advance we have updated all chapters in the book. Many concepts are well established and remain a cornerstone of the book. Our tradition of noting areas of controversy in the field of neonatology continues. In order to maintain balance, contributors and editors represent a cross section of neonatal practice in the United States.

I would like to thank all contributors to this and previous editions of the book, the editorial staff at McGraw-Hill, and my family for their continued support of this project. In particular, Dr. George Dover, Chairman of Pediatrics at Johns Hopkins is acknowledged for his academic support.

I welcome suggestions and comments about this manual. Letters should be addressed to:

Tricia Gomella, MD
c/o McGraw-Hill Medical Publishers
Two Penn Plaza, 12th Floor
New York, NY 10121-2298

Tricia Lacy Gomella, MD
August, 2003

1 Prenatal Testing

PRENATAL DIAGNOSIS

I. **First-trimester screening.** Maternal serum can be analyzed for certain biochemical markers that, in combination with ultrasound measurement of the fetal nuchal translucency, can be used to calculate a risk assessment for trisomies 18 and 21. In the first trimester, these serum markers are the free β-human chorionic gonadotropin (hCG) and pregnancy-associated plasma protein A (PAPP-A). It is an effective screening tool, with a detection rate of 87–92% for trisomy 21 and fewer false-positive results than the traditional triple-screen test (alpha-fetoprotein [AFP], unconjugated estriol, and hCG). First-trimester screening is performed between 10 and 13 weeks' gestation and requires confirmation of a chromosomal abnormality by an invasive genetic test (usually chorionic villus sampling [CVS]).

II. **Second-trimester screening.** Two common second-trimester tests are the maternal serum AFP (MSAFP) and the triple-screen test. The MSAFP is a sensitive marker for open neural tube defects, whereas the triple-screen test yields a risk assessment for open neural tube defects as well as trisomies 18 and 21. These tests are usually performed between 15 and 20 weeks' gestation and require an invasive test to confirm the diagnosis of a chromosomal abnormality (usually amniocentesis). The usefulness of the triple-screen test is limited by its high number of false-positive test results.

III. **Ultrasound testing.** Ultrasound examination is used in the following circumstances.

   A. **Calculation of gestational age.** Measurement of the crown-rump length between 8 and 12 weeks' gestation allows for the most accurate assessment of gestational age, to within 5–7 days. After the first trimester, a combination of biparietal diameter, head circumference, abdominal circumference, and femur length is used to estimate gestational age and fetal weight. Measurements in the second trimester are accurate to within approximately 2 weeks and in the third trimester to within 3 weeks.

   B. **Anatomic survey.** A large number of congenital anomalies can be diagnosed reliably by ultrasonography, including anencephaly, hydrocephalus, congenital heart disease, gastroschisis, omphalocele, spina bifida, renal anomalies, diaphragmatic hernia, cleft lip and palate, and skeletal dysplasia. Identification of these anomalies before birth can help determine the safest type of delivery and the support personnel needed. Ultrasonography can also aid in determining fetal gender.

   C. **Assessment of growth and fetal weight.** Ultrasonography is useful to detect and monitor both intrauterine growth restriction (IUGR) and fetal macrosomia. Estimation of fetal weight is also important in counseling patients regarding expectations after delivering a premature infant.

   D. **Assessment of amniotic fluid volume**
      1. **Oligohydramnios (decreased amniotic fluid).** This is associated with a major anomaly in 15% of cases. Rupture of membranes is the most common cause of oligohydramnios. Other causes include placental insufficiency, renal anomalies, bladder outlet obstruction, karyotypic abnormalities, and severe cardiac disease. The kidneys and the bladder can be seen with ultrasonography at ~14 weeks' gestation.
      2. **Polyhydramnios (hydramnios) (excess of amniotic fluid).** Polyhydramnios is associated with major anomalies in 15% of cases. It is associated with gestational diabetes, anencephaly, neural tube defects, bowel ob-

struction such as duodenal atresia, multiple gestation, nonimmune hydrops fetalis, and exstrophy of the bladder.
   E. **Assessment of placental location and presence of retroplacental hemorrhage.** This is useful in suspected cases of placenta previa or abruptio placentae.
   F. **Diagnosis of multiple pregnancy and determination of chorionicity.** The determination of chorionicity is made by examination of the fetal membranes and is best done by 14 weeks' gestation.
   G. **Determination of pregnancy viability.** This is important in the first trimester, when fetal heart motion can be detected at 6–7 weeks' gestation. It is also important in the case of a suspected fetal demise later in pregnancy.
   H. **Assessment of fetal well-being:**
      1. **Biophysical profile.** Ultrasonography is used to assess fetal movements and breathing activity.
      2. **Doppler studies.** Doppler ultrasonography of fetal vessels, particularly the umbilical artery, is a useful adjunct in the management of high-risk pregnancies, especially those complicated by IUGR. Changes in the vascular Doppler pattern (ie, absent or reversed end-diastolic flow in the umbilical artery) signal a deterioration in placental function and possibly a worsening fetal condition. The use of Doppler ultrasonography has been associated with a 38–50% decrease in perinatal mortality in high-risk pregnancies; however, no benefit in using this technique to screen a low-risk population has been proven.
   I. **Visual guidance for procedures such as amniocentesis, CVS, percutaneous umbilical blood sampling (PUBS), and some fetal surgeries (eg, placement of bladder or chest shunts).**
IV. **Amniocentesis.** Amniotic fluid can be analyzed for prenatal diagnosis of karyotypic abnormalities, in fetuses diagnosed with congenital defects, to determine fetal lung maturity, to monitor the degree of isoimmunization by measurement of the content of bilirubin in the fluid, and for the diagnosis of chorioamnionitis. Testing for karyotypic and congenital abnormalities is usually done at 16–20 weeks' gestation. A sample of amniotic fluid is removed under ultrasound guidance. Fetal cells in the fluid can be grown in tissue culture for genetic study. With visual guidance from the ultrasonogram, the pregnancy loss rate related to amniocentesis is usually quoted at between 0.3% and 0.5%. Early amniocentesis (before 13 weeks) is associated with a higher rate of fetal loss. This is indicated

   • In women older than 35 years, because of the increased incidence of aneuploidy (ie, trisomies 13, 18, and 21).
   • In those who have already had a child with a chromosomal abnormality.
   • In those in whom X-linked disorders are suspected.
   • To rule out inborn errors of metabolism.

V. **Chorionic villus sampling.** CVS is a technique for first-trimester genetic studies. Chorionic villi are withdrawn either through a needle inserted through the abdomen and into the placenta or through a catheter inserted through the vagina and cervix into the placenta. The cells obtained are identical to those of the fetus and are grown and analyzed. CVS can be performed in the first trimester (usually between 10 and 12 weeks' gestation). Results can be obtained more quickly than with other methods via fluorescence in situ hybridization (FISH) rapid chromosome analysis, thus enabling the patient to have a diagnosis before the end of the first trimester. Indications are the same as for amniocentesis. Reported complications after CVS can include pregnancy loss and limb abnormalities; however, if CVS is performed after 70 days' gestation, there is no increased incidence of limb reduction defects. Pregnancy loss rates after CVS are usually quoted as ranging from 0.6–0.8% but are highly operator dependent.
VI. **Percutaneous umbilical blood sampling.** Under ultrasound guidance, a needle is placed transabdominally into the umbilical vein. Samples of fetal blood can be obtained for karyotype, viral studies, fetal blood type, and hematocrit. This also

provides a route for in utero transfusion. This technique is most often used in cases of fetal hydrops.

ANTEPARTUM TESTS OF FETAL WELL-BEING

I. **Nonstress test.** The nonstress test (NST) is used to detect intact fetal brainstem function. Fetal well-being is confirmed if the baseline heart rate is normal and there are periodic increases in the fetal heart rate. These accelerations are often associated with fetal movement. The following guidelines can be used, although there may be variations between institutions.
   A. **Reactive NST.** In a 20-min monitoring period, there are at least two accelerations of the fetal heart rate 15 beats/min above the baseline fetal heart rate; each acceleration lasts at least 15 s.
   B. **Nonreactive NST.** Fetal heart rate does not meet the criteria just mentioned during a prolonged period of monitoring (usually at least 1 h). *Note:* There are many causes of a nonreactive NST besides fetal compromise, including a fetal sleep cycle, chronic maternal smoking, and exposure to medications such as central nervous system depressants and propranolol. Because of this low specificity, a nonreactive NST should be followed by more definitive testing such as a biophysical profile or a contraction stress test.
II. **Biophysical profile.** The biophysical profile (Table 1–1) is another test used to assess fetal well-being, often when the NST has been nonreactive. An NST is performed along with an ultrasound examination to evaluate fetal breathing movements, gross body movements, tone, and amniotic fluid volume. A score of 8–10 is considered normal, 4–6 indicates possible fetal compromise, and 0–2 predicts high perinatal mortality. This test has not been adequately assessed at early gestational ages.
III. **Contraction stress test.** The contraction stress test (CST) is used to assess a fetus at risk for uteroplacental insufficiency. A monitor is placed on the mother's abdomen to continuously record the fetal heart rate and uterine contractions. An adequate test consists of at least three contractions, each lasting at least 40–60 s, within a period of 10 min. If sufficient contractions do not occur spontaneously, the mother is instructed to perform nipple stimulation or oxytocin is administered by intravenous pump. If oxytocin is needed to produce contractions for the CST, it is called an oxytocin challenge test (OCT). Normally, the fetal heart rate increases in response to a contraction, and no decelerations occur during or after the contraction. If late decelerations occur during or after contractions, uteroplacental insufficiency may be present. The CST is contraindicated in patients with placenta previa, those who have had a previous cesarean section with a vertical incision, and those with high-risk factors for preterm delivery (ie, premature rupture of membranes or incompetent cervix). Test results are interpreted as follows:

TABLE 1–1. BIOPHYSICAL PROFILE SCORING SYSTEM USED TO ASSESS FETAL WELL-BEING

Variable	Normal (2)	Abnormal (0)
Fetal breathing	One episode >30 s in 30 min	None or episode <30 s in 30 min
Body movement	Three or more movements in 30 min	Two or less movements in 30 min
Fetal tone	One episode or active limb or trunk extension with flexion	No movement
Nonstress test	Reactive	Nonreactive
Amniotic fluid	One pocket of amniotic fluid 1 cm or more	No fluid pockets or pocket <1 cm

Based on guidelines from Manning FA et al: Fetal biophysical profile scoring: a prospective study in 1184 high-risk patients. *Am J Obstet Gynecol* 1981;140:289. Reprinted with permission from Elsevier Science

A. **Negative (normal) test.** No late decelerations occur during adequate uterine contractions. The baseline fetal heart rate is normal. This result is associated with a very low perinatal mortality rate in the week after the test.
B. **Positive (abnormal) test.** Late decelerations occur with at least two of three contractions over a 10-min interval. This result can signify poor fetal outcome, and depending on gestational age, delivery is usually recommended.
C. **Equivocal (suspicious) test.** A late deceleration occurs with one of three contractions over a 10-min interval. Prolonged fetal monitoring is usually recommended.

INTRAPARTUM TESTS OF FETAL WELL-BEING

I. **Fetal heart rate monitoring.** Continuous fetal heart rate monitoring has been the standard clinical practice since the 1970s. However, it has not been shown to improve perinatal mortality compared with intermittent auscultation of the fetal heart rate. The only clear benefit to continuous fetal monitoring in labor is a decrease in neonatal seizures. An abnormal fetal heart rate pattern is 50% predictive of low Apgar scores. Fetal heart rate monitoring may be internal, with an electrode attached to the fetal scalp, or external, with a monitor attached to the maternal abdomen. The baseline heart rate, beat-to-beat variability, and long-term variability are measured.
   A. **Baseline fetal heart rate.** The baseline fetal heart rate is the rate that is maintained apart from periodic variations. The normal fetal heart rate is 110–160 beats/min. Fetal tachycardia is present at 160 beats/min or more. Causes of fetal tachycardia include maternal or fetal infection, fetal hypoxia, thyrotoxicosis, and maternal use of drugs such as parasympathetic blockers or beta-mimetic agents. Moderate fetal bradycardia is defined as a heart rate of 90–110 beats/min with normal variability. Severe fetal bradycardia is a heart rate of <90 beats/min. Common causes of bradycardia include hypoxia, complete heart block, and maternal use of drugs such as β-blockers.
   B. **Variability.** Fetal heart rate variability has traditionally been broken down into categories of short-term (beat-to-beat) and long-term variability, although for most practical purposes they are assessed together. In the normal mature fetus, there are slight rapid fluctuations in the interval between beats (beat-to-beat variability). This indicates a functioning sympathetic–parasympathetic nervous system interaction. An amplitude range (baseline variability) >6 beats/min indicates normal beat-to-beat variability and suggests the absence of fetal hypoxia. Absence of variability may be caused by severe hypoxia, anencephaly, complete heart block, and maternal use of drugs such as narcotics or magnesium sulfate. Long-term variability refers to fluctuations in the fetal heart rate over longer periods of time (minutes rather than seconds).
   C. **Accelerations.** Accelerations are often associated with fetal movement and are an indication of fetal well-being.
   D. **Decelerations.** There are three types of decelerations (Figure 1–1).
      1. **Early decelerations.** Early decelerations (decelerations resulting from physiologic head compression) occur secondary to vagal reflex tone, which follows minor, transient fetal hypoxic episodes. These are benign and are not associated with fetal compromise.
      2. **Late decelerations.** Two types of late decelerations exist.
         a. **Late decelerations with maintained beat-to-beat variability.** These are seen in the setting of normal fetal heart rate variability. They are associated with a sudden insult (eg, maternal hypotension) that affects a normally oxygenated fetus and signifies uteroplacental insufficiency. The normal variability of the fetal heart rate signifies that the fetus is physiologically compensated.
         b. **Late decelerations with decreased beat-to-beat variability.** These are associated with decreased or absent fetal heart rate variability.

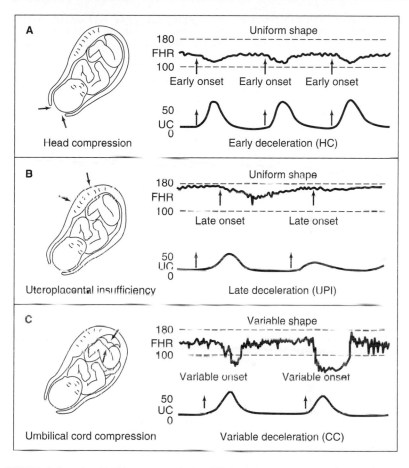

FIGURE 1-1. Examples of fetal heart rate monitoring. FHR, Fetal heart rate (beats per minute); UC, uterine contraction (mm Hg); HC, head compression; UPI, uteroplacental insufficiency; CC, cord compression. *(Modified and reproduced, from McCrann JR, Schifrin BS: Fetal monitoring in high-risk pregnancy. Clin Perinatol 1974;1:149 with permission from Elsevier Science.)*

They may represent fetal hypoxia resulting from uteroplacental insufficiency. Maneuvers such as maternal oxygen supplementation and maternal positioning in the left lateral decubitus position may improve fetal oxygenation and placental circulation and should be attempted.

3. **Variable decelerations.** These are most frequently associated with umbilical cord compression. They are classified as severe when the fetal heart rate decreases to <60 beats/min, the deceleration is longer than 60 s in duration, or the fetal heart rate is 60 beats/min below baseline. If beat-to-beat variability is maintained, the fetus is compensated physiologically and oxygenated normally.

II. **Fetal scalp blood sampling.** Fetal scalp blood sampling is used during labor to determine the fetal acid-base status when the fetal heart rate tracing is non-reassuring or equivocal. This procedure can be performed only after rupture of membranes. It is contraindicated in cases of possible blood dyscrasias in the fetus and with maternal infections caused by herpesvirus or HIV. A blood sample is obtained from the fetal presenting part (usually the scalp but sometimes the buttocks), and the fetal blood pH is determined. A pH of ≥7.25 has been shown to correlate (with 92% accuracy) with a 2-min Apgar score of ≥7. The protocol for interpreting fetal scalp blood pH varies among institutions. Complications of this test are scalp infections (in <1% of infants) and soft tissue damage to the scalp. An example of one such protocol is as follows.

A. pH ≥7.20. Fetus is not acidotic; no intervention required.

B. pH 7.10–7.19. Fetus is preacidotic. Repeat sampling in 15–20 min.

C. pH <7.10. Fetus may be acidotic. Delivery is indicated.

III. **Scalp stimulation/vibroacoustic stimulation.** An acceleration in fetal heart rate in response to either manual stimulation of the fetal presenting part or vibroacoustic stimulation through the maternal abdomen has been associated with a fetal pH of >7.20. These tests are often used in labor to determine fetal well-being in lieu of a scalp blood sampling; however, a lack of fetal response to stimulation is not predictive of acidemia.

IV. **Fetal pulse oximetry.** This promising new technique is designed as an adjunct to nonreassuring fetal heart rate tracings in order to reduce the number of unnecessary interventions. A normal fetal oxygen saturation as measured by pulse oximetry (Spo_2) is 30–70%. A pulse oximetry reading of at least 30% has good correlation with a fetal pH of at least 7.20. Long-term studies are still needed to evaluate this technique.

TESTS OF FETAL LUNG MATURITY

I. **Lecithin-sphingomyelin (L-S) ratio.** Lecithin, a saturated phosphatidylcholine (the condensation product of a phosphatidic acid and choline), can be measured specifically in amniotic fluid and is a principal active component of surfactant. It is manufactured by type II alveolar cells. Sphingomyelin is a phospholipid found predominantly in body tissues other than the lungs. The L-S ratio compares levels of lecithin, which increase in late gestation, with levels of sphingomyelin, which remain constant. The L-S ratio is usually 1:1 by 31–32 weeks' gestation and 2:1 by 35 weeks' gestation. The following are guidelines to L-S ratios.

• L-S ≥ 2:1: Lungs are mature (98% accuracy). Only 2% of these infants will experience respiratory distress syndrome (RDS).
• L-S = 1.5–1.9:1: 50% of infants will experience RDS.
• L-S <1.5:1: 73% of infants will experience RDS.

Some disorders are associated with delayed lung maturation, and higher than normal L-S ratios may be needed before fetal lung maturity is ensured. The two most common disorders are diabetes mellitus (an L-S ratio of 3:1 is usually accepted as indicating maturity) and Rh isoimmunization associated with hydrops fetalis. Acceleration of fetal lung maturity is seen in sickle cell disease, maternal narcotic addiction, prolonged rupture of membranes, chronic maternal hypertension, intrauterine growth restriction, and placental infarction. Differences may also occur in various racial groups.

II. **Phosphatidylglycerol.** Phosphatidylglycerol appears in amniotic fluid at ~35 weeks, and levels increase at 37–40 weeks. This substance is a useful marker for lung maturation late in pregnancy. It is reported as either present or absent.

III. **TDx fetal lung maturity (TDx FLM).** This test (Abbott Laboratories, North Chicago, IL) measures the relative concentrations of surfactant and albumin (milligrams of surfactant per gram of albumin) in amniotic fluid and gives a result that helps assess fetal lung maturity. TDx FLM has several advantages over L-S ratio: (1) Less technical expertise is required; (2) this test can be performed more easily; and (3) results are obtained more quickly. Results are interpreted in the following ways.

- 30–70 mg/g: The infant is at risk for immature lungs. Other conditions may weigh more heavily on the decision to deliver early.
- >70 mg/g: The likelihood of RDS is small.

REFERENCES

Boehm FH: Intrapartum fetal heart rate monitoring. *Obstet Gynecol Clin North Am* 1999;26:623.

Dildy GA: Fetal pulse oximetry: current issues. *J Perinat Med* 2001;29:5.

Krantz DA et al: First-trimester Down syndrome screening using dried blood chemistry and nuchal translucency. *Obstet Gynecol* 2000;96:207.

Manning FA et al: Fetal biophysical profile scoring: a prospective study in 1184 high-risk patients. *Am J Obstet Gynecol* 1981;140:289.

Porter TF et al: Vibroacoustic and scalp stimulation. *Obstet Gynecol Clin North Am* 1999;26:657.

Russell JC et al: Multicenter evaluation of TDx test for assessing fetal lung maturity. *Clin Chem* 1989;35:1005.

Wilson RD: Amniocentesis and chorionic villus sampling. *Curr Opin Obstet Gynecol* 2000;12:81.

2 Delivery Room Management

OBSTETRIC ANESTHESIA AND THE NEONATE

During birth, the status of the fetus can be influenced by obstetric analgesia and anesthesia. Care in choosing analgesic and anesthetic agents can often prevent respiratory depression in the newborn, especially in high-risk deliveries.

I. **Placental transfer of drugs.** Drugs administered to the mother may affect the fetus via placental transfer or, less commonly, may cause a maternal disorder that affects the fetus (eg, maternal drug-induced hypotension may cause fetal hypoxia). All anesthetic and analgesic drugs cross the placenta to some degree. Flow-dependent passive diffusion is the usual mechanism.

Most anesthetic and analgesic drugs have a high degree of lipid solubility, a low molecular weight (<500), and variable protein-binding and ionization capabilities. These characteristics lead to rapid transfer across the placenta. Local anesthetics and narcotics (lipid-soluble, un-ionized) cross the placenta easily, whereas neuromuscular blocking agents (highly ionized) are transferred slowly.

II. **Analgesia in labor**
   A. **Inhalation analgesia.** Inhalation analgesia is rarely used in the United States. Entonox (50% oxygen and 50% nitrous oxide) is widely used in other countries.
   B. **Pudendal block and paracervical block.** Paracervical block may be associated with severe fetal bradycardia caused by uterine vasoconstriction and is now rarely used. If a paracervical block is performed, the fetal heart rate must be monitored. Pudendal blocks have little direct effect on the fetus. However, seizures have been reported after both pudendal and paracervical blocks. Paracervical blocks are used in the first stage of labor and pudendal blocks in the second stage.
   C. **Opioids.** All intravenously administered opioids are rapidly transferred to the fetus and cause dose-related respiratory depression and alterations in the Apgar and neurobehavioral scores.
      1. **Meperidine (Demerol)** can cause severe neonatal depression (measured by Apgar scoring) if the drug is administered 2–3 h before delivery (Kuhnert, 1979). Depression is manifested as respiratory acidosis, decreased oxygen saturation, decreased minute ventilation, and increased time to sustained respiration. Fetal normeperidine (a meperidine metabolite that may cause significant respiratory depression) increases with longer intervals between drug administration and delivery. Levels are highest 4 h after intravenous administration of the drug to the mother. The half-life of meperidine is 13 h in neonates, whereas that of normeperidine is 62 h (Kuhnert, 1985b).
      2. **Morphine** has a delayed onset of action and may cause greater neonatal respiratory depression than meperidine (Jouppila, 1982).
      3. **Butorphanol (Stadol)** and **nalbuphine (Nubain)** are agonist-antagonist narcotic agents that cause less respiratory depression than morphine, particularly when used in high doses.
   D. **Opioid antagonist (naloxone [Narcan]).** Naloxone should never be administered to neonates of women who have received chronic opioid therapy over a long period because it may precipitate acute withdrawal symptoms. Naloxone may be used to reverse respiratory depression caused by acute maternal opioid administration during labor.
   E. **Sedatives and tranquilizers**
      1. **Barbiturates.** Barbiturates cross the placenta rapidly and can have pronounced neonatal effects (eg, somnolence, flaccidity, hypoventilation, and failure to feed) lasting for days. Effects are intensified if opioids are used

simultaneously. This is usually not an issue when barbiturates are used as an induction to general anesthesia for an emergent cesarean delivery.
2. **Benzodiazepines (diazepam [Valium], lorazepam [Ativan], and midazolam [Versed]).** These agents cross the placenta rapidly and equilibrate within minutes after intravenous administration. Fetal levels are often higher than maternal levels. Diazepam given in low doses (<10 mg) may cause decreased beat-to-beat variability and tone but has little effect on Apgar scores and blood gas levels. Larger doses of diazepam may persist for days and can cause hypotonia, lethargy, decreased feeding, and impaired thermoregulation, with resulting hypothermia. All benzodiazepines share these features; however, diazepam is the most thoroughly studied of the benzodiazepine series. In addition, benzodiazepines are less frequently used because they induce childbirth amnesia in the mother. Midazolam may be used to induce general anesthesia. Anesthetic induction with midazolam is safe for the mother, although low 1-min Apgar scores and transient neonatal hypotonia may be seen (Ravlo, 1989).
3. **Phenothiazines.** Phenothiazines are rarely used today, because they may induce hypotension via central alpha blockade. Phenothiazines are sometimes combined with a narcotic (neuroleptanalgesia). Innovar, a combination drug containing the narcotics fentanyl and droperidol, may be safe because of the relatively short half-life of the agents.
4. **Ketamine (Ketaject and many others).** Ketamine may be used for dissociative analgesia. Doses >1 mg/kg may cause neonatal depression and uterine hypotonia. Doses normally used in labor (0.1–0.2 mg/kg) are relatively safe, producing minimal effects in the mother and the neonate.

F. **Lumbar epidural analgesia.** Lumbar epidural analgesia is the most frequently used invasive anesthetic technique for childbirth. Maternal pain and catecholamine levels are reduced (catecholamines cause prolonged incoordinate labor and decreased uterine blood flow), which may lead to diminished maternal hyperventilation and improved fetal oxygen delivery. Vasospasm of uterine arteries in pregnancy-induced hypertension may be corrected (Jouppila, 1982; Shnider, 1979). Labor epidural analgesia lasting longer than 4 h is associated with maternal temperature increases of up to 1 °C. This may lead to neonatal sepsis evaluation and antibiotic treatment if these treatments are done on the basis of intrapartum maternal temperature (Lieberman, 1997).

Local anesthetic (eg, bupivacaine, lidocaine) is usually continuously infused through an epidural catheter placed in the L2–L3 interspace. Alternatively, repeated injections through the catheter may be used. Small doses of an opioid may be added; these have no effect on the neonate. Maternal hypotension caused by sympathetic blockade is easily treated with fluid administration or intravenous ephedrine.

G. **Intrathecal opioid analgesia.** Intrathecal opioids (sufentanil or fentanyl with or without morphine) provide first-stage labor analgesia with minimal motor and sympathetic nerve block. Intrathecal opioids are frequently administered when the fetal head is still high in the pelvis. Transient fetal heart rate changes occur in 10–15% of cases, usually without adverse neonatal outcome (Cohen, 1993), although cesarean delivery has been necessary in some cases (Gambling, 1998).

H. **Caudal epidural analgesia.** Caudal epidural analgesia blocks the sacral nerve roots and provides excellent pain relief in the second stage of labor. Caudal analgesia is not used during the first stage of labor because the large doses needed to block the T11–T12 nerve roots increase pelvic muscle relaxation and impair fetal head rotation. Because fetal intracranial local anesthetic injection can occur, this technique is now rarely used.

I. **Local anesthetics.** All of the regional anesthetic/analgesic techniques (eg, epidural or spinal) and local blocks (eg, pudendal) depend on the use of local anesthetic agents. Bupivacaine is the most commonly used agent because of its longer half-life.

1. **Lidocaine (Xylocaine).** Placental transfer of lidocaine is significant, but Apgar scores are not affected in healthy neonates (Abboud, 1982). Acidotic fetuses accumulate larger amounts of lidocaine through pH-induced ion trapping.

2. **Bupivacaine (Marcaine).** Bupivacaine is theoretically less harmful than lidocaine for the fetus because it has a higher degree of ionization and protein binding than lidocaine. Maternal toxicity leading to convulsions and cardiac arrest has been reported after inadvertent intravascular injection. Bupivacaine, in very low concentrations, is the most commonly used local anesthetic agent for continuous labor analgesia.

3. **Chloroprocaine (Nesacaine).** After systemic absorption, chloroprocaine is rapidly broken down by pseudocholinesterase; thus, very little reaches the placenta or fetus. Neurobehavioral studies indicate no difference between controls and neonates whose mothers were given chloroprocaine. However, because of its short duration and significant motor blockade, chloroprocaine is not useful for continuous labor analgesia.

4. **Ropivacaine (Naropin).** Ropivacaine, a new agent, is similar to bupivacaine but produces less motor block and maternal cardiotoxicity. Neurologic and adaptive capacity scores are somewhat better in infants whose mothers received epidural ropivacaine rather than bupivacaine for labor analgesia (Stienstra, 1995).

J. **Psychoprophylaxis.** The **Lamaze technique** of prepared childbirth involves class instruction for prospective parents. The process of childbirth is explained, and exercises, breathing techniques, and relaxation techniques are taught to relieve labor pain. However, the popular assumption that the neonate benefits if the mother receives no drugs during childbirth may not be true. Pain and discomfort may cause psychological stress and hyperventilation in the mother, which can negatively impact the neonate; supplemental anesthesia may be needed. Approximately 50–70% of women who have learned the Lamaze method request drugs or an anesthetic block during labor. **Other analgesic techniques** include transcutaneous electric nerve stimulation (TENS), hypnosis, and acupuncture.

III. **Anesthesia for cesarean delivery.** Aortocaval compression may decrease placental perfusion; the mother should be positioned supine with the bed tilted left side down. Regional anesthesia is the technique of choice for most cesarean deliveries because it is generally safer for both mother and baby. If *immediate* delivery is indicated, general anesthesia is often used because it has the shortest induction time, although neonates do as well with regional anesthesia (Marx, 1984).

A. **Spinal anesthesia.** Spinal anesthesia (injection of local anesthetic directly into the cerebrospinal fluid) requires one tenth the drug needed for epidural anesthesia (drug injection into the epidural space). Maternal and fetal drug levels are low. Hypotension may occur rapidly but can be attenuated by administering 1.5–2.0 L of balanced salt solution intravenously or infusing prophylactic intravenous ephedrine. Anesthesia is induced more rapidly with spinal than with epidural anesthesia. Abnormalities in Early Neonatal Neurobehavioral Scores (ENNS) (see p 12) are more common after general anesthesia than spinal anesthesia for cesarean delivery.

B. **Lumbar epidural anesthesia.** Placental transfer of local anesthetics occurs, but drug effects can be detected only by neurobehavioral testing. Maternal hypotension may occur but to a lesser extent than with spinal anesthesia.

C. **General anesthesia.** General anesthesia is used in the following circumstances: strong patient preference, emergency delivery (eg, in cases of hemorrhage or fetal bradycardia), and contraindications to regional anesthesia (eg, maternal coagulopathy, maternal neurologic problems, sepsis, or infection). After induction of anesthesia, the mother is maintained on a combination of nitrous oxide and oxygen with low doses of inhaled halogenated agents or intravenous drugs. Opioids or benzodiazepines are rarely given until the cord is clamped.

1. **Agents used in general obstetric anesthesia**
   a. **Premedication.** Cimetidine (Tagamet) or ranitidine (Zantac) (H_2 receptor antagonists) may be used to decrease gastric volume and increase gastric pH to help prevent aspiration pneumonitis. Metoclopramide (Reglan) may be given to speed gastric emptying. The neonate is not affected by these agents. Premedications traditionally used in surgery (eg, atropinics, opioids, and benzodiazepines) are rarely given.
   b. **Thiopental (Pentothal).** Thiopental (4 mg/kg) may be used to induce general anesthesia. Peak fetal concentrations occur within 2–3 min. Apgar scores are not affected by thiopental at the 4-mg/kg dose. Metabolites may affect the neonatal electroencephalogram (EEG) for several days and depress the sucking response.
   c. **Ketamine.** Ketamine (1 mg/kg) is used to induce anesthesia, although it is usually reserved for severe asthmatics (because of its bronchodilator properties) and patients with mild to moderate hypovolemia when cesarean delivery is emergent. Neonatal neurobehavioral test scores after ketamine administration are slightly better than those after thiopental administration.
   d. **Muscle relaxants.** Muscle relaxants, which are highly ionized, cross the placenta in small amounts and have little effect on the neonate.
      i. **Succinylcholine (Anectine and many others)** crosses the placenta in minimal amounts. In twice-normal doses, it is detectable in the fetus, but no respiratory effects are seen until the dose is 5 times normal or both mother and fetus have abnormal pseudocholinesterase.
      ii. **Atracurium (Tracrium), cisatracurium (Nimbex), vecuronium (Norcuron), and rocuronium (Zemuron)** are medium-duration nondepolarizing muscle relaxants. In clinical doses, an insufficient amount of drug crosses the placenta to affect the neonate.
      iii. **Pancuronium (Pavulon) and tubocurarine (Tubarine)** are long-duration muscle relaxants that do not affect the neonate when administered in clinical doses.
   e. **Nitrous oxide** has rapid placental transfer. Prolonged administration of high (>50%) concentrations of nitrous oxide can result in low Apgar scores because of neonatal anesthesia and diffusion hypoxia. Concentrations up to 50% are safe, but neonates may need supplemental oxygen after delivery, especially if the interval between anesthetic induction and delivery is long.
   f. **Halogenated anesthetic agents** (isoflurane [Forane], enflurane [Ethrane], sevoflurane [Ultane], desflurane [Suprane], and halothane [Fluothane]) are used to maintain general anesthesia. Beneficial effects include decreased catecholamines, increased uterine blood flow, and improved maternal anesthesia compared with nitrous oxide alone. Low concentrations of these agents rarely cause neonatal anesthesia. If anesthesia occurs, it is transient because these volatile agents are readily exhaled. High concentrations may decrease uterine contractility. The lowest effective concentration is chosen, and the agent is promptly discontinued after delivery to decrease uterine atony and prevent excessive blood loss.
2. **Neonatal effects of general anesthesia.** Maternal hypoxia resulting from aspiration or failed endotracheal intubation can cause fetal hypoxia. Maternal hyperventilation ($Paco_2$ <20 mm Hg) decreases placental blood flow and shifts the maternal oxyhemoglobin curve to the left, which can lead to fetal hypoxia and acidosis. Fetal oxygen saturation increases with increases in maternal oxygen partial pressure up to a maternal Pao_2 of 300 mm Hg.
3. **Interval between incision of the uterus and delivery.** Incision and manipulation of the uterus cause reflex uterine vasoconstriction, resulting in

fetal asphyxia. Long intervals between uterine incision and delivery (>90 s) are associated with significant lowering of Apgar scores. If the interval is longer than 180 s, low Apgar scores and fetal acidosis result (Datta, 1981). Regional anesthesia decreases reflex vasoconstriction; therefore, the incision-to-delivery interval is less important. The interval may be prolonged with breech, multiple, or preterm delivery; if there is uterine scarring; or if the fetus is large.

4. **Regional versus general anesthesia**
   a. **Apgar scores.** Early studies showed that neonates were less depressed on 1- and 5-min Apgar scores with regional compared with general anesthesia. New general anesthetic techniques lower Apgar scores at 1 min only. This represents transient sedation (ie, temporary neonatal general anesthesia) rather than asphyxia. If the interval between induction and delivery is short, there is less difference between the effects of regional and general anesthesia. If a prolonged delivery time is anticipated, regional anesthesia is preferred because the neonate is less sedated. It is important to note that low Apgar scores secondary to sedation do not have the negative prognostic value of low Apgar scores secondary to asphyxia, provided that the neonate is adequately resuscitated.
   b. **Acid-base status.** The differences in acid-base status are minimal and probably not significant. Infants of diabetic mothers may be less acidotic with general than with regional anesthesia because regional anesthesia-induced hypotension may exacerbate any existing uteroplacental insufficiency.
   c. **Neurobehavioral examinations** are used to detect subtle changes in the neonate in the first few hours after birth. After delivery, there is a 1-h period of alertness, followed by a 3- to 4-h period of deep sleep and decreased responsiveness. The **ENNS** was initially developed to detect neurobehavioral changes 2–8 h after birth (the half-life of most local anesthetics). These changes are usually manifested as decreased tone in an otherwise alert infant. The **Neonatal Neurologic and Adaptive Capacity Score (NNACS)** uses portions of the ENNS, Brazelton Neonatal Behavioral Assessment Scale, and Amiel-Tison Neurologic Examination. This score is more weighted toward assessment of neonatal tone and is helpful in differentiating abnormalities caused by birth trauma rather than drug effects. Early neurobehavioral examinations show clear-cut advantages of regional compared with general anesthesia. Although infants of mothers receiving spinal and epidural anesthesia had similar results at 15 min, by 2 h the epidural group had lower scores. This probably reflects higher local anesthetic uptake. There are no significant differences in long-term studies comparing regional and general anesthesia of meperidine on the newborn.

RESUSCITATION OF THE NEWBORN

Approximately 4 million infants are born in the United States each year in about 5000 hospitals with delivery services. Resuscitation is required for the majority of the 30,000 preterm infants with a birth weight <1500 g and for an unspecified number of additional infants weighing >1500 g with a variety of problems. This results in approximately 10% of all newborns requiring some resuscitative effort at birth (Kattwinkel, 2000). Newborn resuscitation cannot always be anticipated in time to transfer the mother before delivery to a facility with specialized neonatal support. Therefore, every hospital with a delivery suite should have an organized, skilled resuscitation team and appropriate equipment available (Table 2–1) (Ballard, 1998; Kattwinkel, 2000).

TABLE 2-1. EQUIPMENT FOR NEONATAL RESUSCITATION

STANDARD EQUIPMENT SETUP
Radiant warmer
Stethoscope
Oxygen source with warmer and humidifier
Suction source, suction catheter, and meconium "aspirators"
Nasogastric tubes
Apparatus for bag-and-mask ventilation
Ventilation masks
Laryngoscope (handles, blades, and batteries)
Endotracheal tubes (2.5, 3.0, 3.5, and 4.0 mm)
Intravenous fluids (10% dextrose, normal saline, and Ringer's lactate)
Drugs
    Epinephrine (1:10,000 solution)
    Naloxone hydrochloride (0.4 or 1.0 mg/mL)
    Sodium bicarbonate (0.5 mEq/mL)
    Volume expanders (5% albumin, 0 negative whole blood [cross-matched against the mother's blood])
Clock
Syringes, hypodermic needles, and tubes for collection of blood samples
Equipment for umbilical vessel catheterization
Micro–blood gas analysis availability
Warm blankets
ADDITIONAL EQUIPMENT SETUP
All of the above plus the following:
    Pressure manometer for use during ventilation
    Oxygen blender
    Heart rate and blood gas monitoring equipment
    Umbilical vessel catheter setup (ready to insert)
    Transcutaneous oxygen tension or saturation monitor
    Blood gas laboratory immediately available
    Apgar timer
    Camera
    Plastic bags for "micro-preemies"
    Humidified gas

I. **Normal physiologic events at birth.** Normal transitional events at birth begin with initial lung expansion, generally requiring large, negative intrathoracic pressures, followed by a cry (expiration against a partially closed glottis). Umbilical cord clamping is accompanied by a rise in blood pressure and massive stimulation of the sympathetic nervous system. With onset of respiration and lung expansion, pulmonary vascular resistance decreases, followed by a gradual transition (over minutes to hours) from fetal to adult circulation, with closure of the foramen ovale and ductus arteriosus.

II. **Abnormal physiologic events at birth.** The asphyxiated newborn undergoes an abnormal transition. A rhesus monkey model has been used to study changes in physiologic parameters during asphyxiation and resuscitation (Dawes, 1968). Shortly after acute asphyxiation (the cord is clamped while the head is held in a bag filled with saline), the monkey fetus has primary apnea, during which spontaneous respirations can be induced by appropriate sensory stimuli. This lasts for ~1 min, and the fetus then begins deep gasping for 4–5 min, ending with the "last gasp." This is followed by a period of **secondary apnea,** during which spontaneous respirations cannot be induced by sensory stimuli. Death occurs if secondary apnea is not reversed by vigorous ventilatory support within several minutes. Because one can never be certain whether an apneic newborn has primary or secondary apnea, resuscitative efforts should proceed as though secondary apnea is present. This experimental model of acute total asphyxia is comparable to an umbilical cord prolapse. A more common clinical occurrence is prolonged partial asphyxia (eg, with maternal hemorrhage or severe placental insufficiency).

Resuscitative measures are the same for both clinical scenarios, but the outcome is often worse after prolonged partial asphyxia in utero.

III. **Preparation for high-risk delivery.** Preparation for a high-risk delivery is often the key to a successful outcome. Cooperation between the obstetric and pediatric staff is important. Knowledge of potential high-risk situations and appropriate interventions is essential (Table 2–2). It is useful to have an estimation of weight and gestational age, so that drug dosages can be calculated and the appropriate endotracheal tube and umbilical catheter size can be chosen (Table 2–3). While waiting for the infant to arrive, it is useful to think through potential problems, steps that may be undertaken to correct them, and which member of the team will handle each step. Provided there is both time and opportunity, resuscitative measures should be discussed with the parents. This is particularly important when the fetus is at the limit of viability or when life-threatening anomalies are anticipated (On-Call Problem 32 "Counseling parents before high risk delivery").

IV. **Assessment of the need for resuscitation.** The Apgar score (Appendix B) is assigned at 1, 5, and, occasionally, 10–20 min after delivery. It gives a fairly objective retrospective idea of how much resuscitation a term infant required at birth and the infant's response to resuscitative efforts. It is not particularly useful during resuscitation. During those long, tense moments, simultaneous assessment of heart rate, skin color, and respiratory activity provides the quickest and most accurate evaluation of the need for continuing resuscitation. For preterm infants, Apgar scores may be particularly misleading (even in assessment of the response to resuscitation) because of developmental differences in tone and response to stimulation.

A. **Heart rate.** The heart rate is ideally monitored by a cardiotachometer via electrodes taped to the chest. Most often, however, evaluation is done by listening to the apical beat or feeling the pulse by lightly grasping the base of the umbilical cord. The evaluator should tap out each beat so that all team members can hear it. If no heart rate can be heard or felt, ventilatory efforts should be halted for a few seconds so that this finding can be verified by another team member.

B. **Skin color.** Assessment of skin color may be difficult when there is severe bruising, especially in preterm infants. Marked acrocyanosis may also complicate the picture. Looking at the mucous membranes of the mouth may be helpful under these circumstances. Bluish coloring indicates central cyanosis, and oxygen supplementation or assisted ventilation is needed. Pinkish membranes indicate normal oxygen levels, and resuscitation may not be needed.

C. **Respiratory activity.** Respiratory activity is assessed by observing chest movement or listening for breath sounds. If there is no respiratory effort or the effort is poor, the infant needs respiratory assistance by either manual stimulation or bag-and-mask ventilation.

V. **Technique of resuscitation.** The American Heart Association (AHA) and American Academy of Pediatrics' (AAP) *Textbook of Neonatal Resuscitation* (Kattwinkel, 2000) provides the standard of care used in most neonatal intensive care units (NICUs) for the resuscitation of newborns.

TABLE 2–2. SOME HIGH-RISK SITUATIONS FOR WHICH RESUSCITATION MAY BE ANTICIPATED

High-risk situation	Primary intervention
Preterm delivery	Intubation, lung expansion
Thick meconium	Endotracheal suction
Acute fetal or placental hemorrhage	Volume expansion
Use of narcotics in labor	Administration of naloxone
Hydrops fetalis	Intubation, paracentesis, or thoracentesis
Polyhydramnios: gastrointestinal obstruction	Nasogastric suction
Oligohydramnios: pulmonary hypoplasia	Intubation, lung expansion
Maternal infection	Administration of antibiotics
Maternal diabetes	Early glucose administration

TABLE 2-3. EXPECTED BIRTH WEIGHT (50TH PERCENTILE) AT 24-38 WEEKS' GESTATION

Gestational age (weeks)	Birth weight (g)
24	700
26	900
28	1100
30	1350
32	1650
34	2100
36	2600
38	3000

Based on data published in Battaglia FC, Lubchenco LO: A practical classification of newborn infants by weight and gestational age. J Pediatr 1967;71:159.

A. Ventilatory resuscitation

1. General measures

a. **Suctioning.** First, nasal and oropharyngeal secretions should be partially removed with a brief period of suctioning using either a bulb syringe or a suction catheter. More prolonged suctioning delays resuscitation and may cause a profound vagal response in the infant (Cordero, 1971).

b. **Mechanical ventilation.** Most infants can be adequately ventilated with a bag and mask provided that the mask is the correct size with a close seal around the mouth and nose and there is appropriate flow of oxygen to the bag (Figure 2-1). The stomach should be emptied during and after prolonged bag-and-mask ventilation.

c. **Endotracheal intubation.** Endotracheal intubation should be performed when indicated. However, multiple unsuccessful attempts at intubation by inexperienced persons may make a difficult situation worse. In these cases, it may be best to continue mask ventilation until experienced help arrives. Absolute indications for aggressive ventilatory support with endotracheal intubation are difficult to list here because institutional guidelines and clinical situations vary widely. The procedure for endotracheal intubation and some general guidelines are discussed in Chapter 20. Table 2-4 provides guidelines for endotracheal tube selection.

2. Specific measures

a. **Term infant with meconium staining.** Infants born through thick meconium may aspirate this inflammatory material in utero (gasping), during delivery, or immediately after birth. The sickest of these infants have usually aspirated in utero and generally also have reactive pulmonary vasoconstriction. Gregory and associates (1974) were among the first to show that endotracheal suctioning at birth was beneficial. More recently, the AAP and the AHA recommended endotracheal suctioning when meconium is present in the amniotic fluid and the infant is not vigorous (eg, without good muscle tone, good respirations, and heart rate >100 beats/min). **Clinical judgment** is always important in deciding whether or not aggressive endotracheal suctioning is necessary. Meconium aspiration is discussed in detail in Chapter 74.

    i. **Hypopharyngeal suctioning should be started as soon as the head is delivered, before the infant has started to cry.** Deep suctioning should be avoided because it may result in acute laryngospasm.

    ii. **Endotracheal suctioning.** Subsequently, **endotracheal intubation is performed, and suction is applied directly to the endotracheal tube.** Suctioning with a negative pressure of 80-100 mm Hg can be done directly from the wall unit via a connector (meco-

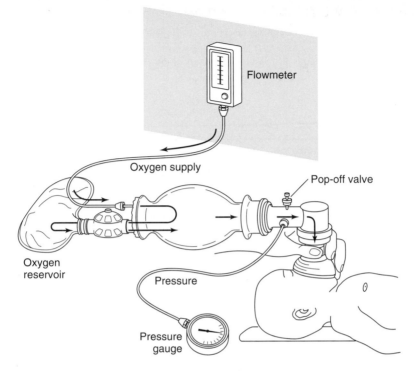

FIGURE 2-1. Bag-and-mask ventilation of the neonate.

nium aspirator) to the endotracheal tube. Suction is applied as the endotracheal tube is slowly withdrawn (Kattwinkel, 2000).

iii. **If meconium has been suctioned "below the cords," suctioning should be repeated after reintubation.** Prolonged or repeated suctioning is not recommended because it will exacerbate the pre-existing asphyxial insult.

iv. **The procedures just described may be continued for up to 2 min after delivery, but then other resuscitative measures (particularly ventilation and oxygenation) must be started.**

TABLE 2-4. GUIDELINES FOR ENDOTRACHEAL TUBE SIZE AND DEPTH OF INSERTION BASED ON WEIGHT AND GESTATIONAL AGE

Weight (g)	Gestational age (weeks)	Endotracheal tube size, inside diameter (mm)	Depth of insertion (cm from upper lip)
<1000	<28	2.5	6–7
1000–2000	28–34	3.0	7–8
2000–3000	34–38	3.5	8–9
>3000	>38	3.5–4.0	9–10

Based on guidelines from Bloom RS, Cropley C: *Textbook of Neonatal Resuscitation.* American Heart Association/American Academy of Pediatrics, 1995.

v. **Supplemental oxygen.** Infants born through thick meconium may have experienced prolonged partial asphyxia in utero as well as pulmonary vascular constriction, leading to pulmonary hypertension after delivery. It is wise, therefore, to provide generous amounts of supplemental oxygen to these infants.

vi. **If meconium-stained fluid** is reported at <34 weeks' gestation, one of the following situations should be suspected.

- The fetus is a growth-retarded term infant.
- The fluid may actually be purulent (consider *Listeria* or *Pseudomonas*).
- The fluid may actually be bile stained (consider proximal intestinal obstruction)

b. **Term infant with perinatal asphyxia**

i. **A term infant with a heart rate of <100 beats/min and no spontaneous respiratory activity requires immediate lung expansion and supplemental oxygen provided by bag-and-mask ventilation.** Initially, the lungs should be **slowly** expanded (5–10 breaths) with high peak inflating pressures (30–40 cm H_2O). If this is not successful in stimulating spontaneous respiratory effort or an improved heart rate, the ventilation rate should be increased to 40–60 breaths/min and peak inflating pressures should be adjusted as necessary to expand the lungs. If bag-and-mask ventilation is ineffective or prolonged positive-pressure ventilation is necessary, endotracheal intubation is indicated. If effective spontaneous respiratory effort results, the infant may be extubated and closely observed while breathing supplemental oxygen.

ii. **A term infant with a heart rate of >100 beats/min but with poor skin color and weak respiratory activity requires stimulation (rubbing the back is often effective), supplemental oxygen blown across the face, and occasionally bag-and-mask ventilation to expand the lungs.** Most of these infants will respond with improved skin color and good spontaneous respiratory effort by 5 min of age.

c. **Preterm infant.** Preterm infants weighing <1200 g most often require immediate lung expansion in the delivery room. Ventilatory support measures should proceed as described for the asphyxiated term infant, with several important differences.

i. If intubation is required, a smaller (2.5- or 3-mm internal diameter) endotracheal tube is selected.

ii. Although high peak inflating pressures may initially be needed to expand the lungs, as soon as the lungs "open up" the pressure should be quickly decreased to as low as 10–15 cm H_2O by the end of the resuscitation if the clinical course permits.

iii. If available, one of several forms of liquid surfactant may be administered intratracheally as prophylaxis for hyaline membrane disease (see Chapters 6 and 74). However, surfactant is not a resuscitative medication and should be administered only to a stable neonate with a correctly placed endotracheal tube.

B. **Cardiac resuscitation.** During delivery room resuscitation, efforts should be directed first to assisting ventilation and providing supplemental oxygen. A sluggish heart rate will usually respond to these efforts.

1. **If the heart rate continues to be <60 beats/min by 30 s of age in spite of ventilatory assistance, chest compression should be initiated.** The thumbs are placed on the midsternum just below a line connecting the nipples, while the palms of the hands encircle the torso and support the back (Figure 2–2). The sternum is compressed ½–¾ in (1.3–1.9 cm) at a regular rate of 90 compressions/min, while ventilating the infant at 30 breaths/min.

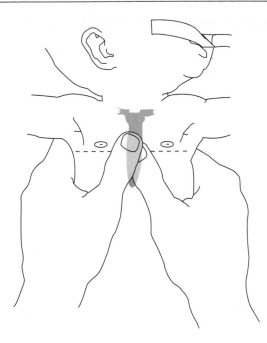

FIGURE 2–2. Technique of external cardiac massage (chest compression) in the neonate. Note the position of the thumbs on the midsternum, just below the midline.

The heart rate should be checked periodically and chest compression discontinued when the heart rate is >60 beats/min.

2. **An infant with no heart rate (a true Apgar of 0) who does not respond to ventilation and oxygenation may be considered stillborn.** Prolonged resuscitative efforts are a matter for ethical consideration (Jain, 1991; Kattwinkel, 2000).

C. **Drugs used in resuscitation.** (See also Emergency Medications and Therapy for Neonates, inside the front and back covers.) The *Textbook of Neonatal Resuscitation* recommends giving medications if the heart rate remains <60 beats/min despite adequate ventilation and chest compressions for a minimum of 30 s.

1. **Route of administration**
   a. **The endotracheal tube** is the fastest route for administration of epinephrine in the delivery room (Lindemann, 1982). Absorption may be impaired if the tube is obstructed or malpositioned.
   b. **The umbilical vein** is the preferred route for drug administration in the delivery room. A No. 3.5 or 5 French umbilical catheter should be inserted just until blood is easily withdrawn (usually <5 cm); this should avoid inadvertent placement in the hepatic or portal vein.
   c. **Alternate routes** of administration include peripheral venous and interosseous routes.

2. **Drugs**
   a. **Epinephrine** may be necessary during resuscitation when adequate ventilation, oxygenation, and chest compression have failed and the heart rate is still <60 beats/min. This drug causes peripheral vasoconstriction, enhances cardiac contractility, and increases heart rate. The

dose is 0.1–0.3 mL/kg of 1:10,000 solution given intravenously or by endotracheal tube. This may be repeated every 3–5 min. If an endotracheal tube is used, the solution should be diluted 1:1 with normal saline.
   b. **Volume expanders.** Hypovolemia should be suspected in any infant requiring resuscitation, particularly when there is evidence of acute blood loss with extreme pallor despite adequate oxygenation, poor peripheral pulse volume despite a normal heart rate, long capillary refill times, or poor response to resuscitative efforts. Appropriate volume expanders include O-negative whole blood (cross-matched against the mother's blood), 10 mL/kg; Ringer's lactate, 10 mL/kg; and normal saline, 10 mL/kg. All are given intravenously over a 5- to 10-min period.
   c. **Naloxone hydrochloride.** Naloxone (Narcan) is a narcotic antagonist and should be administered to an infant with respiratory depression unresponsive to ventilatory assistance whose mother has received narcotics within 4 h before delivery. One major exception to this recommendation is the newborn infant of a drug-addicted mother. These infants should never receive Narcan because acute withdrawal symptoms may develop. The intravenous or intratracheal dosage for Narcan is 0.1 mg/kg. Two concentrations of naloxone are available: 0.4 mg/mL and 1.0 mg/mL. The dose may be repeated every 5 min as necessary (AAP Committee on Drugs, 1989). It should be emphasized that the half-life of Narcan is shorter than that of narcotics.
   d. **Dextrose.** The blood glucose concentration should be checked within 30 min after delivery in asphyxiated term infants, infants of diabetic mothers, and preterm infants, especially those whose mothers received tocolysis with ritodrine. Large boluses of dextrose should be avoided, even when the blood sugar is <25 mg/dL. To avoid wide swings in blood glucose, give a small bolus of 10% dextrose in water (1–2 mL/kg intravenously) and then begin an intravenous infusion of 10% dextrose at a rate of 4–6 mg/kg/min (80–100 mL/kg/day).
   e. **Sodium bicarbonate** is usually not useful during the acute phase of neonatal resuscitation. Without adequate ventilation and oxygenation, it will not improve the blood pH. After prolonged resuscitation, however, sodium bicarbonate may be useful in correcting documented metabolic acidosis. Give 1–2 mEq/kg intravenously (usually over a period of 30 min).
   f. **Atropine and calcium.** Although previously used during resuscitation of the asphyxiated newborn, atropine and calcium are no longer recommended by the AAP or the AHA. Current evidence does not support their effectiveness during delivery room resuscitation.
D. **Other supportive measures**
   1. **Temperature regulation.** Although some degree of cooling in a newborn infant is desirable because it provides a normal stimulus to respiratory effort, excessive cooling increases oxygen consumption and exacerbates acidosis. This is a problem especially for preterm infants, who have thin skin, decreased stores of body fat, and increased body surface area. Heat loss may be prevented by the following measures.
      a. **Dry the infant thoroughly immediately after delivery.**
      b. **Maintain a warm delivery room.**
      c. **Place the infant under a prewarmed radiant warmer.** (See also Chapter 5.) Cover preterm infants with plastic wrap or a plastic bag up to the neck.
   2. **Preparation of the parents for resuscitation.** Initial resuscitation usually occurs in the delivery room with one or both parents present. It is helpful to prepare the parents in advance, if possible. Describe what will be done, who will be present, who will explain what is happening, where the resuscitation will take place, where the father should stand, why crying may not be heard, and where the infant will be taken after stabilization.

REFERENCES

Abboud TK et al: Maternal, fetal, and neonatal responses after epidural anesthesia with bupivacaine, 2-chloroprocaine, or lidocaine. *Anesth Analg* 1982;61:638.

American Academy of Pediatrics Committee on Drugs: Emergency drug doses for infants and children and naloxone use in newborns: clarification. *Pediatrics* 1989;83:803.

Ballard RA: Resuscitation in the delivery room. In Taeusch HW, Ballard RA (eds): *Avery's Diseases of the Newborn*, 7th ed. WB Saunders, 1998.

Benson RC et al: Fetal compromise during elective cesarean section. *Am J Obstet Gynecol* 1965;91:645.

Bland BAR et al: Comparison of midazolam and thiopental for rapid sequence induction for elective cesarean section. *Anesth Analg* 1987;66:1165.

Caritis SN et al: Fetal acid-base state following spinal or epidural anesthesia for cesarean section. *Obstet Gynecol* 1980;56:610.

Cohen SE et al: Intrathecal sufentanil for labor analgesia—sensory changes, side effects, and fetal heart rate changes. *Anesth Analg* 1993;77:1155.

Cordero L Jr, Hon EH: Neonatal bradycardia following nasopharyngeal stimulation. *J Pediatr* 1971;78:441.

Datta S et al: Neonatal effect of prolonged anesthetic induction for cesarean section. *Obstet Gynecol* 1981;58:331.

Dawes GS: *Foetal & Neonatal Physiology*. Year Book, 1968.

Dubowitz LM et al: Clinical assessment of gestational age in the newborn infant. *J Pediatr* 1970;77:1.

Gambling DA et al: A randomized study of combined spinal-epidural analgesia versus intravenous meperidine during labor. *Anesthesiology* 1998;89:1336.

Gregory GA et al: Meconium aspiration in infants: a prospective study. *J Pediatr* 1974;85:848.

Jain L et al: Cardiopulmonary resuscitation of apparently stillborn infants: survival and long-term outcome. *J Pediatr* 1991;118:778.

Jouppila P et al: Lumbar epidural analgesia to improve intervillous blood flow during labor in severe preeclampsia. *Obstet Gynecol* 1982;59:158.

Kang YG et al: Prophylactic intravenous ephedrine infusion during spinal anesthesia for cesarean section. *Anesth Analg* 1982;61:839.

Kattwinkel J: *Textbook of Neonatal Resuscitation*, 4th ed. American Heart Association and American Academy of Pediatrics, 2000.

Kuhnert BR et al: Disposition of meperidine and normeperidine following multiple doses during labor: II. Fetus and neonate. *Am J Obstet Gynecol* 1985a;151:410.

Kuhnert BR et al: Effects of low doses of meperidine on neonatal behavior. *Anesth Analg* 1985b;64:335.

Kuhnert BR et al: Meperidine and normeperidine levels following meperidine administration during labor: II. Fetus and neonate. *Am J Obstet Gynecol* 1979;133:909.

Lieberman E et al: Epidural analgesia, intrapartum fever and neonatal sepsis evaluation. *Pediatrics* 1997;99:415.

Lindemann R: Endotracheal administration of epinephrine during cardiopulmonary resuscitation (letter). *Am J Dis Child* 1982;136:753.

Marx GF et al: Fetal-neonatal status following cesarean section for fetal distress. *Br J Anaesth* 1984;56:1009.

Moore J et al: The placental transfer of pentazocine and pethidine. *Br J Anaesth* 1973;45(suppl):798.

Ravlo O et al: A randomized comparison between midazolam and thiopental for elective cesarean section anesthesia: II. Neonates. *Anesth Analg* 1989;68:234.

Sepkoski CM: Neonatal neurobehavior: development and its relation to obstetric anesthesia. *Clin Anaesthesiol* 1986;4:209.

Shnider SM, Moya F: Effects of meperidine on the newborn infant. *Am J Obstet Gynecol* 1964;89:1009.

Shnider SM et al: Uterine blood flow and plasma norepinephrine changes during maternal stress in the pregnant ewe. *Anesthesiology* 1979;50:524.

Stienstra R et al: Ropivacaine 0.25% vs. bupivacaine 0.25% for continuous epidural analgesia in labor: a double-blind comparison. *Anesth Analg* 1995;80:285.

Usher R et al: Judgment of fetal age: II. Clinical significance of gestational age and objective measurement. *Pediatr Clin North Am* 1966;13:835.

Wiswell TE et al: Delivery room management of the apparently vigorous meconium stained neonate: Results of the multicenter, international collaborative trial. *Pediatrics* 2000;105:1.

3 Assessment of Gestational Age

Gestational age can be determined prenatally by the following techniques: date of last menstrual period, date of first reported fetal activity (quickening usually occurs at 16–18 weeks), first reported heart sounds (10–12 weeks by Doppler ultrasound examination), and ultrasound examination (very accurate if obtained before 20 weeks' gestation). The American Academy of Pediatrics recommends that all newborns be classified by birth weight and gestational age. The most common techniques for determining gestational age in the immediate postnatal period are discussed in this chapter.

I. **Classification.** Infants are classified as **preterm** (<37 weeks), **term** (37–41½ weeks), or **postterm** (>42 weeks). Refinements developed in neonatal assessment have provided additional classifications based on a combination of features.

A. **Small for gestational age (SGA)** is defined as 2 standard deviations below the mean weight for gestational age or below the 10th percentile (see Appendix F). (For a full discussion, see Chapter 69.) SGA is commonly seen in infants of mothers who have hypertension or preeclampsia or who smoke. This condition has also been associated with TORCH (*t*oxoplasmosis, *o*ther, *r*ubella, *c*ytomegalovirus, and *h*erpes simplex virus) infections (see Chapter 68), chromosomal abnormalities, and other congenital malformations.

B. **Appropriate for gestational age (AGA).** See Appendix F.

C. **Large for gestational age (LGA)** is defined as 2 standard deviations above the mean weight for gestational age or above the 90th percentile (see Appendix F). LGA can be seen in infants of diabetic mothers (see Chapter 66), infants with Beckwith's syndrome, constitutionally large infants with large parents, or infants with hydrops fetalis.

II. **Methods of determining postnatal gestational age**

A. **Rapid delivery room assessment.** The most useful clinical signs in differentiating among premature, borderline mature, and full-term infants are (in order of usefulness): creases in the sole of the foot, size of the breast nodule, nature of the scalp hair, cartilaginous development of the ear lobe, and scrotal rugae and testicular descent in males. These signs and findings are listed in Table 3–1, which enables one to make a rapid assessment at delivery.

B. **New Ballard Score.** The Ballard maturational score has been expanded and updated to include extremely premature infants. It has been renamed the New Ballard Score (NBS). The score now spans from 10 (correlating with 20 weeks' gestation) to 50 (correlating with 44 weeks' gestation). It is best performed at <12 h of age if the infant is <26 weeks' gestation. If the infant is >26 weeks' gestation, there is no optimal age of examination up to 96 h.

1. **Accuracy.** The examination is accurate whether the infant is sick or well to within 2 weeks of gestational age. It overestimates gestational age by 2–4 days in infants between 32 and 37 weeks' gestation.

2. **Criteria.** The examination consists of six neuromuscular criteria and six physical criteria. The neuromuscular criteria are based on the understanding that passive tone is more useful than active tone in indicating gestational age.

3. **Procedure.** The examination is administered twice by two different examiners to ensure objectivity, and the data are entered on the chart (Figure 3–1). This form is available in most nurseries. The examination consists of two parts: neuromuscular maturity and physical maturity. The 12 scores are totaled, and maturity rating is expressed in weeks of gestation, estimated by using the chart provided on the form. Part 2 of the form (Figure 3–2) is then used to plot gestational assessment against length, height, and head circumference to determine whether the infant is SGA, AGA, or LGA. These are the so-called **Lubchenco charts.**

TABLE 3–1. CRITERIA FOR RAPID GESTATIONAL ASSESSMENT AT DELIVERY

Feature	36 Weeks and earlier	37–38 Weeks	39 Weeks and beyond
Creases in soles of feet	One or 2 transverse creases; posterior three-fourths of sole smooth	Multiple creases; anterior two-thirds of heel smooth	Entire sole, including heel, covered with creases
Breast nodule[a]	2 mm	4 mm	7 mm
Scalp hair	Fine and woolly; fuzzy	Fine and woolly; fuzzy	Coarse and silky; each hair single-stranded
Ear lobe	No cartilage	Moderate amount of cartilage	Stiff ear lobe with thick cartilage
Testes and scrotum	Testes partially descended; scrotum small, with few rugae	?	Testes fully descended; scrotum normal size, with prominent rugae

[a]The breast nodule is not palpable before 33 weeks. Underweight full-term infants may have retarded breast development.
Modified and reproduced with permission from Elsevier Science, Usher R et al: Judgment of fetal age: II. Clinical significance of gestational age and objective measurement. *Pediatr Clin North Am* 1966;13:835.

MATURATIONAL ASSESSMENT OF GESTATIONAL AGE (New Ballard Score)

Name _____ Date/Time of birth _____ Sex _____

Hospital No. _____ Date/Time of exam _____ Birth weight _____

Race _____ Age when examined _____ Length _____

Apgar score: 1 minute _____ 5 minutes _____ 10 minutes _____ Head circ. _____

Examiner _____

SCORE

Neuromuscular _____

Physical _____

Total _____

Maturity rating

Score	Weeks
-10	20
-5	22
0	24
5	26
10	28
15	30
20	32
25	34
30	36
35	38
40	40
45	42
50	44

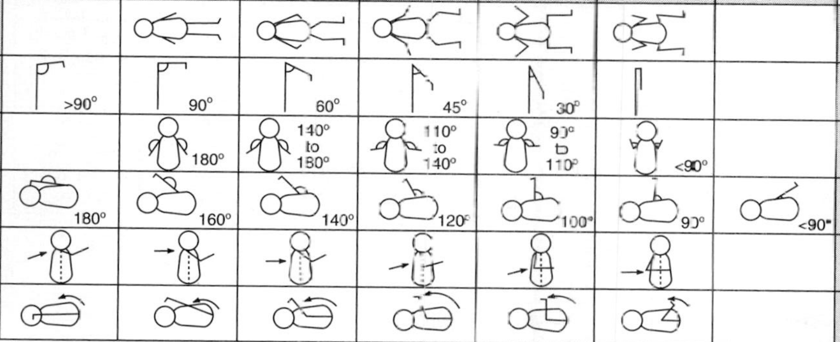

Neuromuscular maturity

Neuromuscular maturity sign	-1	0	1	2	3	4	5	Record score here
Posture								
Square window (wrist)	>90°	90°	60°	45°	30°	0°		
Arm recoil		180°	140° to 180°	110° to 140°	90° to 110°	<90°		
Popliteal angle	180°	160°	140°	120°	100°	90°	<90°	
Scarf sign								
Heel to ear								
						Total neuromuscular maturity score		

FIGURE 3–1. Maturational assessment of gestational age (New Ballard Score) (Reproduced, with permission, from Ballard JL et al: New Ballard Score, expanded to include extremely premature infants. J Pediatr 1991;119:417.)

23

Physical maturity

Physical maturity sign	Score							Record score here
	−1	0	1	2	3	4	5	
Skin	sticky friable transparent	gelatinous red translucent	smooth pink visible veins	superficial peeling &/or rash, few veins	cracking pale areas rare veins	parchment deep cracking no vessels	leathery cracked wrinkled	
Lanugo	none	sparse	abundant	thinning	bald areas	mostly bald		
Plantar surface	heel-toe 40–50 mm: −1 <40 mm: −2	>50 mm no crease	faint red marks	anterior transverse crease only	creases ant. 2/3	creases over entire sole		
Breast	imperceptible	barely perceptible	flat areola no bud	stippled areola 1–2 mm bud	raised areola 3–4 mm bud	full areola 5–10 mm bud		
Eye/ear	lids fused loosely: −1 tightly: −2	lids open pinna flat stays folded	sl. curved pinna; soft slow recoil	well curved pinna; soft but ready recoil	formed and firm, instant recoil	thick cartilage ear stiff		
Genitals (male)	scrotum flat, smooth	scrotum empty, faint rugae	testes in upper canal rare rugae	testes descending few rugae	testes down good rugae	testes pendulous deep rugae		
Genitals (female)	clitoris prominent & labia flat	prominent clitoris & small labia minora	prominent clitoris & enlarging minora	majora & minora equally prominent	majora large minora small	majora cover clitoris & minora		
							Total physical maturity score	

Gestational age
(weeks)

By dates _____
By ultrasound _____
By exam _____

FIGURE 3–1. Continued

Classification of newborns (both sexes) by intrauterine growth and gestational age

Name _____ Date of exam _____

Hospital No. _____ Sex _____ Length _____

Race _____ Birth weight _____ Head circ _____

Date of birth _____ Gestational age _____

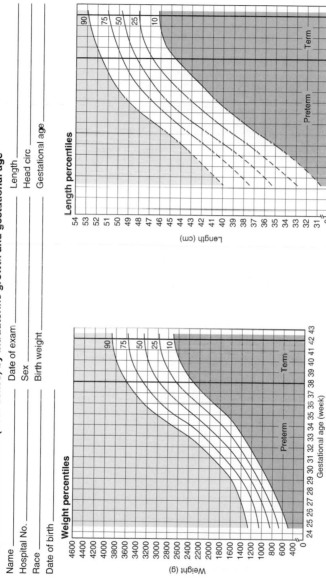

FIGURE 3–2. Classification of newborns (both sexes) by intrauterine growth and gestational age. (Reproduced, with permission, from Battaglia FC, Lubchenco LO: A practical classification for newborn infants by weight and gestational age. J Pediatr 1967;71:159; and Lubchenco LO et al: intrauterine growth in length and head circumference as estimated from live births at gestational ages from 26 to 42 weeks. Pediatrics 1966;37:403. Courtesy of Ross Laboratories, Columbus, Ohio 43216.)

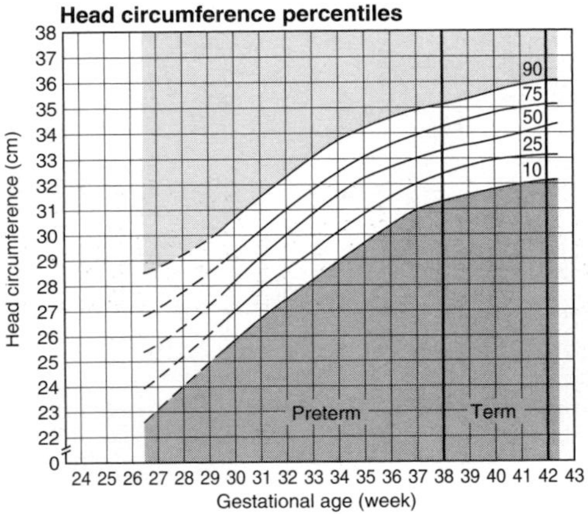

Head circumference percentiles

Head circumference (cm): 22 23 24 25 26 27 28 29 30 31 32 33 34 35 36 37 38

Gestational age (week): 24 25 26 27 28 29 30 31 32 33 34 35 36 37 38 39 40 41 42 43

Percentiles: 90 75 50 25 10

Preterm | Term

Classification of infant*	Weight	Length	Head circ.
Large for Gestational Age (LGA) (>90th percentile)			
Appropriate for Gestational Age (AGA) (10th to 90th percentile)			
Small for Gestational Age (SGA) (<10th percentile)			

*Place an "X" in the appropriate box (LGA, AGA, or SGA) for weight, for length, and for head circumference.

FIGURE 3-2. Continued

a. Neuromuscular maturity

   i. Posture. Score 0 if the arms and legs are extended, and score 1 if the infant has beginning flexion of the knees and hips, with arms extended; determine other scores based on the diagram.

   ii. Square window. Flex the hand on the forearm between the thumb and index finger of the examiner. Apply sufficient pressure to achieve as much flexion as possible. Visually measure the angle between the hypothenar eminence and the ventral aspect of the forearm. Determine the score based on the diagram.

   iii. Arm recoil. Flex the forearms for 5 s; then grasp the hand and fully extend the arm and release. If the arm returns to full flexion, give a score of 4. For lesser degrees of flexion, score as noted on the diagram.

   iv. Popliteal angle. Hold the thigh in the knee-chest position with the left index finger and the thumb supporting the knee. Then extend the leg by gentle pressure from the right index finger behind the ankle. Measure the angle at the popliteal space and score accordingly.

   v. Scarf sign. Take the infant's hand and try to put it around the neck posteriorly as far as possible over the opposite shoulder and score according to the diagram.

   vi. Heel to ear. Keeping the pelvis flat on the table, take the infant's foot and try to put it as close to the head as possible without forcing it. Grade according to the diagram.

b. Physical maturity. These characteristics are scored as shown in Figure 3–1.

   i. Skin. Carefully look at the skin and grade according to the diagram. Extremely premature infants have sticky, transparent skin and receive a score of −1.

   ii. Lanugo hair is examined on the infant's back and between and over the scapulae.

   iii. Plantar surface. Measure foot length from the tip of the great toe to the back of the heel. If the results are <40 mm, then give a score of −2. If it is between 40 and 50 mm, assign a score of −1. If the measurement is >50 mm and no creases are seen on the plantar surface, give a score of 0. If there are creases, score accordingly.

   iv. Breast. Palpate any breast tissue and score.

   v. Eye and ear. This section has been expanded to include criteria that apply to the extremely premature infant. Loosely fused eyelids are defined as closed, but gentle traction opens them. Score this as −1. Tightly fused eyelids are defined as inseparable by gentle traction. Base the rest of the score on open lids and the examination of the ear.

   vi. Genitalia. Score according to the diagram.

C. Direct ophthalmoscopy. Another method for determination of gestational age uses direct ophthalmoscopy of the lens. Before 27 weeks, the cornea is too opaque to allow visualization; after 34 weeks, atrophy of the vessels of the lens occurs. Therefore, this technique allows for accurate determination of gestational age at 27–34 weeks only. This method is reliable to ±2 weeks. The pupil must be dilated under the supervision of an ophthalmologist, and the assessment must be performed within 48 h of birth before the vessels atrophy. The following grading system is used, as shown in Figure 3–3.

- **Grade 4 (27–28 weeks):** Vessels cover the entire anterior surface of the lens or the vessels meet in the center of the lens.
- **Grade 3 (29–30 weeks):** Vessels do not meet in the center but are close. Central portion of the lens is not covered by vessels.
- **Grade 2 (31–32 weeks):** Vessels reach only to the middle-outer part of the lens. The central clear portion of the lens is larger.
- **Grade 1 (33–34 weeks):** Vessels are seen only at the periphery of the lens.

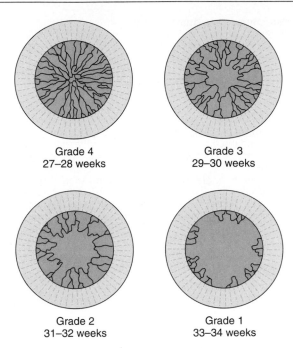

Grade 4
27–28 weeks

Grade 3
29–30 weeks

Grade 2
31–32 weeks

Grade 1
33–34 weeks

FIGURE 3–3. Grading System for assessment of gestational age by examination of the anterior vascular capsule of the lens. *(Reproduced, with permission, from Hittner HM et al: Assessment of gestational age by examination of the anterior vascular capsule of the lens.* J Pediatr *1977;91:455.)*

REFERENCES

Amiel-Tison C: Neurological evaluation of the maturity of newborn infants. *Arch Dis Child* 1968;43:89.

Ballard JL et al: New Ballard Score, expanded to include extremely premature infants. *J Pediatr* 1991;119:417.

Ballard JL et al: A simplified score for assessment of fetal maturation of newly born infants. *J Pediatr* 1979;95:769.

Dodd V: Gestational age assessment. *Neonatal Network* 1996;15:1.

Dubowitz LM et al: Clinical assessment of gestational age in the newborn infant. *J Pediatr* 1970;77:1.

Farr V et al: The definition of some external characteristics used in the assessment of gestational age in the newborn infant. *Dev Med Child Neurol* 1966;8:657.

Fletcher MA: Ch. 3 *Assessment of Gestational Age* p. 55–66. *Physical Diagnosis of Neonatology,* 1st ed. Lippincott Raven, 1998.

Hittner HM et al: Assessment of gestational age by examination of the anterior vascular capsule of the lens. *J Pediatr* 1977;91:455.

Usher R et al: Judgment of fetal age: II. Clinical significance of gestational age and objective measurement. *Pediatr Clin North Am* 1966;13:835.

4 Newborn Physical Examination

The newborn infant should undergo a complete physical examination within 24 h of birth. It is easier to listen to the heart and lungs first when the infant is quiet. Warming the stethoscope before using it decreases the likelihood of making the infant cry.

I. **Vital signs**
   A. **Temperature.** Indicate whether the temperature is rectal (which is usually 1° higher than oral), oral, or axillary (which is usually 1° lower than oral).
   B. **Respirations.** The normal respiratory rate in a newborn is 40–60 breaths/min.
   C. **Blood pressure.** Blood pressure correlates directly with gestational age, postnatal age of the infant, and birth weight. (For normal blood pressure curves, see Appendix C.)
   D. **Pulse rate.** The normal pulse rate is 100–180 beats/min in the newborn (usually 120–160 beats/min when awake, 70–80 beats/min when asleep). In the healthy infant, the heart rate increases with stimulation.

II. **Head circumference, length, weight, and gestational age**
   A. **Head circumference and percentile.** (For growth charts, see Appendix F.) Place the measuring tape around the front of the head (above the brow [the frontal area]) and the occipital area. The tape should be above the ears. This is known as the occipitofrontal circumference, which is normally 32–37 cm at term.
   B. **Length and percentile.** For growth charts, see Appendix F.
   C. **Weight and percentile.** For growth charts, see Appendix F.
   D. **Assessment of gestational age.** See Chapter 3.

III. **General appearance.** Observe the infant and record the general appearance (eg, activity, skin color, and obvious congenital abnormalities).

IV. **Skin**
   A. **Color**
      1. **Plethora (deep, rosy red color).** Plethora is more common in infants with polycythemia but can be seen in an overoxygenated or overheated infant. It is best to obtain a central hematocrit on any plethoric infant. Erythema neonatorum is a condition in which an infant has an overall blush or reddish color. It usually appears in the transition period and can occur when the infant has been stimulated. This is a normal phenomenon and lasts only several hours.
      2. **Jaundice (yellowish color if secondary to indirect hyperbilirubinemia, greenish color if secondary to direct hyperbilirubinemia).** With jaundice, bilirubin levels are usually >5 mg/dL. This condition is abnormal in infants <24 h old and may signify Rh incompatibility, sepsis, and TORCH (*t*oxoplasmosis, *o*ther, *r*ubella, *c*ytomegalovirus, and *h*erpes simplex virus) infections (see Chapter 68). After 24 h, it may result either from these diseases or from such common causes as ABO incompatibility or physiologic causes.
      3. **Pallor (washed-out, whitish appearance).** Pallor may be secondary to anemia, birth asphyxia, shock, or patent ductus arteriosus. Ductal pallor is the term sometimes used to denote pallor associated with patent ductus arteriosus.
      4. **Cyanosis (desaturation of 5 g of hemoglobin usually necessary for one to note a bluish color)**
         a. **Central cyanosis (bluish skin, including the tongue and lips).** Central cyanosis is caused by low oxygen saturation in the blood. It may be associated with congenital heart or lung disease.

    b. Peripheral cyanosis (bluish skin with pink lips and tongue). Peripheral cyanosis may be associated with **methemoglobinemia,** which occurs when hemoglobin oxidizes from the ferrous to the ferric form; the blood actually can have a chocolate hue. Methemoglobin is incapable of transporting oxygen or carbon dioxide. This disorder can be caused by exposure to certain drugs or chemicals (eg, nitrates or nitrites) or may be hereditary (eg, NADH-methemoglobin reductase deficiency or hemoglobin M disease [NADH is the reduced form of nicotinamide adenine dinucleotide]). Treatment for infants is with methylene blue.

    c. Acrocyanosis (bluish hands and feet only). Acrocyanosis may be normal for an infant who has just been born (or within the first few hours after birth) or for one who is experiencing cold stress. If the condition is seen in an older infant with a normal temperature, decreased peripheral perfusion secondary to hypovolemia should be considered.

  5. Extensive bruising (ecchymoses) may be associated with a prolonged and difficult delivery and may result in early jaundice. Petechiae (pinpoint hemorrhages) can be limited to one area and are usually of no concern. If they are widespread and progressive, then they are of concern and a workup for coagulopathy should be considered.

  6. "Blue on pink" or "pink on blue." Whereas some infants are pink and well perfused and others are clearly cyanotic, some do not fit either of these categories. They may appear bluish with pink undertones or pink with bluish undertones. This coloration may be secondary to poor perfusion, inadequate oxygenation, inadequate ventilation, or polycythemia.

  7. Harlequin coloration (clear line of demarcation between an area of redness and an area of normal coloration). The cause is usually unknown. The coloration can be benign and transient (lasting usually <20 min) or can be indicative of shunting of blood (persistent pulmonary hypertension or coarctation of the aorta). There can be varying degrees of redness and perfusion. The demarcating line may run from the head to the belly, dividing the body into right and left halves, or it may develop in the dependent half of the body when the newborn is lying on one side.

  8. Mottling (lacy red pattern) may be seen in healthy infants and in those with cold stress, hypovolemia, or sepsis. Persistent mottling, referred to as **cutis marmorata,** is found in infants with Down syndrome, trisomy 13, or trisomy 18.

  9. Vernix caseosa. This is a greasy white substance that covers the skin until the 38th week of gestation. Its purpose is to provide a moisture barrier. It is completely normal.

  10. Collodion infant. In this condition, the skin resembles parchment, and there can be some restriction in growth of the nose and ears. This may be a normal condition or can be a manifestation of another disease.

  11. Dry skin. Most term infants do not have dry skin. Postdate or postmature infants can exhibit excessive peeling of skin. Congenital syphilis and candidiasis can present with peeling skin at birth.

B. Rashes

  1. Milia. Milia is a rash in which tiny, sebaceous retention cysts are seen. The whitish, pinhead-sized concretions are usually on the chin, nose, forehead, and cheeks. No erythema is seen. These benign cysts disappear within a few weeks after birth. These are seen in approximately 33% of infants. Pearls are large single milia that can occur on the genitalia and areola.

  2. Erythema toxicum. In erythema toxicum, numerous small areas of red skin with a yellow-white papule in the center are evident. Lesions are most noticeable 48 h after birth but may appear as late as 7–10 days.

Wright's staining of the papule reveals eosinophils. This benign rash, which is the most common type, resolves spontaneously. If suspected in an infant younger than 34 weeks' gestation, it is best to rule out other causes because this rash is more common in term infants.

3. **Candida albicans rash.** C. albicans diaper rash appears as erythematous plaques with sharply demarcated edges. Satellite bodies (pustules on contiguous areas of skin) are also seen. Usually, the skinfolds are involved. Gram's stain of a smear or 10% potassium hydroxide preparation of the lesion reveals budding yeast spores, which are easily treated with nystatin ointment or cream applied to the rash 4 times daily for 7–10 days.

4. **Transient neonatal pustular melanosis** is characterized by three stages of lesions, which may appear over the entire body:

   • Pustules.
   • Ruptured vesicopustules with scaling/typical halo appearance.
   • Hyperpigmented macules.

   This benign, self-limiting condition requires no specific therapy.

5. **Acne neonatorum.** The lesions are typically seen over the cheeks, chin, and forehead and consist of comedones and papules. The condition is usually benign and requires no therapy; however, severe cases may require treatment with mild keratolytic agents.

6. **Herpes simplex.** One can see a pustular vesicular rash, vesicles, bullae, or denuded skin. The rash is most commonly seen at the fetal scalp monitor site, occiput, or buttocks (presentation site at time of delivery). Tzanck smear will reveal multinucleated giant cells.

C. **Nevi.** Hemangiomas near the eyes, nose, or mouth that interfere with vital functions or sight may need surgical intervention.

1. **Macular hemangioma ("stork bites").** A macular hemangioma is a true vascular nevus normally seen on the occipital area, eyelids, and glabella. The lesions disappear spontaneously within the first year of life.

2. **Port-wine stain (nevus flammeus)** is usually seen at birth, does not blanch with pressure, and does not disappear with time. If the lesion appears over the forehead and upper lip, then **Sturge-Weber syndrome** (port-wine stain over the forehead and upper lip, glaucoma, and contralateral jacksonian seizures) must be ruled out.

3. **Mongolian spot.** Mongolian spots are dark blue or purple bruise-like macular spots usually located over the sacrum. Usually present in 90% of blacks and Asians, they occur in <5% of white children and disappear by 4 years of age. They are the most common birthmark.

4. **Cavernous hemangioma.** A cavernous hemangioma usually appears as a large, red, cyst-like, firm, ill-defined mass and may be found anywhere on the body. The majority of these lesions regress with age, but some require corticosteroid therapy. In more severe cases, surgical resection may be necessary. If associated with thrombocytopenia, **Kasabach-Merritt syndrome** (thrombocytopenia associated with a rapidly expanding hemangioma) should be considered. Transfusions of platelets and clotting factors are usually required in patients with this syndrome.

5. **Strawberry hemangioma (macular hemangioma).** Strawberry hemangiomas are flat, bright red, sharply demarcated lesions that are most commonly found on the face. Spontaneous regression usually occurs (70% disappearance by 7 years of age).

V. **Head.** Note the general shape of the head. Inspect for any cuts or bruises secondary to forceps or fetal monitor leads. Transillumination can be done for severe hydrocephalus and hydranencephaly. Check for microcephaly or macrocephaly.

A. **Anterior and posterior fontanelles.** The anterior fontanelle usually closes at 9–12 months and the posterior fontanelle at 2–4 months. A large anterior fontanelle is seen with hypothyroidism and may also be found in infants with skeletal disorders such as osteogenesis imperfecta, hypophosphatasia, and chromosomal abnormalities and in those who are small for gestational age. A bulging fontanelle may be associated with increased intracranial pressure, meningitis, or hydrocephalus. Depressed (sunken) fontanelles are seen in newborns with dehydration. A small anterior fontanelle may be associated with hyperthyroidism, microcephaly, or craniosynostosis.

B. **Molding.** Molding is a temporary asymmetry of the skull resulting from the birth process. Most often seen with prolonged labor and vaginal deliveries, it can be seen in cesarean deliveries if the mother had a prolonged course of labor before delivery. A normal head shape is usually regained within 1 week.

C. **Caput succedaneum.** Caput succedaneum is a diffuse edematous swelling of the soft tissues of the scalp that may extend across the suture lines. It is secondary to the pressure of the uterus or vaginal wall on areas of the fetal head bordering the caput. Usually, it resolves within several days (Figure 4–1).

D. **Cephalhematoma** is a subperiosteal hemorrhage that *never* extends across the suture line. It can be secondary to a traumatic delivery or forceps delivery. X-ray films or computed tomography (CT) scans of the head should be obtained if an underlying skull fracture is suspected (<5% of all cephalhematomas). Hematocrit and bilirubin levels should be monitored in these patients. Most cephalhematomas resolve in 2–3 weeks. Aspiration of the hematoma is rarely necessary (see Figure 4–1).

E. **Subgaleal hematoma.** Hemorrhage bleeding occurs below the epicranial aponeurosis. It can cross over the suture line and onto the neck or ear. It may be necessary to replace blood volume lost and correct coagulopathy if present (see Figure 4–1).

F. **Increased intracranial pressure.** The following signs are evident in an infant with increased intracranial pressure.

- Bulging anterior fontanelle
- Separated sutures
- Paralysis of upward gaze (setting-sun sign)
- Prominent veins of the scalp
- Increasing macrocephaly

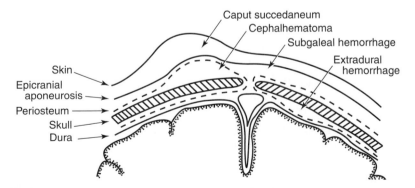

FIGURE 4–1. Types of extradural fluid collections seen in newborn infants. Volpe J.J. Neurology of the Newborn. 3rd ed. Philadelphia: WB Saunders 1995 and Based on data from Pape K.E., Wigglesworth J.S. Haemorrhage, Ischemia and the Perinatal Brach. Philadelphia: J.B. Lippincott, 1979.

The increased pressure may be secondary to hydrocephalus, hypoxic-ischemic brain injury, intracranial hemorrhage, or subdural hematoma.

G. **Craniosynostosis.** Craniosynostosis is the premature closure of one or more sutures of the skull. It should be considered in any infant with an asymmetric skull. On palpation of the skull, a bony ridge over the suture line may be felt, and inability to freely move the cranial bones may occur. X-ray studies of the head should be performed, and surgical consultation may be necessary.

H. **Craniotabes,** a benign condition, is a softening of the skull that usually occurs around the suture lines and disappears within days to a few weeks after birth. If the area is over most of the skull, it may be secondary to a calcium deficiency, and osteogenesis imperfecta and syphilis should be ruled out.

I. **Plagiocephaly.** Plagiocephaly is an oblique shape of a head, which is asymmetric and flattened. It can be seen in preemies and infants whose heads stay in the same position.

VI. **Neck.** Eliciting the rooting reflex (see p 38) causes the infant to turn the head and allows easier examination of the neck. Palpate the sternocleidomastoid for a hematoma and the thyroid for enlargement, and check for thyroglossal duct cysts. A short neck is seen in Turner's, Noonan's, and Klippel-Feil syndromes.

VII. **Face.** Look for obvious abnormalities. Note the general shape of the nose, mouth, and chin. The presence of hypertelorism (eyes widely separated) or low-set ears should be noted.

A. **Facial nerve injury.** Unilateral branches of the facial (eighth) nerve are most commonly involved. There is facial asymmetry with crying. The corner of the mouth droops, and the nasolabial fold is absent in the paralyzed side. The infant may be unable to close the eye, move the lip, and drool on the side of the paresis. If the palsy is secondary to trauma, most symptoms disappear within the first week of life, but sometimes resolution may take several months. If the palsy persists, absence of the nerve should be ruled out.

VIII. **Ears.** Look for an unusual shape or an abnormal position. The normal position is determined by drawing an imaginary horizontal line from the inner and outer canthi of the eye across the face, perpendicular to the vertical axis of the head. If the helix of the ear lies below this horizontal line, the ears are designated as low set. Low-set ears are seen with many congenital anomalies (most commonly Treacher Collins, triploidy, and trisomy 9 and 18 syndromes as well as fetal aminopterin effects). Preauricular skin tags (papillomas), which are benign, are often seen. Hairy ears are seen in infants of diabetic mothers. Gross hearing can be assessed when an infant blinks in response to loud noises.

IX. **Eyes.** Check the red reflex with an ophthalmoscope. If a cataract is present, opacification of the lens and loss of the reflex are apparent. Congenital cataracts require early evaluation by an ophthalmologist. The sclera, which is normally white, can have a bluish tint if the infant is premature because the sclera is thinner in these infants than in term infants. If the sclera is deep blue, **osteogenesis imperfecta** should be ruled out.

A. **Brushfield's spots** (salt-and-pepper speckling of the iris) are often seen with Down syndrome.

B. **Subconjunctival hemorrhage.** Rupture of small conjunctival capillaries can occur normally but is more common after a traumatic delivery. This condition is seen in 5% of newborn infants.

C. **Conjunctivitis.** See Chapter 35.

X. **Nose.** If unilateral or bilateral choanal atresia is suspected, verify the patency of the nostrils with gentle passage of a nasogastric tube. Infants are obligate nose breathers; therefore, if they have bilateral choanal atresia, they will have severe respiratory distress. Nasal flaring is indicative of respiratory distress.

Sniffling and discharge are typical of congenital syphilis. Sneezing can be a response to bright light or drug withdrawal.

XI. Mouth. Examine the hard and soft palates for evidence of a cleft palate. A short lingual frenulum (tongue-tie) may require surgical treatment (especially if tongue mobility is limited).

    A. Ranula. A ranula is a cystic swelling in the floor of the mouth. Most disappear spontaneously.

    B. Epstein's pearls. These keratin-containing cysts, which are normal, are located on the hard and soft palates and resolve spontaneously.

    C. Mucocele. This small lesion on the oral mucosa occurs secondary to trauma to the salivary gland ducts. It is usually benign and subsides spontaneously.

    D. Natal teeth are usually lower incisors. X-ray films are needed to differentiate the two types because management of each is different.

        1. Predeciduous teeth. Supernumerary teeth are found in 1 in 4000 births. They are usually loose, and the roots are absent or poorly formed. Removal is necessary to avoid aspiration.

        2. True deciduous teeth. These teeth are true teeth that erupt early. They occur in <1 in 2000 births. They should not be extracted.

    E. Macroglossia. Enlargement of the tongue can be congenital or acquired. Localized macroglossia is usually secondary to congenital hemangiomas. Macroglossia can be seen in **Beckwith's syndrome** (macroglossia, gigantism, omphalocele, and severe hypoglycemia) and **Pompe's disease** (type II glycogen storage disease).

    F. Frothy or copious saliva is commonly seen in infants with an esophageal atresia with tracheoesophageal fistula.

    G. Thrush. Oral thrush, which is common in newborns, is a sign of infection resulting from *C. albicans.* Whitish patches appear on the tongue, gingiva, or buccal mucosa. Thrush is easily treated with nystatin suspension (0.1–1.0 mL) applied to each side of the mouth, often with a cotton-tipped swab, 3–4 times per day for 7 days.

XII. Chest

    A. Observation. First, note whether the chest is symmetric. An asymmetric chest may signify a tension pneumothorax. Tachypnea, sternal and intercostal retractions, and grunting on expiration indicate respiratory distress.

    B. Breath sounds. Listen for the presence and equality of breath sounds. A good place to listen is in the right and left axillae. Absent or unequal sounds may indicate pneumothorax or atelectasis. Absent breath sounds with the presence of bowel sounds indicates a diaphragmatic hernia; an immediate x-ray film and emergency surgical consultation are recommended.

    C. Pectus excavatum. Pectus excavatum is a sternum that is altered in shape. Usually, this condition is of no clinical concern.

    D. Breasts in a newborn are usually 1 cm in diameter in term male and female infants. They may be abnormally enlarged (3–4 cm) secondary to the effects of maternal estrogens. This effect, which lasts <1 week, is of no clinical concern. A usually white discharge, commonly referred to as "witch's milk," may be present. Supernumerary nipples are extra nipples and occur as a normal variant.

XIII. Heart. Observe for heart rate, rhythm, quality of heart sounds, active precordium, and presence of a murmur. The position of the heart may be determined by auscultation. Abnormal situs syndromes are described in Chapter 62, pp. 358–359.

    A. Murmurs may be associated with the following conditions.

        1. Ventricular septal defect (VSD), the most common heart defect, accounts for ~25% of congenital heart disease. Typically, a loud, harsh, blowing pansystolic murmur is heard (best heard over the lower left sternal border). Symptoms such as congestive heart failure usually do not begin until after 2 weeks of age and typically are present from

6 weeks to 4 months. The majority of these defects close spontaneously by the end of the first year of life.

2. **Patent ductus arteriosus (PDA)** is a harsh, continuous, machinery-
type, or "rolling thunder," murmur that usually presents on the second
or third day of life, localized to the second left intercostal space. It may
radiate to the left clavicle or down the left sternal border. A hyperactive
precordium is also seen. Clinical signs include wide pulse pressure and
bounding pulses.

3. **Coarctation of the aorta,** a systolic ejection murmur, radiates down
the sternum to the apex and to the interscapular area. It is often loudest
in the back.

4. **Peripheral pulmonic stenosis.** A systolic murmur is heard bilaterally
in the anterior chest, in both axillae, and across the back. It is secondary to the turbulence caused by disturbed blood flow because the
main pulmonary artery is larger than the peripheral pulmonary arteries.
This usually benign murmur may persist up to 3 months of age. It may
also be associated with rubella syndrome.

5. **Hypoplastic left heart syndrome.** A short, midsystolic murmur usually
presents anywhere from day 1 to 21. A gallop is usually heard.

6. **Tetralogy of Fallot** typically is a loud, harsh systolic or pansystolic
murmur best heard at the left sternal border. The second heart sound is
single.

7. **Pulmonary atresia**
   a. **With VSD.** An absent or soft systolic murmur with the first heart
   sound is followed by an ejection click. The second heart sound is
   loud and single.
   b. **With intact intraventricular septum.** Most frequently, there is no
   murmur and a single second heart sound is heard.

8. **Tricuspid atresia.** A pansystolic murmur along the left sternal border
with a single second heart sound is typically heard.

9. **Transposition of the great vessels** is more common in males than females.
   a. **Isolated (simple).** Cardiac examination is often normal, but
   cyanosis and tachypnea are present along with a normal chest x-ray
   film and electrocardiogram.
   b. **With VSD.** The murmur is loud and pansystolic and is best heard at
   the lower left sternal border. The infant typically has congestive
   heart failure at 3–6 weeks of life.

10. **Ebstein's disease.** A long, systolic murmur is heard over the anterior
portion of the left chest. A diastolic murmur and gallop may be present.

11. **Truncus arteriosus.** A systolic ejection murmur, often with a thrill, is
heard at the left sternal border. The second heart sound is loud and
single.

12. **Single ventricle.** A loud, systolic ejection murmur with a loud, single
second heart sound is heard.

13. **Atrial septal defects (ASDs)**
   a. **Ostium secundum defect** rarely presents with congestive heart
   failure in infancy. A soft systolic ejection murmur is best heard at the
   upper left sternal border.
   b. **Ostium primum defect** rarely occurs in infancy. A pulmonary ejection murmur and early systolic murmur are heard at the lower left
   sternal border. A split second heart sound is heard.
   c. **Common atrioventricular canal** presents with congestive heart failure in infancy. A harsh, systolic murmur is heard all over the chest. The
   second heart sound is split if pulmonary flow is increased.

14. **Anomalous pulmonary venous return**
   a. **Partial.** Findings are similar to those for ostium secundum defect
   (see Section XIII. A.13.a.).

   b. **Total.** With a severe obstruction, no murmur may be detected on examination. With a moderate degree of obstruction, a systolic murmur is heard along the left sternal border, and a gallop murmur is heard occasionally. A continuous murmur along the left upper sternal border over the pulmonary area may also be audible.

15. **Congenital aortic stenosis.** A coarse, systolic murmur with a thrill is heard at the upper right sternal border and can radiate to the neck and down the left sternal border. If left ventricular failure is severe, the murmur is of low intensity. Symptoms that occur in infants only when the stenosis is severe are pulmonary edema and congestive heart failure.

16. **Pulmonary stenosis (with intact ventricular septum).** If the stenosis is severe, a loud, systolic ejection murmur is audible over the pulmonary area and radiates over the entire precordium. Right ventricular failure and cyanosis may be present. If the stenosis is mild, a short pulmonary systolic ejection murmur is heard over the pulmonic area along with a split second heart sound.

B. **Palpate the pulses (femoral, pedal, radial, and brachial).** Bounding pulses can be seen with patent ductus arteriosus. Absent or delayed femoral pulses are associated with coarctation of the aorta.

C. **Check for signs of congestive heart failure.** Signs may include hepatomegaly, gallop, tachypnea, wheezes and rales, tachycardia, and abnormal pulses.

XIV. **Abdomen**

A. **Observation.** Obvious defects may include an **omphalocele,** in which the intestines are covered by peritoneum and the umbilicus is centrally located, or a **gastroschisis,** in which the intestines are not covered by peritoneum (the defect is usually to the right of the umbilicus). A **scaphoid abdomen** may be associated with a diaphragmatic hernia.

B. **Auscultation.** Listen for bowel sounds.

C. **Palpation.** Check the abdomen for distention, tenderness, or masses. The abdomen is most easily palpated when the infant is quiet or during feeding. In normal circumstances, the liver can be palpated 1–2 cm below the costal margin and the spleen tip at the costal margin. Hepatomegaly can be seen with congestive heart failure, hepatitis, or sepsis. Splenomegaly is found with cytomegalovirus (CMV) or rubella infections or sepsis. The kidneys (especially on the right) can often be palpated. Kidney size may be increased with polycystic disease, renal vein thrombosis, or hydronephrosis. Abdominal masses are more commonly related to the urinary tract.

XV. **Umbilicus.** Normally, the umbilicus has two arteries and one vein. The absence of one artery occurs in 5–10 of 1000 singleton births and in 35–70 of 1000 twin births. The presence of only two vessels (one artery and one vein) could indicate renal or genetic problems (most commonly trisomy 18). If there is a single umbilical artery, there is an increased prevalence of congenital anomalies and intrauterine growth retardation and a higher rate of perinatal mortality. If the umbilicus is abnormal, ultrasonography of the abdomen is recommended. In addition, inspect for any discharge, redness, or edema around the base of the cord that may signify a patent urachus or omphalitis. The cord should be translucent; a greenish-yellow color suggests meconium staining, usually secondary to fetal distress.

XVI. **Genitalia.** Any infant with ambiguous genitalia should not undergo gender assignment until a formal endocrinology evaluation has been performed (see Chapter 60). A male with any question of a penile abnormality should not be circumcised until he is evaluated by a urologist or a pediatric surgeon.

A. **Male.** Check for dorsal hood, hypospadias, epispadias, and chordee. Normal penile length at birth is >2 cm. Newborn males always have a marked phimosis. Determine the site of the meatus. Verify that the testicles are in the scrotum and examine for groin hernias. Undescended testicles are more common in premature infants. Hydroceles are common and usually disappear by 1 year of age. Observe the color of the scrotum. A bluish color may suggest testicular torsion and requires immediate urologic/surgical consultation. Infants will have well-developed scrotal rugae at term. A smooth scrotum suggests prematurity.

B. Female. Examine the labia and clitoris. A mucosal tag is commonly attached to the wall of the vagina. Discharge from the vagina is common and is often blood tinged secondary to maternal estrogen withdrawal. If the labia are fused and the clitoris is enlarged, adrenal hyperplasia should be suspected. A large clitoris can be associated with maternal drug ingestion. Labia majora at term are enlarged.

XVII. Lymph nodes. Palpable lymph nodes, usually in the inguinal and cervical areas, are found in ~33% of normal neonates.

XVIII. Anus and rectum. Check for patency of the anus to rule out imperforate anus. Check the position of the anus. Meconium should pass within 48 h of birth for term infants. Premature infants are usually delayed in passing meconium.

XIX. Extremities. Examine the arms and legs, paying close attention to the digits and palmar creases.

A. Syndactyly, or abnormal fusion of the digits, most commonly involves the third and fourth fingers and the second and third toes. A strong family history exists. Surgery is performed when the neonates are older.

B. Polydactyly is supernumerary digits on the hands or the feet. This condition is associated with a strong family history. An x-ray film of the extremity is usually obtained to verify whether any bony structures are present in the digit. If there are no bony structures, a suture can be tied around the digit until it falls off. If bony structures are present, surgical removal is necessary. Axial extra digits are associated with heart anomalies.

C. Simian crease. A single transverse palmar crease is most commonly seen in Down syndrome but is occasionally a normal variant.

D. Talipes equinovarus (clubfoot) is more common in males. The foot is turned downward and inward, and the sole is directed medially. If this problem can be corrected with gentle force, it will resolve spontaneously. If not, orthopedic treatment and follow-up are necessary.

E. Metatarsus varus is adduction of the forefoot. This condition usually corrects spontaneously.

XX. Trunk and spine. Check for any gross defects of the spine. Any abnormal pigmentation or hairy patches over the lower back should increase the suspicion that an underlying vertebral abnormality exists. A sacral or pilonidal dimple may indicate a small meningocele or other anomaly.

XXI. Hips. Congenital hip dislocation occurs in ~1 in 800 live births. More common in white females, this condition is more likely to be unilateral and to involve the left hip. Two clinical signs of dislocation are asymmetry of the skinfolds on the dorsal surface and shortening of the affected leg.

Evaluate for congenital hip dislocation by using the **Ortolani** and **Barlow maneuvers.** Place the infant in the frog-leg position. Abduct the hips by using the middle finger to apply gentle inward and upward pressure over the greater trochanter (Ortolani's sign). Adduct the hips by using the thumb to apply outward and backward pressure over the inner thigh (Barlow's sign). (Some clinicians suggest omitting the Barlow maneuver because this action may contribute to hip instability by stretching the capsule unnecessarily.) A click of reduction and a click of dislocation are elicited in infants with hip dislocation. If this disorder is suspected, radiographic studies and orthopedic consultation should be obtained.

XXII. Nervous system. First, observe the infant for any abnormal movement (eg, seizure activity) or excessive irritability. Then evaluate the following parameters.

A. Muscle tone

1. Hypotonia. Floppiness and head lag are seen.

2. **Hypertonia.** Increased resistance is apparent when the arms and legs are extended. Hyperextension of the back and tightly clenched fists are often seen.
B. **Reflexes.** The following reflexes are normal for a newborn infant.
   1. **Rooting reflex.** Stroke the lip and the corner of the cheek with a finger and the infant will turn in that direction and open the mouth.
   2. **Glabellar reflex (blink reflex).** Tap gently over the forehead and the eyes will blink.
   3. **Grasp reflex.** Place a finger in the palm of the infant's hand and the infant will grasp the finger.
   4. **Neck-righting reflex.** Turn the infant's head to the right or left and movement of the contralateral shoulder should be obtained in the same direction.
   5. **Moro reflex.** Support the infant behind the upper back with one hand, and then drop the infant back 1 cm or more to—but not on—the mattress. This should cause abduction of both arms and extension of the fingers. Asymmetry may signify a fractured clavicle, hemiparesis, or brachial plexus injury.
C. **Cranial nerves.** Note the presence of gross nystagmus, the reaction of the pupils, and the ability of the infant to follow moving objects with his or her eyes.
D. **Movement.** Check for spontaneous movement of the limbs, trunk, face, and neck. A fine tremor is usually normal. Clonic movements are not normal and may be seen with seizures.
E. **Peripheral nerves**
   1. **Erb-Duchenne paralysis** involves injury to the fifth and sixth cervical nerves. There is adduction and internal rotation of the arm. The forearm is in pronation; the power of extension is retained. The wrist is flexed. This condition can be associated with diaphragm paralysis.
   2. **Klumpke's paralysis** involves the seventh and eighth cervical nerves and the first thoracic nerve. The hand is flaccid with little or no control. If the sympathetic fibers of the first thoracic root are injured, ipsilateral ptosis and miosis can occur.
F. **General signs of neurologic disorders**
   1. **Symptoms of increased intracranial pressure** (bulging anterior fontanelle, dilated scalp veins, separated sutures, and setting-sun sign) (see p 32).
   2. **Hypotonia or hypertonia.**
   3. **Irritability or hyperexcitability.**
   4. **Poor sucking and swallowing reflexes.**
   5. **Shallow, irregular respirations.**
   6. **Apnea.**
   7. **Apathy.**
   8. **Staring.**
   9. **Seizure activity** (sucking or chewing of the tongue, blinking of the eyelids, eye rolling, and hiccups).
   10. **Absent, depressed, or exaggerated reflexes.**
   11. **Asymmetric reflexes.**

5 Temperature Regulation

The chance of survival of neonates is markedly enhanced by the successful prevention of excessive heat loss. For that purpose, the newborn infant must be kept under a **neutral thermal environment.** This is defined as the external temperature range within which metabolic rate and hence oxygen consumption are at a minimum while the infant maintains a normal body temperature (see Figures 5–1 and 5–2 and Table 5–1). The **normal skin temperature** in the neonate is 36.0–36.5 °C (96.8–97.7 °F). The **normal core (rectal) temperature** is 36.5–37.5 °C (97.7–99.5 °F). **Axillary temperature** may be 0.5–1.0 °C lower (95.9–98.6 °F). A normal body temperature implies only a balance between heat production and heat loss and should not be interpreted as the equivalent of an optimal and minimal metabolic rate and oxygen consumption.

I. **Hypothermia and excessive heat loss.** Preterm infants are predisposed to heat loss because they have little subcutaneous fat, a high ratio of surface area to body weight, and reduced glycogen and brown fat stores. In addition, their hypotonic ("frog") posture limits their ability to curl up to reduce the skin area exposed to the colder environment.
   A. **Mechanisms of heat loss** in the newborn include the following.
      1. **Radiation.** Radiation is heat loss from the infant (warm object) to a colder nearby object.
      2. **Conduction.** Conduction is direct heat loss from the infant to the surface with which he or she is in direct contact.
      3. **Convection.** Convection is heat loss from the infant to the surrounding air.
      4. **Evaporation.** Heat may be lost by water evaporation from the skin of the infant (this is especially likely immediately after delivery).
   B. **Consequences of excessive heat loss.** Those related to the compensatory augmentation in heat production through the increase in metabolic rate include the following:
      1. **Insufficient oxygen supply and hypoxia from increased oxygen consumption.**
      2. **Hypoglycemia secondary to depletion of glycogen stores.**
      3. **Metabolic acidosis caused by hypoxia and peripheral vasoconstriction.**
      4. **Decreased growth.**
      5. **Apnea.**
      6. **Pulmonary hypertension as a result of acidosis and hypoxia.**
   C. **Consequences of hypothermia.** As the capacity to compensate for the excessive heat loss is overwhelmed, hypothermia will ensue.
      1. **Clotting disorders: Disseminated intravascular coagulation and pulmonary hemorrhage can accompany severe hypothermia.**
      2. **Shock with resulting decreases in systemic arterial pressure, plasma volume, and cardiac output.**
      3. **Intraventricular hemorrhage.**
      4. **Severe sinus bradycardia.**
      5. **Increased neonatal mortality.**
   D. **Treatment of hypothermia.** Rapid versus slow rewarming continues to be *controversial,* although more clinicians are leaning toward more rapid rewarming. Rewarming may induce apnea and hypotension; therefore, the hypothermic infant should be continuously and closely monitored regardless of the rewarming method. One recommendation is to rewarm at a rate of 1 °C/h unless the infant weighs <1200 g, the gestational age is <28 weeks, or the temperature is <32.0 °C (89.6 °F) and the infant can be rewarmed more slowly (with a rate not to exceed 0.6 °C/h). Another recommendation is that, during rewarm-

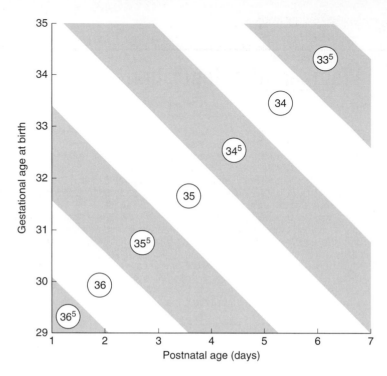

FIGURE 5–1. Neutral thermal environment during the first week of life, based on gestational age. *(Reproduced, with permission, from Sauer PJJ et al: New standards for neutral thermal environment of healthy very low birthweight infants in week one of life. Arch Dis Child 1984;59:18.)*

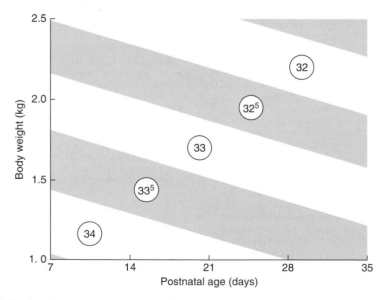

FIGURE 5–2. Neutral thermal environment from days 7 to 35 (in °C), based on body weight. *(Reproduced, with permission, from Sauer PJJ et al: New standards for neutral thermal environment of healthy very low birthweight infants in week one of life. Arch Dis Child 1984;59:18.)*

TABLE 5–1. APPROXIMATE NEUTRAL THERMAL ENVIRONMENT IN INFANTS WHO WEIGH >2500 g OR ARE >36 WEEKS' GESTATION[a]

Age	Temperature (°C)
0–24 h	31.0–33.8[b]
24–48 h	30.5–33.5
48–72 h	30.1–33.2
72–96 h	29.8–32.8
4–14 days	29.0–32.6
>2 weeks	Data not established[b]

[a]For infants <2500 g or <36 weeks, see Figures 5–1 and 5–2.
[b]In general, the smaller the infant is, the higher is the temperature.
Based on data from Scopes J, Ahmed I. Range of initial temperatures in sick and premature newborn babies. *Arch Dis Child* 1966;41:417.

ing, the skin temperature should not be >1 °C warmer than the coexisting rectal temperature.

1. **Equipment**
   a. **Closed incubator.** Incubators are usually used for infants who weigh <1800 g. Closed incubators are convectively heated (heated airflow); therefore, they do not prevent radiant heat loss unless they are provided with double-layered walls. Similarly, evaporation loss will be compensated for only when additional humidity is added to the incubator. One disadvantage of incubators is that they make it difficult to closely observe a sick infant or to perform any type of procedure. Body temperature changes associated with sepsis may be masked by the automatic temperature control system of closed incubators. Such changes will hence be expressed in the variations of the incubator's environmental temperature. An infant can be weaned from the incubator when his or her body temperature can be maintained at an environmental temperature of <30.0 °C (usually when the body weight reaches 1600–1800 g). Enclosed incubators maintain a neutral thermal environment by using one of the following devices:

   i. **Servocontrolled skin probe attached to the abdomen of the infant.** If the temperature falls, additional heat is delivered. As the target skin temperature is reached, the heating unit turns off automatically. A potential disadvantage is that overheating may occur if the skin sensor is detached from the skin.

   ii. **Air temperature control device.** With this device, the temperature of the air in the incubator is increased or decreased depending on the measured temperature of the infant. Use of this mode requires constant attention from a nurse and is usually used in older infants.

   iii. **Air temperature probe.** This probe hangs in the incubator near the infant and maintains a constant air temperature. There is less temperature fluctuation with this kind of probe.

   b. **Radiant warmer.** The radiant warmer is typically used for very unstable infants or during the performance of medical procedures. Heating is provided by radiation and, therefore, does not prevent convective and evaporative heat loss. The temperature can be maintained in the "servo mode" (ie, by means of a skin probe) or the "nonservo mode" (also called the "manual mode"), which maintains a constant radiant energy output regardless of the infant's temperature. If the radiant warmer is used in the manual mode, the infant should be observed very carefully to avoid overheating; this warmer should be used only for a limited period, such as in the delivery room. Insensible water loss may be extremely large in the very low birth weight (VLBW) infant (up to

7 mL/kg/h). Covering of the skin with semipermeable dressing or the use of a water-based ointment (eg, Aquaphor) may help to reduce insensible transepidermal water loss.

2. **Temperature regulation in the healthy term infant (weight >2500 g)**
   a. **Place the infant under a preheated radiant warmer immediately after delivery.**
   b. **Dry the infant completely to prevent evaporative heat loss.**
   c. **Cover the infant's head with a cap.**
   d. **Place the infant, wrapped in blankets, in a crib.**
      Note: Studies have shown that a healthy term infant can be wrapped in warm blankets and placed directly into the mother's arms without any significant heat loss.
3. **Temperature regulation in the sick term infant.** Follow the same procedure as for the healthy term infant, except place the infant under a radiant warmer with temperature servoregulation.
4. **Temperature regulation in the premature infant (weight 1000–2500 g)**
   a. **For an infant who weighs 1800–2500 g with no medical problems,** use of a crib, cap, and blankets is usually sufficient.
   b. **For an infant who weighs 1000–1800 g:**
      i. **A well infant should be placed in a closed incubator with servo-control.**
      ii. **A sick infant** should be placed under a radiant warmer with servo-control.
5. **Temperature regulation in the VLBW infant (weight <1000 g)**
   • **In the delivery room:** considerable evaporative heat loss occurs immediately after birth. Consequently, speedy drying of the infant has been emphasized as a very important aspect of the management of the VLBW infant. A more efficient and different approach has been advocated whereby an occlusive polyethylene wrap is applied from shoulder to feet, without drying, immediately at birth.
   • **In the nursery:** either the radiant warmer or the incubator can be used, depending on the institutional preference.

   a. **Radiant warmer**
      i. **Use servocontrol** with the temperature for abdominal skin set at 36.5–37.0 °C.
      ii. **Cover the infant's head** with a cap.
      iii. **To reduce convective heat loss,** place plastic wrap (eg, Saran Wrap) loosely over the infant below the neck. Prevent this wrap from directly contacting the infant's skin. Avoid placing the warmer in a drafty area.
      iv. **Maintain an inspired air temperature** of the hood or ventilator of ≥34.0–35.0 °C.
      v. **Place under the infant** a heating pad (K-pad) that has an adjustable temperature within 35.0–38.0 °C. To maintain thermal protection, it can be set between 35.0 and 36.0 °C. If the infant is hypothermic, the temperature can be increased to 37.0–38.0 °C (this is *controversial*).
      vi. **If the temperature cannot be stabilized,** move the infant to a closed incubator (in some institutions).
   b. **Closed incubator**
      i. **Use servocontrol,** with the temperature for abdominal skin set at 36.0–36.5 °C.
      ii. **Use a double-walled incubator** if possible.
      iii. **Cover the infant's head** with a cap.
      iv. **Keep the humidity level** at ≥40–50%.
         Note: Excessive humidity and dampness of the clothing and incubator can lead to excessive heat loss or accumulation of fluid and possible infections.

v. **Keep the temperature** of the ventilator at ≥34.0–35.0 °C.

vi. **Place under the infant** a heated mattress (K-pad) that has an adjustable temperature within 35.0–38.0 °C. For thermal protection, the temperature can be set between 35.0 and 36.0 °C. For warming a hypothermic infant, it can be set as high as 37.0–38.0 °C.

vii. **If the temperature is difficult to maintain,** try increasing the humidity level or use a radiant warmer (in some institutions).

II. **Hyperthermia.** *Hyperthermia* is defined as a temperature that is greater than the normal core temperature of 37.5 °C.

A. **Differential diagnosis**

1. **Environmental causes.** Some causes include excessive environmental temperature, overbundling of the infant, placement of the incubator in sunlight, a loose temperature skin probe with an incubator or radiant heater on a servocontrol mode, or a servocontrol temperature set too high.

2. **Infection.** Bacterial or viral infections (eg, herpes).

3. **Dehydration.**

4. **Maternal fever in labor.**

5. **Drug withdrawal.**

6. **Unusual causes.**

   a. **Hyperthyroid crisis or storm.**

   b. **Drug effect (eg, prostaglandin E₁).**

   $ $

   b. **Drug effect (eg, prostaglandin E_1).**

   c. **Riley-Day syndrome** (periodic high temperatures secondary to defective temperature regulation).

B. **Consequences of hyperthermia.** Hyperthermia, like cold stress, increases metabolic rate and oxygen consumption, resulting in tachycardia, tachypnea, irritability, apnea, and periodic breathing. If severe, it may lead to dehydration, acidosis, brain damage, and death.

C. **Treatment**

1. **Defining the cause of the elevated body temperature is the most important initial issue.** Mainly, one needs to determine whether the elevated temperature is the result of a hot environment or an increased endogenous production, such as is seen with infections. In the former case, one may find a loose temperature probe, an elevated incubator air temperature, and the extremities of the infant as high as the rest of the body. In the case of "true fever," one expects a low incubator air temperature as well as cold extremities secondary to peripheral vasoconstriction.

2. **Other measures** include turning down any heat source and removing excessive clothing.

3. **Additional measures for older infants** with significant temperature elevation

   a. **A tepid water sponge bath.**

   b. **Acetaminophen** (5–10 mg/kg per dose, orally or rectally, every 4 h).

REFERENCES

Sarman I et al: Rewarming preterm infants on a heated, water-filled mattress. *Arch Dis Child* 1989;64:687.

Sauer PJJ et al: New standards for neutral thermal environment of healthy very low birthweight infants in week one of life. *Arch Dis Child* 1984;59:18.

Scopes J, Ahmed I: Range of initial temperatures in sick and premature newborn babies. *Arch Dis Child* 1966;41:417.

Tafari N, Gentz J: Aspects on rewarming newborn infants with severe accidental hypothermia. *Acta Paediatr Scand* 1974;63:595.

Vohra S et al: Effect of polyethylene occlusive skin wrapping on heat loss in very low birth weight infants at delivery: a randomized trial. *J Pediatr* 1999;134:547.

6 Respiratory Management

Management of infants with respiratory distress is a basic function of neonatal intensive care. Skillful use of the ever-increasing range of mechanical devices and pharmacologic agents in the treatment of respiratory disease depends on a sound knowledge of respiratory physiology and pathology. Optimal treatment continues to be difficult to define, and considerable variability exists in assessing the risk–benefit ratio of various management strategies. This section provides an overview of current techniques used for neonatal respiratory support.

I. **General physiologic support**
   A. **Fluid therapy.** Most neonatal pulmonary disease is associated with increased pulmonary vascular permeability and is best managed with fluid restriction. Furthermore, excessive fluid administration may lead to prolonged patency of the ductus arteriosus and pulmonary edema. Depletion of intravascular volume leading to a decrease in cardiac output is also deleterious to pulmonary function.
   B. **Environment.** Normal body temperature of 36.5–37.5 °C (97.7–99.5 °F) is essential to respiratory management. Loss of normal body temperature profoundly affects acid-base balance, resulting in metabolic acidosis and increased oxygen consumption. Increased ambient humidity can ameliorate excessive losses of water and heat through immature skin.
   C. **Skin care.** The integrity of the skin is important for maintenance of both fluid balance and body temperature. Loss of intact skin also leads to increased risk for systemic infection. Minimal use of adhesives (tapes, leads, or patches) and careful protection of skin over bony prominences are essential.
   D. **Body position.** Positioning of respiratory care patients is important for optimal management. Unplanned changes of body position may alter endotracheal tube placement. Prolonged supine positioning ultimately leads to posterior lung segment atelectasis. Lateral positioning during mechanical ventilation can assist in improving atelectatic lobes or regions of interstitial emphysema. Finally, prone positioning of infants has been shown to greatly enhance ventilation by allowing greater total lung expansion and facilitating drainage of secretions.
   E. **Airway management.** Adequate measures for maintaining patency of the airways include positioning, suctioning of secretions, postural drainage, chest vibration, and gentle percussion. Chest physiotherapy should nevertheless be avoided in the first days of life of the very low birth weight infant because of increased risk of intraventricular hemorrhage. Excessive suctioning may also lead to airway trauma. Securing of the endotracheal tube and comfortable placement of nasal prongs are important.
   F. **Gastrointestinal.** Decompression of the stomach improves diaphragmatic excursion. An indwelling nasogastric or orogastric tube for gastric decompression and decreased bowel gas may be needed.
   G. **Calories.** Parenteral alimentation can begin as soon as acid-base balance is achieved and normal renal function is verified. Although adequate calorie intake is not possible early in the course of respiratory distress, early feedings by gavage of small volumes (1–2 mL every 3–4 h) are possible for most infants receiving mechanical ventilation. Early enteral feeds stimulate alimentation and set the stage for steady advancement of feedings.
II. **Monitoring.** Multiple means of monitoring cardiovascular and pulmonary status are available and are required for adequate management of infants in respiratory distress.

A. Blood gases. Management of ventilation, oxygenation, and changes in acid-base status are most accurately determined by arterial blood gas studies.

1. **Arterial blood gas studies** are the most standardized and accepted measure of respiratory status, especially for the oxygenation of low birth weight infants. They are considered invasive monitoring and require arterial puncture or an indwelling arterial catheter. Access via the umbilical artery or peripherally in the radial or posterior tibial artery is now considered routine.

2. **Arterial blood gases** may vary according to gestational age, age at the time of sampling, and ongoing ventilatory care. Examples of normal values for infants are given in Table 6–1.

3. **Calculated arterial blood gas indexes** for determining progression of respiratory distress are as follows:

   a. **Alveolar-to-arterial oxygen gradient (AaDo$_2$)** of >600 mm Hg for successive blood gases over 6 h is associated with >80% mortality in most infants if treatment and ventilation do not become effective. The formula for AaDo$_2$ is

$$AaDo_2 = \left[(Fio_2)(Pb - 47) - \frac{Paco_2}{R} \right] - Pao_2$$

   where Pb = barometric pressure (760 mm Hg at sea level), 47 = water vapor pressure, Paco$_2$ is assumed to be equal to alveolar Pco$_2$, and R = respiratory quotient (usually assumed to be 1 in neonates).

   b. **Arterial-to-alveolar oxygen ratio (a/A ratio)** is also an index for effective respiration. The a/A ratio is the index most often used for evaluation of response to surfactant therapy and is used as an indicator for inhaled nitric oxide therapy for pulmonary hypertension. The formula for the a/A ratio is

$$a / A = Pao_2 \Big/ \left[(Fio_2)(Pb - 47) - \frac{Paco_2}{R} \right]$$

B. Venous blood gases. Determination of values is the same as for arterial blood gases, but interpretation is different. The pH values are slightly lower and Pvco$_2$ values are slightly higher, whereas Pvo$_2$ values are of no value in assessing oxygenation.

C. Capillary blood gases. Arterializing of capillary blood is simply warming of the infant's heel just before sampling. The pH and Pco$_2$ values are usually slightly lower than arterial values, but this may vary considerably depending on the sampling technique. Po$_2$ data are of no value.

TABLE 6–1. NORMAL RANGE OF ARTERIAL BLOOD GAS VALUES FOR TERM AND PRETERM INFANTS AT NORMAL BODY TEMPERATURE AND ASSUMING NORMAL BLOOD HEMOGLOBIN CONTENT[a]

Gestational age	Pao$_2$ (mm Hg)	Paco$_2$ (mm Hg)	pH	Hco$_3$ (mEq/L)	BE/BD
Term	80–95	35–45	7.32–7.38	24–26	±3.0
Preterm (30–36 weeks' gestation)	60–80	35–45	7.30–7.35	22–25	±3.0
Preterm (<30 weeks' gestation)	45–60	38–50	7.27–7.32	19–22	±4.0

Hco$_3$, bicarbonate; BE, base excess, BD, base deficit.
[a]Values for Pao$_2$, Paco$_2$, and pH are measured directly by electrodes. Hco$_3$ and BE/BD values are calculated from nomograms of measured values at normal (14.8–15.5 mg/dL) hemoglobin content and body temperature (37 °C) and assuming hemoglobin saturation of ≥88%.

D. Noninvasive blood gas monitoring. Use of these technologies is strongly encouraged. They allow for continuous monitoring and can dramatically reduce the frequency of blood gas sampling, reducing iatrogenic blood loss and decreasing cost. Blood gas sampling is still necessary for calibrating noninvasive measures, determining acid-base status, and detecting hyperoxia.

    1. Pulse oximetry (Sao$_2$). The pulse oximeter uses a photo sensor on the skin to measure the percentage of oxygen saturation of hemoglobin available for oxygen transport. It is affected by the oxyhemoglobin dissociation curve. A higher saturation for a given oxygen tension (a curve shifted to the left) occurs with alkalosis, hypothermia, fetal hemoglobin, high altitude, and hypometabolism. A lower saturation for a given oxygen tension (a curve shifted to the right) occurs with acidosis, hyperthermia, hypermetabolism, and hypercarbia. Figure 6–1 compares hemoglobin saturation in adults and infants at birth, whereas Figure 6–2 illustrates a series of infant pulse oximetry studies correlating Sao$_2$ and Pao$_2$. Table 6–2 shows oxygen saturation of arterial blood (Sao$_2$) as a function of Pao$_2$ and pH and is useful in the interpretation of pulse oximeter readings.

        a. Limitations include poor correlation of Sao$_2$ to Pao$_2$ at upper and lower Pao$_2$ values. Sao$_2$ of 88–93% corresponds to Pao$_2$ of 50–80 mm Hg. For infants with high or low saturations, arterial blood gas correlation is needed.

        b. Advantages include minimal damage to the skin and no required manual calibration. Sao$_2$ by pulse oximetry is less affected by skin temperature and perfusion than transcutaneous oxygen.

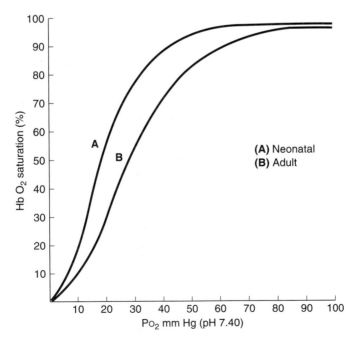

FIGURE 6–1. Comparison between normal mean oxyhemoglobin dissociation curves of **(A)** term infants at birth and **(B)** adults. The pH is 7.40. *(Modified and reproduced, with permission, from Sherwood WC, Cohen A [editors]: Transfusion Therapy: The Fetus, Infant, and Child. Masson. 1980.)*

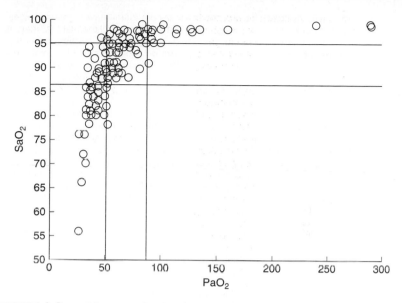

FIGURE 6-2. Range of Sao_2 versus Pao_2 by pulse oximetry on a group of monitored neonates. *Adapted, with permission, from Cunningham MD et al: Clinical experience with pulse oximetry in managing oxygen therapy in neonatal intensive care.* J Perinatol *1988;8:333.*)

TABLE 6-2. Sao_2 AS A FUNCTION OF Po_2 AND pH[a,b]

	pH				
Po_2	7.30	7.35	7.40	7.45	7.50
120	98	98	98	98	99
100	97	97	97	98	98
90	96	96	97	97	97
80	95	95	96	96	97
70	92	93	94	95	95
65	91	92	93	94	94
60	88	90	91	92	93
55	85	87	89	90	91
50	81	83	85	87	88
45	76	78	80	83	85
40	69	71	74	77	79
35	61	63	66	69	72
30	51	54	57	60	62
20	29	32	34	36	39
10	7	8	9	10	11

[a]Assuming a temperature of 37 °C, normal levels of 2,3 diphosphoglycerate, a $Paco_2$ of 40 mm Hg, and adult hemoglobin.
[b]This table is merely a reference tool and is not to be used for deriving precise values of Po_2 or pH from the Ohmeda Biox saturation readings. Courtesy the Ohmeda Company, Boulder, Colorado.

    c. Disadvantages include the tendency of patient movement and excessive external lighting to interfere with readings and the fact that there is no correction of Sao_2 for abnormal hemoglobin (eg, methemoglobin).

  2. Transcutaneous oxygen ($tcPo_2$) monitoring measures the partial pressure of oxygen from the skin surface by an electrochemical sensor known as the Clark polarographic electrode. The electrode heats the skin to 43–44 °C, and contact is maintained through a conducting electrolyte solution and an oxygen-permeable membrane.

    a. Limitations include the need for daily recalibration, relocation to different skin sites every 4–6 h, and irritation or injury to a premature infant's skin secondary to adhesive rings and thermal burns. Poor skin perfusion caused by shock, acidosis, hypoxia, hypothermia, edema, or anemia may prevent accurate measurements.

    b. Other disadvantages are related to the high cost of technician time and materials for relocation of the electrode and recalibration. Also, $tcPo_2$ has limited or no use in extremely low birth weight infants because it may result in skin injury.

    c. Advantages are that $tcPo_2$ is noninvasive and may provide indication of excessively high Pao_2 (>100 mm Hg).

  3. Transcutaneous carbon dioxide monitoring ($tcPco_2$) is usually accomplished simultaneously by a single lead enclosed with a $tcPo_2$ electrode. The $tcPco_2$ electrode (Stowe-Severinghaus) operates by tissue CO_2 equilibration across the skin and generation of an electrical charge proportional to the change in pH of the contact electrolyte solution.

    a. Limitations of $tcPco_2$ include all of those associated with $tcPo_2$ monitoring. Calibration and response times are longer for $tcPo_2$.

    b. Advantages. $tcPco_2$ is noninvasive and relatively accurate. Determination of $tcPco_2$ does not require the high electrode temperatures necessary for $tcPo_2$. The combination of $tcPo_2$ and pulse oximetry can dramatically decrease the frequency of arterial blood gas sampling.

    c. Disadvantages include the need for frequent technical support as well as skin injury in extremely low birth weight infants.

  4. End-tidal CO_2 monitoring ($Petco_2$). Expired breath analysis by infrared spectroscopy for CO_2 content gives close correlation to $Paco_2$. This technique is increasingly available for neonates. It gives rapid information about changes in CO_2, unlike the slow response time of $tcPco_2$.

    a. Limitations. An adapter to the endotracheal tube is often required, which may significantly increase the dead space of the patient's circuit. Accuracy is limited when the respiratory rate is >60 breaths/min or if the humidity of inspired air is excessive. Current devices are of limited use for premature infants.

    b. Advantages are that it is a noninvasive technique that may correlate well with arterial $Paco_2$.

    c. Disadvantages are related to various disease states. High ventilation-perfusion mismatches such as intrapulmonary shunts, uneven ventilation, or increased dead space are conditions that would give unreliable $Petco_2$ values. Generally, a/A ratios of <0.3 negate $Petco_2$ monitoring.

E. Monitoring of vital signs and other physiologic parameters. The infant with respiratory distress may have derangements of other organ functions. Comprehensive monitoring requires that physical measurements as well as biochemical and electrophysical monitoring be incorporated into the overall patient data.

  1. Physical examination for color and respiratory effort as well as auscultation of the lungs for equality of breath sounds is important. Additionally, cardiac, neurologic, and abdominal examinations are required. Abdominal distention cannot be overlooked in an infant with respiratory distress.

2. **Blood pressure** requires frequent monitoring. Vasopressor therapy is often required for neonates with severe respiratory distress. Standard nomograms for blood pressure (see Appendix C) are available for comparative data.

3. **Urine output** is a critical value in the overall assessment of a neonate in respiratory failure. A urine output of 1.5–3.0 mL/kg/h signifies good cardiac output, adequate intravascular volume with normal central venous pressure, and normal mean blood pressure values. Also of importance is urine specific gravity; fluctuating values of 1.008–1.015 are indicators of normal fluid balance.

4. **Central venous pressure.** The umbilical vein catheter at the level of the right atrium may be used for central venous pressure monitoring. Levels of 4–6 cm H_2O are generally taken as normal; however, the range is 2–8 cm H_2O. Use of umbilical vein catheters for this purpose is controversial because of the risk of air embolism and infection.

5. **Monitoring blood studies** for hemoglobin, hematocrit, calcium, sodium, potassium, chloride, blood urea nitrogen, and creatinine is related to managing respiratory failure and maintaining satisfactory cardiovascular and renal function.

F. **Monitoring mechanical ventilation.** Although there are many different types of infant ventilators, only a few devices and means for monitoring events during mechanical breath cycles are available.

1. **Inspired oxygen.** Fraction of inspired oxygen (F_{IO_2}) is a percentage of oxygen available for inspiration. It is expressed as either a percentage (21–100%) or a decimal (0.21–1.00). Battery-operated oxygen analyzers are standard for monitoring oxygen therapy for infants. They consist of electrochemical cells calibrated by ambient or inspired oxygen concentrations up to 100%. During mechanical ventilation, an in-line oxygen analyzer with a ventilator circuit for continuous readout of the oxygen concentration flowing to the infant is preferable. Further management of oxygen therapy requires:

   a. **Calibration of the analyzer** every 8–12 h.

   b. **Blending of air and oxygen** to ensure the least amount of oxygen required to maintain desired blood oxygen saturation.

   c. **Humidification** of all inspired oxygen and air mixtures.

   d. **Warming** of inspired gases to 34–35 °C through a humidification device gives ~96% water vapor saturation.

2. **Mean airway pressure (Paw).** $\overline{Paw}$ is an average of the proximal pressure applied to the airway throughout the entire respiratory cycle (Figure 6–3). The ventilator settings of rate (R), inspiratory time (IT), peak inspiratory pressure (PIP), and positive end-expiratory pressure (PEEP) can be expressed as $\overline{Paw}$ by the formula

$$\overline{Paw} = \frac{(R)(IT)(PIP) + \left[60 - (R)(IT) \times PEEP\right]}{60}$$

   a. $\overline{Paw}$ correlates well with mean lung volume for a given mode and strategy of mechanical ventilation.

   b. $\overline{Paw}$ >10–15 cm H_2O during conventional ventilation is associated with an increased risk of air leaks (pneumothorax or pulmonary interstitial emphysema).

   c. $\overline{Paw}$ **of high-frequency ventilation** is not strictly comparable with that of conventional mechanical ventilation.

   d. **Oxygen index** (OI) is a frequently used calculation that incorporates F_{IO_2}, $\overline{Paw}$, and Pao_2.

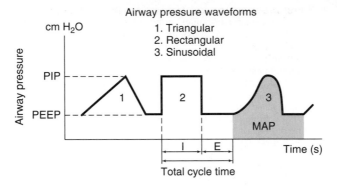

FIGURE 6–3. Graphic representation of ventilator airway pressure waveforms and other ventilator terminology. See Glossary for explanations.

$$OI = \frac{F_{IO_2} \times \overline{Paw} \times 100}{Pao_2}$$

OI values of 30–40 are indicative of severe respiratory distress. If OI is found to increase steadily over a 6-h period from 30 to 40, profound respiratory failure on conventional mechanical ventilation is apparent. Mortality may exceed 80%.

3. **Pulmonary functions.** New flow sensors allow for frequent or continuous monitoring of mechanical and spontaneous breath mechanics for flow, airway pressure, and volume. With flow sensors, or pneumotachygraphs, additional pulmonary function testing is possible. Occluded breath techniques provide passive mechanics for compliance and resistance as well as determination of time constants.

   a. **$\overline{Paw}$** is determined in the proximal airway from a differential pressure transducer. Transpulmonary pressure is a measure of the difference between $\overline{Paw}$ and esophageal pressure taken from an indwelling esophageal catheter or balloon.

   b. **Tidal volume (V_T)**, a function of PIP during mechanical ventilation, is integrated from flow (mL/s) and measured as mL/breath. By convention, V_T is expressed as breath volume adjusted to body weight (mL/kg). Several devices are now available for continuous bedside V_T monitoring. V_T varies from 5 to 7 mL/kg for most newborn infants.

   c. **Minute ventilation (MV).** Respiratory rate and V_T combine to give MV as

$$MV = Rate \times V_T$$

   Example: 40 breaths/min $\times$ 6.5 mL/kg = 260 mL/kg/min.
   Normal MV values for newborns are 240–360 mL. Monitoring of V_T and MV simultaneously with Paw provides for graded adjustments of PIP, PEEP, and IT. Optimal V_T should be determined on the basis of adequate MV at the least PIP and balanced by achieving acceptable blood gases.

   d. **Pressure-volume (P-V) and flow-volume (F-V) loops** are a visualization of breath-to-breath dynamics. Flow, volume, and pressure signals combine to give P-V and F-V loops. Loops give inspiratory and expiratory limits of the breath cycle. F-V loops provide information regarding airway resistance, especially restricted expiratory breath flow. P-V loops primarily reflect a changing lung dynamic compliance.

  e. **Compliance** (C_L) values of <1.0 cm H_2O/mL are consistent with interstitial or alveolar lung disease such as respiratory distress syndrome (RDS). Lung compliance of 1.0–2.0 mL/cm H_2O reflects recovery, as in postsurfactant therapy.

  f. **Resistance** (R_L) of >100 cm H_2O/L/s is suggestive of airway disease with restricted airflow such as in bronchopulmonary dysplasia.

  g. **Time constant** (K_t) is the product of $C_L \times R_L$ (in seconds). Normal values are 0.12–0.15 s. K_t is a measure of how long it takes for alveolar and proximal airway pressures to equilibrate. At the end of 3 time constants, 95% of the V_T has entered (during inspiration) or left (during expiration) the alveoli. To avoid gas trapping, the measured expiratory time should be >3 times K_t (0.36–0.45 s).

III. **Ventilatory support.** Infants with respiratory distress may need only supplemental oxygen, whereas those with respiratory failure and apnea require mechanical ventilatory support. This section reviews the spectrum of available means for ventilatory support, with the exception of high-frequency ventilation (see section VI). Mechanical ventilatory support offers great benefits but also incurs significant risks. Considerable controversy still exists concerning the proper use of any mode or strategy of assisted ventilation.

  A. **Oxygen supplementation without mechanical ventilation.** Hypoxic infants able to maintain an adequate minute ventilation are assisted with free-flow oxygen or air-oxygen mixtures.

   1. **Oxygen hoods** provide an enclosure for blended air-oxygen supply, humidification, and continuous oxygen concentration monitoring. Hoods are easy to use and provide access to and visibility of the infant. Pulse oximetry is recommended while hoods are in use.

   2. **Mask oxygen** is not suitable for infants because of poor control and lack of monitoring of oxygen supply.

   3. **Nasal cannulas** are well suited for infants needing low concentrations of oxygen. Delivery can be controlled by flowmeters delivering as little as 0.025 L/min. Flow rates of >1 L/min may impart distending airway pressure. Table 6–3 gives approximate percentages of nasal cannula oxygen based on flow rates of 0.25–1.0 L/min at blended Fio_2 settings of 40–100%. Pulse oximeter monitoring is recommended while nasal cannulas are in use.

  B. **Continuous positive airway pressure (CPAP).** A mask, nasal prongs, or an endotracheal tube can be used to apply CPAP. It improves Pao_2 by stabilizing the airway and allowing alveolar recruitment. CO_2 retention may result from excessive distending airway pressure.

   1. **Full-face mask CPAP** is rarely used. A new nasal mask CPAP device has become available. This technique may reduce trauma to the nares compared with prongs or nasopharyngeal CPAP.

TABLE 6–3. NASAL CANNULA CONVERSION TABLE

Flow rate (L/min)	Fio_2			
	100%	80%	60%	40%
0.25	34%	31%	26%	22%
0.50	44%	37%	31%	24%
0.75	60%	42%	35%	25%
1.00	66%	49%	38%	27%

General guideline only; numbers are not exact.

2. **Nasal CPAP prongs** are the most commonly applied means of delivering CPAP and are used for respiratory assistance in infants with mild RDS. The prongs are also used postextubation to maintain airway and alveolar expansion in the process of weaning from mechanical ventilation and recovery from respiratory diseases. This treatment maintains upper airway patency and, as such, is useful in infants with apnea of infancy. CPAPs may range from 2–8 cm H_2O, although 2–6 cm H_2O is most often used. Overdistention of the airway can lead to excessive CO_2 retention or air leak (pneumothorax). Gastric distention may be a complication of nasal CPAP, and an orogastric tube for decompression should be used. Infants can be fed by nasogastric tube during nasal CPAP therapy with close monitoring of abdominal girth.

3. **Nasopharyngeal CPAP** is an alternative to nasal prongs. An endotracheal tube is passed nasally and advanced to the nasopharynx. A ventilator or CPAP device is used to deliver continuous distending pressure as with nasal prongs. This approach is slightly more secure in active infants and may cause less trauma to the nasal septum.

4. **Endotracheal tube CPAP** has nearly the same effect as nasal prongs. It is often an intermediate measure after weaning from mechanical ventilation. It is also a means of assisted ventilation when minute ventilation is adequate but secretions are excessive and tracheal suctioning is required. Because of the increased airway resistance from the endotracheal tube, endotracheal CPAP may increase the work of breathing to the extent that apneas may ensue. CPAP is usually abandoned for mechanical ventilation when a/A ratios have fallen <0.22 or apneic episodes occur.

C. **Mechanical ventilation.** The decision to initiate mechanical ventilation is complex. The severity of respiratory distress, severity of blood gas abnormalities, natural history of the specific lung disease, and degree of cardiovascular and other physiologic instabilities must be considered. Because mechanical ventilation may result in serious complications, the decision to intubate and ventilate should not be taken lightly.

1. **Bag-and-mask or bag-to-endotracheal tube hand-held assemblies** allow for emergency ventilatory support. Portable manometers are always required for monitoring peak airway pressures during hand-bag ventilation. Bags may be self-inflating or flow-dependent anesthesia-type bags. All hand-held assemblies must have pop-off valves to avoid excessive pressures to the airway.

2. **Pressure-control infant ventilators.** These are the most commonly used ventilators in neonatal care. They are time-cycled for initiating and limiting the inspiratory cycle of ventilation and pressure-limited to control the flow and volume for each delivered breath. Delivered breath volume and P̄aw are determined by ventilator settings. Air-oxygen mixtures are heated and humidified for delivery through the continuous-flow circuit attached to the airway. Establishing effective ventilatory settings is the key to successful ventilatory support. Table 6–4 gives basic ventilator setting changes and expected blood gas responses.

   a. **Support rates may vary** from 1 to 150, but most commonly they are 20–60 breaths/min. The rate is adjusted to combine with V_T to provide adequate minute ventilation.

   b. **IT varies** from 0.2 to 1 s, but most commonly it is 0.25–0.5 s. IT must allow for adequate expiratory time (ET). For example, at a rate of 60 breaths/min, an IT of 0.35 s gives an ET of 0.65 s.

   c. **PIP.** Delivered V_T depends on PIP. Initial choice of PIP is dependent on observation of chest wall movement during hand-bag ventilation, manometer readings during hand-bag ventilation, and auscultation of breath sounds. Subsequently, PIP should be adjusted to achieve optimal V_T (5–7 mL/kg), minute ventilation, and effective gas exchange

TABLE 6–4. CHANGES IN BLOOD GAS LEVELS CAUSED BY CHANGES IN VENTILATOR SETTINGS

Variable	Rate	PIP	PEEP	IT	F_{IO_2}
To increase Pa_{CO_2}	Decr.	Decr.	NA	NA	NA
To decrease Pa_{CO_2}	Incr.	Incr.	NA[a]	NA[b]	NA
To increase Pa_{O_2}	NA	Incr.	Incr.	Incr.	Incr.
To decrease Pa_{O_2}	NA	Decr.	Decr.	NA	Decr.

PIP, peak inspiratory pressure; PEEP, positive end-expiratory pressure; IT, inspiratory time; F_{IO_2}, fraction of inspired oxygen; Decr., decrease; NA, not applicable; Incr., increase.
[a]In severe pulmonary edema and pulmonary hemorrhage, increased PEEP can decrease Pa_{CO_2}.
[b]Not applicable unless the inspiratory:expiratory ratio is excessive.

based on satisfactory blood gas determinations. Optimal V_t may vary according to specific disease.

   d. **PEEP.** Like CPAP, PEEP is a distending pressure that stabilizes the airway and prevents alveolar derecruitment. Settings for PEEP range from 2–6 cm H_2O pressure, although most commonly pressures are 2–4 cm H_2O.

   e. **Pāw.** The ventilator settings just discussed determine Pāw (see Section II,F,2). Pāw of 4–20 cm H_2O is used with pressure-control ventilators. If settings result in Pāw >15 cm H_2O, without improved ventilation, a change to high-frequency ventilation should be considered.

3. **Volume-control infant ventilators.** Previously, volume ventilation was not considered for infants because measurement and monitoring of optimal V_T were not possible. With the development of variable orifice and hot-wire continuous-flow sensors, volume monitoring and thus volume-control ventilation have become available for newborn care.

   a. **Rate varies as it does for pressure-control ventilation.** Because volume is preset, monitoring of both mechanical and spontaneous breath V_T allows for determination of volume-control ventilator-derived minute ventilation versus the infant's own minute ventilation.

   b. **IT** must be set to allow for adequate volume delivery. Exceedingly short IT (<0.32 s) reduces volume delivery.

   c. **PIP** varies automatically for the delivery of preset V_T in accordance with changing lung compliance. Improving compliance, especially after surfactant therapy, may lead to excessive volume delivery with pressure-control ventilators. Volume-control ventilation, however, minimizes the risk for lung overdistention.

   d. **PEEP** usage is the same for volume- and pressure-control ventilation.

   e. **Pāw** should be monitored as in pressure-control ventilation, and the same upper limits (10–15 cm H_2O) suggest high-frequency ventilation if Pāw increases >15 cm H_2O.

4. **Synchronized intermittent mechanical ventilation (SIMV).** Mechanical ventilation of the alert, nonsedated, nonparalyzed infant imparts automated breaths irrespective of the infant's own respiratory cycle. The result is repeated bouts of interrupted or "bucked" breaths, causing patient agitation and poor ventilation (Figure 6–4). Technical developments have resulted in synchronized ventilation for both pressure-control and volume-control ventilators. SIMV is also available with assist-control modes for those ventilators that allow for preset rates if an infant becomes apneic on intermittent mechanical ventilation. Advantages of SIMV include lower PIP settings while achieving optimal V_T and maintenance of adequate minute ventilation at a lower Pāw. SIMV also allows for greater patient comfort during mechanical ventilation, less agitation, and much less need for sedation. Four different types of SIMV are now available.

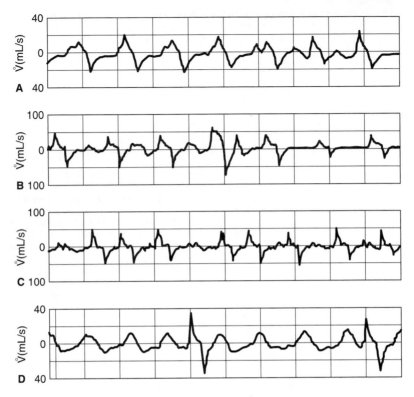

FIGURE 6–4. Waveforms A and B are of infants with interrupted breaths on mechanical ventilation without synchronized intermittent mechanical ventilation (SIMV). Waveforms C are reflective of SIMV at mechanical rates of 40 bpm with an infant respiratory rate of 50–60 bpm. Waveforms D are of SIMV for an infant on a ventilator with a rate of 15 bpm and a spontaneous infant breathing rate of 55–60 bpm.

    a. Synchronizing ventilation with abdominal wall movement using a Graseby capsule. Abdominal wall movement requires optimal capsule placement (Infant Star/Star Sync, Infrasonics, San Diego, CA).

    b. Airway flow sensing by hot-wire anemometer allows for flow-synchronized ventilation based on the airway flow signal originating with the first phase of inspiration (Bear Cub/NVM1, Bear Medical, Riverside, CA). A similar anemometer is also available as a built-in unit with the ventilator (Baby Log 8000, Draeger, Lubeck, Germany).

    c. Variable orifice pneumotachometers for flow-synchronized ventilation use the inspiratory flow signal to synchronize spontaneous breaths with mechanical breaths (VIP Bird, Palm Springs, CA).

    d. Patient-triggered synchronized ventilation uses chest wall impedance leads to signal chest wall movement (Sechrist IV/SAVI, Sechrist, Anaheim, CA).

  D. Fine-tuning mechanical ventilation. The usual goal of mechanical ventilation is to supplement the patient's spontaneous efforts sufficiently to achieve adequate gas exchange. Adequate gas exchange must be determined for each patient because goals vary depending on diagnosis, gestational age, and level of support required. For example, in a 600-g premature infant with RDS, excessive V_T and hyperoxia are associated with significant long-term morbidity. In this patient, ventilation to provide a Pco_2 of 55 mm Hg with supplemental oxygen to maintain Po_2 of 50–70 mm Hg would be considered optimal by many practitioners. In a term infant with meconium aspiration and pulmonary hypertension, a Pco_2 of 25 mm Hg and a Po_2 of 150 mm Hg may be desired, even if large V_Ts and high pressures are required.

Neonatal lung disease is rarely static, necessitating frequent adjustments to ventilatory parameters. A list of basic ventilator setting changes and effects is found in Table 6–4.

1. **Weaning from mechanical ventilation and extubation.** As lung function improves with disease resolution, mechanical support should be decreased as quickly as tolerated. Most patients do not need to be "weaned" from mechanical support; they need support decreased to match their need. Continuous monitoring with pulse oximetry and $tcPco_2$ aids in weaning and limits the need for blood gas sampling. A reduced oxygen requirement and improved compliance (decrease in PIP to maintain V_T) usually herald the weaning phase.

   Although *controversial*, pretreatment of infants with aminophylline is believed by some clinicians to enhance infant response to progressive weaning efforts. Disease state, gestational age, and caloric support influence response to weaning process.

   a. **PIP is usually weaned first** because overinflation injury is more deleterious than providing a greater rate than necessary. PIP is decreased to maintain normal V_T (or chest excursion).

   b. **Fio_2 is weaned whenever possible** as determined by pulse oximetry or blood gases. Decreases in PIP decrease $\overline{Paw}$ and may transiently increase oxygen requirements during weaning.

   c. **Weaning to extubation.** Three methods are being used, and their indications are "institutionally" based.

      i. **Progressive rate wean.** Rate settings should be decreased frequently. Infants ready to be weaned tolerate the rate wean and do not require more Fio_2. An infant should be able to maintain adequate minute ventilation without experiencing hypercarbia or apnea. When the ventilator rate is <10–15 breaths/min, the infant should be extubated. Some infants may require several hours to wean, whereas others need several days to 1 week or more.

      ii. **CPAP weaning.** The rate should be weaned down to 5–10 breaths/min. If this condition is tolerated for 1 h, endotracheal CPAP should be set at 3–4 cm H_2O for 2–4 h. If the infant tolerates this step with acceptable blood gases and no respiratory distress, he or she should be started on 5 min of CPAP and then given 55 min of full ventilatory support. The interval on CPAP should be increased by 5 min/h. Once 60 full min of CPAP is tolerated, continuous CPAP can be attempted. Extubation is performed in 2–4 h if CPAP continues to be well tolerated. This form of weaning is *controversial*. Breathing with endotracheal CPAP may increase the work of breathing, and some clinicians believe that the potential benefits of CPAP are lost because the infant tires unnecessarily.

      iii. **Weaning assist-control ventilation.** Because all spontaneous breaths are mechanically supported by this mode of ventilation, reduction of the rate below the patient's spontaneous rate has no effect on the level of support. Weaning is accomplished by successive decreases in PIP. When adequate ventilation is maintained with minimal pressures (10–12 cm H_2O), extubation may be attempted.

2. **Care after extubation.** Continued monitoring of blood gases, respiratory effort, and vital signs is required. Additional oxygen support is often needed in the immediate postextubation period.

a. **Supplemental oxygen** may be given by hood or by nasal cannulas. The oxygen concentration should be increased by >5% over the last oxygen level obtained while the infant was on the ventilator.

b. **Nasal CPAP** may be especially helpful in preventing reintubation secondary to postextubation atelectasis.

c. **Chest physical therapy** (every 3–4 h) after extubation helps to maintain a clear airway. Postural drainage with percussion and suction procedures should be monitored routinely. Aerosol treatments with bronchodilators also help to maintain airway patency.

d. **If the infant has had an increasing oxygen requirement** or has clinically deteriorated, an anteroposterior chest x-ray film should be obtained 6 h postextubation to monitor for atelectasis.

IV. **Pharmacologic respiratory support and surfactant.** Numerous medications are available for improvement of respiration. They represent a broad range of therapeutics, of which the bronchodilators and anti-inflammatory drugs are the oldest and most common. The use of mixtures of inhaled gases such as helium and nitric oxide are recent forms of treatment. Sedatives and paralyzing agents remain *controversial* in neonatal respiratory management. Finally, surfactant replacement therapy has rapidly become a major adjunct in the care of preterm infants, and its use has expanded to disease states other than RDS (hyaline membrane disease), for which it was originally intended. All medications are discussed with regard to dosage and side effects in Table 6–5 but are briefly reviewed here for the purpose of incorporating their use into respiratory management strategies.

A. **Bronchodilators (inhaled agents).** Most of these drugs are sympathomimetic agents that stimulate β_1-, β_2-, or α-adrenergic receptors. They have both inotropic and chronotropic effects and provide bronchial smooth muscle and vascular relaxation. Albuterol is probably the most commonly used aerosolized bronchodilator. Other bronchodilators are presented in Table 6–5. Two anticholinergic agents (atropine and ipratropium) are also used as inhaled bronchodilators for inhibition of acetylcholine at lung receptor sites and bronchial smooth muscle relaxation. All are used to minimize airway resistance and allow decreased $\overline{Paw}$ needed for mechanical ventilation.

B. **Bronchodilators (systemic).** Aminophylline (parenteral) and theophylline (enteral) are methylxanthines with considerable bronchial dilating action. Neonatal use includes bronchodilatation and stimulation of respiratory effort.

C. **Anti-inflammatory agents**

1. **Steroid therapy** has been widely used in the treatment or prevention of chronic lung disease. Although steroid therapy results in significant short-term improvement in pulmonary function, long-term benefit remains unproved. The substantial adverse effects of steroid therapy have led the American Academy of Pediatrics and the Canadian Pediatric Society to issue a joint recommendation against the routine use of steroid therapy.

2. **Cromolyn** prevents mast cells from releasing histamine and leukotriene-like substances. Its actions are slow but progressive over 2–4 weeks. Indications for its use in neonates have not been established. This agent is considered for use in infants with progressive reactive airway disease, prolonged mechanical ventilatory support, and minimal response to attempts to wean from the ventilator.

D. **Inhaled gas mixtures**

1. **Heliox** (helium, 78–80%; oxygen, 20–22%) produces an inspired gas less dense than nitrogen-oxygen mixtures or oxygen alone. Use of heliox reduces the increased resistive load of breathing, improves distribution of ventilation, and creates less turbulence in narrow airways. Limited neonatal use has indicated that heliox has been associated with lower inspired oxygen requirements and shorter duration of mechanical ventilatory support.

2. **Nitric oxide** (NO) is a potent gaseous vasodilator produced by endothelial cells. NO is rapidly bound by hemoglobin, limiting its action to the site

TABLE 6-5. AEROSOL THERAPY IN NEONATES, INDICATING DOSING, RECEPTOR EFFECTS, AND COMMON SIDE EFFECTS

Drug	Receptors	Side effects
Isoproterenol (Isuprel): 0.1–0.25 mL (0.5–1.25 mg) of 0.5% solution. Dilute with NS to 3 mL. Dose: every 3–4 h.	β_1: chronotropic, inotropic β_2: relax airways and vasculature, smooth muscle	Tachycardia Arrhythmias Hypertension Hyperglycemia Tolerance, tremor Excessive smooth muscle relaxation = airway collapse
Albuterol (Salbutamol, Ventolin): 0.04 mL/kg/dose of 0.5% solution. Dilute with NS to 3 mL. Dose: every 4–6 h.	β_2: long lasting (duration, 3–8 h) Fewer side effects than isoproterenol or metaproterenol	Tachycardia (potentiated by methylxanthines) Hypertension Hyperglycemia Tremor
Metaproterenol: 0.1–0.25 mL (5–12.5 mg) of 5% solution. Dilute with NS to 3 mL. Dose: every 6 h.	β_2: less specific for airways than albuterol	Same as isoproterenol Cardiac arrhythmias potentiated by hypoxia
Cromolyn (Intal): 20 mg. Dilute with NS to 3 mL. Dose: every 6–8 h.	Anti-inflammatory by stabilizing mast cells	Anaphylaxis Caution in patients with liver or renal disease Bronchospasm from inflammatory response Upper airway irritation
Terbutaline (Brethine): 0.01–0.02 mg/kg. Dilute with NS to 3 mL. Dose: every 2–8 h. Minimum dose: 0.1 mg.	β_2: peripheral dilation	Hypertension Hyperglycemia Tachycardia
Atropine: 0.03–0.05 mg/kg. Dilute with NS to 2.5 mL. Dose: every 6–8 h.	Vagolytic	Tachycardia Arrhythmia Hypotension Ileus, airway dryness Thick secretions, suggest use in combination with albuterol
Ipratropium (Atrovent): 175 mcg. Dilute with NS to 3 mL. Dose: every 8 h.	Antagonizes acetylcholine at parasympathetic sites	Nervousness Dizziness Nausea, blurred vision Cough, palpitations Rash, urinary difficulties
Epinephrine, racemic (Vaponefrin): 0.1–0.3 mL. Dilute with NS to 3 mL. Dose: every 30 min–2 h 4 times. (Racemic epinephrine, 2 mg = L-epinephrine, 1 mg) L-Epinephrine 1:1000: 0.05–0.15 mL. Dilute with NS to 3 mL. Dose: 30 min–2 h 4 times.	α receptor	Tachycardia Tremor Hypertension

NS, normal saline.

of production or administration. Delivered in the ventilatory gas, NO produces vasodilation only in the vascular bed of well-ventilated regions of the lung, thereby reducing intrapulmonary shunt as well as pulmonary vascular resistance. Furthermore, there is no systemic effect.

a. Actions. NO diffuses rapidly across alveolar cells to vascular smooth muscle, where it causes an increase in cyclic guanosine monophosphate (GMP), resulting in smooth muscle relaxation.

b. Dosage. NO is administered at low concentration, 2–80 ppm. The dose is titrated to effect (improved oxygenation being the most common). Rarely do concentrations >20–40 ppm yield additional benefit.

c. Administration. NO is blended into the ventilatory gases, preferably close to the patient connector to avoid excessive dwell time with high oxygen concentrations, which may result in excessive NO_2 concentrations. In-line sensors are used to measure delivered NO and nitrogen dioxide (NO_2) concentrations. Scavenging of expiratory gases is often performed, although the amount of NO and NO_2 released into room air rarely results in detectable concentrations. Techniques for use with high-frequency ventilators have also been developed. Co-oximetry measurement of methemoglobin is required. The NO dose should be decreased if methemoglobin is >4% or if the NO_2 concentration is >1–2 ppm.

d. Indications for use. NO is currently under investigation for use in a variety of lung diseases in which inappropriate pulmonary vascular constriction adversely affects oxygenation. The resultant vasodilation may either decrease pulmonary vascular resistance in general, thereby reducing right-to-left shunting, or result in less intrapulmonary shunt, or both. Use of NO in cases of severe respiratory failure suggests that it may reduce the need for extracorporeal membrane oxygenation (ECMO) in 30–45% of eligible patients.

e. Adverse effects. Systemic vascular effects are not seen with NO use. NO_2 poisoning and methemoglobinemia are the most likely complications. Use of NO in centers that do not provide ECMO is controversial.

E. Sedatives and paralyzing agents. Agitation is a common problem for infant mechanical ventilation. Infants may have interrupted respiratory cycles and respond by "bucking" or "fighting" the ventilator breaths. The agitation that results is often associated with hypoxic episodes. Sedation or muscle relaxation by paralysis may be required. It should be noted, however, that with the use of ventilators with either flow-sensed or patient-triggered synchronized ventilation (SIMV) much less sedation is required and paralysis is rarely needed.

1. Sedatives include lorazepam, phenobarbital, fentanyl, and morphine. Each agent has advantages and side effects.

2. Paralyzing agents include pancuronium and vecuronium. Muscle relaxation by paralysis results in considerable third spacing of fluid, requiring added volume expanders to maintain blood pressure and urine output.

F. Surfactant replacement therapy. The availability of surfactant treatment has dramatically changed the care of infants with RDS (hyaline membrane disease). Surfactant administration early in the course of RDS restores pulmonary function and prevents tissue injury that otherwise results from ventilation of surfactant-deficient lungs. As a result, mortality from RDS has dropped dramatically.

1. Composition. Three natural surfactant preparations are available in the United States. Beractant (Survanta) was the first approved by the Food and Drug Administration (FDA) and is produced from purified minced bovine lung, with the addition of phospholipids and spreading agents. Calfactant (Infasurf) is a purified extract of calf surfactant. Poractant alfa (Curosurf) is a purified extract of porcine surfactant. All contain the hydrophobic surfactant-associated proteins SP-B and SP-C, which are necessary for spreading and surface layer formation (Table 6–6). Clinical comparison trials are underway.

2. Actions. All surfactant preparations are intended to replace the missing or inactivated natural surfactant of the infant. Surface tension reduction and stabilization of the alveolar air–water interface are the basic functions of surfactant compounds. Air–water interface stability imparts lower

TABLE 6-6. COMPOSITION OF PULMONARY SURFACTANT (% BY WEIGHT)

Phospholipids	85%
PC	80%
PG	7%
PI + PS	5%
PE	4%
Sph	2%
Other	2%
Neutral lipids (cholesterol, free fatty acids)	7%
Surfactant-associated proteins (SP-A, SP-B, SP-C)	8%

PC, phosphatidylcholine; PG, phosphatidylglycerol; PI, phosphatidylinositol; PS, phosphatidylserine; PE, phosphatidylethanolamine; Sph, sphingomyelin; SP-A, -B, and -C, surfactant proteins A, B, and C.

alveolar surface tension and prevents atelectasis, or alternating areas of atelectasis and hyperinflation.

3. **Dosage and administration.** Each preparation has specific dosage and dosing procedures. Direct tracheal instillation is involved in all preparations. Surfactants are given both by continuous infusion via side port on the endotracheal tube adapter and by aliquots via a catheter placed through the endotracheal tube. Changes in body position during dosing aid in more uniform delivery of surfactant. The relative advantages of these methods of administration are currently being studied.

    a. **Prophylactic dosing at birth.** This form of treatment is used less often and only when resuscitation and surfactant administration can be safely pursued simultaneously.

    b. **Administration of surfactant preparations** after respiratory distress is established. Currently, surfactant therapy occurs once the patient has been stabilized and the diagnosis of RDS has been established.

    c. **Repeat dosing** may follow at 6- to 12-h intervals. Repeat doses should follow loss of response after initial improvement has been seen. Repeat dosing after the second dose is *controversial*

    d. **Airway obstruction** may occur during surfactant administration because of the viscosity of the surfactant preparations. Increased mechanical support may be required until the surfactant is spread from the airways to the alveoli.

4. **Efficacy of surfactant treatment** can be observed for both immediate and long-term clinical conditions.

    a. **Early effects** include a reduction of FIO_2 need and improved PaO_2, $PaCO_2$, and a/A ratio. Likewise, improved V_T and compliance should be noted with improved lung function and decreased ventilator PIPs.

    b. **Long-term effects** should result in decreased necessity for mechanical ventilation and less severe chronic lung disease of infancy. Complications of patent ductus arteriosus, necrotizing enterocolitis, and intraventricular hemorrhage have not been significantly influenced by surfactant therapy to date.

5. **Side effects**

    a. **Small risk for pulmonary hemorrhage.**

    b. **Secondary pulmonary infections.**

    c. **Air leak (pneumothorax) after bolus administration of surfactant compounds.** Rapid changes in V_T require immediate reduction of PIPs. Failure to do so while also decreasing FIO_2 may lead to air leaks.

6. **Surfactant therapy for diseases other than RDS (hyaline membrane disease).** Encouraging preliminary reports of surfactant therapy have been noted in cases of pneumonia, meconium aspiration syndrome, per-

sistent pulmonary hypertension, and adult respiratory distress syndrome (ARDS), but no protocols for treatment are available at this time. Dilute surfactant solutions are being studied for use as lung lavage fluids for meconium aspiration.

V. **Strategies for respiratory management of certain newborn diseases**
   A. **RDS (hyaline membrane disease)**
      1. **Clinical presentation.** Patients are premature with immature lungs and surfactant deficiency. Blood gases reflect poor oxygenation, declining a/A ratios (<0.5), and CO_2 accumulation. Monitoring of lung mechanics reveals poor compliance and diminished V_T but near-normal airway resistance. Progressive atelectasis resulting from surfactant deficiency worsens the compliance (lung stiffness), and the work of breathing increases to maintain minute ventilation. All of the these result in exhaustion of the infant and, ultimately, apnea.
      2. **Management.** Oxygen supplementation is required to maintain Pao_2 at 50–80 mm Hg. The goal of ventilation is to increase the Pao_2 and decrease the $Paco_2$. Ventilator settings begin with PIPs to allow even movement of the chest wall and provide a V_T of 5–7 mL/kg. If V_T cannot be measured, an estimate of adequate PIP can be made based on a chest x-ray film showing expansion to 8 ribs. Rates can be determined by a decline in CO_2 or by calculating minute ventilation. For the more hypercarbic infants, rates of 50–60 breaths/min and V_Ts of 5–6 mL/kg will give minute ventilation of ~360. PEEP of 4–5 cm H_2O is most often required. ITs vary from 0.30–0.38 s. As soon as optimal lung expansion, V_T, and minute ventilation have been achieved, surfactant therapy by tracheal instillation should begin (at 2–4 h of life). This should result in a 30% reduction of Fio_2 and a 30% increase in the a/A ratio. The improvement should allow for a decreased PIP while maintaining an adequate V_T and minute ventilation.
   B. **Group B β-hemolytic streptococcal (GBS) disease** of the newborn with pneumonia and hypotension
      1. **Clinical presentation.** Infants may be of any gestational age but are often near or at term. The disease represents interstitial inflammation, atelectasis caused by inflammatory debris, and surfactant deficiency. Mild respiratory distress with tachypnea rapidly becomes severe, with marked cyanosis and hypoxemia. Ventilatory support is needed as soon as blood gases confirm a poor a/A ratio or $AaDo_2$. Natural surfactant production is suppressed, and alveolar surfactant is inactivated by inflammatory proteins.
      2. **Management.** After endotracheal intubation, mechanical ventilation should be at a rate that is synchronized with the infant's spontaneous rate (SIMV). Increased PIPs to achieve V_Ts of 5–8 mL/kg and minute ventilation of 300–360 mL/kg are required in larger infants. Systemic hypotension often accompanies GBS. Excessive PEEP (5–6 cm H_2O) may impede venous return. PEEP of 2–4 cm H_2O is recommended. Because GBS patients may experience severe hypoxia from persistent pulmonary hypertension, OI monitoring should begin early. With Fio_2 at 100%, a calculated OI of >30 suggests the need for more advanced respiratory support. High-frequency ventilation should be considered along with inhaled NO therapy. If there is no response to high-frequency ventilation and the OI is >40, ECMO may also be considered. A trial of surfactant therapy and inhaled NO may be performed before ECMO. Additional support includes the use of vasopressors, colloid infusions, antibiotics, intravenous immune globulins, glucose, and electrolyte solutions.
   C. **Chronic lung disease of infancy**
      1. **Clinical presentation.** Infants are usually 2–3 weeks old and ventilator dependent and require supplemental oxygen. Lung mechanics reveal marginal compliance of 0.8–1.0 mL/cm H_2O and marked increases of re-

sistance to 120–140 cm $H_2O/L/s$. Airway resistance is most increased on expiration.

2. **Management.** Many parameters must be addressed in infants with chronic lung disease of infancy. Careful fluid management, minimal use of diuretics, and maximal caloric intake are required. Respiratory care includes chest physical therapy and appropriate airway humidification. Hypoxia must be avoided by administering supplemental oxygen to continuously maintain Sao_2 at 92–95%. Bronchodilators, both systemic and aerosol, are helpful. Steroid therapy has been associated with marked improvement in many infants. Cromolyn therapy may be of use but remains controversial. Ventilator management seeks to maintain adequate V_T (6–8 mL/kg) delivered over longer ITs (>0.4 s). PIP is dictated by achieving adequate V_T and minute ventilation. Synchronized ventilation is particularly helpful in patients with chronic lung disease of infancy. $Paco_2$ may be accepted at higher values (55–60 mm Hg) with adequate acid-base balance from renal compensation. Ventilatory support should take into account that airway resistance and consequently respiratory time constant are markedly elevated. Slow respiratory rates are to be preferable to high rates. A short expiratory time does not allow for adequate expiratory flow and will produce air trapping with cystic or bullous changes of the lungs.

VI. **Overview of high-frequency ventilation.** High-frequency ventilation refers to a variety of ventilatory strategies and devices designed to provide ventilation at rapid rates and very low V_Ts. The ability to provide adequate ventilation in spite of reduced V_T (equal to or less than dead space) may reduce the risk of barotrauma. Rates during high-frequency ventilation are often expressed in hertz. A rate of 1 Hz (1 cycle/s) is equivalent to 60 breaths/min.

All methods of high-frequency ventilation should be administered with the assistance of well-trained respiratory therapists and after comprehensive education of the nursing staff. Furthermore, because rapid changes in ventilation or oxygenation may occur, continuous monitoring is highly recommended. Optimal utilization of these ventilators is evolving, and different strategies may be indicated for a particular lung disease.

A. **Definitive indications for high-frequency ventilation support**
1. **Pulmonary interstitial emphysema (PIE).** A multicenter trial has demonstrated high-frequency jet ventilation to be superior to conventional ventilation in patients with early PIE as well as in neonates who do not respond to conventional ventilation.
2. **Severe bronchopleural fistula.** In severe bronchopleural fistula not responsive to thoracostomy tube evacuation and conventional ventilation, high-frequency jet ventilation may provide adequate ventilation and decrease fistulas.
3. **Hyaline membrane disease.** High-frequency ventilation has been used with success. It is usually implemented at the point of severe respiratory failure with maximal conventional ventilation (a rescue treatment). Earlier treatment has been advocated. No advantages have yet been demonstrated for a very early intervention (in the first hours of life) when infants are pretreated with surfactant.
4. **Patients qualifying for ECMO.** Pulmonary hypertension with or without associated parenchymal lung disease (eg, meconium aspiration, pneumonia, hypoplastic lung, diaphragmatic hernia) can result in intractable respiratory failure and high mortality unless the patient is treated by ECMO. The prior use of high-frequency ventilation among ECMO candidates has been successful and eliminated the need for ECMO in 25–45% of cases.
B. **Possible indications.** High-frequency ventilation has been used with success in infants with other disease processes. Further study is needed to de-

velop clear indications and appropriate ventilatory strategies before this treatment can be recommended for routine use in infants with these diseases.
1. **Pulmonary hypertension.**
2. **Meconium aspiration syndrome.**
3. **Diaphragmatic hernia with pulmonary hypoplasia.**
4. **Postoperative Fontan procedures.**
VII. **High-frequency ventilators, techniques, and equipment.** Three types of high-frequency ventilators are currently in use: high-frequency jet ventilators (HFJVs), high-frequency flow interrupters (HFFIs), and high-frequency oscillatory ventilators (HFOVs).
   A. **HFJVs.** The HFJV injects a high-velocity stream of gas into the endotracheal tube, usually at frequencies between 240 and 600 bpm and V_Ts equal to or slightly greater than dead space. During high-frequency jet ventilation, expiration is passive. The only FDA-approved HFJV is the Bunnell Life Pulse ventilator (Bunnell, Salt Lake City, UT), which is discussed here.
      1. **Indications.** Mostly used for PIE, the Bunnell ventilator has been used for the other indications described for all types of high-frequency ventilation.
      2. **Equipment**
         a. **Bunnell Life Pulse ventilator.** The PIP, jet valve "on time," and respiratory frequency are entered into a digital control panel on the jet. PIPs are servocontrolled by the Life Pulse from the pressure port. The ventilator has an elaborate alarm system to ensure safety and to help detect changes in pulmonary function. It also has a special humidification system.
         b. **Conventional ventilator.** A conventional ventilator is needed to generate PEEP and sigh breaths. PEEP and background ventilation are controlled with the conventional ventilator.
      3. **Procedure**
         a. **Initiation**
            i. **Replacement of the endotracheal tube adapter with a jet adapter or reintubation with a special triple-lumen jet tube.**
            ii. **Settings on the jet ventilator**
               (a) **Default jet valve "on time":** 0.020 s.
               (b) **Frequency of jet:** 420/min.
               (c) **PIP on the jet:** 2–3 cm H_2O below that on the conventional ventilator. Frequently, infants require considerably less PIP during high-frequency jet ventilation.
            iii. **Settings on the conventional ventilator**
               (a) **PEEP:** PEEP is maintained at 3–5 cm H_2O.
               (b) **Rate:** As the jet ventilator comes up to pressure, the rate is decreased to 5–10 breaths/min.
               (c) **PIP:** Once at pressure, the PIP is adjusted to a level 1–3 cm H_2O below that on the jet (low enough not to interrupt the jet ventilator).
            iv. **Close observation is required at all times, especially during initiation.**
      4. **Management.** Management of high-frequency jet ventilation is based on the clinical course and radiographic findings.
         a. **Elimination of CO_2.** Alveolar ventilation is much more sensitive to changes in V_T than in respiratory frequency during high-frequency ventilation. As a result, the delta pressure (PIP – PEEP) is adjusted to attain adequate elimination of CO_2, whereas jet valve "on time" and respiratory frequency are usually not readjusted during high-frequency jet ventilation.
         b. **Oxygenation.** Oxygenation is often better during high-frequency jet ventilation than during conventional mechanical ventilation in neonates with PIE. However, if oxygenation is inadequate and the infant

is already on 100% oxygen, an increase in $P\overline{aw}$ usually results in improved oxygenation. It can be accomplished by:
   i. Increasing PEEP.
   ii. Increasing PIP.
   iii. Increasing background conventional ventilator (either rates or pressure).
   c. **Positioning of infants.** Positioning infants with the affected side down may speed resolution of PIE. In bilateral air leak, alternating placement on dependent sides may be effective. Diligent observation and frequent radiographs are necessary to avoid hyperinflation of the nondependent side.
5. **Weaning.** When weaning, the following guidelines are used.
   a. **PIP is reduced as soon as possible** ($Paco_2$ <35–40 mm Hg). Because elimination of CO_2 is very sensitive to changes in VT, PIP is weaned 1 cm H_2O at a time.
   b. **Oxygen concentration is weaned** if oxygenation remains good (Pao_2 >70–80 mm Hg).
   c. **Jet valve "on time" and frequency are usually kept constant.**
   d. **Constant attention is paid to the infant's clinical condition** and radiographs to detect early atelectasis or hyperinflation.
   e. **Air leaks are resolved.** Continuation of high-frequency jet ventilation occurs until the air leak has been resolved for 24–48 h, which often corresponds to a dramatic decrease in ventilator pressures and oxygen requirement.
   f. **If no improvement in the condition occurs,** a trial of conventional ventilation is used after 6–24 h on jet ventilation.
6. **Special considerations**
   a. **Airway obstruction.** When a stiff triple-lumen endotracheal tube is used, the bevel of the tube may become lodged against the tracheal wall, resulting in airway obstruction. This problem can usually be recognized quickly. Chest wall movement is decreased, although breath sounds may be adequate. The servopressure (driving pressure) is usually very low. (An obstruction in the endotracheal tube proximal to the distal pressure port results in a high servopressure alarm.) Positioning the tube with the jet port facing anteriorly usually maintains good tube position.
   b. **Inadvertent PEEP (air trapping).** In larger infants, the flow of jet gases may result in inadvertent PEEP. Decreasing the background flow on the conventional ventilator may correct the problem, or it may be necessary to decrease the respiratory frequency to allow more time for expiration.
7. **Complications**
   a. **Tracheitis.** Necrotizing tracheobronchitis was a frequent complication in the early days of jet ventilation. This problem is much less frequent with the recognition of the critical importance of proper humidification of the jet gases. If tracheitis occurs, emergent bronchoscopy may be indicated. The clinical signs include the following.
      i. **Increased airway secretions.**
      ii. **Evidence of airway obstruction (including air trapping).**
      iii. **Acute respiratory acidosis.**
   b. **Intraventricular hemorrhage.** There has been no increase in the incidence or severity of intraventricular hemorrhage with the use of the HFJV.
   c. **Bronchopulmonary dysplasia.** There has been no apparent decrease in the incidence of bronchopulmonary dysplasia with the use of the HFJV.
B. **HFFIs.** The HFFI shares some characteristics with the HFOV and the HFJV. It operates at frequencies as high as those for the HFOV but does not have

active exhalation. Bursts of gas approximate those of the HFJV, but a standard endotracheal tube can be used. The only FDA-approved HFFI is the Infrasonics Infant Star ventilator (Infrasonics, San Diego, CA), which is discussed here.

1. **Indications.** The indications are the same as those for the HFJV. The Infrasonics Infant Star ventilator may not be effective in infants whose birth weight is >1800 g. If an infant of this size qualifies for high-frequency ventilation, the HFJV or the HFOV may prove to be more effective.

2. **Equipment**
   a. **The Infrasonics Infant Star ventilator.** The manufacturer prefers to call this ventilator a flow oscillator because of the ventilation technique used and its flow characteristics. It can be termed a hybrid oscillator because it has features of both a flow interrupter (jet) and an oscillator.
      i. The bursts of gas are 18 ms in duration (preset at the factory). The sudden expansion of gas after the burst creates a rebound negative-pressure deflection that closely approximates the active exhalation of oscillatory ventilation.
      ii. The user-defined parameters are frequency (10–20 Hz), $\overline{Paw}$, and amplitude, which is a function of volume of gas per burst.
   b. **Conventional ventilator.** The high-frequency mode on the Infant Star ventilator must be used in combination with the conventional ventilator. Rate, PEEP, and PAP are set on the conventional ventilator.
   c. **Endotracheal tube.** A regular endotracheal tube is used.

3. **Procedure: Initiation of Infant Star ventilation**
   a. **Conventional ventilator settings**
      i. **Rate** is set at 5 breaths/min. It is extremely important to have a conventional rate set during high frequency so that atelectasis does not develop. V_Ts are very small during high frequency.
      ii. **PIP and PEEP** are not changed from the original settings.
   b. **HFFI settings**
      i. **Frequency** is always maintained at 15 Hz (900 breaths/min). It is not adjusted during high-frequency ventilation.
      ii. **$\overline{Paw}$** is determined by the PEEP level and initially should be set to match the $\overline{Paw}$ before initiation of HVF. That is, if $\overline{Paw}$ was 15 on conventional ventilatory support, it should be set on the high-frequency ventilator by means of setting the PEEP at 15.
      iii. **Amplitude.** After the frequency and the $\overline{Paw}$ are set, the amplitude should be adjusted. It should be increased until the chest wall of the infant begins to vibrate visually. This setting is the most difficult and arbitrary to determine. The range is 10–30 mL.
   c. **After the high-frequency device is initially set, arterial blood gas values and chest x-ray studies are used to adjust settings.** Chest x-ray studies are usually done every 6 h until the infant is stabilized.

4. **Management on the Infant Star.** It is important to note that the $\overline{Paw}$ controls oxygenation and the amplitude controls elimination of CO_2.
   a. **If Pao$_2$ is low,** $\overline{Paw}$ should be increased on the Infant Star. PEEP is the main determinant of $\overline{Paw}$ and lung volume; therefore, PEEP levels should be increased until oxygenation is adequate. The conventional rate can be increased, but this is a less effective means of increasing oxygenation.
   b. **If Paco$_2$ is high**
      i. Poor oxygenation as well as high Paco$_2$ indicates decreased lung volume; a chest x-ray study at this time often reveals a hypoventilated lung with atelectasis. PEEP should be increased.
      ii. If adequate oxygenation exists, amplitude should be increased until adequate CO_2 removal is achieved.

iii. Hyperoxygenation may be an indication of air trapping, and PEEP should be decreased. A chest x-ray film reveals lung hyperinflation.

5. **Weaning.** Once adequate gas exchange has been achieved and oxygenation is adequate, careful weaning should begin. In general, weaning should follow the pattern described next.

   a. **If Pao_2 is acceptable** and a chest x-ray film does not show hyperexpansion, wean the Fio_2. (If hyperexpansion is present, PEEP is weaned, follow by steps c, d, and e below.)

   b. **When the Fio_2 has been weaned to 60%,** wean the PEEP.

   c. **If $Paco_2$ elimination is good** ($Paco_2$ <40 mm Hg), wean the amplitude.

   d. **When the amplitude has reached low levels** (~10 mL), conventional breaths may be added to ventilatory strategy.

   e. **Frequency does not need to be decreased during weaning.** *Note:* It is necessary to perform serial chest x-ray studies to rule out atelectasis and underinflation while weaning is in progress. The x-ray films may indicate that PEEP has been decreased too much or that amplitude needs to be increased.

6. **Complications.** The main complication is gas trapping, resulting in hyperexpansion, which can be prevented by meticulously monitoring serial chest x-ray studies and arterial blood gas values and by using appropriate weaning procedures.

C. **HFOVs.** The HFOV generates V_T less than or equal to dead space by means of an oscillating piston or diaphragm. This mechanism creates active exhalation as well as inspiration. The SensorMedics (Yorba Linda, CA) HFOV is currently approved by the FDA for use in neonates.

1. **Indications.** Respiratory failure: High-frequency oscillatory ventilation is indicated when conventional ventilation does not result in adequate oxygenation or ventilation or requires the use of very high airway pressures. Like other forms of high-frequency ventilation, success is more likely when increased airway resistance is not the dominant pulmonary pathophysiology. Best results are seen when parenchymal disease is homogeneous. Some clinicians advocate high-frequency oscillatory ventilation as the primary method of assisted ventilation in premature infants with RDS.

2. **Equipment.** The SensorMedics HFOV is a piston oscillator. It is not used in conjunction with a conventional ventilator. The user-defined parameters are frequency, $\overline{Paw}$, and power applied for piston displacement.

3. **Procedure: initiation**

   a. **Conventional ventilator is discontinued.**

   b. **Settings**

      i. **Frequency** is usually set at 15 Hz for premature infants with RDS. Larger infants and those with a significant component of increased airway resistance (meconium aspiration) should be started at 5–10 Hz.

      ii. **$\overline{Paw}$** is set higher (2–5 cm H_2O) than on the previous conventional ventilation. If overdistention or air leaks were present before initiation of high-frequency oscillatory ventilation, a lower $\overline{Paw}$ should be considered.

      iii. **Amplitude** (analogous to PIP on conventional ventilation) is regulated by the power of displacement of the piston. This power is increased until there is visible chest wall vibration.

   c. **After high-frequency oscillatory ventilation has been initiated,** careful and frequent assessment of lung expansion and adequate gas exchange is necessary. Air trapping is a continuous potential threat in this form of treatment. Signs of overdistention, such as descended and flat diaphragms and small heart shadow, are monitored with frequent chest x-ray films.

4. Management
   a. **If Pao_2 is low,** an increase in $\overline{Paw}$ may be necessary. Chest radiographs may be helpful in determining the adequacy of lung expansion.
   b. **If $Paco_2$ is high**
      i. **If oxygenation is poor,** the $\overline{Paw}$ may be too high or too low, resulting in either hyperinflation or widespread collapse, respectively. Again, chest x-ray films are necessary to differentiate between these two conditions.
      ii. **If oxygenation is adequate,** the amplitude (power) should be increased.

5. Weaning
   a. **In the absence of hyperinflation,** Fio_2 is weaned before $\overline{Paw}$ for adequate Pao_2. Below 40% Fio_2, wean $\overline{Paw}$ exclusively.
   b. **$\overline{Paw}$** should be weaned as the lung disease improves with the goal of maintaining optimal lung expansion. Excessively aggressive early weaning of $\overline{Paw}$ may result in widespread atelectasis and the need for significant increases in $\overline{Paw}$ and Fio_2.
   c. **Amplitude** should be weaned for acceptable $Paco_2$.
   d. **Frequency** is usually not adjusted during weaning. A decrease in frequency is necessary when signs of lung overdistention cannot be eliminated by a reduction in $\overline{Paw}$.
   e. **The neonate may be switched** to conventional ventilation at a low level of support or may be extubated directly from an HFOV.

6. Complications. See section VII,B.

VIII. Liquid ventilation. Perfluorocarbon liquids (PFCs) are biochemically inert, colorless, odorless liquids that have a high capacity for respiratory gases. Using a liquid for gas exchange eliminates problems associated with the air–liquid interface, providing even inflation of the lungs. PFCs are almost twice as dense as water and result in a redistribution of pulmonary blood flow because of the intrapulmonary pressure gradient present in a fluid-filled lung. PFCs also have relatively low surface tension. Laboratory work suggests that PFCs may decrease inflammatory injury in the lungs, although the mechanisms are not well defined. At this time, liquid ventilation is used experimentally in severe pulmonary failure. Two methods of liquid ventilation are being studied: total liquid ventilation (TLV) and partial liquid ventilation (PLV; also known as perfluorocarbon-assisted gas exchange [PAGE]).

A. TLV is technically extraordinarily complex. Unlike gaseous ventilation, both inspiration and expiration must be active because of the high viscosity of PFC. Respiratory rates of 5–6 breaths/min optimize CO_2 elimination. Because liquids are incompressible, inspiratory and expiratory volumes must be precisely matched to prevent massive injury from either overinflation or suction. Common use of TLV requires both the development of a commercial liquid ventilator and identification of a patient population that will be well served by this technique.

B. PLV is a much less technologically challenging modality. In PLV, the lungs are filled to functional residual capacity (FRC) gradually while conventional ventilation is maintained. Once FRC is reached (usually determined by the appearance of a fluid meniscus in the endotracheal tube at end expiration), additional PFC is added only to make up for evaporative losses. Gaseous ventilation is managed in the usual manner. In severely injured lungs, PLV can improve oxygenation, even in those patients not responsive to surfactant. When PLV is no longer needed, the PFC is allowed to evaporate. PLV is currently being studied in adults and children with ARDS. Likely neonatal candidates include those infants with respiratory failure who are not ECMO candidates. Further understanding of the anti-inflammatory actions of PFCs may suggest other indications for PLV.

C. **Other respiratory uses of PFCs.** PFCs are being investigated for use in the delivery of drugs to the lungs. Because of their low surface tension, PFCs distribute evenly throughout the lungs, perhaps causing more uniform drug delivery than aerosolization or tracheal instillation. PFCs may also be useful as a lavage fluid.

GLOSSARY OF TERMS USED IN RESPIRATORY SUPPORT

Alveolar-to-arterial oxygen ratio (a/A ratio). See section II,A,3,b.

Assist. A setting at which the infant initiates the mechanical breath, triggering the ventilator to deliver a preset V_T or pressure.

Assist-control. The same as assist, except that if the infant becomes apneic, the ventilator delivers the number of mechanical breaths per minute set on the rate control.

Continuous positive airway pressure (CPAP). A spontaneous mode in which the ambient intrapulmonary pressure that is maintained throughout the respiratory cycle is increased.

Control. A setting at which a certain number of mechanical breaths per minute is delivered. The infant is unable to breathe spontaneously between mechanical breaths.

End-tidal CO_2 (etCO$_2$). A measure of the Pco_2 of end expiration.

Expiratory time (ET). The amount of time set for the expiratory phase of each mechanical breath.

Flow rate. The amount of gas per minute passing through the ventilator. It must be sufficient to prevent rebreathing (ie, 3 times the minute volume) and to achieve the PIP during IT. Changes in the flow rate may be necessary if changes in the airway waveform are desired. The normal range is 6–10 L/min; 8 L/min is commonly used.

Fraction of inspired oxygen (Fio_2). The percentage of oxygen concentration of inspired gas expressed as decimals (room air = 0.21).

I:E ratio. Ratio of inspiratory time to expiratory time. The normal values are 1:1, 1:1.5, or 1:2.

Inspiratory time (IT). The amount of time set for the inspiratory phase of each mechanical breath.

Intermittent mechanical ventilation (IMV). Mechanical breaths are delivered at intervals. The infant breathes spontaneously between mechanical breaths.

Minute ventilation. V_T (proportional to PIP) multiplied by rate.

Oxyhemoglobin dissociation curve. A curve showing the amount of oxygen that combines with hemoglobin as a function of Pao_2 and $Paco_2$. The curve shifts to the right when oxygen uptake by the blood is less than normal at a given Po_2, and it shifts to the left when oxygen uptake is greater than normal.

Oxygen index (OI). See section II,F,2,d.

Pao_2. Partial pressure of arterial oxygen.

PAP. The total airway pressure. In the Siemens Servo 900-C, it is the PIP plus the PEEP.

$P\overline{a}w$. The average proximal pressure applied to the airway throughout the entire respiratory cycle.

Pco_2. Carbon dioxide partial pressure.

Peak inspiratory pressure (PIP). The highest pressure reached within the proximal airway with each mechanical breath. *Note:* In the Siemens Servo 900-C, the PIP is defined as the inspiratory pressure above the PEEP.

Po_2. Oxygen partial pressure.

Positive end-expiratory pressure (PEEP). The pressure in the airway above ambient pressure during the expiratory phase of mechanical ventilation.

Rate. Number of mechanical breaths per minute delivered by the ventilator.

Sao_2. Oxygen saturation of arterial blood.
Tidal volume (V_r). The volume of gas inspired or expired during each respiratory cycle.
Total cycle time (Tc). IT plus ET.
Waveform. A pattern of change in airway pressure during the entire respiratory cycle. The three types of waveforms are square, sine, and triangular. The sine and square forms are the most common. The square wave indicates that the volume is being delivered at a constant rate; the sine wave indicates that the volume is being delivered at a variable rate (see Figure 6–4).

REFERENCES

American Academy of Pediatrics Committee on Fetus and Newborn and Canadian Paediatric Society Fetus and Newborn Committee: Postnatal corticosteroids to treat or prevent chronic lung disease in preterm infants. *Pediatrics* 2002;109:330.

Bernstein CT: Synchronous and patient-triggered ventilation in newborns. *Neonatal Respir Dis* 1993;3:1.

Carter JM et al: High-frequency oscillatory ventilation for the treatment of acute neonatal respiratory distress failure. *Pediatrics* 1990;85:159.

Clark RH et al: Lung injury in neonates: causes, strategies for prevention, and long-term consequences. *J Pediatr* 2001;139:478.

Clark RH et al: Prospective randomized comparison of high frequency oscillatory and conventional ventilation in respiratory distress syndrome. *J Pediatr* 1993;122:609.

Cunningham MD: Assessing pulmonary function in the neonate. In Pomerance J, Richardson CJ (eds): *Neonatology for the Clinician.* Appleton & Lange, 1993.

Cunningham MD et al: Clinical experience with pulse oximetry in managing oxygen therapy in neonatal intensive care. *J Perinatol* 1988;8:333.

Cunningham MD: Intensive care monitoring of pulmonary mechanics for preterm infants undergoing mechanical ventilation. *J Perinatol* 1989;9:56.

Davis JM et al: Drug therapy for bronchopulmonary dysplasia. *Pediatr Pulmonol* 1990;8:117.

Dunn MS et al: Bovine surfactant replacement therapy in neonates of less than 30 weeks' gestation: a randomized controlled trial of prophylaxis versus treatment. *Pediatrics* 1991; 87:377.

Ellean C et al: Helium-oxygen mixture in respiratory distress syndrome: a double-blind study. *J Pediatr* 1993;122:132.

Flynn JT et al: A cohort study of transcutaneous oxygen tension and the incidence and severity of retinopathy of prematurity. *N Engl J Med* 1992;326:1050.

Freeman RK, Poland RL: *Guidelines for Perinatal Care,* 35th ed. American Academy of Pediatrics/American College of Obstetricians and Gynecologists, 1992.

Gerstmann DR et al: High-frequency ventilation: issues of strategy. *Clin Perinatol* 1991;18:563.

HiFO Study Group: Randomized study of high-frequency oscillatory ventilation in infants with severe respiratory distress syndrome. *J Pediatr* 1993;122:609.

Jobe AH: Pulmonary surfactant therapy. *N Engl J Med* 1993;328:861.

Kezler M et al: Multicenter controlled trial comparing high-frequency jet ventilation and conventional mechanical ventilation in newborn infants with pulmonary interstitial emphysema. *J Pediatr* 1991;119:85.

Kinsella JP, Abman SH: Clinical approach to inhaled nitric oxide therapy in the newborn with hypoxia. *J Pediatr* 2000;136:717.

Kinsella JP et al: Clinical responses to prolonged treatment of persistent pulmonary hypertension of the newborn with low doses of inhaled nitric oxide. *J Pediatr* 1993;123:103.

Peris LV et al: Clinical use of arterial/alveolar oxygen tension ratio. *Crit Care Med* 1983;11:888.

Primak RA: Factors associated with pulmonary air leak in preterm infants receiving mechanical ventilation. *J Pediatr* 1983;102:764.

Sinha SK, Donn SM (eds): *Manual of Neonatal Respiratory Care,* Futura, 2000.

Spitzer AR et al: Ventilatory response to combined high-frequency jet ventilation and conventional mechanical ventilation for the rescue treatment of severe neonatal lung disease. *Pediatr Pulmonol* 1989;7:244.

Wilkie RA, Bryan MH: Effect of bronchodilators on airway resistance in ventilator-dependent neonates with chronic lung disease. *J Pediatr* 1987;111:278.

7 Fluids and Electrolytes

Fluid and electrolyte therapy plays an important role in the early medical management of preterm neonates, especially extremely low birth weight (ELBW) infants. Fluid management in the first several days of life has been shown to be a factor in the development of morbidities such as intraventricular hemorrhage, necrotizing enterocolitis, symptomatic patent ductus arteriosus, and bronchopulmonary dysplasia (Costarino & Baumgart, 1986). It is, therefore, crucial that the clinician pay close attention to details regarding fluid therapy, especially in the first several days of life.

FLUID AND ELECTROLYTE BALANCE

Fluid balance is a function of the distribution of water in the body, water intake, and water losses. Fluid distribution in the body changes with increasing gestation. Water losses also change with gestational age, with differences in renal function and insensible water loss (IWL) between term and preterm infants. The clinician must account for these variables in deciding the amount of fluid to administer to the patient.

I. **Total body water (TBW).** TBW accounts for nearly 75% of the body weight in term newborns and even more in preterm infants. TBW is divided into two large parts: intracellular fluid (ICF) and extracellular fluid (ECF). In more premature infants, TBW and ECF volumes both increase, whereas ICF decreases. Both term and preterm infants experience an acute expansion of the ECF by shifts of fluid from the ICF during the first few days of life.

Antenatal events sometimes play a role in the distribution of body water. Isoimmune diseases or other conditions that lead to hydrops fetalis can cause ECF expansion. Maternal indomethacin therapy can also lead to volume expansion, and maternal diuretic therapy or placental insufficiency can lead to decreased hydration.

II. **Renal function.** Both term and preterm infants have low glomerular filtration rates (GFRs), and the GFR is even lower in preterm infants. Infant kidneys are able to produce dilute urine, and any limitation of the neonatal kidney in excreting excess water results from a low GFR. The low GFR in preterm infants results from a relatively low renal blood flow, which increases after 34 weeks' gestation.

In term neonates, the kidneys can concentrate urine up to 800 mOsm/L compared with 1500 mOsm/L in an adult kidney. The preterm infant's kidney is even less able to concentrate urine secondary to a relatively low interstitial urea concentration, an anatomically shorter loop of Henle, and a distal tubule and collecting system that is less responsive to antidiuretic hormone (ADH).

III. **Insensible water loss.** IWL is the evaporation of water through the skin and mucous membranes. In term infants, maintenance fluid requirements can be expressed as a function of metabolism (Table 7–1). In newborn infants, one third of the IWL occurs through the respiratory tract and the remaining two thirds through the skin.

The relationship between metabolism and maintenance fluid requirements does not hold true for infants who weigh <800 g at birth or who are <27 weeks' gestational age. The most important variable influencing IWL is the maturity of the infant. The higher IWL in preterm, low birth weight infants results from greater water permeability through a relatively immature epithelial layer, a larger surface area–body weight ratio, and a relatively greater skin vascularity. The average IWL in preterm infants according to birth weight is listed in Table 7–2.

IWL is also influenced by respiratory status and environmental factors such as the type of warming unit used (radiant warmer vs incubator), phototherapy, room

TABLE 7-1. RELATIONSHIP BETWEEN METABOLISM AND MAINTENANCE FLUIDS

Route	Loss/gain	Fluid replacement (mL/100 kcal metabolized energy)
Insensible		
Skin	Loss	25
Respiration	Loss	15
Urine	Loss	60
Stool	Loss	10
Water of oxidation	Gain	10
Total for maintenance		100

Modified and reproduced, with permission, from Winters RW (ed): Maintenance fluid therapy. In *The Body Fluids in Pediatrics.* Little, Brown, 1973;113.

humidity, and ambient temperature. Table 7–3 summarizes the effect of 10 different factors on IWL. In general, for healthy premature infants who weigh 800–2000 g and are nursed in closed incubators, IWL increases linearly as body weight decreases. However, for sick infants of similar weight nursed on an open radiant warmer and undergoing assisted ventilation, IWL increases exponentially as body weight decreases.

When assessing appropriate fluid management in individual cases, birth weight, type of warmer, ambient humidity (ideally, 40–90%), phototherapy, and respiratory status must be taken into account. High-humidity incubators that can provide relative humidity up to 90% decrease the IWL in ELBW infants significantly.

FLUID THERAPY

Suggested fluid recommendations, discussed next, are based on historically averaged values for infants managed in single-walled incubators (Baumgart et al, 1982; Bell & Oh, 1979; Costarino & Baumgart, 1986); however, the advantage of using humidified incubators dictates a new fluid management strategy for preterm infants (Gaylord et al, 2001).

Fluid replacement in preterm neonates must be carefully calculated to allow for normal loss of ECF and weight while preventing dehydration from IWL, which can lead to hypotension, acidosis, and hypernatremia. It is important to avoid excessive fluid therapy, which has been associated with increased incidence of patent ductus arteriosus, bronchopulmonary dysplasia, intraventricular hemorrhage, and necrotizing enterocolitis. Fluid recommendations for preterm infants are from Shaffer et al (1992a). For estimated adjustments for environmental variables, see Table 7–3.

TABLE 7-2. INSENSIBLE WATER LOSS (IWL) IN PRETERM INFANTS

Birth weight (g)	Average IWL (mL/kg/day)
>750–1000	64
1001–1250	56
1251–1500	38
1501–1750	23
1751–2000	20
2001–3250	20

TABLE 7–3. FACTORS IN THE NURSERY ENVIRONMENT THAT AFFECT INSENSIBLE WATER LOSS

Increases IWL	Decreases IWL
1. Severe prematurity, 100–300%	1. Humidification in incubator, 50–100%
2. Open warmer bed, 50–100%	2. Plastic head shield in incubator, 30–50%
3. Forced convection, 30–50%	3. Plastic blanket under radiant warmer, 30–50%
4. Phototherapy, 30–50%	4. Tracheal intubation with humidification, 20–30%
5. Hyperthermia, 30–50%	
6. Tachypnea, 20–30%	

Estimates of percent change represent empirical data. IWL, insensible water loss.
Modified and reproduced, with permission, from Costarino A, Baumgart S: Modern fluid and electrolyte management of the critically ill premature infant. *Pediatr Clin North Am* 1986;33:153. Appears with permission from Elsevier Science.

I. **Suggested fluids and electrolytes**
   A. **Term infants**
      1. **Day 1.** Give dextrose 10% in water ($D_{10}W$) at a rate of 60–80 mL/kg/day. This amount provides ~6–7 mg/kg/min of glucose. Although guidelines for calcium (Ca^{2+}) supplementation in this time frame are variable, it is our practice not to supplement calcium unless specifically indicated.
      2. **Days 2–7.** Once tolerance of fluid therapy has been established and urine output is satisfactory (1–2 mL/kg/h), the rate and composition of the solution can be modified. The goals of fluid and electrolyte administration during this period include the following:
         • Loss of expected weight during the first 3–5 days (10–15% of birth weight).
         • Maintenance of normal serum electrolytes.
         • Avoidance of oliguria.
         • Transition to enteral intake.
         a. **Fluid volume (range, 80–120 mL/kg/day).** Depending on the tolerance of the previous day's fluid therapy, estimations of IWL, and clinical status of the infant (patent ductus arteriosus, congenital heart failure, and pulmonary edema), increases of 10–20 mL/kg/day may be considered.
         b. **Glucose.** Once a glucose load is established and tolerated, increasing the load by 10–15% per day is appropriate.
         c. **Sodium.** Sodium (Na^+) requirements range from 2–4 mEq/kg/day; however, in some infants, a larger sodium supplement may be necessary to compensate for sodium diuresis. After the first few days of life, sodium intake should be adjusted to keep serum sodium levels between 135 and 145 mEq/L.
         d. **Potassium.** Potassium (K^+) requirements range from 1–2 mEq/kg/day. Potassium supplementation is usually not required on the first day of life, and sometimes it is not necessary until the third day. Extreme care should be taken to document renal function before adding potassium (determination of urine output is usually adequate). Normal serum potassium levels are 4.0–5.5 mEq/L.
         e. **Nutrition.** Enteral feedings should be started as soon as possible. If such feedings supply inadequate caloric intake or a required nothing-by-mouth (NPO) period is prolonged, total parenteral nutrition (TPN) may be necessary. TPN may begin as early as 36–48 h of life if electrolyte and fluid requirements are stable. When enteral feedings are begun, intravenous fluids are progressively decreased as enteral fluid intake is slowly increased. A combined fluid intake of ~120 mL/kg/day should be maintained. Enteral feedings supply adequate electrolytes,

vitamins, trace elements, and the basic proteins, fats, and carbohydrates when appropriate volumes are given.
B. **Preterm infants**
1. **Day 1.** During the immediate postnatal period, critically ill premature infants may require volume resuscitation for shock or acidosis. Fluids administered during stabilization should be considered when planning subsequent fluid management.
2. **Days 1–3**
   a. **Fluid volume and glucose requirements.** Preterm infants, particularly those weighing <1000 g, require more fluids and are less tolerant of glucose. For preterm infants of ≥800–1000 g, begin fluids at a rate of 80–100 mL/kg/day, adding the appropriate amount of glucose to provide 5–6 mg/kg/min (approximately $D_{7.5}W$).

   Inadequate hydration can lead to hyperosmolarity and may be a risk factor for intraventricular hemorrhage. Infants admitted to a radiant warmer should be transferred to incubators as soon possible to minimize IWL. The fluid management of ELBW infants should be guided by close observation of weight and serum sodium levels. During the first week of life fluids should be adjusted to allow a gradual weight loss (<4% per day), with an anticipated overall maximum weight loss of 15–20% by 7 days of life.

   During the first week of life, fluid therapy should be managed by increments or decrements of 20–40 mL/kg/day, depending on weight and serum sodium levels, to keep sodium at a normal range of 135–145 mmol/L.

   D_5W provides a more suitable glucose load at these increased rates, and insulin infusions may be needed in ELBW infants with large IWLs. These infants are also at risk for hyperosmolarity secondary to hyperglycemia.

   Infants weighing <800 g may require additional fluids until the skin becomes more mature (at 5–7 days). High fluid supplementation (at even >160 mL/kg/day) may be required in ELBW infants.
   b. **Electrolyte supplementation.** Sodium, potassium, and chloride supplementation are usually not necessary during this time, while the newborn adjusts from the fetal to the extrauterine environment. The infant undergoes an isotonic contraction of the ECF compartment, with excretion of excess water.

   Appropriate fluid therapy will prevent both hyponatremia and hypernatremia. Costarino et al (1992) showed that restriction of sodium intake during the first 3–5 days of life led to more normal serum osmolarity. He also found a decrease in the incidence of bronchopulmonary dysplasia.

   Potassium supplementation, at 1–3 mEq/kg/day, can be initiated once urine output is established.

   Calcium should be supplemented in preterm infants because their body stores are relatively low. During gestation, the rate of calcium accretion in the fetus is greatest in the third trimester. Calcium supplementation at 20–30 mg/kg/day is recommended.
3. **Days 3–7.** After the transitional phase of volume contraction, the preterm infant enters a maintenance phase, and fluid administration can be decreased as the skin becomes more mature and IWLs through the skin decrease. Fluid therapy then begins to resemble that outlined previously for term infants, with advancing volumes and transition over to enteral intake. Enteral nutrition must be introduced gradually because of the risks for necrotizing enterocolitis.

   Electrolyte supplementation can be initiated as the fluid status stabilizes, using guidelines similar to those for term infants.

   ELBW infants and other preterm infants may need additional sodium supplementation. A syndrome of "late hyponatremia" has been described in these infants and is likely a result of limited renal conservation, along with accelerated incorporation of sodium into bone during rapid growth. These infants then grow poorly until they are given sodium supplementation and a correction of their hyponatremia occurs.

II. Monitoring of fluid and electrolyte status. Fluid and electrolyte replacement therapy should be monitored by daily weight measurements, vital sign determinations, and specific urine and serum laboratory studies.

  A. Body weight. The body weight should be recorded daily for term and larger preterm infants. The expected weight loss during the first 3–5 days of life is 10–15% of birth weight in term infants (15–20% of birth weight in preterm infants). A loss of >20% of birth weight during the first week of life is extreme and suggests uncompensated IWL. If the weight loss is <2% per day for the first 4–5 days, fluid administration is probably excessive. For ELBW infants, body weights should be checked 2 or more times daily to more closely monitor fluid status. An in-bed scale for measuring body weight is an extremely useful tool in the care of these infants.

  Postnatal growth curves, such as that of Shaffer et al (1992b), can be useful in adjusting fluid therapy based on weight measurements (Figure 7–1).

  B. Serum levels. Tests for serum hematocrit (Hct), sodium, potassium, blood urea nitrogen (BUN), creatinine, acidosis, and base deficit should be performed. Serum osmolality can also be measured. Increases in any of these parameters may indicate inadequate fluid therapy. Hyponatremia, a falling Hct, or a low BUN may be signs of overhydration

  The total potassium balance cannot be measured effectively in the serum because potassium is mainly an intracellular ion. Hyperkalemia may become a life-threatening problem in infants weighing <800 g; thus, electrolytes should be monitored frequently (every 4–6 h) in these infants.

  C. Fluid intake and output. Fluid status should be measured by accurate fluid intake and output. Urine output measuring <1.0 mL/kg/h may indicate a need for increased fluid intake, whereas urine output >3.0 mL/kg/h may indicate overhydration and the need for restriction. Urine specific gravity, electrolytes, and osmolality may be useful in the further assessment of fluid status, although reduced function of the immature kidney in the preterm infant may make these parameters less useful.

  D. General appearance and vital signs. Hypotension, poor perfusion, tachycardia, and poor pulses may all be signs of inadequate intake.

FLUID CALCULATIONS

  I. Environmental factors. Sick infants under radiant warmers or receiving phototherapy have dramatically increased IWL. To compensate, additional fluids must be given (see Table 7–3).

  II. Glucose. The normal glucose requirement is 6–8 mg/kg/min. Intake can be slowly increased to 12–15 mg/kg/min as tolerated, however, to allow for growth. Glucose intake can be calculated as follows:

Glucose requirement (mg/kg/min) =

$$\frac{(\text{Percentage of glucose} \times \text{Rate [mL/h]} \times 0.167)}{\text{Weight (kg)}}$$

The alternate method is:

Glucose requirement (mg/kg/min) =

$$\frac{(\text{Amount of glucose/mL [from Table 7–4]} \times \text{Total fluids})}{\text{Weight (kg)/(60 min)}}$$

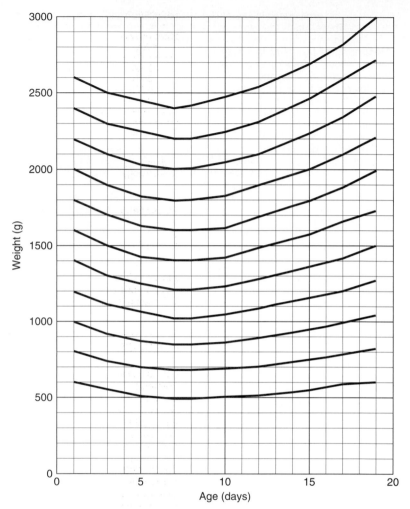

FIGURE 7–1. Postnatal weight changes according to birth weight. Appears with permission from Elsevier Science. *Modified and reproduced with permission, from Shaffer SG et al: fluid requirements in the preterm infant.* Clin Perinatol *1992;19:233.)* Appears with permission from Elsevier Science.

TABLE 7–4. GLUCOSE CONCENTRATION IN COMMONLY USED INTRAVENOUS FLUIDS

Solution (%)	Glucose concentration (mg/mL)
D_5W	50
$D_{7.5}W$	75
$D_{10}W$	100
$D_{12.5}W$	125
$D_{15}W$	150

D_5W, dextrose 5% in water; $D_{7.5}W$, dextrose 7.5% in water; $D_{10}W$, dextrose 10% in water; $D_{12.5}W$, dextrose 12.5% in water; $D_{15}W$, dextrose 15% in water.

TABLE 7-5. SODIUM CONTENT OF COMMONLY USED INTRAVENOUS FLUIDS

Solution	Sodium concentration (mEq/mL)
3% normal saline	0.500
Normal saline	0.154
½ normal saline	0.075
¼ normal saline	0.037
⅛ normal saline	0.019

III. Sodium. The normal sodium requirement in infants is 2–3 mEq/kg/day. The following calculations can be used to determine the amount of sodium the infant is receiving.

Amount of Na^+/mL (from Table 7–5) × Total fluids / day = Amount of Na^+/day

$$\frac{\text{Amount of } Na^+/\text{day}}{\text{Weight (kg)}} = \text{Amount of } Na^+(\text{kg/day})$$

IV. Potassium. The normal requirement for potassium in infants is 1–2 mEq/kg/day. The potassium intake can be easily calculated and added to the intravenous fluids as potassium chloride. Potassium should be supplemented only after urine output is established.

MODIFIERS OF FLUID AND ELECTROLYTE REQUIREMENTS

I. IWL. As mentioned previously (see pp 69–70), physiologic and environmental factors influence IWL and thus total fluid requirements.

II. Diabetes insipidus. Secondary to either a central (decreased production) or a nephrogenic (unable to be used by the kidneys) cause, the activity of ADH is decreased. This leads to an increased urine output. Hydration is best maintained by replacement of urine volume and sodium loss in addition to IWL. Frequent measurements of body weight (every 12 h) and sodium (every 6–8 h) are necessary to gauge the efficacy of therapy. With diabetes insipidus of central nervous system origin, 1-deamino-8-D-arginine vasopressin (DDAVP) therapy may be helpful.

III. Syndrome of inappropriate ADH (SIADH) secretions. An inappropriate increase in the secretion of ADH results in a decreased urine output with urine osmolality >100 mOsm/L, decreased serum osmolality, and hyponatremia (usually on the basis of volume expansion). SIADH is treated by restriction of fluid to ~50–60 mL/kg/day or less.

IV. Renal failure. Renal failure in the neonate is usually secondary to hypoxia or shock. Fluids should be adjusted to compensate only for IWL and replacement of urine volume, if any. Potassium supplementation should be avoided.

REFERENCES

Baumgart S et al: Fluid, electrolyte, and glucose maintenance in the very low birth weight infant. *Clin Pediatr* 1982;4:199.

Bell E, Oh W: Fluid and electrolyte balance in very low birth weight infants. *Clin Perinatol* 1979; 6:139.

Bell E et al: Effect of fluid administration on the development of symptomatic patent ductus arteriosus and congestive heart failure in premature infants. *N Engl J Med* 1980;320:598.

Costarino A, Baumgart S: Modern fluid and electrolyte management of the critically ill premature infant. *Pediatr Clin North Am* 1986;33:153.

Costarino AT, Baumgart S: Water as nutrition. In Tsang RC (ed): *Nutritional Needs of the Preterm Infant.* Williams & Wilkins, 1993.

Costarino AT et al: Sodium restriction versus daily maintenance replacement in very low birth weight premature neonates: a randomized, blind therapeutic trial. *J Pediatr* 1992;120:99.

Day GM et al: Electrolyte abnormalities in very low birth weight infants. *Pediatric Res* 1976; 10:522.

Gaylord SM et al: Improved fluid management utilizing humidified incubator in extremely low birth weight infants. *J Perinatol* 2001;21:438.

Kavvadia V et al: Randomized trial of two levels of fluid input in the perinatal period—effect on fluid balance, electrolyte and metabolic disturbances in ventilated VLBW infants. *Acta Paediatr* 2000;89:237.

Lorenz JM et al: Phases of fluid and electrolyte homeostasis in the extremely low birth weight infant. *Pediatrics* 1995;96:484.

Lorenz JM et al: Water balance in very low birth weight infants: relationship to water and sodium intake and effect on outcome. *J Pediatr* 1982;101:423.

Meyer M et al: A clinical comparison of radiant warmer and incubator care for preterm infants from birth to 1800 grams. *Pediatrics* 2001;108:395.

Oh W: Fluid and electrolyte management. In Fanaroff A, Martin RJ (eds): *Neonatal-Perinatal Medicine—Diseases of the Fetus and Infant,* 6th ed. Mosby-Year Book, 1996.

Omar S et al: Effects of prenatal steroids in extreme low birth weight infants. *Pediatrics* 1999;104:482.

Shaffer SG et al: Fluid requirements in the preterm infant. *Clin Perinatol* 1992a;19:233.

Shaffer SG et al: Hyperkalemia in very low birth weight infants. *J Pediatr* 1992b;121:275.

Zenk K: Calculating dextrose infusion in mg/kg/min. *PeriScope* 1984;Aug 5.

8 Nutritional Management

GROWTH ASSESSMENT OF THE NEONATE

I. **Anthropometrics.** Serial measurements of weight, length, and head circumference allow for evaluation of growth patterns.
   A. **Weight.** During the first week of life, weight loss of 10–15% of birth weight is expected because of changes in body water compartments. Preterm infants regain their birth weight slower than term infants. Weight gain generally begins by the second week of life. Average daily weight gain based on normal intrauterine growth is 10–20 g/kg/day or 20–30 g/day (1–3% of body weight/day). Infants should be weighed daily.
   B. **Length.** Weekly assessment of length is recommended. Average length gain in preterm infants is 0.8–1.0 cm/week, whereas term infants average 0.69–0.75 cm/week.
   C. **Head circumference.** Intrauterine growth is 0.5–0.8 cm/week. This is used as an indicator of brain growth. Premature infants exhibit catch-up growth in head circumference that may exceed normal growth rate, but an increase in head circumference >1.25 cm/week may be abnormal and associated with hydrocephalus or intraventricular hemorrhage.

II. **Classification**
   A. **Measurements** of weight, length, and head circumference are plotted on growth charts to facilitate comparison to established norms. This can help to identify special needs.
   B. **Normal growth** customarily falls between the 10th and 90th percentiles when plotted on growth charts based on intrauterine growth curves and adjusted for gestational age.
      1. **Appropriate for gestational age (AGA).** AGA is indicative of appropriate intrauterine growth.
      2. **Large for gestational age (LGA).** This often occurs in infants of diabetic mothers. The common nutritional concern is prevention and control of hypoglycemia. Other causes of LGA infants include postmaturity and Beckwith-Wiedemann syndrome.
      3. **Small for gestational age (SGA).** If all parameters fall below the 5th percentile, higher caloric requirements are often needed to achieve appropriate growth.

NUTRITIONAL REQUIREMENTS IN THE NEONATE

I. **Calories**
   A. **To maintain weight,** give 50–60 kcal/kg/day (60 nonprotein kcal/kg/day).
   B. **To induce weight gain,** give 100–120 kcal/kg/day to a term infant (gain: 15–30 g/day) and 110–140 kcal/kg/day to a premature infant (70–90 nonprotein kcal/kg/day). Growth in premature infants is assumed to be adequate when it approximates the intrauterine rate (ie, 15 g/kg/day).

II. **Carbohydrates.** Approximately 10–30 g/kg/day (7.5–15g/kg/day) are needed to provide 40–50% of total calories. Lesser amounts of carbohydrates should provide total energy requirements in infants with chronic lung disease.

III. **Proteins.** Adequate protein intake has been estimated at 2.25–4.0 g/kg/day (7–16% of total calories, or 2–3 g/100 kcal for efficient utilization). Protein intake in low birth weight infants should not exceed 4.0 g/kg/day.

IV. Fats. Fat requirements are 5–7 g/kg/day (limit: 40–55% of total calories, or keto-sis may result). To meet essential fatty acid requirements, 2–5% of nonprotein calories should be in the form of linoleic acid and 0.6% in the form of linolenic acid (together comprising 3% of total energy requirements). Linoleic and linolenic acids are precursors for arachidonic acid (AA) and docosahexanoic acid (DHA), important in neural and retinal maturation. Breast milk contains long-chain polyunsaturated fatty acids (LCPUFAs) that are absent in formula milk. LCPUFAs may be important in retinal and brain development.

V. Vitamins and minerals. Vitamin requirements for preterm infants are not clearly established. Guidelines are provided in Table 8–1 for low birth weight infants. Caution is required with vitamin supplementation because toxicity may occur with both water- and fat-soluble vitamins as a result of immature renal and hepatic function. Vitamin supplementation may be needed with certain types of formula (Table 8–2).

A. Vitamin A may be useful in attenuating chronic lung disease in preterm infants at a dose of 5000 IU IM 3 times/week for 12 doses.

B. In infants with **osteopenia of prematurity,** various amounts of calcium, phosphorus, and vitamin D may be supplemented.

C. For infants receiving **recombinant human erythropoietin therapy,** additional iron supplementation is necessary. Although recommended doses vary, it is generally agreed that a dose in excess of maintenance therapy is needed. These doses may approach 6–10 mg/kg/day. For infants on high doses of iron, monitoring for hemolytic anemia is important and vitamin E supplementation (15–25 IU/day) may be required. The addition of iron to parenteral nutrition remains controversial. Preterm infants should receive iron supplementation (2–4 mg/kg/day, maximum 15 mg/day) by 2 months of age or when birth weight is doubled, whichever comes first. All term infant formulas have supplemental iron.

VI. Fluids. See Chapter 7 for fluid requirements.

PRINCIPLES OF INFANT FEEDING

I. Criteria for initiating infant feeding. Term healthy infants should be breast-fed as soon as possible within the first hour. The following criteria should usually be met before initiating infant feedings.

A. No history of excessive oral secretions, vomiting, or bilious-stained gastric aspirate.

B. Nondistended, soft abdomen, with normal bowel sounds. If the abdominal examination is abnormal, an abdominal x-ray film should be obtained.

C. Respiratory rate <60 breaths/min for oral feeding and <80 breaths/min for gavage feeding. Tachypnea increases the risk of aspiration.

D. Prematurity. Considerable controversy surrounds the timing of initial enteral feeding for the preterm infant. However, it is now believed that feedings should be initiated as soon as clinically possible. Early enteral feedings are associated with better endocrine adaptation, enhanced immune functions, and earlier discharge. Institutional practices may vary, however. In general, enteral feeding is started in the first 3 days of life with the objective of reaching full enteral feeding in 2–3 weeks. Parenteral nutrition, including amino acids and lipids, should be initiated within 1–3 days to provide adequate protein and caloric intake. Early parenteral nutrition is also associated with better weight gain.

1. For the **stable, larger premature neonate** (>1500 g), the first feeding may be given within the first 24 h of life. Early feeding may allow the release of enteric hormones, which exert a trophic effect on the intestinal tract.

2. On the other hand, apprehension about **necrotizing enterocolitis (NEC),** primarily in the very low birth weight (VLBW) infant, has meant that initia-

TABLE 8-1. DAILY ENTERAL VITAMIN AND MINERAL REQUIREMENTS

Nutrient	Term infant (per day)	Stable preterm LBW infant (dose/kg)
Daily enteral requirements		
Vitamins		
Vitamin A (with lung disease)	700 mcg	700–1500 mcg
Vitamin D	400 IU	400 IU
Vitamin E	7 IU	6–12 IU
Vitamin K	200 mcg	8–10 mcg
Vitamin C	80 mg	18–24 mg
Thiamine	1.2 mg	0.18–0.24 mg
Riboflavin	1 4 mg	0.25–0.36 mg
Niacin	17 mg	3.6–4.8 mg
Pyridoxine	1.0 mg	0.15–0.20 mg
Vitamin B_{12}	1.0 mcg	0.3 mcg
Folic acid	140 mcg	25–50 mcg
Biotin	20 mcg	3.6–6.0 mcg
Pantothenate	5 mg	1.2–1.7 mg
Minerals		
Calcium	250 mg	120–330 mg
Phosphorus	150 mg	60–140 mg
Magnesium	20 mg	7.9–15 mg
Sodium	1–2 mEq/kg	2.0–3.0 mEq
Potassium	2–3 mEq/kg	2.0–3.0 mEq
Iron	1 mg/kg	2–3 mg
Copper	20 mcg/kg	120–150 mcg
Zinc		1000 mcg
Manganese	5 mcg/100 kcal	0.75–7.5 mcg
Molybdenum	0.75–7.5 mcg	0.3 mcg
Selenium	2 mcg/kg	1.3–3.0 mcg
Chromium	0.20 mcg/kg	0.1–0.5 mcg
Iodide	1 mcg/kg	30–60 mcg

Nutrient	Term infant (per day)	Preterm infant (dose/kg)	Stable preterm infant (dose/kg)
Daily parenteral requirements			
Vitamins			
Vitamin A (with lung disease)	700 mcg	500 mcg	700–1500 mcg
Vitamin D	400 IU	160 IU	40–160 IU
Vitamin E	7 mg	2.8 mg	3.5 mg
Vitamin K	200 mcg	80 mcg	8–10 mcg
Vitamin C	80 mg	25 mg	15–25 mg
Thiamine	1.2 mg	0.35 mg	0.2–0.35 mg
Riboflavin	1.4 mg	0.15 mg	0.15–0.20 mg
Niacin	17 mg	6.8 mg	4.0–6.8 mg
Pyridoxine	1.0 mg	0.18 mg	0.15–0.20 mg
Vitamin B_{12}	1.0 mcg	0.3 mcg	0.3 mcg
Folic acid	140 mcg	56 mcg	56 mcg
Biotin	20 mcg	6 mcg	5–8 mcg
Pantothenate	5 mg	2 mg	1–2 mg
Minerals			
Calcium		75–90 mcg	
Phosphorus		48–67 mcg	
Magnesium		6–10.5 mcg	
Sodium	1–2 mEq/kg	2.5–3.5 mEq < 1.5 kg: 4–8 mEq	
Potassium	2–3 mEq/kg	2–3 mEq	
Iron		2–4 mcg (after 6–8 weeks)	
Copper[a]	20 mcg/kg	20 mcg	
Zinc	250 mcg/kg	1200–1500 mcg	

(*continued*)

TABLE 8–1. DAILY VITAMIN AND MINERAL REQUIREMENTS *(continued)*

Nutrient	Term infant (per day)	Preterm infant (dose/kg)	Stable preterm infant (dose/kg)
Manganese	1 mcg/kg	10–20 mcg	
Molybdenum	0.25 mcg	0.3 mcg	
Selenium[b]	2 mcg/kg	2 mcg	
Chromium	0.20 mcg/kg	0.2 mcg	
Iodide	1 mcg/kg	1 mcg	
Conditionally essential nutrients[c]			
Cystine	225–395 mmol/100 kcal		
Taurine	30–60 mmol/100 kcal		
Tyrosine	640–800 mmol/100 kcal		
Inositol	150–375 mmol/100 kcal		
Choline	125–225 mmol/100 kcal		

LBW, low birth weight.
[a]Omit in cholestatic jaundice.
[b]Start supplementation at 2–4 weeks. Omit in renal dysfunction.
[c]Nutrients that are normally synthesized by humans but for which premature infants may have a reduced synthetic capability to produce.

tion of enteral feeding is often precluded in infants with the following associated conditions:
   a. **Perinatal asphyxia.**
   b. **Mechanical ventilation.**
   c. **Hemodynamic instability (use of pressors).**
   d. **Sepsis.**
   e. **Frequent episodes of apnea and bradycardia.**
   f. **Absent end-diastolic flow in the umbilical artery on antenatal Doppler studies.**
   g. **Presence of umbilical catheters (controversial).**
   h. **Feeding in the presence of patent ductus arteriosus and indomethacin therapy (controversial).**
II. **Feeding guidelines and choice of formula.** Human milk is preferred for feeding term, preterm, and sick infants. If a commercial infant formula is chosen, generally no special considerations apply to healthy, full-term newborn infants. Preterm infants may require more careful planning. Many different, highly specialized formulas are available. Iron-fortified formula has become the formula of choice for term infants because its use has contributed to a decreased rate of anemia. Table 8–2 outlines indications for various formulas. The compositions of commonly used infant formulas and breast milk can be found in Table 8–3.
   A. **Formulas**
      1. **Iso-osmolar formulas (270–300 mOsm/kg water).** The majority of infant formulas are iso-osmolar (Similac 20 or Enfamil 20 [with and without iron]). These are the formulas used most often for healthy infants. Premature formulas that contain 24 cal/oz (Similac Special Care 24 or Enfamil Premature Formula 24) are also iso-osmolar and are indicated for rapidly growing premature infants.
      2. **Hypo-osmolar formulas** (<270 mOsm/kg water) have a lower osmolality, which can improve feeding tolerance.
         a. **Similac 13,** with an osmolality of 200 mOsm/kg water, was specifically designed as a conservative initial feeding for infants who have not been fed enterally for several days or weeks. It is not suitable for long-term feeding because it does not meet the nutrient needs of most infants.
         b. **Other hypo-osmolar formulas** include most of the premature formulas that contain 20 cal/oz (Similac Special Care 20 or Enfamil Premature

TABLE 8-2. INFANT FORMULA INDICATIONS AND USES

Formula	Indications	Vitamin and mineral supplement[a]
Human milk	All infants	MV; iron if >1500 g; fluoride
Breast milk fortifiers	Preterm infant (<1500 g and <34 weeks)	at 40 weeks; folate until 2000 g
Term Formulas		
Iso-osmolar		
Enfamil 20	Full-term infants: as supplement to breast milk	MV if <32 oz/day
Similac 20	Preterm infants >1800–2000 g	
Higher osmolality		
Enfamil 24	Term infants: for infants on fluid	
Similac 24 & 27	restriction or who cannot handle required volumes of 20-cal formula to grow	
Low osmolality		
Similac 13	Preterm and term infants: for conservative initial feeding in infants who have not been fed orally for several days or weeks. *Not for long-term use.*	
Soy formulas		
ProSobee (lactose and sucrose free)	Term infants: milk sensitivity, galactosemia, carbohydrate intolerance	MV if <32 oz/day
Isomil (lactose free)	*Do not use in preterm infants. Phytates can bind calcium and cause rickets.*	
Protein hydrolysate formulas		
Nutramigen	Term infants: gut sensitivity to proteins, galactosemia, multiple food allergies, persistent diarrhea	MV if <32 oz/day
Pregestimil	Preterm and term infants: disaccharidase deficiency, diarrhea, GI defects, cystic fibrosis, food allergy, celiac disease, transition from TPN to oral feeding	
Alimentum	Term infants: protein sensitivity, pancreatic insufficiency, diarrhea, allergies, colic, carbohydrate and fat malabsorption	
Neocate	Term infants: cow's milk protein allergies; contains 100% free amino acids (elemental formula)	
Special Formulas		
Portagen	Preterm and term infants: pancreatic or bile acid insufficiency, intestinal resection	MV if <32 oz/day; calcium needed
Similac PM 60/40	Preterm and term infants: problem feeders on standard formula; infants with renal, cardiovascular, or digestive diseases that require decreased protein and mineral levels; breast-feeding supplement, initial feeding	MV and Fe if standard formula weight >1500 g
Carnation Good Start	Term infants: whey protein; moderate mineral content; may be more palatable	
Lactofree	Preterm and term infants: lactose free, milk sensitivity	
Premature formulas		
Low osmolality		
Similac Special Care 20 Enfamil Premature 20	Premature infants (<1800–2000 g) who are growing rapidly. These formulas promote growth at intrauterine rates. Vitamin and mineral concentrations are higher to meet the needs of growth. Usually started on 20 cal/oz and advanced to 24 cal/oz as tolerated.	
Iso-osmolar		
Similac Special Care 24	Same as for low-osmolality premature formulas	
Enfamil Premature 24	Preterm infants >1800 g. Promotes catch-	
Neocare	up growth and improved bone mineralization	

(*continued*)

TABLE 8–2. INFANT FORMULA INDICATIONS AND USES (continued)

Formula	Indications	Vitamin and mineral supplement[a]
Transitional formulas Enfacare Neosure	Preterm infants; promotes better mineralization	

Fe, iron; GI, gastrointestinal; MV, multivitamin; TPN, total parenteral nutrition.
[a]Such as Poly-Vi-Sol (Mead Johnson).

Formula 20), which are designed to be better tolerated by premature infants and satisfy nutritional requirements.

3. **Hyperosmolar formulas** (>300 mOsm/kg water) are 24- and 27-cal/oz formulas, with the exception of the iso-osmolar, 24-cal/oz premature formulas. Formulas such as Similac 24, Enfamil 24, and Similac 27 are hypercaloric formulas designed to provide a greater percentage of the calories as protein and to provide increased mineral concentrations. They are used to provide nutritional needs for infants on fluid restriction.

4. **Transitional formulas.** Preterm infants continue to need nutritional supplementation after discharge. These have higher protein and mineral contents than the term formulas. Infants discharged on special formulas (Neosure, Enfacare, see Table 8–3) have better somatic growth, weight gain, and bone mineralization. Supplementation should be continued until a corrected age of 9 months.

B. **General guidelines**

1. **Initial feedings.** Use maternal breast milk for initiating feedings. In the absence of maternal breast milk, donor breast milk (see later discussion of breast milk) may be used in VLBW infants (after obtaining parental consent) to initiate feeds. Sterile water, dextrose 5% in water (D_5W), or dextrose 10% in water ($D_{10}W$) should be avoided as initial feeds. The use of formula feeds is associated with a 6–10 times higher incidence of NEC in preterm low birth weight infants than breast milk and 3 times higher when breast milk and formula are used together versus breast milk alone.

2. **Subsequent feedings.** Feedings with breast milk should be advanced gradually if the initial feeds are tolerated. Feedings should be advanced 10–30 mL/kg/day. Feedings may be advanced once to twice a day. Some clinicians advance feeds in small volume with each feeding. Particular care should be taken in intrauterine growth retardation (IUGR) infants, those with absent end-diastolic flow on antenatal Doppler ultrasonography, and those at risk for NEC (see prior discussion of NEC). Some clinicians advocate diluting formulas with sterile water and advancing as tolerated. Other practitioners believe that this is unnecessary and that full-strength formula can be used if the infant tolerates the initial feeding without difficulty. Breast milk is never diluted.

3. **Minimal enteral feedings ("trophic feeding").** Trophic feeds are subnutritional quantities of milk feeds, based on the concept of minimal enteral feedings. This practice—also called hypocaloric, trophic, trickle feedings, low-volume enteral substrate, or gastrointestinal priming—is characterized by a small-volume feeding to supplement parenteral nutrition. Studies focus on use in infants <1500 g at birth. This method has been accepted because of benefits such as improved feeding tolerance, prevention of gastrointestinal atrophy, and facilitation of gastrointestinal tract maturation leading to a shorter time required to attain full enteral feedings. Other benefits include decreased incidences of cholestasis, nosocomial infections, metabolic bone disease, and decreased hospital stay without an increase in the incidence of NEC. There is no standard method of minimal enteral feeding, and a wide variety of feeding techniques and formulas exist.

TABLE 8–3. COMPOSITION OF INFANT FORMULAS

Characteristics	Mature human breast milk	Preterm human breast milk	Enfamil 20, Enfamil 20 with iron	Similac 20, Similac 20 with iron
Calories/100 mL	68	67	67	68
Osmolality (mOsm/kg H_2O)	290	290	278	300
Osmolarity (mOsm/L)	255	255	270	270
Protein				
Grams/100 mL	1.05	1.4	1.42	1.39
% Total calories	6	8	8	8
Source			Cow's milk, whey	Nonfat milk, whey
Fat				
Grams/100 mL	3.9	3.9	3.9	3.65
% Total calories	52	52	48	49
Source			Soy and coconut oils	Soy and coconut oils
Linoleic acid (mcg)	374	369	860	675
Carbohydrates				
Grams/100 mL	7.2	6.6	8.1	7.3
% Total calories	42	40	44	43
Source	Lactose	Lactose	Lactose	Lactose
Minerals (mg/100 mL)				
Calcium (mg)	28	25	53	52
Phosphorus (mg)	14	13	36	28
Iodine (mcg)	11	11	7	4.1
Iron (mg)	0.03	0.12	1.22	1.22
Magnesium (mg)	3.5	3.1	5.4	4.1
Sodium (mg)	18	25	18	16.2
Potassium (mg)	52	57	73	71
Chloride (mg)	42	55	43	43
Zinc (mg)	0.12	0.34	0.68	0.51
Copper (mcg)	25	65	56	61
Manganese (mcg)	0.6	0.6	11.1	3.4
Selenium (mcg)	1.5	1.5	2	1.5
Vitamins/100 mL				
Vitamin A (IU)	223	389	203	203
Vitamin D (IU)	2	2	41	41
Vitamin E (IU)	0.3	1.1	1.4	1
Vitamin K (mcg)	0.2	0.2	5.4	5.4
Thiamine/B_1 (mcg)	21	21	54	68
Riboflavin/B_2 (mcg)	35	48	95	101
Niacin/B_3 (mcg)	150	150	676	709
Vitamin B_6 (mcg)	20	15	41	41
Vitamin B_{12} (mcg)	0.05	0.05	0.20	0.17
Folic acid (mcg)	5	3.3	10.8	10.1
Vitamin C (mg)	4.1	11	8.1	6.1
Pantothenic acid (mcg)	180	120	338	304
Biotin (mcg)	0.4	0.4	2.2	3
Choline (mg)	9.2	9.4	8.9	11
Inositol (mg)	15	15	4.5	3.2

(continued)

TABLE 8–3. COMPOSITION OF INFANT FORMULAS (*continued*)

Characteristics	Similac Special Care 20	Enfamil Premature Formula 20	Similac Special Care 24	Enfamil Premature Formula 24
Calories/100 mL	68	68	81	81
Osmolality (mOsm/kg H_2O)	235	240	280	300
Osmolarity (mOsm/L)	211	220	246	260
Protein				
Grams/100 mL	1.83	2.2	2.19	2.7
% Total calories	11	12	11	12
Source	Nonfat milk and whey	Nonfat milk and whey	Nonfat milk and whey	Nonfat milk and whey
Fat				
Grams/100 mL	3.67	3.8	4.38	4.7
% Total calories	49	44	49	44
Source	MCTs, soy and coconut oils	MCTs, soy and coconut oils	MCTs, soy and coconut oils	MCTs, soy and coconut oils
Linoleic acid (mcg)	473	796	564	981
Carbohydrates				
Grams/100 mL	7.2	8.3	8.5	10.7
% Total calories	42	44	42	44
Source	Lactose, glucose polymers	Lactose, corn syrup solids	Lactose, glucose polymers	Lactose, corn syrup solids
Minerals/100 mL				
Calcium (mg)	122	111	145	133
Phosphorus (mg)	67	56	81	67
Iodine (mcg)	4	17	5	20
Iron (mg)	1.22	1.22	1.45	1.45
Magnesium (mg)	8.1	4.6	9.7	5.5
Sodium (mg)	29	26	35	31
Potassium (mg)	87	70	104	83
Chloride (mg)	55	57	65	69
Zinc (mg)	1.01	1.01	1.21	1.21
Manganese (mcg)	8.1	4.7	9.7	5.8
Copper (mcg)	169	94	202	115
Selenium (mcg)	1.2		1.45	
Vitamins/100 mL				
Vitamin A (IU)	845	845	1008	1008
Vitamin D (IU)	101	182	121	218
Vitamin E (IU)	2.7	4.3	3.2	5.1
Vitamin K (mcg)	8.1	5.4	9.7	6.5
Thiamine/B_1 (mcg)	169	135	202	161
Riboflavin/B_2 (mcg)	419	203	500	242
Niacin/B_3 (mcg)	3378	2703	4032	3226
Vitamin B_6 (mcg)	169	101	202	121
Vitamin B_{12} (mcg)	0.37	0.17	0.44	0.20
Folic acid (mcg)	25	23.6	29.8	28.2
Vitamin C (mg)	25	13.5	29.8	16.1
Pantothenic acid (mcg)	1284	811	1532	968
Biotin (mcg)	25	3	30	3.7
Choline (mg)	6.8	9	8.1	11.1
Inositol (mg)	4	12.7	4.9	15.7

(*continued*)

TABLE 8–3. COMPOSITION OF INFANT FORMULAS (*continued*)

Characteristics	Isomil 20	ProSobee 20	Lactofree	Isomil DF
Calories/100 mL	68	68	68	68
Osmolality (mOsm/kg H$_2$0)	250	200	200	240
Osmolarity (mOsm/L)	220	170	220	220
Protein				
Grams per 100 mL	1.66	1.9	1.49	1.8
% Total calories	11	12	9	11
Source	Soy protein	Soy protein	Milk protein	Soy protein
Fat				
Grams/100 mL	3.69	3.9	3.72	3.69
% Total calories	49	48	50	49
Source	Soy and coconut oils	Soy and coconut oils	Palm, soy, coconut, and sunflower oils	Soy and coconut oils
Linoleic acid (mcg)	675	646	646	878
Carbohydrates				
Grams/100 mL	7	7.9	7	6
% Total calories	49	48	42	49
Source	Corn syrup, sucrose	Corn syrup solids	Glucose polymers	Corn syrup solids, sucrose
Minerals/100 mL				
Calcium (mg)	71	71	55	71
Phosphorus (mg)	51	56	37	51
Iodine (mcg)	10	7	10	10
Iron (mg)	1.22	1.27	1.22	1.22
Magnesium (mg)	5.1	7.4	5.4	5.1
Sodium (mg)	30	24	20	30
Potassium (mg)	73	81	74	73
Chloride (mg)	42	54	45	42
Zinc (mg)	0.51	0.81	0.68	0.51
Copper (mcg)	51	56	56	51
Manganese (mcg)	17	18.6	11.1	20
Selenium (mcg)	1.4	2.0	2.0	1.4
Vitamins/100 mL				
Vitamin A (IU)	203	203	203	203
Vitamin D (IU)	41	41	41	41
Vitamin E (IU)	2	1.4	1.4	2
Vitamin K (mcg)	10.1	5.4	5.4	10.1
Thiamine/B$_1$ (mcg)	41	54	54	41
Riboflavin/B$_2$ (mcg)	61	61	61	61
Niacin/B$_3$ (mcg)	912	676	676	912
Vitamin B$_6$ (mcg)	41	41	41	41
Vitamin B$_{12}$ (mcg)	0.3	0.21	0.2	0.3
Folic acid (mcg)	10.1	10.8	10.8	10.1
Vitamin C (mg)	6.1	8.1	8.1	6.1
Pantothenic acid (mcg)	507	338	338	507
Biotin (mcg)	3	2.2	2.2	3
Choline (mg)	5.4	9	9	5.4
Inositol (mg)	3.4	4.4	4.4	3.4

(continued)

TABLE 8-3. COMPOSITION OF INFANT FORMULAS (*continued*)

Characteristics	Similac PM 60/40	Similac 27	Carnation Good Start	Protagen	Enfamil AR
Calories/100 mL	68	91	68	68	67
Osmolality (mOsm/kg H_2O)	280	430			
Osmolarity (mOsm/L)	250	370		210	
Protein					
Grams/100 mL	1.49	2.46	1.62	2.36	1.67
% Total calories	9	11	9	14	10
Source	Whey, casein	Cow's milk	Hydrolyzed whey	Sodium caseinate	Whey, nonfat milk
Fat					
Grams/100 mL	3.78	4.79	3.45	3.24	
% Total calories	41	42	46	43	46
Source	Soy and coconut oils	Soy and coconut oils	Palm, soy, coconut, and safflower oils	85% MCTs, 15% corn oil	Palm, olein; coconut, and high oleic sun-flower oils
Linoleic acid (mcg)	878			646	
Carbohydrates					
Grams/100 mL	6.9	9.5	7.4	7.8	7.3
% Total calories	41	42	44	46	44
Source	Lactose, malto-dextrin	Lactose solids, sucrose	Lactose, maltodextrin	Corn syrup solids, sucrose	Rice starch, lactose, malto-dextrin
Minerals/100 mL					
Calcium (mg)	38	82	43	64	52
Phosphorus (mg)	19	64	24	47	35
Iodine (mcg)	4	8	10	5	6.7
Iron (mg)	0.15	0.2	1.01	1.27	1.2
Magnesium (mg)	4.1	6.4	4.5	13.5	5.3
Sodium (mg)	16	31	16	37	27
Potassium (mg)	58	120	66	84	72
Chloride (mg)	40	74	40	58	50
Zinc (mg)	0.51	0.68	0.51	0.64	0.67
Copper (mcg)	61			56	100
Manganese (mcg)	3.4			11.1	80
Selenium (mcg)	1.3			2.0	0.33
Vitamins/100 mL					
Vitamin A (IU)	203	273	203	527	200
Vitamin D (IU)	41	55	41	53	40
Vitamin E (IU)	1.7	2.7	0.8	2.1	1.33
Vitamin K (mcg)	5.4	7.3	5.5	10.5	5.3
Thiamine/B_1 (mcg)	68	91	41	105	53
Riboflavin/B_2 (mcg)	101	136	91	127	93
Niacin/B_3 (mcg)	709	955	507	1419	667
Vitamin B_6 (mcg)	41	55	51	142	40
Vitamin B_{12} (mcg)	0.17	0.23	0.15	0.43	0.2
Folic acid (mcg)	10.1	13.6	6.1	10.5	10.6
Vitamin C (mg)	6.1	8.2	5.4	5.5	8
Pantothenic acid (mcg)	304	409	304	709	333
Biotin (mcg)	3			2.2	5
Choline (mg)	8.1			9	8.5
Inositol (mg)	16.2			4.4	3

(continued)

TABLE 8-3. COMPOSITION OF INFANT FORMULAS (*continued*)

Characteristics	Similac 13	Similac, Similac with iron 24	Enfamil, Enfamil with iron 24	NeoSure 22	EnfaCare
Calories/100 mL	44	81	81	74	68
Osmolality (mOsm/kg H_2O)	200	380	360	250	320
Osmolarity (mOsm/L)	190	340	320	224	290
Protein					
Grams/100 mL	1.19	2.19	1.77	1.9	1.89
% Total calories	11	11	9	10	11
Source	Cow's milk	Cow's milk	Nonfat milk, whey	Nonfat milk, whey	Casein, whey
Fat					
Grams/100 mL	2.32	4.25	4.52	4.1	3.4
% Total calories	47	47	50	49	45
Source	Soy and coconut oils	Soy and coconut oils	Soy and coconut oils	MCTs, soy, coconut oils	Soy, MCTs, high oleic sunflower oil, coconut oils
Linoleic acid (mcg)		1048	646	559	715
Carbohydrates					
Grams/100 mL	4.62	8.5	8.3	7.7	8
% Total calories	42	42	41	41	43
Source	Lactose	Lactose	Lactose	Lactose, corn syrup solids	Glucose poly- mers, lactose
Minerals/100 mL					
Calcium (mg)	40	73	63	77	90
Phosphorus (mg)	58	56	43	46	49
Iodine (mcg)	6	7	5	11	11.1
Iron (mg)	0.1	1.45	1.52	1.32	1.33
Magnesium (mg)	0.31	5.6	6.3	6.7	6
Sodium (mg)	15	27	22	24	26
Potassium (mg)	58	106	87	106	79
Chloride (mg)	36	65	51	56	58
Zinc (mg)	0.33	0.60	0.63	0.9	0.92
Copper (mcg)		72	50	89	90
Manganese (mcg)		4	10	7.5	11
Selenium (mcg)		2	2	1.7	1.7
Vitamins/100 mL					
Vitamin A (IU)	132	242	250	343	330
Vitamin D (IU)	26	48	51	52	59
Vitamin E (IU)	1.3	2.4	1.6	2.6	3
Vitamin K (mcg)	3.5	6.5	6.5	8	5.9
Thiamine/B_1 (mcg)	44	81	63	164	148
Riboflavin/B_2 (mcg)	66	121	121	112	148
Niacin/B_3 (mcg)	462	847	1008	1455	1480
Vitamin B_6 (mcg)	26	48	51	74	74
Vitamin B_{12} (mcg)	0.11	0.20	0.19	0.29	0.22
Folic acid (mcg)	6.6	12.1	12.6	18.3	19.2
Vitamin C (mg)	40	7.3	6.5	11	11.8
Pantothenic acid (mcg)	198	363	379	597	630
Biotin (mcg)		3.5		6.7	4.5
Choline (mg)		13		12	11.2
Inositol (mg)		3.8		4.5	2.2

(continued)

TABLE 8–3. COMPOSITION OF INFANT FORMULAS (*continued*)

Characteristics	Pregestimil	Nutramigen	Alimentum	Neocate
Calories/100 mL	68	68	68	67
Osmolality (mOsm/kg H$_2$0)	320	320	370	342
Osmolarity (mOsm/L)	290	290	330	
Protein				
Grams/100 mL	1.89	1.89	1.86	2.08
% Total calories	11	11	11	12
Source	Casein hydrolysate	Casein hydrolysate	Casein hydrolysate	L-Amino acids
Fat				
Grams/100 mL	3.78	3.38	3.74	3.01
% Total calories	50	45	50	41
Source	55% MCTs, corn, soy, safflower oils	Palm, soy, coconut, sunflower oils	MCTs, soy, sunflower oils	Soy, coconut oil, safflower oils
Carbohydrates				
Grams/100 mL	3.78	3.38	3.74	7.84
% Total calories	41	44	41	47
Source	Modified corn-starch, corn syrup	Modified corn-starch, corn syrup	Tapioca starch, sucrose	Corn syrup solids
Minerals/100 mL				
Calcium (mg)	64	64	71	83
Phosphorus (mg)	43	43	51	62
Iodine (mcg)	5	10	10	10
Iron (mg)	1.27	1.22	1.22	1.24
Magnesium (mg)	7.4	7.4	5.1	8.3
Sodium (mg)	26	32	30	25
Potassium (mg)	74	74	80	104
Chloride (mg)	58	58	54	52
Zinc (mg)	0.64	0.68	0.51	1.13
Copper (mcg)	50	50	50	
Manganese (mcg)	16.7	16.7	5.4	
Selenium (mcg)	1.9	1.9	1.4	
Vitamins/100 mL				
Vitamin A (IU)	257	203	203	274
Vitamin D (IU)	51	41	30	58
Vitamin E (IU)	2.6	1.4	2.0	0.8
Vitamin K (mcg)	12.7	5.4	10.1	5.9
Thiamine/B$_1$ (mcg)	53	54	41	62
Riboflavin/B$_2$ (mcg)	64	61	61	92
Niacin/B$_3$ (mcg)	845	676	912	1034
Vitamin B$_6$ (mcg)	43	41	41	83
Vitamin B$_{12}$ (mcg)	0.21	0.20	0.30	0.11
Folic acid (mcg)	10.5	10.8	10.1	6.8
Vitamin C (mg)	7.9	8.1	6.1	6.2
Pantothenic acid (mcg)	318	338	507	415
Biotin (mcg)	2	2	3	
Choline (mg)	9	9	5.4	
Inositol (mg)	11.3	11.3	3.4	

MCTs, medium-chain triglycerides; Isomil DF, Isomil Diarrhea Formula.
[a]Similac 20 low iron contains 0.15 mg iron/100 mL; Enfamil 20 low iron contains 0.11 mg iron/100 mL.

Mother's breast milk should be preferred over donor breast milk or preterm formula for trophic feedings.

a. **Type of formula.** Breast milk is the preferred feeding; however, positive results have been achieved using preterm infant formulas.

b. **Feeding method.** Orogastric or nasogastric routes are used for feeding. Nasogastric tubes in small infants may increase airway resistance. Both continuous and bolus feedings have been used. The most effective method remains to be identified, but a trend exists toward bolus feedings. Enteral feedings should be advanced as clinically tolerated.

c. **Volume.** Volumes studied have varied from 0.1–24 mL/kg/day.

d. **Minimal enteral feedings for extremely low birth weight infants (<1000 g, <28 weeks)** should start at 10–20 mL/kg/day divided as q2h feeds, advance as tolerated. Alternatively, start at 0.5–2 mL every 6 h; advance to every 4 h and then every 2 h. If continuous feeds are used, up to 0.5–1 mL/kg/h volume may be used.

4. **Weight-specific guidelines** are based on **birth weight** and **gestational age** (GA) as presented in this section. For an infant presumed to be at risk for NEC, the rate of enteral feeding advancement should not exceed 20 mL/kg/day and 10 cal/kg/day. Protocols vary by institution.

a. **Weight: <1200 g; GA: <30 weeks.** Gavage feeding through an orogastric or nasogastric tube is appropriate.

  i. **Initial feeding:** breast milk or donor breast milk (see prior discussion); preterm infant formulas.

  ii. **Maintenance feeding:** breast milk (with or without human milk fortifier, see indications presented later) or preterm formulas (20 or 24 cal/oz). Donor breast milk should not be used for maintenance because it does not provide adequate proteins and minerals for long-term growth.

  iii. **Subsequent feedings**

    (a) **Volume.** Bolus feeds, 10–20 mL/kg/day in divided volumes every 2 h. Advance feeds by 10–20 mL/kg/day. Alternatively, give 0.5–1.0 mL/h continuously and increase by 0.5–1.0 mL every 12–24 h. When 10 mL/h is tolerated, change feedings to every 2 h and advance as tolerated.

    (b) **Strength.** Use expressed breast milk or preterm formula. Once full feedings of 20 cal/oz are tolerated, consider advancing to 24-cal/oz feedings or adding human milk fortifier to breast milk.

b. **Weight: 1200–1500 g; GA: <32 weeks.** Gavage feeding through a nasogastric tube should be used.

  i. **Initial feeding.** Give breast milk or preterm formula every 2–3 h.

  ii. **Subsequent feedings**

    (a) **Volume.** Bolus feeds, 10–20 mL/kg/day in divided volumes, every 3 h. Advance feeds by 10–20 mL/kg/day. Alternatively, give 2 mL/kg every 2 h, and increase by 1 mL every 12 h up to 20 mL every 2 h. Then change to feedings every 3 h.

    (b) **Strength.** Use breast milk or preterm formulas. Once full feedings of 20 cal/oz are tolerated, advance to 24 cal/oz if desired or add human milk fortifier (22 or 24 cal/oz).

c. **Weight: 1500–2000 g.** Use gavage feeding through an orogastric or nasogastric tube. Breast-feeding or bottle-feeding can be attempted if the infant is >1600 g, >34 weeks' gestation, and neurologically intact. Initiation of early nursing is associated with earlier time to achieve full enteral feeds.

  i. **Initial feeding.** Use expressed breast milk or preterm infant formulas. For infants >1800 g (>36 weeks), term infant formulas may be considered *(controversial)*.

    Breast milk or preterm infant formula should be used.

      ii. Subsequent feedings. Give 2.5–5 mL/kg every 3 h, and advance 10–20 mL/kg/day as tolerated.

  d. Weight: 2000–2500 g; GA: >36 weeks. Nursing or bottle-feeding should be tried if the infant is neurologically intact.

      i. Initial feeding. Begin breast milk or term infant formula.

      ii. Subsequent feedings. Give 5 mL/kg every 3–4 h, and advance 10–20 mL/kg/day as tolerated.

  e. Weight: >2500 g. Breast-feed or use a bottle if the infant is neurologically intact.

      i. Initial feeding. See Section II,B,4,d,i above.

      ii. Subsequent feedings. Feed every 3–4 h, and advance as tolerated. Use 5 mL/kg; advance 20 mL/kg/day.

III. Management of feeding intolerance. If feeding is initiated but not tolerated, a complete abdominal examination should be performed. Consider abdominal x-ray studies if the physical findings are suspicious. If the abdominal evaluation is normal:

  A. Attempt continuous feedings with a nasogastric or orogastric tube. Check the gastric aspirate, and follow the recommendations presented in Chapter 36.

  B. Use breast milk preferably or special formula (eg, Similac PM 60/40 or Pregestimil) because they may be better tolerated.

IV. Nutritional supplements. Supplements are sometimes added to feedings, primarily to increase caloric intake (Table 8–4). They provide additional energy supplies with no concomitant increase in fluid volume. Protein supplementation results in increase in short-term weight gain, linear growth, and head growth. Long-term effects on growth and neurodevelopment are not conclusive. There are insufficient data to evaluate the effects of carbohydrate or fat supplementation on long-term growth and development in preterm infants.

    Some clinicians strongly believe that any necessary caloric supplementation should be given as a high-calorie formula (ie, 24 kcal/oz) instead of as a supplement because all nutrients in such a formula are in proportion to one another and allow maximum absorption. Nutritional supplements are often used in infants with bronchopulmonary dysplasia who are not gaining weight and need additional calories with no increase in protein, fat, or water intake.

BREAST-FEEDING

I. Advantages

  A. Protein quality. The predominance of whey and the mixture of amino acids are compatible with the metabolic needs of low birth weight infants.

  B. Digestion and absorption are improved with breast milk.

  C. Immunologic benefits. Breast-feeding provides immunologic protection against bacterial and viral infections (particularly upper respiratory tract and gastrointestinal infections). Studies of infants breast-fed for >6 months show that they have a decreased incidence of cancer.

  D. Promotion of bonding between the mother and her infant.

  E. Lower renal solute load, which facilitates better tolerance.

  F. Other advantages. Breast-feeding in preterm infants has been associated with a decreased risk for NEC and a significantly higher intelligence quotient (IQ) at the age of 8 years. The risk of breast and ovarian cancers in the mother also appears to be lower. Breast milk contains linoleic acid (LA) and α-linolenic acid (ALA) from which other essential long-chain polyunsaturated fatty acids (LCPUFA), docosahexaenoic acid (DHA), and arachidonic acid (AA) are produced. These play an important role in retinal and neurologic development. Most formulas are deficient in LCPUFAs. Supplementation with DHA and AA has not resulted in consistent outcomes. Formulas with DHA and AA will soon be available in the United States.

TABLE 8-4. NUTRITIONAL SUPPLEMENTS USED IN INFANTS

Supplement	Nutrient content	Calories	Indications and contraindications	Amount to use
Carbohydrate				
Polycose	Glucose polymers	3.8 kcal/g powder; 2 kcal/mL liquid	Calorie supplementation[a]	**Powder:** 0.5 g/oz of 20-cal formula = 22 cal/oz; 1 g/oz of 20-cal formula = 24 cal/oz **Liquid:** 1 mL to 1 oz of 20-cal formula = 22 cal/oz
Infant rice cereal	Rice	15 cal/tbsp	Thickens feedings	1 tsp/4 oz of formula
Fat				
Medium-chain triglyceride	Lipid fraction of coconut oil	8.3 kcal/g, 7.7 cal/mL	Limit to 50% calories from fat to prevent ketosis; may cause diarrhea; do not use in BPD because of risk of aspiration pneumonia[b]	0.5 mL/4 oz of formula = 21 cal/oz; 1 mL/4 oz of formula = 22 cal/oz 1 mL/2 oz of formula = 22 xal/oz
Vegetable oil	Soy, corn oil	9.0 cal/g (120 cal/tbsp)	To increase calories if fat absorption is normal[c]	0.5 mL/4 oz of formula = 21 cal/oz; 1 mL/4 oz of formula = 22 cal/oz
Microlipid	Safflower oil Soy lecithin Ascorbic acid Linoleic acid	4.5 cal/mL 5.9 g/tbsp	To increase caloric density, fluid restriction	1 mL/2 oz of formula = 22 cal/oz
Protein				
Casec	Calcium caseinate	3.4 cal/g (4 g of protein/tbsp); calcium = 62 mg/tbsp, sodium = 4.4 mg/tbsp, calories = 17/tbsp	Useful in chronic fluid restriction and as breast milk supplement; do not use in premature infants because of high solute load	

BPD, bronchopulmonary dysplasia.
[a]Limiting formula intake while increasing calories may compromise protein, vitamin, and mineral intake, which may also lead to hyperglycemia and diarrhea.
[b]Always mix with formula to avoid the possibility of lipid aspiration or pneumonia.
[c]Vitamin E may need to be increased to at least 1 IU/g of linoleic acid.

II. **Contraindications and disadvantages**
   A. **Active tuberculosis** in the mother.
   B. **Certain viral and bacterial infections** in the mother. For specific recommendations, see Appendix G, Isolation Guidelines.
   C. **Use of medications** that are passed in significant amount in the breast milk, which may harm the infant. For the effects of medications and substances on lactation and breast-feeding, see Chapter 81.
   D. **An infant with a cleft lip or palate** may have difficulty in nursing. Expressed breast milk can be fed to the infant using specially designed bottles (relative contraindication).
   E. **IUGR infants (<1500 g)** may require greater amounts of protein, sodium, calcium, phosphorus, and vitamin D than some formulas contain. These requirements should be monitored routinely and supplemented as necessary. *Note:* Temporary problems in the mother, such as sore or cracked nipples that resolve with treatment or mastitis treated with antibiotics, do not preclude nursing.

III. **Donor breast milk.** The use of donor breast milk is both regional and *controversial.* Historically, donor breast milk has been used for centuries; however, current practice tends toward limited use. In recent years, concerns regarding the transmission of infectious processes such as HIV, cytomegalovirus, and tuberculosis have led to questions regarding the safety of its use. If donor breast milk or milk banks are to be used, donor screening, heat treatment (pasteurization) of the milk, and parental counseling on these potential risks are recommended. Donor milk is deficient in protein, minerals, and calories to meet long-term requirements of preterm infants for growth and development.

IV. **Storage.** Breast milk can be stored frozen at –20 °C for up to 6 months and refrigerated at 4 °C for up to 24 h.

V. **Breast milk fortifiers (supplements).** The breast milk fortifiers (Table 8–5) are designed as a supplement to mother's milk for rapidly growing premature infants. Use of human milk beyond the second and third weeks in preterm infants may provide insufficient amounts of protein, calcium, phosphorus, and possibly copper, zinc, and sodium. Clinical experience has shown that the addition of human milk fortifier to a preterm mother's milk resulted in increased somatic growth related to increased protein and energy intake but no regular improvement in mineral retention. Periodic monitoring of urine osmolality, serum blood urea nitrogen, creatinine, and calcium is required. Three fortifiers are currently available in the United States.
   A. **Indications.** Breast milk fortifiers are indicated for those premature infants who tolerate unfortified human milk at full feedings, usually at 2–4 weeks of age, up to the time of discharge or at a birth weight of 2500–3000 g. Criteria for use include <34 weeks' gestation at birth and <1500 g at birth. In addition, breast milk fortifiers are indicated for fluid-restricted infants who require an increase in calories. Fortifiers can be added when 100 mL/kg/day of enteral feeding is reached.
      1. **Enfamil Human Milk Fortifier (EHMF)**
         a. **Composition.** The protein is 60% whey protein and 40% casein, which is similar to breast milk. The carbohydrate is 75% glucose polymers and 25% lactose. The fat is negligible. This fortifier comes in powder form.
         b. **Calories.** One packet of fortifier added to 50 mL of human milk provides an additional 2 cal/fl oz. The same amount of fortifier added to 25 mL of human milk supplies an additional 4 cal/fl oz. Once the powder is added to the milk, the container should be capped and mixed well. It can be covered and stored under refrigeration but should be used within 8 h.
         c. **Hypercalcemia** has been reported in some extremely low birth weight (<1000 g) infants receiving fortified breast milk. For these infants,

TABLE 8–5. COMPARISON OF 3 COMMERCIALLY AVAILABLE BREAST MILK SUPPLEMENTS

Variable	Similac Natural Care[a]	Enfamil HMF[b]	Similac HMF[b]
Volume	100 mL	100 mL	100 mL
Total calories	73 (24 cal/oz)	81 (24 cal/oz)	79 (24 cal/oz)
Osmolality (mOsm/kg H_2O)	300	365	385
Variables supplemented			
Calories	9	14	14
Protein (g)	0.1	0.7	1
Fat (g)	0.4	0.04	0.36
Carbohydrates (g)	1.3	2.7	1.8
Minerals			
Calcium (mg)	71	60	117
Chloride (mg)	9	17.7	38
Copper (μg)	62	40	170
Iron (mg)	0.1		0.35
Magnesium (mg)	3.4	4	7.0
Phosphorus (mg)	36	33	67
Potassium (mg)	28	15.6	63
Sodium (mg)	8	7	15
Vitamins/L			
Vitamins A (IU)	150	780	620
Vitamin B_1 (μg)	96	187	233
Vitamin B_2 (μg)	233	250	417
Vitamin B_6 (μg)	99	193	211
Vitamin B_{12} (μg)	0.2	0.21	0.64
Vitamin C (mg)	12.8	24	25
Vitamin D (IU)	58.8	210	120
Vitamin E (IU)	1.0	3.4	3.2
Vitamin K (μg)	4.0	9.1	8.3
Folic acid (μg)	12.8	23	23
Niacin (μg)	1920	3100	3570
Panthenic acid (μg)	640	790	1500
Biotin (μg)			26

HMF: human milk fortifier (4 packets/100 mL breast milk)
[a]50 mL breast milk plus 50 mL fortifier.
[b]4 packets of fortifier plus 100 mL of breast milk

serum calcium must be monitored. Fortification of breast milk should start beyond 2 weeks' postnatal age at a ratio not exceeding 1 packet/25 mL of breast milk.

2. **Similac Human Milk Fortifier (SHMF)**
   a. **Composition.** The protein is whey predominant with 2% soy lecithin. The carbohydrate is lactose and corn syrup solids. The fat is predominantly coconut oil (MCT).
   b. **Calories.** The fortifier provides 24 kcal/fl oz, when added in the ratio of 1 packet/25 mL of breast milk.

3. **Similac Natural Care (SNC)**
   a. **Composition.** The protein is whey predominant. The carbohydrate is lactose and glucose polymers in equal amounts. The fat is a mixture of 50% medium-chain triglycerides, 30% soy oil, and 20% coconut oil. This fortifier is a ready-to-use liquid formula that can be mixed with human milk.
   b. **Calories.** Similac Natural Care contains 24 cal/floz. It is most commonly diluted with human milk in a 1:1 proportion. Storage requirements are the same as for EHMF discussed previously.

TOTAL PARENTERAL NUTRITION

Total parenteral nutrition (TPN) is intravenous administration of all nutrients (fats, carbohydrates, proteins, vitamins, and minerals) necessary for metabolic requirements and growth. Parenteral nutrition (PN) is supplemental intravenous administration of nutrients. Enteral nutrition (EN) is oral or gavage feedings.

I. **Intravenous routes used in PN**
   A. **Central PN.** Central PN is usually reserved for patients requiring long-term (>2 weeks) administration of most calories. Basically, this type of nutrition involves infusion of a hypertonic nutrient solution (15–25% dextrose, 5–6% amino acids) into a vessel with rapid flow through an indwelling catheter, the tip of which is in the vena cava just above or beyond the right atrium. Disadvantages include increased risk of infection and complications from placement. Two methods are commonly used for placement.
      1. **A percutaneous catheter,** positioned in the antecubital or external jugular vein or saphenous vein, is advanced into the superior or inferior vena cava. This technique avoids surgical placement and results in fewer complications. (For details of the procedure, see Chapter 27.)
      2. **A central catheter (Broviac)** can be placed through a surgical cutdown in the internal or external jugular or subclavian vein. The proximal portion of the catheter (which has a polyvinyl cuff to promote fibroblast proliferation for securing the catheter) is tunneled subcutaneously to exit some distance from the insertion site, usually the anterior chest. This protects the catheter from inadvertent dislodgement and reduces the risk of contamination by microorganisms. The anesthesia and surgery needed for placement of the catheter are disadvantages to this method.
   B. **Peripheral PN.** This route, which uses a peripheral vein, may also be used in the neonatal intensive care unit (NICU) and is usually associated with fewer complications. The concentration of the amino acids and the dextrose solution limit the amount of solution that can be infused. The maximum concentration of dextrose that can be administered is 12.5% and the maximum concentration of amino acids, 3.5%.
      Note: PN can be given through an umbilical artery catheter, a route that has been used in some centers; however, the umbilical artery is not a preferred site and should be used with caution. The maximum dextrose concentration that can be administered using this method is 15%.

II. **Indications.** PN is used as a supplement to enteral feedings or as a complete substitution (TPN) when adequate nourishment cannot be achieved by the enteral route. Common indications in neonates include congenital malformation of the gastrointestinal tract, gastroschisis, meconium ileus, short bowel syndrome, NEC, paralytic ileus, respiratory distress syndrome, extreme prematurity, sepsis, and malabsorption. PN is usually started on day 2 or 3 of life, depending on the severity of the patient's illness. In preterm VLBW infants, 1–1.5 g/kg/day of amino acids should be started on day 1 and is associated with better outcomes and growth.

III. **Caloric concentration.** Caloric densities of various energy sources are as follows.

   • Dextrose (anhydrous): 3.4 kcal/g
   • Protein: 4 kcal/g
   • Fat: 9 kcal/g
   • 10% fat emulsion: 1.1 kcal/mL
   • 20% fat emulsion: 2 kcal/mL

IV. **Composition of PN solutions**
   A. **Carbohydrates**
      1. **The only commercially available carbohydrate source is dextrose (glucose).** A solution of 5.0–12.5 g/dL is used in peripheral PN and up to

25 g/dL in central PN. Dextrose concentrations should be calculated as milligrams per kilograms per minute.

2. **To allow for an appropriate response of endogenous insulin** and to prevent the development of osmotic diuresis secondary to glucosuria, neonates should not routinely be started on >6–8 mg/kg/min of dextrose. Frequent testing of urine for the presence of glucose is required. Infusion rates can be increased by 0.5–1 mg/kg/min each day as tolerated to achieve adequate caloric intake in the presence of stable blood sugar levels. See Chapter 7 for the formula used to calculate the amount of glucose, in milligrams per kilogram per minute, that an infant is receiving.

B. **Proteins.** Inadequate protein intake may result in failure to thrive, hypoalbuminemia, and edema. Excessive protein can cause hyperammonemia, serum amino acid imbalance, metabolic acidosis, and cholestatic jaundice. Early addition of amino acids to PN may also stimulate endogenous insulin secretion. Low birth weight infants lose 1% of endogenous protein daily unless supplemented.

1. **Crystalline amino acid** solutions are available as nitrogen sources. The standard solutions originally designed for adults are not ideal because they contain high concentrations of amino acids (eg, glycine, methionine, and phenylalanine) that are potentially neurotoxic in premature infants. Pediatric crystalline amino acid solutions (eg, TrophAmine, Aminosyn PF) are available, which contain less of those potentially neurotoxic amino acids as well as additional tyrosine, cystine, and taurine. These pediatric solutions also have a lower pH to allow for the addition of sufficient quantities of calcium (2 mEq/dL) and phosphorus (1–2 mg/dL) in order to meet daily requirements.

   Note: It is no longer necessary, except in VLBW infants, to gradually increase the protein concentration of PN over several days (Kerner, 1900).

2. **Amino acids** should not be started unless >40 cal/kg/day is given as glucose, because the amino acids will be poorly used and acidosis and hyperammonemia will develop. Amino acids can be started at a rate of 0.5 g/kg/day in infants weighing <1500 g and increased by increments of 0.5 g/kg/day. Studies have demonstrated that amino acids can be safely administered at 1.5 g/kg/day on day 1 in premature and VLBW infants and may improve nitrogen balance because of an increased ability to synthesize protein. In term infants, the starting rate can be 1.5 g, with increases of 1 g/kg/day. To avoid hyperammonemia and acidosis, total proteins should not exceed 4 g/kg/day in preterm infants. At most institutions, amino acid solutions are prepared in 1%, 2%, and 3% concentrations. This works out to the following equivalents.

   - 100 mL/kg/day of 1% solution = 1 g/kg/day of protein
   - 100 mL/kg/day of 2% solution = 2 g/kg/day of protein
   - 100 mL/kg/day of 3% solution = 3 g/kg/day of protein

3. **Cysteine hydrochloride** is often added to TPN solutions because cysteine is unstable over time and is omitted from amino acid solutions. The premature infant lacks the ability to convert methionine to cysteine; thus, it is conditionally essential. Cysteine is also converted to cystine and to glutathione, an antioxidant. Addition of cysteine into TPN lowers the pH of the solution, resulting in acidosis. Additional acetate may be required. It may also decrease hepatic cholestasis. The recommended dose is 40 mg of cysteine per gram of protein (72–85 mg/kg/day).

4. **Glutamine** has been identified as a key amino acid, as respiratory fuel for rapidly proliferating cells like enterocytes and lymphocytes, in acid-base balance, and as a nucleotide precursor. Glutamine may play a role in maintaining gut integrity and may decrease the incidence of sepsis. It also attenuates gut atrophy in fasting states. Vernix is a rich source of glutamine. Despite its seeming beneficial properties, routine glutamine supple-

mentation in enteral or parenteral nutrition is not yet recommended for preterm infants pending clinical trial outcomes.

C. **Fats.** Fats are essential for normal body growth and development, in cell structure and function, and in retinal and brain development. Because of their high caloric density, intravenous fat solutions (eg, Intralipid, Lyposyn II, Nutralipid, Soyacal) provide a significant portion of daily caloric needs. Most intravenous fat solutions are isotonic (270–300 mOsm/L) and, therefore, are not likely to increase the risk of infiltration of peripheral lines. When administering fat solutions to neonates with unconjugated hyperbilirubinemia, caution may be needed because of the competitive binding between bilirubin and nonesterified fatty acids on albumin, which may increase significantly during infusion.

1. **Concentrations.** Lipid emulsions are supplied either as 10% or 20% solutions providing 10 or 20 g of triglyceride, respectively. A common regimen is 0.5 g/kg/day on the first day, 1 g/kg/day on the second day, and 2 g/kg/day (maintenance dose) on the third day. The infusion is given continuously over 20–24 h, and the rate should not exceed 0.12 g/kg/h. For example, in an infant weighing 2 kg who is to start at an amount of 0.5 g/kg/day:

   - 2 kg × 0.5 g/kg/day = 1 g/day
   - 1 mL of 10% Intralipid = 0.1 g
   - 1 mL/0.1 g = x mL/g
   - $0.1x = 1$
   - $x = 10$ mL

   This infant should receive a total of 10 mL of 10% Intralipid in a 24-h period to equal 0.5 g/kg/day. The volume (eg, 10 mL) is divided by 24 h. It should run at 0.4 mL/h for 24 h. Use of 20% lipid emulsion is associated with decreased levels of cholesterol, triglycerides, and phospholipids because of its lower phospholipids–triglycerides ratio and lower liposomal contents than 10% lipid emulsions.

2. **Complications.** Fat intolerance (hyperlipidemia) may be seen. Periodic determination of blood triglyceride levels is recommended. Levels should be <150 mg/dL when the infant is jaundiced and <200 mg/dL otherwise. The infusion of fats should be decreased or stopped when these levels are exceeded.

3. **Carnitine supplementation** *(controversial).* Carnitine synthesis and storage are not well developed in infants <34 weeks' gestation. Carnitine is a carrier molecule necessary for oxidation of long-chain fatty acids. An exogenous source of carnitine is available from human milk and infant formulas; however, studies have shown that preterm infants on TPN become deficient in 6–10 days. Carnitine can be added to TPN solutions at a safe initial dose of 10 mg/kg/day. Carnitine-deficient infants may experience hypotonia, nonketotic hypoglycemia, cardiomyopathy, encephalopathy, and recurrent infections.

D. **Vitamins.** Vitamins are added to intravenous solutions in the form of a pediatric multivitamin suspension (MVI Pediatric) based on recommendations by the Nutritional Advisory Committee of the American Academy of Pediatrics. The dose of parenteral vitamins for preterm infants should be 2 mL/kg of the 5-mL reconstituted MVI Pediatric sterile lyophilized powder.

E. **Trace elements.** Trace elements are added to the solution based on weight and total volume: 0.5 mL/kg/week for infants on short-term TPN and 0.5 mL/kg/day for those on long-term TPN. Increased amounts of zinc (1–2 mg/day) are often given to help promote healing in patients who require gastrointestinal surgery. At many institutions, a prepared solution is available. For recommended doses of trace elements, see Table 8–6.

F. **Electrolytes.** Electrolytes can be added according to specific needs, but for low birth weight infants, requirements are usually satisfied by standard amino acid solution formulations that contain electrolytes (Table 8–7).

TABLE 8-6. RECOMMENDATIONS FOR TRACE ELEMENT SUPPLEMENTATION IN TPN SOLUTIONS FOR NEONATES

Element (mcg/kg/day)	Full term	Premature
Zinc	250	400
Copper	20	20
Chromium[a]	0.2	0.2
Manganese[a]	1	1
Fluoride	500[b]	—
Iodine	1	1
Molybdenum[a]	0.25	0.25
Selenium	2.0	2.0

TPN, total parenteral nutrition.
[a]For TPN greater than 4 weeks.
[b]Not well defined in the premature infant. Indicated only in prolonged TPN therapy (eg, more than 3 months).

G. **Heparin.** Heparin should be added to PN (0.5–1 U/mL TPN) to maintain catheter patency. In addition, there is a decreased risk for phlebitis and an increase in lipid clearance as a result of release of lipoprotein lipase.

V. **Monitoring of PN.** Hyperalimentation can cause many alterations in biochemical function. Thus, compulsive anthropometric and laboratory monitoring is essential for all patients. Recommendations are given in Table 8-8.

VI. **Complications of PN.** Most complications of PN are associated with the use of central hyperalimentation and primarily involve infections and catheter-related problems. However, metabolic difficulties can occur with both central and peripheral TPN. The major complication of peripheral hyperalimentation is accidental infiltration of the solution, which causes sloughing of the skin.

A. **Infection.** Sepsis can occur in infants receiving central hyperalimentation. The most common organisms include coagulase-positive and coagulase-negative *Staphylococcus, Streptococcus viridans, Escherichia coli, Pseudomonas* spp, *Klebsiella* spp, and *Candida albicans.* Contamination of the central catheter can occur as a result of infection at the insertion site or use of the catheter for blood sampling or administration of blood. It is best not to open the catheter.

B. **Catheter-associated problems.** Complications associated with placement of central catheters (specifically in the subclavian vein) occur in ~4–9% of pa-

TABLE 8-7. COMPOSITION OF AMINO ACID SOLUTIONS FOR LOW BIRTH WEIGHT INFANTS (STANDARD FORMULATION)

Electrolytes (mEq/L)	Amino acid concentration					
	1.0%		2.0%		3.0%	
	A	T	A	T	A	T
Na+	20	20	20	20	20	20
Cl−	20	20	20	20	20	20
K+	15	15	15	15	15	15
Mg2+	11	11	11	11	11	11
Ca2+	15	15	15	15	15	15
Acetate	7.6	9.3	15.3	18.6	22.8	27.9
Phosphorus (mmol/L)	10	10	10	10	10	10

A, Aminosyn PF; T, TrophAmine.

TABLE 8–8. MONITORING SCHEDULE FOR NEONATES RECEIVING PARENTERAL NUTRITION

Measurement	Baseline study	Frequency of measurement
Anthropometric		
Weight	Yes	Daily
Length	Yes	Weekly
Head circumference	Yes	Daily
Metabolic		
Glucose	Yes	Daily
(Dextrostix when changing dextrose concentrations)		
Calcium and phosphorus	Yes	Twice per week initially, then weekly
Electrolytes (Na, Cl, K, CO_2)	Yes	Once a day for 3 days, then twice a week; 3 times a week if <1000 g
Magnesium	Yes	Weekly
Hematocrit	Yes	Every other day for 1 week, then weekly
BUN and creatinine	Yes	Twice a week, then weekly
Bilirubin	Yes	Weekly
Ammonia	Yes	Weekly if using high protein
Total protein and albumin	Yes	Weekly
SGOT or SGPT	Yes	Weekly
Triglycerides	Yes	Weekly for patients on intravenous fat
Urine		
Specific gravity and glucose	Yes	For first week, test each urine sample, then once per shift

BUN, blood urea nitrogen; SGOT, serum glutamic-oxaloacetic transaminase; SGPT, serum glutamate pyruvate transaminase.

tients. Complications include pneumothorax, pneumomediastinum, hemorrhage, and chylothorax (caused by injury to the thoracic duct). Thrombosis of the vein adjacent to the catheter tip, resulting in "superior vena cava syndrome" (edema of the face, neck, and eyes), may be seen. Pulmonary embolism can also occur secondary to thrombosis. Malpositioned catheters may result in collection of fluid in the pleural cavity, causing hydrothorax, or the pericardial space, causing tamponade.

C. **Metabolic complications**

1. **Hyperglycemia** resulting from excessive intake or change in metabolic rate, such as infection or glucocorticoid administration.
2. **Hypoglycemia** from sudden cessation of infusion (secondary to intravenous infiltration).
3. **Azotemia** from excessive protein (nitrogen) uptake.
4. **Hyperammonemia.** All currently available amino acid mixtures contain adequate arginine (>0.05 mmol/kg/day). Therefore, if there is an increase in blood ammonia, symptomatic hyperammonemia does not occur.
5. **Abnormal serum and tissue amino acid pattern.**
6. **Mild metabolic alkalosis.**
7. **Cholestatic liver disease.** With prolonged administration of intravenous dextrose and protein and absence of enteral feeding, cholestasis usually occurs. The incidence ranges from as high as 80% in VLBW infants receiving TPN for >30 days (with no enteral feeding) to 15% or lower in neonates weighing >1500 g receiving TPN for >14 days. Monitoring for abnormalities in liver function and the development of direct hyperbilirubinemia is important in long-term TPN.
   a. **Bacterial infection** may play a significant role in the occurrence of cholestatic liver disease.
   b. **The use of amino acid mixtures** designed to maintain normal plasma amino acid patterns and early starting (as soon as possible) of enteral feedings in small amounts may help alleviate this problem.

    c. TPN may be cycled over 10–18 h as opposed to a continuous 24-h infusion. This facilitates a short period of decreased circulating insulin levels, which in turn facilitates mobilization of fat and glycogen stores, decreasing the risk of fatty infiltration of the liver and hepatic dysfunction. This practice is reserved for infants who are stable on TPN and who are expected to remain in need of long-term TPN.

    d. The trace elements copper and manganese should be withheld in the presence of hepatic dysfunction.

8. **Complications of fat administration.** Infusion of fat emulsion has been associated with several metabolic disturbances, hyperlipidemia, platelet dysfunction, acute allergic reactions, deposition of pigment in the liver, and lipid deposition in the blood vessels of the lung. Most metabolic problems apparently occur with rapid rates of infusion and are not seen at infusion rates of <0.12 g/kg/h.

    Exposure of lipids to light, especially phototherapy, may cause increased production of toxic hydroperoxides. Steroids cause elevated triglyceride levels. Thrombocytopenia, increased risk of sepsis, alteration in pulmonary functions, and hypoxemia have also been reported. In sepsis, there is decreased peripheral utilization of lipids. Free fatty acids produced from lipid breakdown compete with bilirubin for binding with albumin, resulting in elevated free bilirubin. Lipid infusion should not exceed 0.5–1 g/kg/day with plasma bilirubin >8–10 mg/dL and albumin levels 2.5–3.0 gm/dL.

9. **Deficiency of essential fatty acids (EFAs)** is associated with decreased platelet aggregation (thromboxane A_2 deficiency), poor weight gain, scaling rash, sparse hair growth, and thrombocytopenia. Essential fatty acid deficiency can occur within 72 h in preterm infants if exogenous fatty acids are not supplemented. Use of only safflower oil to provide lipid emulsions may result in deficiency omega-3 long-chain polyunsaturated fatty acids. EFAs are essential to the developing eyes and brain of the human neonate.

10. **Mineral deficiency.** Most minerals are transferred to the fetus during the last trimester of pregnancy. The following problems may occur.

    a. Osteopenia, rickets, and pathologic fractures (see Chapter 77).

    b. Zinc deficiency occurs if zinc is not added to TPN after 4 weeks. Cysteine and histidine in TPN solution increases urinary losses. Infants with this deficiency can have poor growth, diarrhea, alopecia, increased susceptibility to infection, and skin desquamation surrounding the mouth and anus (acrodermatitis enteropathica). Zinc losses are increased in patients with an ileostomy or colostomy.

    c. Infants with copper deficiency have osteoporosis, hemolytic anemia, neutropenia, and depigmentation of the skin.

    d. Deficiency of manganese, copper, selenium, molybdenum, and iodine may occur if not supplemented after 4 weeks.

CALORIC CALCULATIONS

An infant should receive 100–120 kcal/kg/day for growth. (Infants require fewer calories [80–90 cal/kg/day] if receiving TPN only.) Some hypermetabolic infants may require >120 kcal/kg/day. For maintenance of a positive nitrogen balance, oral intake of 70–90 nonprotein kcal/kg/day is necessary. Equations for calculating the caloric intake for oral formula and TPN follow (see Table 8–9).

I. **Infant formulas.** Most standard infant formulas are 20 cal/oz and contain 0.67 kcal/mL. Specific caloric concentrations of formulas are given in Table 8–3. To calculate total daily calories, use the following equation.

$$kcal\,/\,kg\,/\,day = \frac{\text{Total mL of formula} \times kcal\,/\,mL}{\text{Wt (kg)}}$$

TABLE 8-9. TPN CALCULATIONS

Amino acids:	% Amino acids = $\dfrac{\text{Wt (kg)} \times \text{(g/kg/day)} \times 100}{\text{Vol in 24 h}}$
Dextrose: Glucose utilization rate (mg/kg/min):	$\dfrac{\text{Rate (mL/h)} \times \% \text{ dextrose}}{\text{Wt (kg)} \times 6}$
Lipids:	Rate (mL/h): $\dfrac{\text{g/kg/day} \times 5 \times \text{Wt (kg)}}{24}$
Nonprotein calories/kg/day:	$\dfrac{(\text{mL lipid/24 h} \times 2 \text{ Cal/mL}^a) + (\text{mL TPN/24 h} \times \% \text{ dextrose} \times 0.034)}{\text{Kg}}$

^{a}For 20% lipids only.

II. Carbohydrates. If only dextrose infusion is given, the total daily caloric intake is calculated as follows. (For caloric concentration of common solutions, see Table 8–10.)

$$\text{kcal} / \text{kg} / \text{day} = \frac{\text{mL of solution} / \text{h} \times 24 \text{ h} \times \text{ kcal in solution}}{\text{Wt (kg)}}$$

III. PROTEINS. Use the prior formula given for carbohydrates and the caloric concentrations given in table 8–10.

IV. Fat emulsions. A 10% fat emulsion (Intralipid) contains 1.1 kcal/mL; a 20% emulsion, 2 kcal/mL. Use the following formula to calculate daily caloric intake supplied by Intralipid 20%.

$$\text{kcal} / \text{kg} / \text{day} = \frac{\text{Total mL} / \text{day of solution} \times 2 \text{ kcal} / \text{mL}}{\text{Wt (kg)}}$$

TABLE 8-10. CALORIC CONCENTRATIONS OF VARIOUS PARENTERAL SOLUTIONS

Dextrose solutions (anhydrous) (kcal/mL)

$D_5 = 0.17$
$D_{7.5} = 0.255$
$D_{10} = 0.34$
$D_{12.5} = 0.425$
$D_{15} = 0.51$
$D_{20} = 0.68$
$D_{25} = 0.85$

Protein solutions (g/day)	% Concentration	Caloric concentration (kcal/mL)
0.5	0.5	0.02
1.0	1	0.04
1.5	1.5	0.06
2.0	2.0	0.08
2.5	2.5	0.10
3.0	3.0	0.12

0.5% solution, if given 100 mL/day = 0.5 g of protein/day

REFERENCES

Auestad N et al: Growth and development in term infants fed long-chain polyunsaturated fatty acids. *Pediatrics* 2001;108:372.

Barnes LA (ed): *Pediatric Nutrition Handbook,* 3rd ed. American Academy of Pediatrics, 1993.

Berseth CL: Minimal enteral feedings. *Clin Perinatol* 1995;22:61.

Bonner CM et al: Effects of parenteral L-carnitine supplementation on fat metabolism and nutrition in premature infants. *J Pediatr* 1995;126:287.

Craigo SD, Beach ML, Harvey-Wilkes KB, et al: Ultrasound predictors of neonatal outcome in intrauterine growth restriction. *Am J Perinatol* 1996;13:465.

Denne SC et al: Nutrition and metabolism in the high-risk neonate. In Fanaroff AA, Martin RJ (eds): *Neonatal-Perinatal Medicine—Diseases of the Fetus and Infant,* Vol 1, 7th ed. Mosby-Year Book, 2002.

Gross SJ, Slagle TA: Feeding the low birth weight infant. *Clin Perinatol* 1993;20:193.

Katrine KF: Anthropometric assessment. In Groh-Wargo S et al (eds): *Nutritional Care for the High Risk Newborns.* Precept Press, 2000.

Kerner JA Jr (ed): *Manual of Pediatric Nutrition.* Wiley, 1983.

Krug SK: Parenteral nutrition: Vitamins, minerals and trace elements. In Groh-Wargo S et al (eds): *Nutritional Care for the High Risk Newborns.* Precept Press, 2000.

Kuschel CA, Harding JE: *Carbohydrate Supplementation of Human Milk for Promoting Growth in Preterm Infants.* The Cochrane Library, 2001.

Kuschel CA, Harding JE: *Fat Supplementation of Human Milk for Promoting Growth in Preterm Infants.* The Cochrane Library, 2001.

Kuschel CA, Harding JE: *Protein Supplementation of Human Milk for Promoting Growth in Preterm Infants.* The Cochrane Library, 2001.

Lucas A: Enteral nutrition. In Tsang RC (ed): *Nutritional Needs of the Preterm Infant. Scientific Basis and Practical Guidelines.* Williams & Wilkins, 1993.

Lucas A, Cole TJ: Breast milk and neonatal necrotizing enterocolitis. *Lancet* 1990;336:1519.

McLure RJ: Trophic feeding of the preterm infant. *Acta Paediatr Suppl* 2001;436:19.

Price PT: Parenteral nutrition: administration and monitoring. In Groh-Wargo S et al (eds): *Nutritional Care for the High Risk Newborns.* Precept Press, 2000.

Robertson AF, Bhatia J: Feeding premature infants. *Clin Pediatr* 1993;32:36.

Sapsford AL: Enteral nutrition: human milk and enteral nutrition products. In Groh-Wargo S et al (eds): *Nutritional Care for the High Risk Newborns.* Precept Press, 2000.

Sapsford AL: Enteral nutrition: recommended enteral nutrient intakes. In Groh-Wargo S et al (eds): *Nutritional Care for the High Risk Newborns.* Precept Press, 2000.

Sapsford AL: Parenteral nutrition: energy, carbohydrate, protein, and fat. In Groh-Wargo S et al (eds): *Nutritional Care for the High Risk Newborns.* Precept Press, 2000.

Tubman TRJ, Thompson TW: *Glutamine Supplementation for Prevention of Morbidity in Preterm Infants.* Cochrane Library Review, 2001.

Tyson JE et al: Vitamin A supplementation for extremely low birth weight infants. *N Engl J Med* 1999;340:1962.

Yu VYH: Enteral feeding in the preterm infant. *Early Human Dev* 1999;56:89.

9 Neonatal Radiology

COMMON RADIOLOGIC TECHNIQUES

I. **Radiographic exams.** The need for radiographs must always be weighed against the risks of exposure of the neonate to radiation (eg, 3–5 mrem per chest radiographic view). The infant's gonads should be shielded as much as possible, and any person holding the infant during the x-ray procedure should also wear a protective shield. For the usual vertically oriented radiographic exposure, personnel need be only 1 ft outside the zone of exposure.

A. **Chest radiographs**

1. **The anteroposterior (AP) view** is the single best view for identification of heart or lung disease, verification of endotracheal tube and other line positions, and identification of air leak complications of mechanical ventilation, such as pneumothorax.

2. **The cross-table lateral view** is of limited diagnostic value except to determine whether a pleural chest tube is positioned anteriorly (best for drainage of a pneumothorax) or posteriorly (best for drainage of a pleural fluid collection).

3. **The lateral decubitus view** is best for ruling out a small pneumothorax or one that is difficult to assess on the AP view. For example, if a pneumothorax is suspected on the left, a right lateral decubitus view of the chest should be obtained, with the infant placed right side down. An air collection between lung and chest wall will be visible on the side on which the pneumothorax is present. The disadvantages of the lateral decubitus view are that it is (1) sometimes difficult to perform in unstable infants and (2) more time consuming than a regular AP supine view.

4. **The upright view,** which is rarely used in the neonatal intensive care unit (NICU), can identify abdominal perforation by showing free air under the diaphragm.

B. **Abdominal radiographs**

1. **The AP view** is the single best view for diagnosing abdominal disorders and checking placement of umbilical arterial and venous catheters.

2. **The cross-table lateral view** helps diagnose abdominal perforation, but the left lateral decubitus view is better for this purpose. Abdominal perforations may be missed on the AP and cross-table lateral views if the amount of intraperitoneal air is limited or if the segment of perforated bowel contains only fluid.

3. **The left lateral decubitus view** (with the infant placed left side down) is best for diagnosis of intestinal perforation. Free intra-abdominal air resulting from bowel perforation will be visible as an air collection between the liver and right lateral abdominal wall.

C. **Barium contrast studies (barium swallow or barium enema).** Barium sulfate, an inert compound, is not absorbed from the gastrointestinal tract and results in little or no fluid shift.

1. **Indications.** The use of barium as a contrast agent is recommended for the following.

a. **Gastrointestinal (GI) tract imaging.** Barium enema is used to rule out lower intestinal tract obstruction from a variety of causes.

b. **Suspected esophageal atresia** with or without tracheoesophageal fistula. Most esophageal atresias can be diagnosed by inserting a radiopaque nasogastric tube; the tube will curl up in the blind-ending proximal esophageal pouch. If additional confirmation is required, air can be injected under fluoroscopy to distend the pouch. Barium or other contrast agent injection is rarely required.

c. **Suspected esophageal perforation.** Barium swallow is used only if previous studies using low-osmolality water-soluble contrast agents have been negative.

d. **Suspected gastroesophageal reflux.** Barium swallow is used as the first-line study.

2. **Contraindications.** Barium contrast studies are not recommended in infants with **suspected abdominal perforation** because barium is irritating to the peritoneum and can result in "barium peritonitis."

D. **High-osmolality water-soluble contrast studies**

1. **Advantages** of these agents (eg, Hypaque or Gastrografin) over barium include the following:

   a. **These materials are not toxic to the peritoneum** if they leak from the GI tract, and they are absorbed and cleared from the body.

   b. **Because these agents draw water into the bowel lumen,** they may be used therapeutically to relieve some cases of bowel obstruction or to treat meconium ileus.

2. **Disadvantages**

   a. **Significant fluid shift may occur.** Thus, to avoid inducing hypovolemic shock, fluid and electrolyte status must be monitored closely if these agents are used.

   b. **These materials are very irritating to the lungs** if aspirated.

   c. **Necrotizing enterocolitis** resulting in death has been reported. Bowel necrosis has rarely occurred after the use of these agents for meconium ileus.

3. **Indications**

   a. **Evaluation** of the bowel if perforation is suspected.

   b. **Differentiation** of ileus from obstruction.

   c. **Treatment** of meconium obstruction syndromes.

E. **Low-osmolality water-soluble contrast agents.** These agents have many advantages over barium and the high-osmolality contrast agents.

1. **Advantages**

   a. **These agents do not cause fluid shifts.**

   b. **If bowel perforation is present,** these substances are nontoxic to the peritoneal cavity. In addition, they do not damage the bowel mucosa.

   c. **If aspirated, there is limited irritation (if any) to the lungs.**

   d. **Unlike high-osmolality water-soluble contrast agents, low-osmolality water-soluble contrast agents have very limited absorption** from the normal intestinal tract and thus maintain good opacification throughout the intestinal tract on delayed imaging.

2. **Disadvantages** include a much higher cost than barium and other water-soluble agents.

3. **Indications**

   a. **Suspected H-type tracheoesophageal fistula.**

   b. **Suspected esophageal perforation.**

   c. **Evaluation of the bowel** if perforation is suspected.

   d. **Unexplained pneumoperitoneum.**

   e. **Evaluation of "gasless abdomen"** in a neonate >12 h of age.

F. **Radionuclide studies.** Radionuclide studies provide more physiologic than anatomic information and usually involve a lower radiation dose to the patient compared with radiographic exams.

1. **The reflux scintiscan** is used for documenting and quantitating gastroesophageal reflux. This procedure is comparable to the pH probe examination and superior to the barium swallow. Technetium-99m-labeled pertechnetate in a water-based solution is instilled into the stomach. The patient is then scanned in the supine position for 1–2 h with a gamma camera.

2. **The radionuclide cystogram** is used for documenting and quantitating vesicoureteral reflux. Advantages over the radiographic voiding cystourethrogram (VCUG) is a much lower radiation dose (by 50–100 times) and a longer monitoring period (1–2 h). Disadvantages include much poorer anatomic detail; bladder diverticula, posterior urethral valves, or mild reflux cannot be reliably identified. This technique should not be the initial examination for evaluation of the lower urinary tract, especially in males.

3. **The radionuclide bone scan** is used for evaluation of possible osteomyelitis. This procedure involves a three-phase study (blood flow, blood pool, and bone uptake) after intravenous injection of technetium-99m-labeled methylene diphosphonate.

   a. **Advantages** include a sensitivity to bony changes earlier than with the radiograph.

   b. **Disadvantages** are several. Such a bone scan (1) may not identify the acute phase of osteomyelitis (ie, the first 24–48 h); (2) requires absence of patient motion; (3) gives poorer anatomic detail than radiographs; and (4) has resultant areas of positive uptake ("hot spots") that are nonspecific.

II. **Ultrasonography**

   A. **Ultrasonography of the brain** is performed to rule out intraventricular hemorrhage and to grade the size of ventricles. It can be performed in any NICU with a portable ultrasound unit. No special preparation is needed. However, an open anterior fontanelle must be present and no intravenous catheters should be placed on the scalp. The classification of intraventricular hemorrhage based on ultrasonographic findings as developed by Papile (Dolfin et al, 1983) is given next. Examples are shown in Figures 9–1 through 9–4.

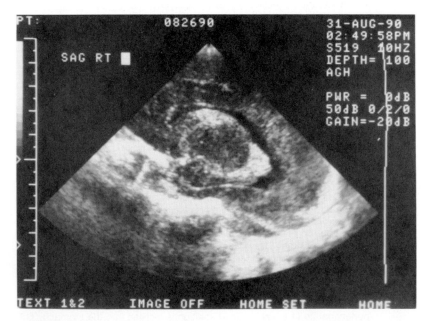

FIGURE 9–1. Ultrasonogram of the head (right sagittal view), showing a small germinal matrix hemorrhage (grade I intraventricular hemorrhage).

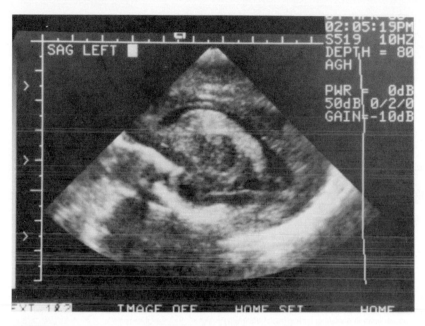

FIGURE 9–2. Ultrasonogram of the head (left sagittal view), showing germinal matrix and intraventricular hemorrhage but minimal ventricular enlargement. Same patient as in Figure 9–3.

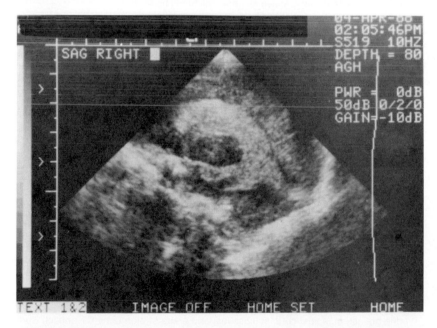

FIGURE 9–3. Ultrasonogram for the same patient as in Figure 9–2 (right sagittal view), demonstrating a large intraventricular hemorrhage with an enlarged ventricle (grade III).

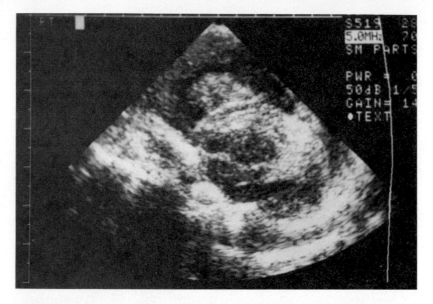

FIGURE 9–4. Ultrasonogram of the head (left sagittal view), demonstrating intraventricular hemorrhage and localized intraparenchymal hemorrhage (grade IV).

- **Grade I:** Subependymal, germinal matrix hemorrhage.
- **Grade II:** Intraventricular extension without ventricular dilatation.
- **Grade III:** Intraventricular extension with ventricular dilatation.
- **Grade IV:** Intraventricular and intraparenchymal hemorrhage.

B. **Abdominal ultrasonography** is useful in the evaluation of abdominal distention, abdominal masses, and renal failure. Abdominal sonography can be performed portably. The addition of duplex and color Doppler evaluation of regional vessels is a supplementary procedure that can identify vascular occlusion resulting from thrombosis.

C. **Power Doppler sonography** better demonstrates amplitude of blood flow compared with color Doppler but does not define direction of blood flow and is very motion sensitive.

III. Computed tomographic (CT) scanning

A. **CT scanning of the head** is more complicated than ultrasonography because the patient must be moved to the CT unit and be adequately sedated. CT scanning provides more global information than ultrasonography of the head, particularly at the periphery of the brain.

B. **This technique can be used to diagnose intraventricular, subdural, or subarachnoid bleeding and cerebral edema or infarction.** To diagnose cerebral infarction, infusion of contrast medium is necessary. If infusion is used, blood urea nitrogen and creatinine levels must be obtained before the CT test to rule out renal impairment, which may be a contraindication to the use of intravenous contrast media. An intravenous catheter must be placed, preferably not in the head.

IV. **Magnetic resonance imaging (MRI).** MRI is now an acceptable mode of imaging in the neonate, and its use is expanding. MRI is superior to CT for imaging the brainstem, spinal cord, soft tissues, and areas of high bony CT artifact. Supplemental magnetic resonance arteriography (MRA) and magnetic resonance venography (MRV) are now available to improve vascular anatomy and flow.

A. **Advantages** are the absence of ionizing radiation and visualization of vascular anatomy without contrast agents.

B. **Disadvantages** are as follows: (1) It cannot always be performed on critically ill infants requiring ventilator support, (2) the scanning time is longer (although rapidly becoming much shorter with newer equipment), and (3) sedation is usually required.

RADIOGRAPHIC EXAMPLES

Invasive life support and monitoring techniques depend on proper positioning of the device being used. Caution is necessary when identifying ribs and correlating vertebrae in the newborn as a means for determining the proper position of a catheter or tube. Errors are occasionally made because it is assumed that infants have 12 ribs, as do older children and adults. In fact, it is not uncommon for infants to have a noncalcified 12th rib; thus, the 11th rib is mistaken for the 12th rib and an incorrect count of the lumbar vertebrae follows.

I. **Endotracheal intubation**

A. The preferred location of the endotracheal tube (ETT) tip is halfway between the thoracic inlet (the medial ends of the clavicles) and the carina. Correct tube placement is shown in Figure 9–5.

B. If the ETT has been placed too low, the tip usually enters the right main bronchus, a straighter line than with the left main bronchus. The chest film may show asymmetric aeration with both hyperinflation and atelectasis. If the tube extends below the carina or does not match the tracheal air column in position, suspect esophageal intubation. Increased proximal intestinal air may

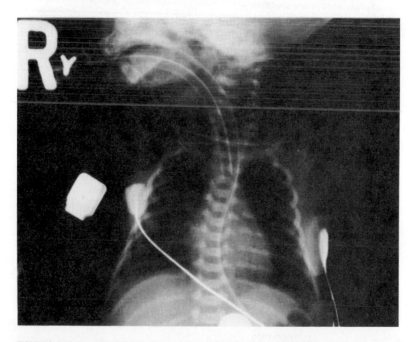

FIGURE 9–5. Chest x-ray film showing proper placement of an endotracheal tube.

also reflect esophageal intubation. An ETT placed too high will have the tip above the clavicle, and the x-ray film may show diffuse atelectasis.

II. **Umbilical vein catheterization (UVC).** The catheter tip should be at the junction of the inferior vena cava and right atrium, projecting just above the diaphragm on the AP chest radiograph. Degree and direction of patient rotation will affect how the UVC appears positioned on the radiograph. Figure 9–6 shows correct UVC tip placement.

III. **Umbilical artery catheterization (UAC).** The use of high versus low UAC placement depends on institutional preference. Some clinicians believe that high catheters are associated with a higher risk of hypertension and that low catheters have a higher risk of vasospasms, but this has not been proved.

    A. **If high placement is desired,** the tip should be between thoracic vertebrae 6 and 9 (above the origin of the celiac axis) (Figure 9–7).

    B. **For low placement,** the tip should be below the third lumbar vertebra, optimally between L3 and L5 (Figure 9–8). A catheter placed below L5 usually does not function well and carries a risk of severe vasospasm in small arteries. Note that the catheter turns downward and then upward on an abdominal x-ray film. The upward turn is the point at which the catheter passes through the internal iliac artery (hypogastric artery).

    Note: If both a UAC and a UVC are positioned and an x-ray study is performed, it is necessary to differentiate the two so that line placement can be

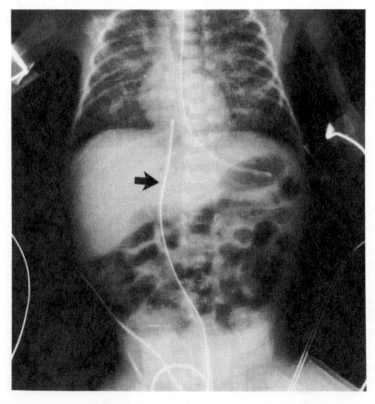

FIGURE 9–6. Abdominal x-ray showing correct placement of an umbilical venous catheter (arrow). The tip of the nasogastric tube is properly positioned in the stomach.

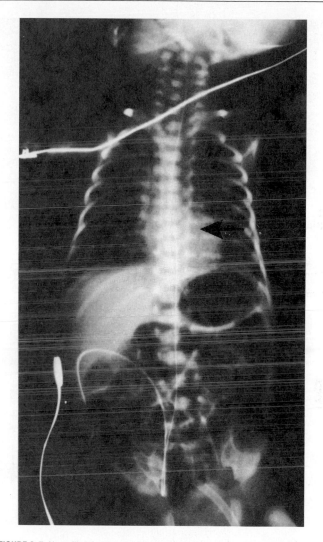

FIGURE 9–7. X-ray film showing correct positioning of a high umbilical artery catheter.

properly assessed. The UAC turns downward and then upward on the x-ray film, whereas the UVC takes only an upward or cephalad direction.

IV. **Extracorporeal membrane oxygenation (ECMO).** ECMO is a type of external life support using a membrane oxygenator that can be applied to a neonate in severe but reversible respiratory or cardiac failure (see Chapter 11). Desaturated blood is removed by a jugular venous cannula (arrows in Figure 9–9), while oxygenated blood is returned to the neonate by a carotid arterial cannula (arrowhead in Figure 9–9).

V. **Partial liquid ventilation (PLV).** PLV using the perfluorocarbon perflubron is an experimental form of temporary support to improve gas exchange in newborns in respiratory failure in whom conventional therapy, including surfactant, or ECMO

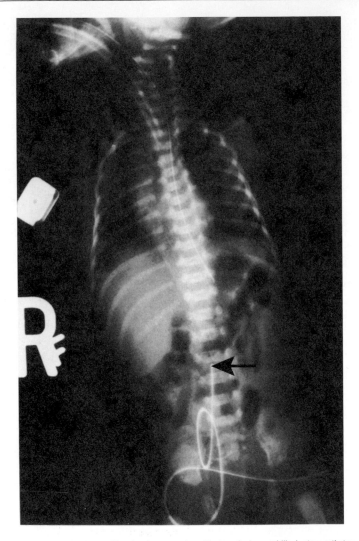

FIGURE 9–8. Abdominal x-ray film showing correct positioning of a low umbilical artery catheter.

has failed. Perflubron is instilled into the lungs via the endotracheal tube in conjunction with continued mechanical ventilation. The chest radiograph demonstrates diffusely opaque lungs (Figure 9–10).

RADIOGRAPHIC PEARLS

I. **Pulmonary diseases**
   A. **Hyaline membrane disease (HMD).** A fine, diffuse reticulogranular pattern is seen secondary to microatelectasis of the alveoli. The chest radiograph re-

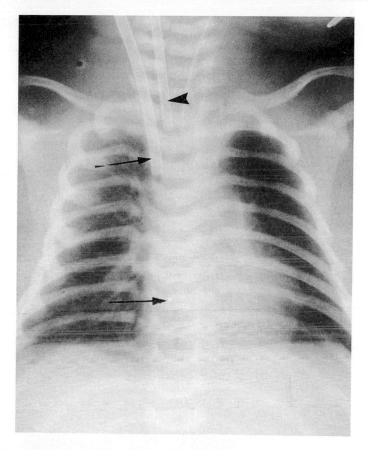

FIGURE 9-9 Chest x-ray film showing well-positioned ECMO venous (arrows) and arterial (arrowhead) cannulas in the right atrium and the aortic arch, respectively, in a patient on extracorporeal membrane oxygenation life support.

veals radiolucent areas known as air bronchograms, produced by air in the major airways and contrasted with the opacified, collapsed alveoli.

B. **Meconium aspiration.** Bilateral, patchy, coarse infiltrates and hyperinflation of the lungs are present.

C. **Pneumonia.** Diffuse alveolar or interstitial disease that is usually asymmetric and localized. Group B streptococcal pneumonia can appear similar to HMD. Pneumatoceles (air-filled lung cysts) can occur with staphylococcal pneumonia. Pleural effusions or empyema may occur with any bacterial pneumonia.

D. **Transient tachypnea of the newborn.** Hyperaeration with symmetric perihilar and interstitial streaky infiltrates are typical. Pleural fluid may occur as well, appearing as widening of the pleural space or as prominence of the minor fissure.

E. **Bronchopulmonary dysplasia.** Many centers no longer rely on the following grading system for this condition, but it is included for historical purposes.

- **Grade I:** X-ray findings are similar to those of severe HMD.
- **Grade II:** Dense parenchymal opacification is seen.

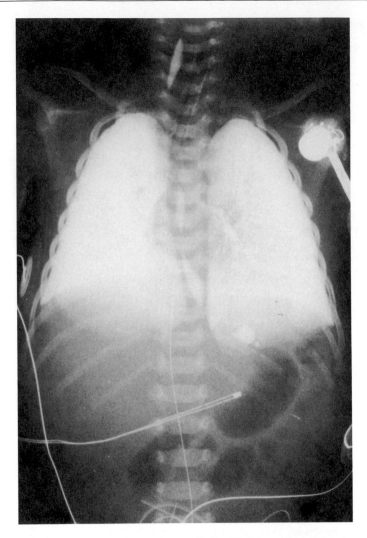

FIGURE 9–10. Chest x-ray film showing complete opacification of both lungs with perflubron in a patient receiving partial liquid ventilation support.

- **Grade III:** A bubbly, fibrocystic pattern is evident.
- **Grade IV:** Hyperinflation is present, with multiple fine, lacy densities spreading to the periphery and with areas of lucency similar to bullae of the lung.

F. **Wilson-Mikity syndrome.** Hyperaeration and a bubbly appearance of the lung are apparent (cystic lesions with thickening of interstitial structures).

G. **Air leak syndromes**
   1. **Pneumopericardium.** Air surrounds the heart, including the inferior border (Figure 9–11).

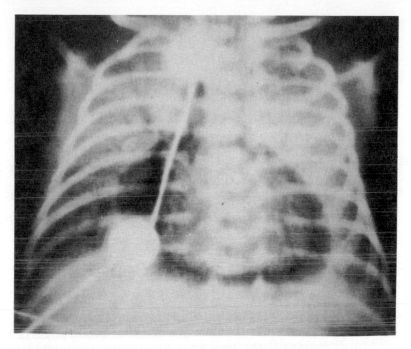

FIGURE 9-11. Chest x-ray film showing pneumopericardium in a 2-day-old infant.

    2. Pneumomediastinum
       a. AP view. A hyperlucent rim of air is present lateral to the cardiac border and thymus. This rim may displace the thymus superiorly away from the cardiac silhouette (angel wing sign) (Figure 9-12).
       b. Lateral view. An air collection is seen either substernally (anterior pneumomediastinum) or in the retrocardiac area (posterior pneumomediastinum) (see Figure 9-12).
    3. Pneumothorax. The lung is typically displaced away from the lateral chest wall by a radiolucent zone of air. The adjacent lung may be collapsed with larger pneumothoraces (Figure 9-13). The small pneumothorax may be very difficult to identify. There is only a subtle zone of air peripherally, a diffusely hyperlucent hemithorax, unusually sharply defined cardiothymic margins, or a combination of these.
    4. Tension pneumothorax. The diaphragm on the affected side is depressed, the mediastinum is shifted to the contralateral hemithorax, and collapse of the ipsilateral lobes is evident (see Figure 9-13).
    5. Pulmonary interstitial emphysema. Single or multiple circular radiolucencies with well-demarcated walls are seen in a localized or diffuse pattern. The volume of the involved portion of the lung is usually increased, often markedly so (Figure 9-14).
  H. Atelectasis. A decrease in lung volume or collapse of part or all of a lung is apparent, appearing as areas of increased opacity. The mediastinum may be shifted toward the side of collapse. Compensatory hyperinflation of the opposite lung may be present.
    1. Microatelectasis. See Chapter 74, HMD.

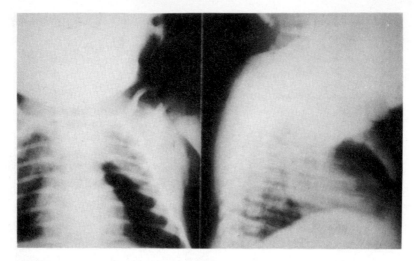

FIGURE 9–12. Pneumomediastinum. **(Left)** Anteroposterior chest x-ray film. **(Right)** Cross-table lateral chest x-ray.

   2. **Generalized atelectasis.** Diffuse increase in opacity ("white-out") of the lungs is visible on the chest film. It may be seen in severe respiratory distress syndrome, airway obstruction, if the endotracheal tube is not in the trachea, and hypoventilation.
   3. **Lobar atelectasis.** Lobar atelectasis is atelectasis of one lobe. The most common site is the right upper lobe, which appears as an area of dense opacity ("white-out") on the chest film. In addition, the right minor fissure is usually elevated. This pattern of atelectasis commonly occurs after extubation.
   I. **Pulmonary hypoplasia.** Small lung volumes and a bell-shaped thorax are seen. The lungs usually appear radiolucent.
   J. **Pulmonary edema.** The lungs appear diffusely hazy with an area of greatest density around the hilum of each lung. Heart size is usually increased.
II. **Cardiac diseases.** The cardiothoracic ratio, which normally should be <0.6, is the width of the base of the heart divided by the width of the lower thorax. An index >0.6 suggests cardiomegaly. The pulmonary vascularity is increased if the diameter of the descending branch of the right pulmonary artery exceeds that of the trachea.
   A. **Cardiac dextroversion.** The cardiac apex is on the right and the aortic arch and stomach bubble are on the left. The incidence of congenital heart disease associated with this finding is high (>90%).
   B. **Congestive heart failure.** Cardiomegaly, pulmonary venous congestion (engorgement and increased diameter of the pulmonary veins), diffuse opacification in the perihilar regions, and pleural effusions (sometimes) are seen.
   C. **Patent ductus arteriosus.** Cardiomegaly, pulmonary edema, ductal haze (pulmonary edema with a patent ductus arteriosus), and increased pulmonary vascular markings are evident.
   D. **Ventricular septal defect.** Findings include cardiomegaly, an increase in pulmonary vascular density, enlargement of the left ventricle and left atrium, and enlargement of the main pulmonary artery.
   E. **Coarctation of the aorta**
      1. **Preductal coarctation.** Generalized cardiomegaly, with normal pulmonary vascularity, is seen.

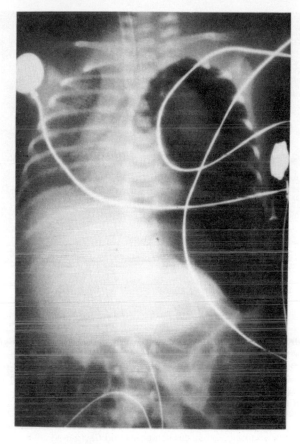

FIGURE 9–13. Left pneumothorax as shown on an anteroposterior chest x-ray film in a ventilated infant on day 2 of life.

2. **Postductal coarctation.** An enlarged left ventricle and left atrium and a dilated ascending aorta are present.

F. **Tetralogy of Fallot.** The heart is boot-shaped. A normal left atrium and left ventricle is associated with an enlarged, hypertrophied right ventricle and small or absent main pulmonary artery. There is decreased pulmonary vascularity. A right aortic arch occurs in 25% of patients.

G. **Transposition of the great arteries.** The chest film may show cardiomegaly, with an enlarged right atrium and right ventricle, narrow mediastinum, and increased pulmonary vascular markings, but in most cases the chest film appears normal.

H. **Total anomalous pulmonary venous return (TAPVR).** Pulmonary venous markings are increased. Cardiomegaly is minimal or absent. Congestive heart failure and pulmonary edema may be present, especially with type 3 (subdiaphragmatic) TAPVR.

I. **Hypoplastic left heart syndrome.** The chest film can be normal at first but then may show cardiomegaly and pulmonary vascular congestion, with an enlarged right atrium and ventricle.

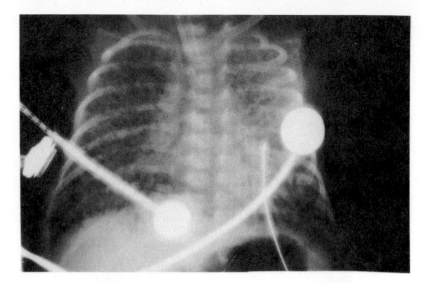

FIGURE 9–14. Chest x-ray film showing bilateral pulmonary interstitial emphysema in a 7-day-old ventilated infant.

    J. Tricuspid atresia. Heart size is usually normal or small, the main pulmonary artery is concave, and pulmonary vascularity is decreased.

    K. Truncus arteriosus. Characteristic findings include cardiomegaly, increased pulmonary vascularity, and enlargement of the left atrium. A right aortic arch occurs in 30% of patients.

    L. Atrial septal defect. Varying degrees of enlargement of the right atrium and ventricle are seen. The aorta and the left ventricle are small, and the pulmonary artery is large. Increased pulmonary vascularity is also evident.

    M. Ebstein's anomaly. Gross cardiomegaly and decreased pulmonary vascularity are apparent. The right heart border is prominent as a result of right atrial enlargement.

    N. Valvular pulmonic stenosis. Heart size and pulmonary blood flow are usually normal unless the stenosis is severe. Dilatation of the main pulmonary artery is the typical chest film finding.

III. Abdominal disorders

    A. Changes in the following normal patterns should raise suspicion of gastrointestinal tract disease.

        1. Air in the stomach should occur within 30 min after delivery.

        2. Air in the small bowel should be seen by 3–4 h of age.

        3. Air in the colon and rectum should be seen by 6–8 h of age.

    B. Intestinal obstruction. Gaseous intestinal distention is present. Gas may be decreased or absent distal to the obstruction. Air-fluid levels are seen proximal to the obstruction.

    C. Ascites. Gas-filled loops of bowel, if present, are located in the central portion of the abdomen. The abdomen may be distended, with relatively small amounts of gas (**"ground-glass" appearance**). A uniform increase in the density of the abdomen, particularly in the flank areas, may be evident.

    D. Calcification in the abdomen is most often seen secondary to meconium peritonitis, which may also cause calcifications in the scrotum in male infants. Calcifications in the abdomen may also be seen in infants with neuroblastoma or teratoma or may signify calcification of the adrenals after adrenal hemorrhage.

E. **Pneumoperitoneum**
   1. **Supine view.** Free air is seen as a central lucency, usually in the upper abdomen (Figure 9–15).
   2. **Upright view.** Free air is present in a subdiaphragmatic location.
   3. **Left lateral decubitus view.** Air collects over the lateral border of the liver, separating it from the adjacent abdominal wall.
F. **Pneumatosis intestinalis.** Intraluminal gas in the bowel wall (produced by bacteria that have invaded the bowel wall) may appear as a string or cluster of bubbles (submucosal) or a curvilinear lucency (subserosal). It is most frequently seen in infants with necrotizing enterocolitis (Figure 9–16).
G. **Situs inversus (complete).** The stomach, aortic arch, and cardiac apex all are right sided. There is only a limited increased incidence of congenital heart disease.
H. **Ileus.** Distended loops of bowel are present. Air-fluid levels may be seen on the upright or cross-table lateral abdominal film.
I. **Absence of gas in the abdomen.** Absence of gas in the abdomen may be seen in patients taking muscle-paralyzing medications (eg, pancuronium) because they do not swallow air. It may also be evident in infants with esoph-

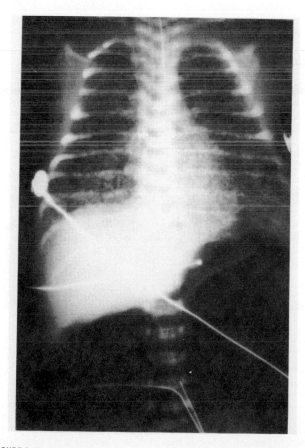

FIGURE 9–15. Abdominal x-ray film showing pneumoperitoneum in a 3-day-old infant.

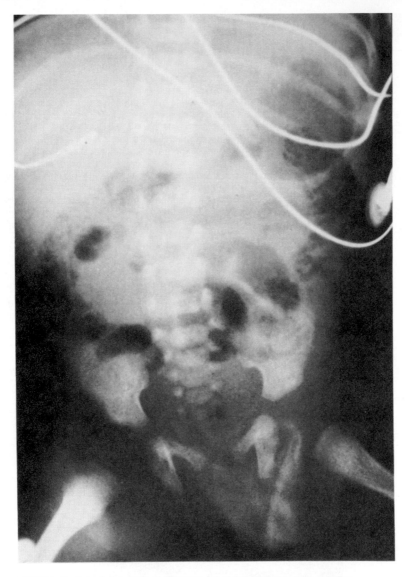

FIGURE 9-16. Abdominal x-ray film showing pneumatosis intestinalis in a 4-day-old infant.

ageal atresia without tracheoesophageal fistula and in cases of severe cerebral anoxia resulting in central nervous system depression and absence of
swallowing.

J. **Portal venous air.** Air is demonstrated in the portal veins (often best seen on
a lateral view). This finding may indicate bowel necrosis, which can occur in
an advanced degree of necrotizing enterocolitis, intestinal infarction secondary to mesenteric vessel occlusion, and iatrogenically introduced gas into

the portal vein, which can occur during umbilical vein catheterization or exchange transfusion.

REFERENCES

Blickman JG: Pediatric Radiology: The Requisites. Mosby, 1994.

Dolfin T et al: Incidence, severity and timing of subependymal and intravascular hemorrhages in preterm infants born in a prenatal unit as detected by serial real-time ultrasound. Pediatrics 1983;71:541.

Greenspan JS et al: Partial liquid ventilation in critically ill infants receiving extracorporeal life support. Pediatrics 1997;99:1.

Gross GW et al: Bypass cannulas utilized in extracorporeal membrane oxygenation in neonates. radiographic findings. Pediatr Radiol 1995;25:337.

Gross GW et al: Thoracic complications of extracorporeal membrane oxygenation: findings on chest radiographs and sonograms. AJR Am J Roentgenol 1992;158:353.

Kirks DR: Practical Pediatric Imaging, 3rd edition. Lippincott-Raven, 1008.

Siegel MJ: Pediatric Sonography. Raven Press, 1991.

Swischuk LE: Imaging of the Newborn, Infant and Young Child, 3rd edition. Williams & Wilkins, 1989.

10 Management of the Extremely Low Birth Weight Infant During the First Week of Life

This chapter addresses the initial care of premature infants of <1000 g birth weight. Many aspects of the care of extremely low birth weight (ELBW) infants are *controversial,* and each institution has developed its own philosophy, style, and techniques for managing these infants. It is of the utmost importance to follow the practices of your own institution. This chapter offers guidelines that the authors have found useful for stabilizing and caring for extremely small infants.

I. **Delivery room management**
   A. **Ethics (see also Chapter 15).** The neonatologist and other health care team members should make every effort to meet with the family before delivery to discuss the treatment options for the ELBW infant. The strategy is to present the multiple treatment options available and to recognize and openly acknowledge the uncertainty of prognosis. The team may provide current survival statistics, by birth weight and gestational age, to help establish realistic expectations.
   B. **Resuscitation**
      1. **Thermoregulation.** Polyethylene wrap (ie, Saran Wrap) applied immediately after birth reduces postnatal fall in temperature by reducing evaporative and convective heat loss. The ELBW infant should not be dried but rather immediately wrapped in Saran Wrap under a radiant warmer. The wrap is removed on admission.
      2. **Respiratory support.** Because of their gestational age, many of these infants will require intubation at delivery. For infants who require intubation, prophylactic surfactant may also be given in the delivery room.
      3. **Transport.** As soon as possible the infant should be transported to the neonatal intensive care unit (NICU). Transport must be in a prewarmed portable incubator. Occlusive wrap should remain in place and the infant should be placed under warmed blankets with a knit hat. Infants transported from referring hospitals should be handled in a similar manner with the addition of an underlying thermal mattress.

II. **Temperature and humidity control.** Because the tiny infant has little subcutaneous fat, relatively large skin surface area, and minimal energy reserves, a **constant neutral thermal environment** is essential for survival. This is defined as the environmental temperature that minimizes heat loss so as not to increase oxygen consumption and incur metabolic stress. To maintain minimal evaporative heat loss, it is best if the environmental humidity is ≥40–80%. Low ambient humidity will require higher ambient temperatures to maintain infant skin temperature; optimal skin temperature is 36.0–36.5 °C.
   A. **Incubators or radiant warmers.** ELBW infants may initially be managed either **in double-walled incubators or under radiant heaters with protective plastic sheeting or covers.** Radiant warmers allow accessibility to the infant but produce large evaporative heat and water losses and slightly higher basal metabolic rates than the incubator. Use of the radiant warmer is dictated by the infant's clinical status and medical needs. In general, the following patients may require radiant warmer beds: those undergoing preparation for surgery or in the immediate postoperative period, recently delivered or transported patients, critically ill or clinically unstable infants re-

quiring multiple interventions, and infants with chest tubes. Hypothermia must be avoided. The definition of *hypothermia* is not readily agreed upon; however, some centers strive for core temperatures of 37.0 °C, whereas others allow infants to be maintained at temperatures as low as 35.5 °C. *Guidelines for Perinatal Care* recommends maintaining either a skin temperature of 36.0–36.5 °C or a core body temperature of 36.0–37.5 °C.

B. Humidification. ELBW infants have increased insensible water loss largely as a result of evaporation. In particular, the ratio of body surface area to body weight is greatly increased with a greater proportion of body water relative to body mass. Furthermore, transcutaneous water loss is enhanced by their thin epidermis and underdeveloped stratum corneum. Using increased environmental humidity can minimize these evaporative losses. **Warm humidification within the incubator or the area beneath the protective plastic cover of a radiant warmer is recommended.**

1. **Use a respiratory care humidification unit,** the same as used with oxygen hoods. The fluids used for the humidification in these systems should be changed every 24 h. If the manufactured humidity reservoirs of the incubators are used, special attention to infection control is needed, especially to avoid skin infection by fungi or bacteria.

2. **Minimize nosocomial infection in humidified environments** by not allowing stuffed toys or other nonmedical items inside the incubator or radiant warmer and by changing linens regularly if the infant's condition is stable.

C. Monitoring and maintenance of body temperature. Infants weighing <1000 g have poor mechanisms for regulation of temperature and depend on environmental support.

1. **Maintain skin temperature of 36.0–36.5 °C.** Rectal thermometers are not to be used for tiny infants. Electronic thermometers are readily available and eliminate concerns for mercury toxicity or accidental glass breakage.

2. **Using a servocontrol skin probe,** record skin temperature and environmental temperature every hour until the skin temperature is stable (36.0–36.5 °C) and follow up thereafter with recordings at 2-h intervals.

3. **Check axillary temperature** only if skin temperature is outside the range of 36.0–36.5 °C. You may need to change from servo- to nonservocontrol (manual) to warm the smallest infants. Use extreme caution while in the manual temperature mode because the danger of hyperthermia does exist with radiant warmer use.

4. **Record the incubator humidity** every hour until it is stable (40–80%) and then every 2 h for maintenance.

5. **If minor surgical procedures are required,** convert the overhead radiant warmer to servocontrol set at 37 °C.

6. **Low birth weight infants must be weighed** at least once daily for management of fluids and electrolytes. The incubator should be equipped with an **in-bed scale for continuous weighing of the infant to minimize handling and loss of thermal-controlled environment. The scale should be preheated** within the incubator before admission and should be calibrated after optimal air temperature and humidity have been established.

7. **Other heat-conserving practices** include the use of knit hats, fetal positioning, and occlusive port sleeves on incubators. Heating pads or thermal mattresses may be useful, but do not place infants directly on heating pads because burns may result.

8. **Accessory items for infant care must be prewarmed.** These items may include intravenous fluids, stethoscope, saline lavages, and any other items that come in direct contact with the infant. Placement of these items in the infant's incubator 30 min before use warms them to avoid heat loss by conduction from the infant.

D. **Slow warming or cooling of infants.** Warming of infants who become hypothermic must be gradual.
   1. **Cooling.** If the infant's skin temperature is >37.0 °C, set the warmer temperature control to 0.4 °C lower than the infant's skin temperature. Continue to reduce the warmer temperature until desired temperature is achieved. If increased temperature persists, consider evaluation for pathologic conditions such as sepsis, intraventricular hemorrhage, or mechanical overheating by exterior lamps. Do not turn off the warmer because this may cause a sudden decrease in the infant's temperature.
   2. **Warming.** If the infant's temperature is <36.0 °C, set the warmer temperature 0.4 °C higher than the infant's temperature. Continue this procedure until the desired temperature is achieved. Continual observation of environmental and skin temperatures are essential to evaluate rewarming efforts.
      Frequent monitoring and observation of the infant are necessary to assess tolerance. **Do not rewarm faster than 1 °C/h.** When skin temperature of 36.5 °C is achieved, rewarming efforts should be gradually discontinued and temperature maintenance by servocontrol should be monitored. Rapid rewarming of ELBW infants must be avoided because core body temperatures >37.5 °C cause increased insensible water losses, increased oxygen consumption, increased incidence of intraventricular hemorrhage, and deviations in vital signs. Do not use radiant warmer heat as additional heat over double-walled incubators because the excess heat may warp or shatter the Plexiglas.
E. **Infants on mechanical ventilation**
   1. For all ELBW infants receiving mechanical ventilation, **humidification and warming of administered ventilatory gases** are important to minimize insensible fluid losses.
   2. **In-line warming of ventilatory gas circuits** minimizes "rain-out" of the humidified air and oxygen and maintains airway temperature as close as possible to 35 °C.
III. **Fluids and electrolytes.** Because of increased insensible water loss and immature renal function, these infants have increased fluid requirements, necessitating **intravenous fluid therapy** or, in some cases, infusion of fluids through umbilical catheters or a percutaneous catheter. (See Chapter 7.)
   A. **Intravenous fluid therapy**
      1. **Insensible water loss.** Extreme insensible body fluid losses occur in tiny infants under direct radiant heat if not shielded by protective plastic sheeting or enclosed in protective plastic hoods or other types of enclosures. However, be aware that excessive fluid intake may contribute to the development of a hemodynamically significant patent ductus arteriosus (PDA) and should be monitored closely.
      2. **First day of life.** Guidelines for total fluids per kilogram of body weight for the first day of life are given in Table 10–1. The table gives suggested volumes (including catheter flushes and medications) for infants in radiant warmers. Fluids may be adjusted with the addition of humidity.
      3. **Second and subsequent days of life.** Fluid management on the second and subsequent days depends on changes in body weight, renal function (blood urea nitrogen [BUN], creatinine, urine output), and serum electrolyte concentrations (see Chapter 7).
      4. **Additional fluid may be required if phototherapy is used.** The fluid volume should be increased by 10–20 mL/kg/day.
   B. **Infusion of fluids**
      1. **Umbilical artery catheter.** Use only for laboratory and hemodynamic monitoring if other intravenous access is available. Infuse ½ normal saline (NS) + ½ unit heparin/mL.
      2. **Umbilical venous catheter.** Use double-lumen if available. Use for all infusions. Add ½ unit heparin/mL to maintenance fluids.

TABLE 10-1. ADMINISTRATION RATES FOR THE FIRST DAY OF LIFE FOR INFANTS ON RADIANT WARMERS

Birth weight (g)	Gestational age (weeks)	Fluid rate (mL/kg/day)
500–600	23	140–200
601–800	24	115–125
801–1000	25–27	90–110

Fluid rates may be adjusted with the addition of humidity as follows:
40% humidity, decrease fluids by 20%;
60% humidity, decrease fluids by 30%;
80% humidity, decrease fluids by 40%.

    3. Broviac/percutaneous infusion catheters. Add ½ unit heparin/mL to maintenance fluids.

    4. Radial arterial line/posterior tibial arterial line. Add 2 units heparin/mL to ½ NS.

    5. Document catheter placement on insertion and monitor for changes.

  C. For catheter flushing, use the same fluids as those being infused as intravenous fluids. Avoid NS as a flush solution because of excessive sodium. In addition, avoid hypotonic solutions (<0.45 NS or <5% dextrose); these solutions may cause red blood cell hemolysis.

  D. Monitoring of fluid therapy. The infant's fluid status should be evaluated at least twice daily and the fluid intake adjusted accordingly. Fluid status is monitored via measurement of body weight, urine output, urine specific gravity, blood pressure measurements, serum sodium, hematocrit, and physical examination.

    1. Body weight. The most important method of monitoring fluid therapy is the measurement of body weight. If an in-bed scale is used, weigh the infant every 12 h. If an in-bed scale is not available, weighing may have to be delayed to every 24–48 h, depending on the stability of the tiny infant, to prevent excessive handling and cold stress. A weight loss of up to 15% of birth weight may be experienced by the end of the first week of life. Greater weight loss is considered excessive, and environmental controls for insensible fluid losses and fluid management must be carefully reviewed.

    2. Urine output and specific gravity. Monitoring urine output is the second most important method of monitoring fluid therapy. For greatest accuracy, diapers should be weighed before use and immediately after urination. In addition to urine volume, urine specific gravity should be determined to check renal function and the state of hydration.

      a. First 12 h. Any amount of urine output is acceptable.

      b. Twelve to 24 h. The minimum acceptable urine output is 0.5 mL/kg/h, with urine specific gravity of 1.008–1.015.

      c. Day 2 and beyond. Normal urine output for the second day is 1–2 mL/kg/h. After the second day of life, urine output may increase to 3.0–3.5 mL/kg/h; 4–5 mL/kg/h is excessive and indicates early fluid overload, which may lead to electrolyte loss. Urine specific gravity should fluctuate between 1.008 and 1.015. Values outside this range warrant reevaluation of fluid management or environmental humidity control.

    3. Hemodynamic monitoring is a valuable tool in assessing fluid status in the infant.

      a. Heart rate. The accelerated heart rate of the tiny infant, which averages 140–160 beats/min, is generally considered within normal limits. Tachycardia, with a heart rate in excess of 160 beats/min, may be a sign of hypovolemia, pain, inadequate ventilation, anemia, or temperature instability.

b. **Arterial blood pressure.** The most accurate measurement of arterial blood pressure is via an indwelling arterial catheter and transducer. Cuff pressures may be difficult to obtain because of the infant's small size and lower systemic pressures. In our institution our goal is to maintain the infant's mean arterial pressure at or equal to the gestational age. Although mean arterial pressures are important, it is also necessary to evaluate the infant's perfusion, urine output, and acid-base balance.

4. **Electrolyte values.** Serum electrolyte levels should be monitored at least twice daily or every 4–8 h for the most immature infants. Sodium is added as diuresis begins, and potassium is added after urination has been established.

a. **Sodium.** Initially, tiny infants have a sufficient sodium level (132–138 mEq/L) and require no sodium intake. However, when the serum sodium level begins to decrease (usually on the third to fifth days of life), sodium should be added to the intravenous fluids (3–8 mEq/kg/day of sodium). In subsequent monitoring of the serum sodium levels:

   i. **If sodium is >142 mEq/L,** consider that the sodium intake is too high or the infant is dehydrated.

   ii. **If sodium is <133 mEq/L,** more sodium may be needed or the infant may have fluid overload. If the decrease in the serum sodium level is believed to be caused by fluid overload, the total daily fluids should be reduced.

   Note: Hypernatremia in the first few days of life may be caused by dehydration or by inadvertent sodium administration from normal saline catheter flushes. Flush catheters only with the intravenous fluids being used for maintenance fluid therapy. If infusion is being done through an umbilical artery catheter, heparinized intravenous fluid can be used for flushing.

b. **Potassium**

   i. **During the first 48 h after birth,** tiny infants are prone to the development of increased serum potassium levels of ≥5 mEq/L (range, 4.0–8.0 mEq/L). The increase is mostly a result of immature renal tubular function. Most clinicians recommend that no potassium be given during this time. Electrocardiographic (ECG) changes are not usually seen until the serum potassium level is >9.0 mEq/L. The following clinical guidelines are offered.

   (a) **Serum potassium 7–8 mEq/L.** Accept the value as the upper limit and observe the infant and the ECG. Repeat serum studies every 4–6 h.

   (b) **Serum potassium 8–9 mEq/L.** Check urine output. The minimal acceptable output is 1–2 mL/kg/h (2–3 mL/kg/h is preferred) with urine specific gravity of 1.006–1.012. Observe for elevated or peaked T-wave changes on the bedside heart rate monitor. Monitor BUN and creatinine.

   (c) **Serum potassium levels >9 mEq/L.** These levels are usually pathologic and are associated with decreasing renal function or cardiac irregularities, or both. Consider administration of sodium bicarbonate, calcium solutions, or glucose/insulin infusions. In our institution, once potassium levels are >9 mEq/L, the utilization of Kayexalate enemas (1 g/kg) along with albuterol metered-dose inhaler (MDI) (4 puffs every 2 h, 1 puff = 90 mcg) have proven to be successful in decreasing potentially high levels. Clinical trials support adult use of albuterol in MDI and intravenous forms for the treatment of hyperkalemia while neonatal use remains controversial.

    ii. Three to 6 days after birth. Usually by days 3 to 6, the initially elevated serum potassium level begins to decrease. As potassium levels approach 4 mEq/L, add supplemental potassium to intravenous fluids. Begin with 1–2 mEq/kg/day. Measure serum potassium every 6–12 h until the level is stabilized.

   IV. Blood glucose. As with larger high-risk infants, ELBW infants should be supported with 4–6 mg/kg/min glucose infusion. This support can usually be achieved by starting with a 5–10% dextrose solution, depending on glucose needs. Meter testing of blood glucose should be performed every 2 h until a stable blood glucose level (50–90 mg/dL) has been established. Urine samples should be checked for glucosuria. Trace glucosuria is acceptable and may occur with a blood glucose level as low as 120 mg/dL, but higher levels of serum glucose and glucosuria require recalculation of glucose administration and total fluid administration.

   V. Calcium. Serum calcium should be monitored once or twice daily. When the serum calcium decreases below 7.5 mg/dL, we institute treatment with calcium gluconate (for dosage, see Chapter 80). This decrease usually happens on the second day of life. Although a few infants may not require calcium therapy, some centers routinely institute daily maintenance calcium supplementation in their intravenous solutions (eg, 2 mg of calcium gluconate/mL intravenous solution).

   VI. Nutrition. If the infant is metabolically stable, **parenteral nutrition** should be started routinely on the first or second day of life and continued until the infant is receiving sufficient enteral feeding to promote growth. In the ELBW infant, **intravenous lipids** (20%) should be started by 48 h of age; one should start with perhaps 0.5 g/kg/day and increase by 0.5 g/kg/day every 24–48 h up to 2 g/kg/day while monitoring triglyceride levels. Most centers have arbitrarily taken 100–200 mg/dL as a safe triglyceride level. **Early feeds of small amounts of breast milk or premature formulas** (0.5–1.0 mL/h by bolus or continuous drip intragastrically) can promote gut development, characterized by increased gut growth, villous hypertrophy, digestive enzyme secretion, and enhanced motility. This approach is called **minimal enteral feedings.** The decision to either advance or maintain minimal enteral feedings at a constant level should take into account the clinical status of the infant. Minimal enteral feeding should be started with maternal or donor breast milk. It has been shown that incidence of infection and retinopathy of prematurity is decreased when breast milk is used. Mothers should be provided information regarding the benefits of breast milk and should be encouraged to pump their breasts regularly. Once feedings are established, the breast milk can be fortified with supplements. If breast milk is not available, premature formulas can be used. In our practice, the initiation of enteral feedings is withheld for 1–3 days after severe perinatal asphyxia, with the expectation that it will decrease the risk of necrotizing enterocolitis.

  VII. Respiratory support. The smaller the infant, the weaker are the muscles of ventilation. Many of these infants initially require **mechanical ventilation.** Although some centers prefer a trial of nasal continuous positive airway pressure (CPAP) before intubation, we have found that it is often prudent to electively intubate these infants in the delivery room. Respiratory support is discussed in detail in Chapter 6.

    A. Endotracheal intubation

      1. Type of endotracheal tube. When possible, use an endotracheal tube with 1-cm markings on the side. The internal diameter (ID) of the tube should routinely be 2.5 or 3.0 mm, according to body weight:

        a. 500–1000 g: 2.5-mm ID.

        b. 1000–1250 g: 3.0-mm ID.

      2. Endotracheal tube placement. (The procedure for endotracheal tube placement is described in detail in Chapter 20.) Confirm proper placement by a chest x-ray study, performed with the infant's head in the midline position, noting the marking at the gum. As a means of subsequently checking proper tube position, on every shift the nurse responsible for the infant should check and record the numbers or letters at the gum line.

B. **Mechanical ventilation.** With the advancement of ventilation technology, various modes are available, including volume ventilation, pressure support, and high-frequency ventilation. This technology assists the clinician in avoiding overexpansion of the lung and lowering mean airway pressures, thereby decreasing the incidence of chronic lung disease in the ELBW infant.

1. **Conventional ventilation.** Tiny infants respond to a wide range of ventilator settings. Some do relatively well on 20–30 cycles/min; others require 50–60 cycles/min, with inspiratory times ranging from 0.28–0.50 s. Use the least airway pressure possible. Seek to maintain mechanical breath tidal volumes of 5–7 mL/kg; this often may be achieved with as little as 8–12 cm inspiratory pressure and 2–3 cm positive end-expiratory pressure. Higher pressures increase the risk of barotrauma and the development of chronic lung disease and must be avoided. We have found that pressures can be kept to a minimum by allowing a mild to moderate respiratory acidosis (pH 7.25–7.32;Pco_2, 45–58 mm Hg). The following conventional ventilatory support guidelines are offered for the initiation of respiratory care. Each tiny infant requires frequent reassessment and revision of settings and parameters. Recommended initial settings for pressure-limited time-cycled ventilators in tiny infants are as follows.

a. **Rate:** 20–60 (usually 30) breaths/min.

b. **Inspiratory time (IT):** 0.3–0.5 (usually 0.33) s.

c. **Peak inspiratory pressure:** 12–20 cm H_2O (select peak inspiratory pressure on the basis of tidal volume if it can be measured; usually 5.0–7.0 mL/kg).

d. **Mean airway pressure:** <8 cm H_2O.

e. **FIO_2:** As required per initial Po_2 values.

f. **Flow rate:** 6–8 L/min.

g. **Synchronized intermittent mandatory ventilation (SIMV) and volume/ pressure control ventilators** have the internal controls that adjust flow delivery. Current ventilators have incorporated enhancements for pressure support, resulting in increased triggering sensitivity, shortened response times, reduced flow acceleration, and improved breath termination parameters.

2. **High-frequency ventilation** uses small (less than dead space) tidal volumes and extremely rapid rates. The advantage of delivering small tidal volumes is that it can be done at relatively low pressures, greatly reducing the risk of barotrauma.

3. **Nasal CPAP (NCPAP).** Some ELBW infants may not require mechanical ventilation. Others may require ventilation for a short period of time for surfactant replacement. These infants may benefit from NCPAP. NCPAP helps maintain lung expansion and improves oxygenation. NCPAP should be used per institutional guidelines.

C. **Monitoring of ventilatory status**

1. **Oxygenation**

a. **Blood gas sampling.** Arterial catheterization (for details, see Chapter 16) should be performed for frequent blood gas sampling. Routinely, these infants require blood gas sampling every 2–4 h. Sampling may need to be done more frequently, possibly as often as every 20 min, but less frequent sampling is desirable as soon as possible to minimize stress and blood loss and the need for blood replacement.

i. **Desirable arterial blood gas values**

(a) **Pao$_2$:** 45–60 mm Hg.

(b) **Paco$_2$:** 45–55 mm Hg. A slightly higher Paco$_2$ is acceptable if the pH remains acceptable.

(c) **pH:** 7.25–7.32 is acceptable.

ii. **Abnormal blood gas values** indicate the need for immediate chest x-ray films (see section VII,C,4 below), chest wall transillumination (see p 293), and repeat blood gas determinations.

b. **Continuous O$_2$ monitoring** should also be performed, preferably by pulse oximetry. Transcutaneous electrode monitoring of O$_2$ and CO$_2$ can be used. To prevent skin tearing and damage, do not use an adhesive disk; instead, use soft restraints to secure the probe to the extremity. Change the Ptcco$_2$/O$_2$ site every 4 h, and use the lowest effective temperature of the transcutaneous probe. The O$_2$ mixture should be adjusted to maintain the pulse oximeter reading between 88% and 95% hemoglobin O$_2$ saturation. Excess oxygenation must be avoided in this group of infants. Failure to regulate the administration of O$_2$ can contribute to the development of retinopathy of prematurity and bronchopulmonary dysplasia.

2. **Flow-volume loops.** Flow-volume loops reflect both inspiratory and expiratory flow limitation. Most notable is the restricted flow of reactive airways during prolonged mechanical ventilation. Computer-assisted breath-to-breath monitoring of pulmonary function with trend analyses facilitates a rapid response to changes in lung mechanics and worsening respiratory status and results in improved matching of ventilatory support as the infant's condition changes.

3. **Infant's appearance.** An abrupt change in the infant's color or the appearance of cyanosis indicates the need for immediate assessment by chest wall transillumination, chest x-ray study, and blood gas sampling. Assess infant for adequate pain control and sedation needs.

4. **Chest x-ray study**

a. **Indications**

i. Abnormal or sudden change in blood gas values.

ii. Adjustment of the endotracheal tube (to confirm proper positioning).

iii. Sudden change in the infant's status.

b. **Technique.** A chest x-ray film should be taken with the infant's head in the midline position to check for endotracheal tube placement; be sure to use gonad shields.

c. **X-ray evaluation.** Check the chest x-ray film for expansion of the lung, chest wall, and diaphragm. Overexpansion (exhibited by hyperlucent lungs and diaphragm below the ninth rib) must be avoided. If overexpansion is present, consider decreasing the peak airway pressure. Some tiny infants do very well with peak inspiratory pressures as low as 8 cm H$_2$O.

D. **Suctioning.** Suctioning should be done on an as-needed basis. The need for suctioning can be determined with the use of flow-loop monitoring, which indicates restricted airflow caused by secretions.

1. **Assessment of the need for suctioning.** To assess the need for suctioning, the nurse or physician should consider the following.

a. **Breath sounds.** Wet or diminished breath sounds may indicate secretions obstructing the airways and the need for suctioning.

b. **Blood gas values.** If the Paco$_2$ increases above 50 mm Hg, suctioning should be considered to clean the airways and avoid the "ball-valve" effect of thick secretions.

c. **Airway monitoring.** By using airflow sensors and continuous computer graphic screen displays, abnormal waveforms indicative of accumulating secretions or airway blockage can be easily seen, and immediate steps can be taken to clear the airway.

d. **Visible secretions** in the endotracheal tube.

e. **Loss of chest wall movement.**
2. **Technique**
   a. **Suctioning should be done** only to the depth of the endotracheal tube. Use a suctioning guide or a marked (1-cm increments) suction catheter.
   b. **Lavage fluid for suctioning** should be sterile normal saline. Use 1–2 drops for each suctioning procedure. Lavage solution should be warmed to 36.0–37.0 °C.
   c. **Suction should be regulated** at 60–80 mm Hg.
   d. **Minimize the effects of suctioning** by preoxygenating with a 5–15% increase in O_2, increasing the baseline ventilatory rate, and using in-line suctioning devices.
E. **Extubation**
   1. **Indications.** When an infant has been weaned to a mean airway pressure of 6 cm H_2O and a low (40%) FIO_2, extubation should be considered. Some experts suggest that extubation to nasal prong or mask CPAP has beneficial effects on respiratory function and the prevention of atelectasis. Other indications for extubation are as follows.
      a. Ventilator rate <10 breaths/min.
      b. Regular spontaneous respiratory rate.
      c. Pulmonary function tests (if available) revealing a compliance of 0.9–1.1 mL/cm H_2O.
   2. **Technique.** Many institutions recommend extubation with positive pressure to prevent atelectasis. Also, to prevent apnea, some will start treatment with **aminophylline or caffeine before extubation** (see Chapter 80). The procedure for tube removal is the same as for larger infants.
   3. **Postextubation care.** Frequent observation of breathing patterns, auscultation of the chest, monitoring of vital signs, and blood gas analysis are mandatory. Immediately after extubation, 0.25 mL of racemic epinephrine may be administered with a micronebulizer for relief of laryngeal edema. This procedure is repeated every 2 h until 3 treatments have been given. After 6 h, the infant is reevaluated for possible further aerosol treatments. After extubation, the infant is placed in an O_2 hood and given FIO_2 that is the same or 5% greater than that administered before extubation.
F. **Vitamin A.** Some institutions are now using intramuscular injections of vitamin A as a mode of therapy to decrease chronic lung disease in ELBW infants. Dosing should begin the first week of life, 5000 IU 3 times/week for 4 weeks.
VIII. **Surfactant.** (See Chapter 6.) Most centers administer surfactant replacement to ELBW infants. It should be administered according to the protocol provided with the specific surfactant replacement product.
IX. **PDA.** Efforts should be made to minimize the risk of PDA. Overhydration must be avoided. If the infant shows any sign of a hemodynamically significant PDA, medical treatment should commence. Several methods are currently being recommended for indomethacin therapy. (For dosage, see Chapter 80.) The first is the originally described method of 3 doses given at 12-h intervals. The second method uses the same total dosage but prolongs the indomethacin treatment over a 5- to 7-day treatment period. A third method involves a slow infusion rate for each dose given over 20–30 min rather than bolus infusion. This method is believed to have less effect for reduced cerebral blood flow. Finally, a fourth method uses continuous infusion. This approach is considered to have less effect for renal vasoconstriction and less PDA recurrence. Continuous IV indomethacin infusion is given at 11 µg/kg/h for a total of 36 h (the same total dose as for other types of infusions). The continuous infusion appears to lessen the problem of decreased cerebral blood flow.
X. **Transfusion.** These infants are usually born anemic, with a hematocrit <40, and they require frequent laboratory specimens. We try to keep the hematocrit

between 35% and 40%. Lower values may be acceptable if the infant is asymptomatic. A cumulative record of blood drawn is also a useful indicator in the decision to transfuse blood. The public is increasingly aware of transfusion issues, and parents should be encouraged to participate in a directed-donor program. Epogen and iron therapy is being used in many centers to stimulate production of red blood cells and to try to limit the use of transfusions.

XI. Skin care. Meticulous skin care is advised. Maintenance of intact skin is the tiny infant's most effective barrier against infection, insensible fluid loss, protein loss, and blood loss and provides for more effective body temperature control. Minimal use of tape is recommended because the infant's skin is fragile, and tears often result with removal. Hypak-zinc-based tape can be used. Alternatives to tape include the use of Op-Site Flexigrid or a hydrogel adhesive, which removes easily with water. Hydrogel adhesive infant care products include electrodes, temperature probe covers, and Bili-Masks. In addition, the very thin skin of the tiny infant allows absorption of many substances. Skin care must focus on maintaining skin integrity and minimizing exposure to topical agents. **Aquaphor ointment** is free of preservatives and decreases chemical exposure and the risk of allergic or irritant contact dermatitis. Aquaphor has been proven to be a successful skin barrier and helps maintain skin integrity. Use of Aquaphor is *controversial*, however; one study demonstrated an increase in late-onset nosocomial infection. Aquaphor may be used per institutional guidelines. Tegaderm can be used over areas of bony prominence, such as the knees or elbows, for hyperactive or irritable infants to prevent skin friction breakdown or under monitoring devices (ie, temperature probe, saturation monitor, or 3IMV probe).

A. **Use hyrogel skin probe or cut servocontrol skin probe covers to the smallest size possible** (try a 2-cm diameter circle) to reduce skin damage resulting from the adhesive.

B. **Monitoring of O_2 therapy is best accomplished by use of a pulse oximeter** for hemoglobin O_2 saturation. The probe must be placed carefully to prevent pressure sores. The site should be rotated a minimum of every 8 h. Alternative means of O_2 monitoring include umbilical catheter blood sampling. The use of transcutaneous O_2 and CO_2 gel electrodes is discouraged. Heated gel electrodes have caused serious skin burns in ELBW infants.

C. **Urine bags and blood pressure cuffs should not be used routinely** because of adhesives and sharp plastic edge cuts. For urine collection, turn the diaper plastic side up. Bladder aspirations are discouraged.

D. **Eye ointment for gonococcal prophylaxis should be applied** per routine admission plan. If the eyelids are fused, apply along the lash line.

E. **When the infant requires a procedure** (eg, placement of an umbilical artery or venous catheter or chest tube) measure 1 mL of chlorhexidine or warm half-strength povidone-iodine solution. One milliliter is sufficient to effectively disinfect 50–60 cm^2 of skin area. After the procedure is completed, the solution should be sponged off immediately with warm sterile water.

F. **Attach ECG electrodes using as little adhesive as possible.** Options include the following.
  1. Consider using limb electrodes.
  2. Consider water-activated gel electrodes.
  3. Use electrodes that have been trimmed down and secured with a flexible dressing material (eg, Kling or Coban).

G. **An initial bath** is not necessary, but if HIV is a consideration, those infants should receive a mild soap bath such as Neutrogena when the infant's temperature has stabilized. Warm sterile water baths are given *only when needed* during the next 2 weeks of life.

H. **Avoid the use of anything that dries out the skin,** such as soaps and alcohol. Bonding agents such as skin prep and Mastisol should be avoided. Solvents such as Detachol should not be used.

I. **Sterile water-soaked cotton balls** are helpful for removing adhesive tape, probe covers, and electrode covers.

   Note: When the skin appears dry, thickened, and no longer shiny or translucent (usually in 10–14 days), these skin care recommendations and procedures may be modified or discontinued.

J. **Environmental.** Use of sheepskins, mattress covers, or blankets in humidified environments helps prevent skin breakdown.

K. **Treatment of skin breakdown**

   1. Clean skin breakdown/excoriated area with warm sterile water.
   2. Apply petroleum-based ointment (ie, Bacitracin) over broken-down infected areas, leaving open to air.
   3. Apply transparent dressings (ie, Tegaderm) over excoriated areas.
   4. Administer intravenous antibiotics if necessary.

XII. **Other special considerations for the ELBW infant**

A. **Infection**

   1. **Cultures.** Many of these infants are born infected or are from an infected environment. Blood and urine cultures should be obtained. Unless there is a strong suspicion of meningitis, lumbar puncture should not be performed.
   2. **Antibiotics.** After obtaining cultures, these infants should be started on **ampicillin** and **cefotaxime** or **aminoglycoside.** Drug levels must be monitored if using aminoglycosides and the dose adjusted accordingly. (See Chapter 80).
   3. **Intravenous gamma globulin therapy.** Studies have suggested that prophylactic treatment with intravenous gamma globulin may prevent infections in ELBW infants. This therapy remains controversial, and one must consult your individual institution for guidelines. (See Chapter 80).

B. **Central nervous system hemorrhage.** Initial cranial ultrasonography is usually performed as soon after birth as practical. For less ill low birth weight infants, an ultrasound scan at 7 days should be routine. Depending on the presence and severity of hemorrhage, follow-up ultrasound scans may be performed.

C. **Hyperbilirubinemia**

   1. **Risk.** There appears to be little risk from mild or moderate hyperbilirubinemia in these infants. Still, efforts should be made to keep the serum bilirubin below 10 mg/dL. Serum bilirubin may need to be monitored twice daily, and an exchange transfusion should be considered when the bilirubin approaches or exceeds 12 mg/dL (see Chapters 38 and 39).
   2. **Phototherapy.** Phototherapy to reduce the serum bilirubin level may be needed and can be used to minimize the need for exchange transfusion. The additional use of the fiberoptic phototherapy blanket may also be useful in reducing bilirubin levels. Some centers start phototherapy immediately after birth. If the infant is treated with phototherapy, the fluid intake should be increased by 10–20 mL/kg/day.

D. **Social problems.** Many families have great difficulty in coping with the issues related to their infant's extreme prematurity and the loss of the idealized infant. Participation in a parent-to-parent support group appears to improve maternal–infant relationships. Experienced nurses and the use of a primary nurse together with ongoing communication from the medical team can decrease the parents' stress and keep them up-to-date on their infant's medical problems. Parents should be invited to participate in the infant's care from the beginning. A social service consultation is mandatory for all of these families. Parent conferences involving the physician, social worker, and primary nurse help the family understand the complex, extended care of their infant. Parent–infant bonding should be promoted, and parents should be encouraged to assist in caring for their child.

E. **Developmental Issues**

1. **Minimal stimulation.** These tiny infants do not tolerate handling and medically necessary procedures. Other stressors include noise, light, and activity such as moving the incubator. Routine tasks should be clustered to allow the infant undisturbed and prolonged periods of rest.
2. **Positioning.** The fetus is maintained in a flexed position. Care should be taken to simulate this positioning in the extremely premature infant. A flexed side-lying or prone posture with supportive boundaries is preferred. A change in position is recommended every 4 h or at the infant's cue.
3. **Kangaroo care** has been shown to promote behavioral state organization as well as parental bonding in the NICU. Temperature, heart rate, respiratory rate, and O_2 saturation have all been found to remain within normal limits during kangaroo care. It has also been shown as a safe practice for intubated infants with central catheters.
4. **Environmental issues.** Decreased noise and light exposure has been shown to foster development of the tiny infant.

REFERENCES

Clifford PA, Barnsteiner J: Kangaroo care and the very low birthweight infant: is it an appropriate practice for all premature babies? *J Neonatal Nurs* 2001;7:14.

Cordero L et al: A comparison of two airway frequencies in mechanically ventilated, very-low birthweight infants. *Respir Care* 2001;46:783.

Edwards WH et al: *The Effect of Aquaphor Original Emollient Ointment on Nosocomial Sepsis Rates and Skin Integrity in Infants of Birth Weight 501 to 1000.* Society for Pediatric Research, 2001.

Hauth J, Merenstein G: *Guidelines for Perinatal Care,* 4th edition. American Academy of Pediatrics/American College of Obstetricians and Gynecologists, 1997.

Hylander MA et al: Association of human milk feedings with a reduction in retinopathy of prematurity among very low birthweight infants. *J Perinatol* 2001;21:356.

Kapoor M, Chan G: Fluid and electrolyte abnormalities. *Crit Care Clin* 2001;17.

Kavvadia V et al: Randomized trial of two levels of fluid input in the perinatal period—effect on fluid balance, electrolyte and metabolic disturbances in ventilated VLBW infants. *Acta Paediatr* 2000;89:237.

Kemper MJ et al: Effective treatment of acute hyperkalaemia in childhood by short-term infusion of salbutamol. *Eur J Pediatr* 1997;156:420.

Lee J et al: Blood pressure standards for very low birthweight infants during the first day of life. *Arch Dis Child* 1999;81:F168.

L'Herault J et al: The effectiveness of a thermal mattress in stabilizing and maintaining body temperature during the transport of very low-birth weight newborns. *Appl Nurs Res* 2001; 14:210.

Mariani G et al: Randomized trial of permissive hypercapnia in preterm infants. *Pediatrics* 1999;104:1082.

Tyson J et al: Vitamin A supplementation for extremely-low-birth-weight infants. *N Engl J Med* 1999;340:1962.

Vohra S et al: Effect of polyethylene occlusive skin wrapping in very low birthweight infants at delivery: a randomized trial *J Pediatrics* 1999;134:547.

Wong SL, Maltz HC: Albuterol for the treatment of hyperkalemia. *Ann Pharmacother* 1999; 33:103.

11 Extracorporeal Membrane Oxygenation

I. **Introduction.** Extracorporeal membrane oxygenation (ECMO) provides cardiopulmonary support by directing venous blood in a nonpulsatile fashion through a membrane oxygenator (artificial lung), where oxygen is added and carbon dioxide removed. The blood is then pumped back into the patient's right atrium (venovenous ECMO) or aorta (venoarterial ECMO) (Figure 11–1). The procedure allows the lungs to rest and avoids continuous high-pressure mechanical ventilation in severe respiratory failure. During ECMO, the lungs continue to function at a low volume to prevent atelectasis and maintain minimal alveolar ventilation. The patient may be entirely dependent on the membrane lung for oxygenation and removal of carbon dioxide or may require only partial support.

II. **Indications.** ECMO is used primarily for critically ill term newborns with reversible respiratory or cardiac failure who have failed maximal medical management. Diseases that have been managed using ECMO include **meconium aspiration syndrome, congenital diaphragmatic hernia, persistent pulmonary hypertension of the newborn (PPHN; usually associated with meconium aspiration or severe asphyxia), cardiac failure after open heart surgery, respiratory distress syndrome, sepsis, and pneumonia.** Improvements in pre-ECMO treatment strategies such as inhaled nitric oxide (iNO), surfactant, and high-frequency oscillatory ventilation (HFOV) have caused a demographic shift in the ECMO population toward more complex pediatric and cardiac cases (Wilson, 1996). Despite increasing pre-ECMO use of these treatment strategies, the length of ECMO treatment has not changed (Roy, 2000). Even with the widespread use of iNO therapy, 22–40% of patients with severe PPHN continue to require ECMO. (Schumacher et al, 2001). The average time on ECMO for respiratory failure is 7.5 days according to the 2001 Extracorporeal Life Support Organization (ELSO) data.

Each ECMO center must establish its own specific criteria for both reversible respiratory failure *and* maximal medical management. These criteria should identify infants who would have a ≥80% mortality or significant morbidity without ECMO. Infants should be identified in time to institute ECMO before severe lung damage occurs.

A. **ECMO entry criteria.** The following general inclusion criteria should be applied only after failure of maximal medical therapy (Short, 1993).
   1. **Weight** >1.8–2 kg; gestational age ≥34 weeks.
   2. **No more than 7 continuous days of assisted ventilation.**
   3. **Reversible lung disease.**
   4. **No major bleeding disorder or major intracranial hemorrhage.**
   5. **No major cardiac lesion.**
   6. **Plus** one or more of the following:
      a. **Alveolar-to-arterial oxygen gradient** (AaDo$_2$) >605–620 mm Hg for 4–12 h. (Normal AaDo$_2$ is <20 mm Hg.)

$$\text{AaDo}_2 = \left[(\text{Fio}_2)(\text{Pb}) - 47) - \frac{(\text{P}_{\text{ACO}_2})}{\text{R}} \right] - \text{Pao}_2$$

where Pb = barometric pressure (760 mm Hg), 47 = water vapor pressure, P$_{\text{ACO}_2}$ = alveolar CO_2 (approximately equivalent to the Paco$_2$), and R = respiratory quotient (0.8).

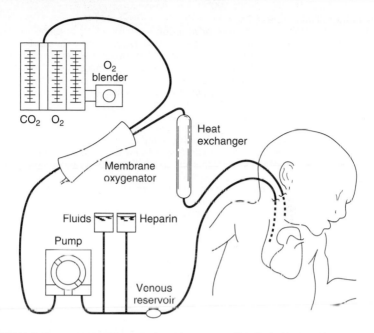

FIGURE 11-1. The venoarterial extracorporeal membrane oxygenation circuit. Blood is withdrawn from the right atrium through a catheter entering the internal jugular vein. Heparin, medications, and fluids are added. The membrane removes CO_2 and adds oxygen. The blood is then warmed and returned to the ascending aorta through a catheter in the internal carotid artery. *(Reproduced with permission from Short: BL, Pearson GD: Journal of Intensive Care Medicine, Volume 1, Number 1, 1986.)*

    b. Pao$_2$ <35-50 mm Hg for 2-12 h.
    c. Oxygenation index (OI) >35-45 for 0.5-6 h.

$$OI = \frac{FiO_2 \times MAP \times 100}{PaO_2}$$

where MAP = mean airway pressure.
    d. Barotrauma.
    e. Acute deterioration with intractable hypoxemia.

TABLE 11-1. CONTRAINDICATIONS TO EXTRACORPOREAL MEMBRANE OXYGENATION (ECMO)

Contraindications	Reason
Gestational age <34 weeks	Risk of intracranial hemorrhage
Birth weight <2000 g	Surgical difficulties with vessel cannulation
Mechanical ventilation > 7-10 days	Irreversible lung disease likely
Intracranial hemorrhage > grade I	High risk of progression of hemorrhage
Coagulopathy	Higher risk of bleeding
Severe perinatal asphyxia with evidence of severe brain damage	Poor neurologic outcome
Severe congenital anomalies	Poor outcome despite ECMO
Cyanotic congenital heart disease without cardiopulmonary failure	Other interventions indicated

III. Contraindications. See Table 11–1.
IV. Procedure. Uniform guidelines have been established to describe essential equipment, procedures, personnel, and training required for neonatal ECMO. A multidisciplinary team approach is necessary because of the variety of diseases treated by ECMO as well as the variety of resulting complications. Venoarterial (VA) ECMO has traditionally been preferred for neonatal patients because it provides both cardiac and respiratory support. Several centers are now using venovenous (VV) ECMO routinely. This method can achieve lung rest and oxygenation while indirectly improving cardiac function.

   A. For VA ECMO the draining venous catheter is placed in the right internal jugular vein and advanced to rest in the right atrium. The arterial catheter is placed in the right common carotid artery and is advanced to the entrance of the aortic arch. (See the sample x-ray film in Figure 9–9.) Blood flow with VA ECMO is nonpulsatile. For VV ECMO the right jugular vein is accessed with a single thin-walled double-lumen catheter, which is then advanced into the right atrium. Blood flow is pulsatile.

   B. During an ECMO "run," the infant's blood must be heparinized to avoid clotting the circuit. Usually a loading dose of 100–150 units of heparin/kg is required during the cannulation procedure, with a heparin drip of 20–70 units/kg/h.

   C. As bypass is achieved, ventilator settings are reduced to final settings: FIO_2, 0.21–0.40; ventilator rate, 10–20 breaths/min; pressure limit, <30 cm H_2O; and positive end-expiratory pressure (PEEP), 5–10 cm H_2O. The infant's oxygenation and ventilation are controlled by the following:

   1. **Adjusting the oxygen,** nitrogen, and carbon dioxide gas through the membrane oxygenator.
   2. **The patient's lungs** through resting ventilator support.
   3. **The percentage of cardiac output** perfusing the membrane oxygenator and the infant's lungs or the ECMO flow. An average ECMO run is 5–7 days but may be as long as 21 days.

   D. Some ECMO centers have been successfully reanastomosing the carotid artery after the procedure, but long-term evaluation of these infants is just beginning.

V. Complications (% reported by ELSO as of January 2002)
   A. Infant
   1. **Intracranial hemorrhage (5.2%).**
   2. **Central nervous system infarction (9.5%).**
   3. **Seizures (12%).**
   4. **Brain death (1%).**
   5. **Pulmonary hemorrhage (4%).**
   6. **Hypertension requiring vasodilators (12.6%).**
   7. **Hypotension requiring inotropes (8.4%).**
   8. **Cardiovascular tamponade (0.3%).**
   9. **Cardiac arrhythmias (4%).**
   10. **Hemolysis (12.8%).**
   11. **Disseminated intravascular coagulation (DIC) (0.8%).**
   12. **Acute renal failure (dialysis required, 3.7%; hemofiltration required, 12.3%).**
   B. Mechanical
   1. **Oxygenator failure (5.7%).**
   2. **Tubing rupture (1.1%).**
   3. **Pump failure (1.8%).**
   4. **Heat exchanger failure (0.9%).**
   5. **Air embolization (5.5%).**
   6. **Membrane lung failure (clots, 18.6%).**
   7. **Cannula problems (11.1%).**
VI. Prognosis. The Neonatal ECMO Registry, established in 1985, lists as of 2001 nearly 17,143 neonatal patients, the first of whom was treated in 1975. Currently,

the overall cumulative neonatal survival rate is 68%. The registry also keeps track of cumulative survival rates for specific diseases, and these data are as follows: meconium aspiration syndrome, 94%; pulmonary hypertension, 79%; hyaline membrane disease, 84%; sepsis, 75%; pneumonia, 58%; and congenital diaphragmatic hernia, 54%.

Long-term follow-up of these high-risk infants has been an integral part of most ECMO programs. Glass et al (1995) reported a 17% incidence of major disability in a cohort of 5-year-old ECMO survivors, a rate comparable to that in other high-risk populations. Cognitive delay was seen in 13%. ECMO survivors without developmental delay had a high rate of behavioral problems and an increased risk of school failure. In 1998 the United Kingdom Collaborative ECMO Group published data from their randomized trial of ECMO versus conventional treatment. Infants with a previous cardiac arrest or intraventricular hemorrhage were excluded from the trial. Thirty-two percent of the ECMO infants died before the age of 1 year and 59% in the conventional group died. Neurologic morbidity was more common in the ECMO group, likely a reflection of the larger number of survivors. Rais-Bahrami (2000) examined the neurodevelopmental outcome in ECMO versus near-miss ECMO patients at 5 years of age. This study showed that the two groups were similar in cognitive outcome, incidence of severe mental handicap, risk of school failure, as well as parent-reported behavioral problems. Approximately 10% of patients in each group were noted to have significant cognitive deficits. Infants with congenital diaphragmatic hernia were noted to be at particular risk. It is essential to recognize that both ECMO and near-miss ECMO patients are at risk for school failure and developmental issues; thus, the ECMO procedure itself does not necessarily further increase the risk for an adverse outcome. Continued comprehensive long-term follow-up is essential before we can be reassured about the outcome of survivors of this high-technology procedure.

REFERENCES

Extracorporeal Life Support Organization: Registry Report, International Summary. Extracorporeal Life Support Organization, 2002.

Glass P et al: Neurodevelopmental status at age five years of neonates treated with extracorporeal membrane oxygenation. J Pediatr 1995;127:447.

Rais-Bahrami K et al: Neurodevelopmental outcome in ECMO vs near-miss ECMO patients at 5 years of age. Clin Pediatr 2000;39:145.

Roy BJ et al: The changing demographics of neonatal extracorporeal membrane oxygenation patients reported to the Extracorporeal Life Support Organization (ELSO) Registry. Pediatr 2000;106:1334.

Schumacher et al: Extracorporeal membrane oxygenation 2001: the odyssey continues. Clin Perinatol 2001;28:629.

Short BL: Pre-ECMO considerations for neonatal patients. In Arensman RM, Cornish JD (eds): Extracorporeal Life Support. Blackwell, 1993.

Short BL et al: Extracorporeal membrane oxygenation in the management of respiratory failure in the newborn. Clin Perinatol 1987;14:737.

United Kingdom Collaborative ECMO Group: The collaborative UK ECMO trial: follow-up to 1 year of age. Pediatr 1998;101:1.

Wilson JM et al: ECMO in evolution: the impact of changing patient demographics and alternative therapies on ECMO. J Pediatr Surg 1996;8:1116.

12 Infant Transport

As regionalization and specialization of care for newborn infants have developed, a special type of team has been created for transport of these infants from a referring hospital to a level III center (neonatal intensive care unit [NICU]). A great deal of planning must take place in order for these teams to function effectively, and clear guidelines must be established regarding personnel, procedures, and equipment needed (American Academy of Pediatrics, 1997). Policies and procedures will reflect the unique characteristics of each region (eg, size, geography, economics, sophistication of medical services). Lines of communication must always be open between the referring hospital and the NICU at all levels (ie, administrators, physicians, nurses) and with ambulance or air services. Ideally, the mother would be transferred to the level III center before delivery of a high-risk infant, but this is not always possible.

I. **Transport team.** The team may include physicians, nurses, respiratory therapists, and perhaps emergency medical technicians (American Academy of Pediatrics Task Force on Interhospital Transport, 1993). Special training must be provided in the care of sick infants. A specific medical protocol is established. The team should be able to contact the attending neonatologist at any time during transport. Appropriate insurance coverage is necessary for team members, and questions of liability must be worked out with legal consultation among hospitals, ambulance services, and aircraft services.

At the referring hospital, team members should conduct themselves as professional representatives of the NICU, avoiding conflict with or criticism of the referring hospital staff. Questions about transport protocol should be worked out directly between the referring physician and the attending neonatologist.

II. **Equipment.** Each transport team should be self-sufficient. Medications and equipment can be chosen according to published lists (American Academy of Pediatrics Task Force on Interhospital Transport, 1993). Special emphasis is placed on maintaining thermal neutrality (eg, plastic swaddling or heated, humidified inspired air mixtures). Noise and vibration often compromise auditory and visual monitoring, and well-calibrated blood pressure and trancutaneous monitors may be useful. An instant camera is a "must" because pictures of the infant may be the mother's only psychological support for days.

III. **Protocol for stabilization and transfer.** The goal of stabilization is to make the transfer uneventful.

   A. **General procedures.** *Attention to the details of stabilization is important!* Unless active resuscitation is underway, the team's first task at the referring hospital is to *listen* to the history and assessment of the infant's status. The vital signs are then obtained. At this point, a precise diagnosis of all the infant's problems may be less important than predicting what the infant will need during transport. It is prudent to initiate anticipated interventions before leaving the referring hospital. For example, an infant with increasing work of breathing and increasing needs for inspired oxygen who faces a 2-h journey probably should be placed on mechanical ventilation and have an intravenous catheter in place before transfer begins. **In most cases, an infant is not ready for transport until basic neonatal needs are met: thermoneutrality, acceptable cardiac and respiratory function, and blood glucose levels in the normal range.** Vital signs must be stable, and catheters and tubes should be appropriately placed. Problems that may occur during transport should be anticipated. The NICU should be given an expected arrival time. The parents should be allowed to see and touch the infant before transport. During transport, vigilant monitoring should continue for unexpected changes in the infant's status. Respiratory rate, heart rate, blood pressure, and oxygen levels should be monitored. After transfer is completed, the team should talk with the parents and, if possible, with the referring physician.

B. Prophylactic antibiotic therapy. Infants at risk for sepsis and those with indwelling catheters should probably receive antibiotic therapy. Culture of blood samples may be performed at the referring hospital or at the NICU. Antibiotic dosages are given in Chapter 80.

C. Gastric intubation. If the infant has a gastrointestinal disorder (including ileus accompanying critical illness) or diaphragmatic hernia or if continuous positive airway pressure is administered through the nose or a mask, venting of the stomach with a nasogastric or orogastric tube is indicated, especially if airplane or helicopter transport will be used. Venting should be performed before transport because the air trapped in the gastrointestinal tract will expand in volume as atmospheric pressure decreases (see Section VI,B).

D. Temperature control and fluid balance. Special attention to temperature and fluid balance is required for infants with open lesions (eg, myelomeningocele or omphalocele). A dry or moist protective dressing over the lesion can be covered by thin plastic wrap to reduce radiant heat loss.

IV. Evaluation of transport. Each transport should have a scoring system that reflects the "before" and "after" status of the infant (Lee et al, 2001). For example, vital signs and glucose oxidase measurements taken when the team first arrives at the referring hospital should be compared with the same measurements taken on admission to the NICU. This system provides quality control of transports and is useful in outreach education to convey constructive criticism to referring hospitals. It is also important to review on a regular basis such things as team response time, referring hospital satisfaction, difficult transports, safety updates, team credentialing, and medical protocols.

V. Outreach education. Transport team members (including neonatologists and administrators) should meet with professionals from each referring hospital. Such a forum for discussion of transport issues and specific transported patients provides mutual feedback and stimulates interhospital protocol decision making (ie, should surfactant be instilled before the transport team arrives).

VI. Special considerations in air transport. Each region should develop protocols for choosing ground or air transport, based on distance, nature of the terrain, location of landing sites, and availability of aircraft and ambulances (American Academy of Pediatrics Task Force on Interhospital Transport, 1993).

A. Safety guidelines. Clear guidelines should be established regarding air transport. Decisions regarding flight safety should be made according to weather and other flight conditions (ie, the pilot should not be given information on the age of the patient or the severity of the illness before making decisions on flight safety). Controlled landing sites familiar to the pilot should be used. Loading and unloading of the aircraft should not take place while engines are running; an idling helicopter is dangerous.

B. Dysbarism. In helicopters and unpressurized aircraft, dysbarism (imbalance between air pressure in the atmosphere and the pressure of gases within the body) causes predictable problems. Partial pressures of inspired gases decrease as altitude increases, so infants will require an increased concentration of inspired oxygen (American Academy of Pediatrics, 1993). Trapped free air in the thorax or intestines will expand in volume and may cause significant pulmonary compromise. A cuffed tube or catheter should be evacuated before takeoff.

Note: Because blood pressure varies with changing gravitational force, fluctuations noted during climbing or descent should not be cause for alarm.

REFERENCES

American Academy of Pediatrics: Interhospital care of the perinatal patient. In *Guidelines for Perinatal Care,* 4th ed. American Academy of Pediatrics, 1997.

American Academy of Pediatrics Task Force on Interhospital Transport: *Guidelines for Air and Ground Transportation of Neonatal and Pediatric Patients.* American Academy of Pediatrics, 1993.

Lee SK et al: Transport risk index of physiologic stability: a practical system for assessing transport care. *J Pediatr* 2001;139:220.

13 Follow-Up of High-Risk Infants

As neonatal intensive care continues to develop as a medical specialty, concern has grown regarding the quality of life of high-risk infants. Follow-up clinics are an important and necessary adjunct to neonatal intensive care because they provide both service to infants and families and feedback to neonatologists and obstetricians.

I. **Goals of the neonatal follow-up clinic**
   A. **Early identification of developmental disability.** Some infants will be referred for further diagnostic evaluation or community services.
   B. **Parent counseling.** Parents of children who do well can be reassured by positive feedback. Anticipatory guidance can help them recognize signs of later school or behavior problems that would require further evaluation. Parents of a child with disabilities will need help in coping with their child's problems. Physical and occupational therapists can provide valuable suggestions regarding positioning, handling, and feeding of infants.
   C. **Identification and treatment of medical complications.** Some disorders may not be anticipated at the time of discharge from the neonatal intensive care unit (NICU).
   D. **Feedback for neonatologists, pediatricians, obstetricians, and pediatric surgeons** regarding developmental progress, medical status, and unusual or unforeseen complications in these infants is essential.
II. **Staff of the neonatal follow-up clinic.** Pediatricians, neurodevelopmental pediatricians, and neonatologists make up the regular staff of the clinic, and many clinics include physical therapists and neuropsychologists. Special consultation may also be needed from audiologists, ophthalmologists, occupational therapists, speech and language specialists, social workers, respiratory therapists, nutritionists, pediatric surgeons, orthopedic surgeons, or other subspecialists.
III. **Risk factors for developmental disability.** It is virtually impossible to diagnose developmental disability with certainty in the neonatal period, but a number of perinatal risk factors have been identified.
   A. **Prematurity.** Although the majority of preterm infants are not significantly handicapped, they do have a higher incidence of cerebral palsy and mental retardation than the general population (5–15% of preterm infants with birth weight <1500 g, 10–40% with birth weight <750 g). Half of all survivors born at the lower limit of viability, <26 weeks gestation, have major disabilities (Wood et al., 2000). Preterm infants also are at greater risk of disorders of higher cortical function, including language disorders, visual perception problems, attention deficits, and learning disabilities. These are also called low-severity high-prevalence conditions. Preterm infants with slow head growth (especially in the postnatal period), asphyxia, sepsis (especially meningitis), chronic lung disease, abnormal neonatal neurodevelopmental examinations, and abnormalities on cranial ultrasonography or magnetic resonance imaging (MRI) have an increased risk of developmental disability. Cranial abnormalities, including intraventricular hemorrhage (especially grades III and IV) and ventricular dilatation (with or without hemorrhage), cortical atrophy, intraparenchymal cysts (periventricular leukomalacia), and other signs of white matter injury, have a poorer prognosis. The incidence of disabilities is very high with intraparenchymal cysts, especially if they are bilateral and large.
   B. **Intrauterine growth retardation (IUGR).** Although full-term infants who are small for gestational age (SGA) appear to have only a slightly higher risk of cerebral palsy and mental retardation, they have an increased incidence of disorders of higher cortical function, especially learning disability. Preterm SGA infants have a high incidence of cerebral palsy and mental retardation,

more similar to appropriate for gestational age (AGA) preterm infants with the same birth weight than to AGA preterm infants with the same gestational age (Pena et al, 1988). The risk of neurodevelopmental disability in SGA infants is usually determined by the cause of IUGR, timing of the insult, and subsequent perinatal complications (eg, asphyxia, hypoglycemia, or polycythemia) (Allen, 1984).

C. **Asphyxia.** Perinatal asphyxia is associated with later developmental disability but is frequently difficult to define. Apgar scores are useful in predicting the outcome only when they are very low (score of 0–3) for extended periods of time (>10 min) in full-term newborns (Nelson & Ellenberg, 1981). Most outcome studies have focused on severely asphyxiated infants who required prolonged resuscitation or who were symptomatic as newborns. The mortality rate for this group is high (50%); however, 75% of the survivors are free of major handicaps. Those with handicaps usually have multiple handicaps, including severe mental retardation, spastic quadriplegia, microcephaly, seizures, and sensory impairment. The degree of abnormality on neonatal examination, electroencephalogram (EEG), and neuroimaging studies predicts neurodevelopmental outcome.

D. **Other risk factors.** Other perinatal factors are less common but are associated with a high risk of disability.

1. **TORCH infections (toxoplasmosis, other, rubella, cytomegalovirus, and herpes simplex virus).** Infants with congenital cytomegalovirus infection, toxoplasmosis, or rubella who are symptomatic at birth have a high incidence (60–90%) of developmental disability. Even if asymptomatic as neonates, they are at risk for sensory impairment and learning disability.

2. **Infection,** especially meningitis, carries a significant risk of later developmental disability.

3. **Hypoglycemia and polycythemia.** The presence of symptomatic hypoglycemia or polycythemia (hyperviscosity) at birth is associated with disability, but outcome studies have not been able to differentiate whether disability is an associated finding or its result.

4. **In utero exposure to drugs.** Maternal use of heroin or methadone during pregnancy can lead to neonatal withdrawal syndrome and a higher rate of attention deficits and behavior problems in preschool and school-age children. Fetal alcohol syndrome includes growth deficiency, dysmorphic features, congenital anomalies, mental retardation, hyperactivity, and fine motor dysfunction. Maternal use of cocaine has been associated with lower birth weights, microcephaly, cerebral infarction, abruptio placentae, fetal distress, and behavioral and EEG abnormalities in newborns, but the long-term effects of cocaine use during pregnancy are still being determined. Other drugs that appear to affect fetal development include phenytoin, trimethadione, valproate, warfarin, aminopterin, and retinoic acid.

IV. **Parameters requiring follow-up**

A. **Growth.** Growth parameters and trends should be carefully monitored at each follow-up visit. These include **length, weight, and head circumference** (see also Appendix F). Although most preterm infants "catch up" in growth during the first year, some SGA infants, extremely immature infants, and infants with severe chronic lung disease may always remain small. Poor head growth is an early indication of developmental disability.

B. **Blood pressure.** A silent sequela of neonatal intensive care that may have serious long-term consequences is high blood pressure. Blood pressure measurements should be performed for all infants on a periodic basis.

C. **Breathing disorders**

1. **Apnea.** Infants requiring home apnea monitors and those receiving theophylline for apnea require close follow-up, with special attention to whether or not resuscitation has been required. When to discontinue monitoring is a matter of debate and is usually decided by the physician and the family. (See Chapter 74.)

2. **Chronic lung disease.** Infants with chronic lung disease require specialized medical and developmental follow-up. The decision to discontinue administration of supplemental oxygen or to taper the amount should be based on pulse oximeter studies during periods of sleep, wakefulness, and feeding and on clinical criteria (ie, growth and exercise intolerance). Poor growth, sleeping or feeding difficulties, rising hematocrit, increasing abnormalities on electrocardiogram and echocardiogram, and plateauing or loss of developmental progress after discontinuing oxygen suggest intermittent hypoxia; oxygen administration should be resumed, the infant should be reexamined. Some infants with chronic lung disease who have done well breathing room air for some time may have problems if upper or lower respiratory tract infections develop.

D. **Hearing.** Because hearing is essential for the acquisition of language, it is important to diagnose hearing impairment as early as possible. All neonates should be screened for hearing impairment using either **brainstem auditory evoked potentials** or **transient evoked otoacoustic emissions.** These tests can identify infants with a high risk of hearing impairment who need careful audiologic follow-up. However, because of the high rate of false-positive results, it is difficult to diagnose hearing loss with certainty in the neonatal period. Infants with a family history of childhood hearing impairment, congenital perinatal hearing (eg, TORCH) infection, congenital malformations of the head or neck, birth weight <1500 g, hyperbilirubinemia requiring exchange transfusion, bacterial meningitis, or severe perinatal asphyxia or who were exposed to ototoxic drugs (eg, furosemide, gentamicin, vancomycin) are at high risk for hearing impairment and should be closely monitored.

E. **Vision.** Retinopathy of prematurity is a disease of the developing retina in preterm infants. An indirect ophthalmoscopic examination should be performed at 5–7 weeks by a pediatric ophthalmologist for all oxygen-exposed premature infants who weigh <1500–1800 g or are delivered at <30–35 weeks' gestation. Infants <1300 g or 30 weeks' gestation require examination regardless of oxygen exposure. Until the retina is fully vascularized, follow-up ophthalmologic examinations should be performed every 2 weeks (or every week if active disease is progressing). Infants with congenital infection and asphyxia should also have ophthalmologic examinations and follow-up. All high-risk infants should have an assessment of visual acuity by 1–5 years of age.

F. **Language and motor skills.** For each infant, a history of language and motor milestones should be obtained and compared with age norms (Capute & Palmer, 1980). Infants with persistent delay, dissociation, or deviance should be carefully assessed for disability by a developmental pediatrician or multidisciplinary team.

1. **Delay** is late acquisition of milestones.

2. **Dissociation** is delay in one area of development compared with other areas and can help diagnose disability. For example, delay in gross and fine motor development with normal language development suggests cerebral palsy, whereas delay in language acquisition with normal motor development suggests mental retardation, language disorder, or hearing impairment.

3. **Deviance** is acquisition of milestones out of normal sequence (eg, the child is able to stand but does not sit well).

G. **Neurologic development** is a dynamic process, and what is normal at a certain age may be abnormal at another. The examiner must know what is normal at each age and must decide whether deviations from normal are significant. Preterm infants are hypotonic at birth and develop flexor tone in a caudocephalad direction. Preterm infants at term and full-term newborns have flexor hypertonia and lose this flexor tone in a caudocephalad direction (ie, at 1–2 months from term, there is more flexor tone in the arms than in the legs). By 4 months from term, muscle tone should be the same in the upper and lower extremities.

1. **Neurodevelopmental examination** of high-risk infants should include assessment of the following.
   a. **Posture.**
   b. **Muscle tone in the extremities.**
   c. **Axial (neck and trunk) muscle tone.**
   d. **Deep tendon reflexes.**
   e. **Pathologic reflexes (eg, Babinski's reflex).**
   f. **Primitive reflexes (eg, Moro or asymmetric tonic neck reflex).**
   g. **Postural reactions (eg, righting or equilibrium response).**
2. **Abnormalities in high-risk infants.** Many high-risk infants have abnormalities during the first year of life that resolve by 1 year of age. Even if they disappear or do not cause significant functional impairment, these early neuromotor abnormalities may signal later dysfunction, including problems with balance, attention deficit, behavior problems, or learning disability. The presence of multiple persistent abnormalities in conjunction with motor delay suggests cerebral palsy. These infants should be referred for multidisciplinary evaluation. Because damage to the central nervous system is seldom focal, infants with motor impairment are likely to have associated deficits (eg, mental retardation, learning disability, or sensory impairment) that eventually may be more debilitating. The following developmental abnormalities are commonly seen in high-risk infants during the first year of life.
   a. **Hypotonia** (generalized or axial) is especially common in preterm infants and infants with chronic lung disease.
   b. **Hypertonia** is seen most often in the lower extremities (hips and ankles) in preterm infants.
   c. **Asymmetry** of function, tone, posture, or reflexes may be seen.
   d. **Neck extensor hypertonia and shoulder retraction** are common in infants with chronic lung disease, tracheostomy, or prolonged intubation and may interfere with head control, hand use, rolling, sitting, and getting in and out of the sitting position.
   e. **Involuntary movements, grimacing, and poor coordination** are indicative of extrapyramidal involvement.
   f. **Feeding problems** may occur.
   H. **Cognitive development.** Language development and visual attention are good early predictors of intelligence and can help identify children with cognitive impairment. Cognitive evaluation may be difficult in infants. High-risk children should have a psychological evaluation at age 1–3 years and before starting school because of the risk of learning disability. An audiologic evaluation should be performed by 6–9 months to rule out hearing impairment.
V. **Correction for prematurity.** Correcting for prematurity when assessing physical or psychological development continues to be *controversial.* Data suggest that motor milestone development proceeds according to age from conception and that one should correct for the degree of prematurity. Recommendations regarding correction for cognitive abilities vary widely: Some correct completely throughout childhood; some correct only to age 1 or 2 years; some use partial correction. We recommend calculating both the child's chronologic age and age corrected for degree of prematurity (the term age equivalent, or adjusted age). A child's language and problem-solving abilities should fall between these two ages. The older a child becomes, the less important this issue is: By the time a child is 5, arithmetically 3 months' difference (eg, 60 vs 57 months) matters little.
VI. **Multidisciplinary evaluation.** The presence of one disability is an indication for careful evaluation in other areas. Brain damage is seldom focal and often diffuse. These infants should be referred for complete multidisciplinary evaluation to identify areas of strength and weakness and to formulate an appropriate rehabilitation program. A comprehensive overview allows for a more realistic determination of prognosis. Appropriate counseling can then be given to the parents.

REFERENCES

Allen MC: After the intensive care nursery: follow-up and outcome. In Rudolph AM et al (eds): *Rudolph's Pediatrics,* 21st ed. Appleton & Lange, 2001.

Allen MC: Developmental implication of intrauterine growth retardation. *Inf Young Child* 1992;5:3.

Allen MC: Developmental outcome and follow-up of the small for gestational age infant. *Semin Perinatol* 1984;8:123.

Allen MC: Limits of viability in the newborn. In Burg FD et al (eds): *Current Pediatric Therapy,* 16th ed. Saunders, 1999.

Allen MC: Outcome and followup of high-risk infants. In Taesch W, Ballard RA (eds): *Schaeffer and Avery's Diseases of the Newborn,* 7th ed. Saunders, 1998.

Allen MC, Alexander GR: Using motor milestones as a multistep process to screen preterm infants for cerebral palsy. *Dev Med Child Neurol* 1997;39:12.

Allen MC, Capute AJ: Neonatal neurodevelopmental examination as a predictor of neuromotor outcome in premature infants. *Pediatrics* 1989;83:498.

Aylward GP: Cognitive and neuropsychological outcomes: more than IQ scores. *Ment Ret Dev Dis Res Rev* 2002;8:234.

Bandstra ES, Burkett G: Maternal-fetal and neonatal effects of in utero cocaine exposure. *Semin Perinatol* 1991;15:288.

Bracewell M, Marlow N: Patterns of motor disability in very preterm children. *Ment Ret Dev Dis Res Rev* 2002;8:241.

Capute AJ, Palmer FB: A pediatric overview of the spectrum of developmental disabilities. *J Dev Behav Pediatr* 1980;1:66.

Capute AJ et al: Clinical linguistic and auditory milestone scale: prediction of cognition in infancy. *Dev Med Child Neurol* 1986;28:762.

Capute AJ et al: Normal gross motor development: the influence of race, sex and socioeconomic status. *Dev Med Child Neurol* 1985;27:635.

de Vries LS, Groenendaal F: Neuroimaging in the preterm infant. *Ment Ret Dev Dis Res Rev* 2002;8:273.

Msall ME, Tremont MR: Measuring functional outcomes after prematurity. developmental impact of very low birth weight and extremely low birth weight status on childhood disability. *Ment Ret Dev Dis Res Rev* 2002;8:258.

Nelson KB, Ellenberg JH: Apgar scores as predictors of chronic neurologic disability. *Pediatrics* 1981;68:36.

Nelson KB, Leviton A: How much of neonatal encephalopathy is due to birth asphyxia? *Am J Dis Child* 1991;145:1325.

Pena IC et al: The premature small for gestational age infant during the first year of life: comparison by birthweight and gestational age. *J Pediatr* 1988;113:1106.

Robertson C, Finer N: Term infants with hypoxic-ischemic encephalopathy: outcome at 3–5 years. *Dev Med Child Neurol* 1985;27:473.

Robertson CMT et al: Eight year school performance and growth of preterm, small for gestational age infants: a comparative study with subjects matched for birth weight or for gestational age. *J Pediatr* 1990;93:636.

Saigal S et al: Cognitive abilities and school performance of extremely low birth weight children and matched term control children at age 8 years: a regional study. *J Pediatr* 1991;118:751.

Wachtel RC et al: A tool for the pediatric evaluation of infants and young children with developmental delay. *Clin Pediatr* 1994;33:410.

Weislas-Kuperus N et al: Neonatal cerebral ultrasound, neonatal neurology and perinatal conditions as predictors of neurodevelopmental outcome in very low birthweight infants. *Early Hum Dev* 1992;31:131.

Wood NS et al: Neurologic and developmental disability after extreme preterm birth. *N Engl J Med* 2000;343:378.

14 Neurologic Evaluation

All studies available in the neonatal period for neurologic evaluation are limited, especially in their ability to accurately predict future intelligence and motor, language, and problem-solving skills. Most tests will provide a gross picture of the brain and its structures without the ability to provide information on function. Also, because of the enormous plasticity of the neonate's brain, even significant defects detectable with these tests may result in "normal" neurodevelopmental outcomes.

I. **Neuroimaging**
  A. **Ultrasonography**
    1. **Definition.** By using the bone window of a fontanelle, sound waves are directed into the brain and reflected according to the echodensity of the underlying structures. The reflected waves are used to create 2- and 3-dimensional images.
    2. **Indication.** Ultrasonography is the preferred tool for identification and observation of germinal matrix/intraventricular hemorrhage and hydrocephalus and is valuable in detecting midline structural abnormalities, hypoxic-ischemic injury, subdural and posterior fossa hemorrhage, ventriculitis, tumors, cysts, and vascular abnormalities. Ultrasonography of the developing cingulate sulcus has been suggested to reflect gestational age. (See sample studies in Chapter 9.)
    3. **Method.** A transducer is placed over the anterior fontanelle, and images are obtained in coronal and parasagittal planes. The posterior fontanelle is the preferred acoustic window for the imaging of the infratentorium, including brainstem and cerebellum (Di Salvo, 2001). Advantages of this technique include high resolution, convenience (performed at the bedside), safety (no sedation, contrast material, or radiation), noninvasiveness, and low cost compared with other imaging studies. Disadvantages include the lack of visualization of nonmidline structures, especially in the parietal regions, and the lack of differentiation between gray and white matter.
    4. **Results.** The integrity of the following structures may be evaluated with ultrasonography: all four ventricles, the choroid plexus, caudate nuclei, thalamus, septum pellucidum, and corpus callosum.
  B. **Doppler ultrasonography**
    1. **Definition.** Like regular ultrasonography, this technique uses a bone window to direct sound waves into the brain. Moving objects (eg, red blood cells) will reflect sound waves with a shift in frequency (Doppler shift) that is proportional to their speed. These changes are measured and expressed as the pulsatility index. The angle of the probe in relation to the flow affects the Doppler shift and requires exact standards for serial measurements.
    2. **Indication.** Knowing the cross-section of the vessel (area), Doppler ultrasonography can provide information on cerebral blood flow (CBF) and resistance.

$$CBF \ (cm^3/time) = CBF \ velocity \ (cm/time) \times Area \ (cm^2)$$

$$Resistance = \frac{(Peak \ systolic \ velocity - Peak \ diastolic \ velocity)}{Peak \ systolic \ velocity}$$

Changes in CBF and resistance have been noted in a variety of pathologic states. Doppler ultrasonography is of clinical value in states of cessation of CBF (eg, brain death or cerebrovascular occlusion), states of altered vascular resistance (eg, hypoxic-ischemic encephalopathy, hydrocephalus, or arteriovenous malformation), and ductal steal syndrome.

3. **Method.** Combined with conventional ultrasonography to identify the blood vessel, Doppler ultrasonography produces a color image indicating flow (red = toward the transducer, blue = away from the transducer). CBF velocity is measured as the area under the curve of velocity waveforms. Small body weight and low gestational ages negatively influence the success rate in visualizing intracranial vasculature.

4. **Results.** Doppler ultrasonography measurements can be compared with age-adjusted norm values for systolic, end-diastolic, and mean flow velocity (Bode & Wais, 1988). Although this technique is not yet a standard bedside tool, it might also prove useful in the evaluation of progressive hydrocephalus and the need for ventriculoperitoneal shunts (decreased CBF secondary to increased intracranial pressure).

C. **Computed tomography (CT)**

1. **Definition.** Using computerized image reconstruction, CT produces 2- and 3-dimensional images of patients exposed to ionizing radiation.

2. **Indication.** CT is the preferred tool for evaluation of the posterior fossa and nonmidline disorders (eg, blood or fluid collection in the subdural or subarachnoid space) as well as parenchymal disorders. It is also helpful in the diagnosis of skull fractures.

3. **Method.** The patient is placed into the scanner and advanced in small increments, and images (cuts) are obtained. Cerebral white matter (more fatty tissue in myelin sheaths around the nerves) and inflammation appear less dense (blacker) than gray matter. Calcifications and hemorrhages appear white. If a patient receives contrast material, blood vessels and vascular structures (eg, falx cerebri and choroid plexus) will appear white. Spaces containing cerebrospinal fluid are clearly shown in black, making it easy to identify diseases that alter their size and shape. Bones also appear white but are poorly defined, and details are better evaluated in a "bone window." Disadvantages include the need for transportation of the neonate, the need for sedation, the potential for hypothermia, and radiation exposure.

4. **Results.** CT provides detailed information on brain structures not accessible by ultrasonography and is superior to magnetic resonance imaging (MRI) in the diagnosis of intracranial calcifications.

D. **MRI**

1. **Definition.** Inside a strong magnetic field, atomic nuclei with magnetic properties (hydrogen protons being most common) align themselves and emit an electromagnetic signal when the field is terminated and the nuclei return to their natural state. Computers reconstruct the signal into 2-dimensional image cuts.

2. **Indication.** MRI is the preferred tool for a number of brain disorders in the neonate that are difficult to visualize by CT, such as disorders of myelination or neural migration, ischemic or hemorrhagic lesions, agenesis of the corpus callosum, arteriovenous malformations, and lesions in the posterior fossa and the spinal cord. Newer functional MRI techniques such as diffusion-weighted imaging (DWI) and blood-oxygenation-dependent (BOLD) imaging provide information on brain physiology but remain controversial at present.

3. **Method.** The patient is placed into the scanner and advanced in small increments, and images (cuts) are obtained. Gray matter appears gray, and white matter, white. Cerebrospinal fluid and bones appear black; however, the fat content in the bone marrow and the scalp appear white. Disadvantages include the need for transportation of the neonate, the potential for hypothermia, difficulties in monitoring the infant during the procedure, and the need for removal of all ferromagnetic objects. Before the advent of ul-

trafast MRI, long procedure times often required sedation. Because of the need for a ferromagnetic-free environment, ventilated infants pose a special problem.

4. **Results.** MRI provides high-resolution images of the brain with exquisite anatomic detail and allows diagnosis of a number of illnesses easily missed by CT. The temporal development of the prenatal brain, including the emergence of sulci and gyri and the myelination process, has been described, allowing for a more meaningful interpretation of MRI in premature infants (Huppi & Inder, 2001). Quantitative volumetric MRI has been used to demonstrate the effects of postnatal dexamethasone on cortical gray matter volume. Diffusion-weighted MRI can be used in the early diagnosis of perinatal hypoxic-ischemic encephalopathy at *any* stage of development. Functional MRI promises new insights into the functional reorganization of the brain after injury. Newer magnetic resonance spectroscopy (MRS) allows the study of metabolic mechanisms through quantitative measurements of certain metabolites.

E. **Near-infrared spectroscopy**
1. **Definition.** Light in the near-infrared range can easily pass through skin, thin bone, and other tissues of the neonate. At selected wavelengths, light absorption is dependent on oxygenated and deoxygenated hemoglobin as well as oxidized cytochrome aa_3, allowing for qualitative measurements of oxygen delivery, cerebral blood volume, and brain oxygen availability and consumption (Volpe, 2001).
2. **Indication.** Although near-infrared spectroscopy is not widely used, it has potential as a bedside tool to follow cerebral oxygen delivery or CBF. It may become a useful technique to assess the effects of new treatments and common interventions (eg, endotracheal suction) on cerebral perfusion and oxygenation.
3. **Method.** A fiberoptic bundle applied to the scalp transmits laser light. Another fiberoptic bundle collects light and transmits it to a photon counter.
4. **Results.** Near-infrared spectroscopy allows qualitative determination of oxygen delivery, cerebral blood volume, and oxygen consumption. In intubated infants near-infrared spectroscopy has been used to identify pressure-passive cerebral circulation, a condition associated with a fourfold increase in periventricular leukomalacia and severe intraventricular hemorrhage.

II. **Electrographic studies**
A. **Electroencephalogram (EEG)**
1. **Definition.** An EEG continuously captures the electrical activity between reference electrodes on the scalp. In the neonatal period, cerebral maturation and development result in significant EEG changes during different gestational ages that must be considered when interpreting results.
2. **Indication.** Indications include documented or suspected seizure activity, events with potential for cerebral injury (eg, hypoxic-ischemic, hemorrhagic, traumatic, or infectious), central nervous system (CNS) malformations, metabolic disorders, developmental abnormalities, and chromosomal abnormalities.
3. **Method.** Several electrodes are attached to the infant's scalp, and the electrical activity is amplified and measured. Recordings can be traced on paper or can be saved electronically. EEG waves are classified into different frequencies: delta (1–3/s), theta (4–7/s), alpha (8–12/s), and beta (13–20/s).
4. **Results.** A number of abnormal findings can be documented on the EEG of the term and preterm infant, including the following:

- Abnormal pattern of development.
- Depression or lack of differentiation.
- Electrocerebral silence ("flat" EEG).

- Burst suppression pattern (depressed background activity alternating with short periods of paroxysmal bursts).
- Persistent voltage asymmetry.
- Sharp waves (multifocal or central).
- Periodic discharges.
- Rhythmic alpha-frequency activity.

Burst suppression patterns are associated with especially high morbidity and mortality and poor prognosis. EEGs are sensitive to a number of external factors, including acute and ongoing illness, medications or drugs, position of the electrodes, and state of arousal.

B. Cerebral function monitor (CFM)

1. **Definition.** CFM or amplitude-integrated EEG records a single EEG channel. The range of the signal amplitude is displayed in microvolts. Discontinuity in the EEG results in a wider trace amplitude and a decreased lower margin.

2. **Indication.** The cerebral function monitor allows for the fast identification of infants at risk for severe hypoxic-ischemic encephalopathy (HIE). Availability of this technique is dependent on institutional practice.

3. **Method.** Three electrodes are attached to the scalp, and the EEG channel is recorded at a speed of 6 cm/h. CFM cannot provide information on EEG frequency or focal lesions. Unlike standard EEG, this technique requires fewer operating and interpreting skills, making it more readily available.

4. **Results.** After asphyxia, the occurrence of a moderately or severely abnormal CFM trace has a positive predictive value >70% for abnormal neurologic outcome.

C. Peripheral nerve conduction velocity

1. **Definition.** Nerve conduction velocity allows the diagnosis of a peripheral nerve disorder by measuring the transmission speed of an electrical stimulus along a peripheral (median, ulnar, peroneal) nerve. Because of smaller nerve fiber diameters affecting the nerve transmission speed, neonates are found to have a lower nerve conduction velocity than adults.

2. **Indication.** In the workup of the weak and hypotonic neonate, nerve conduction velocity is an important tool in diagnosing a peripheral nerve disorder.

3. **Method.** A peripheral nerve is stimulated with a skin electrode, and the corresponding muscle action potential is recorded with another skin electrode. To determine the nerve conduction alone (as opposed to nerve conduction, synaptic transmission, and muscle reaction), the nerve is stimulated at two points and the resulting muscle response times are subtracted. The distance between the two points of stimulation divided by the time difference equals the nerve conduction velocity.

4. **Results.** Nerve conduction velocities are prolonged in disorders of myelination and in axon abnormalities and may have potential clinical value in combination with other tests (eg, muscle biopsy or electromyogram) in these disorders. Initially, infants with anterior horn cell disorders (eg, Werdnig-Hoffmann paralysis) will have normal nerve conduction but may demonstrate decreased velocity later in the course. Neuromuscular junction and muscle disorders do not alter nerve conduction velocity. This test has also been used for gestational age assessment.

D. Evoked potentials. An evoked potential is an electrical response by the CNS to a specific stimulus. Evoked potentials are used to evaluate the intactness and maturity of *ascending* sensory pathways of the nervous system and are relatively unaffected by state, drug, or metabolic effects.

1. **Auditory evoked potential**

   a. **Definition.** An auditory evoked potential is an electrical response by the CNS to an auditory stimulus.

b. Indication. Brainstem auditory evoked potentials may be used to detect abnormalities in threshold sensitivities, conduction time, amplitudes, and shape and may be useful as a hearing screen in high-risk infants.

c. Method. Although neonates respond to an auditory stimulus with brainstem as well as cortical evoked responses, the latter are variable, depending on the state of arousal, and thus difficult to interpret. As a result, auditory evoked potentials (generated by a rapid sequence of clicks or pure tones) traveling along the eighth nerve to the diencephalon are recorded by an electrode over the mastoid and vertex as **brainstem auditory evoked responses,** amplified and digitally stored. The shape (a series of waves) and latency of brainstem auditory evoked potentials depend on gestational age. This technique is sensitive to movement and ambient noise.

d. Results. Injuries in the peripheral pathway (middle ear, cochlea, and eighth nerve) will result in an increased sound threshold and an increase in latency of all waves, whereas central lesions will cause only increased latency of waves originating from distal (in relation to the lesion) structures. Brainstem auditory evoked potentials have been used to demonstrate disorders of the auditory pathways caused by hypoxia-ischemia, hyperbilirubinemia, bacterial meningitis, and other infections (eg, cytomegalovirus [CMV]), intracranial hemorrhage, trauma, systemic illnesses, drugs (eg, aminoglycoside or furosemide), or a combination of these.

When used as a screening procedure at the time of neonatal intensive care unit (NICU) discharge in low birth weight infants, brainstem auditory evoked potentials have a high false-positive rate secondary, in all likelihood, to known gestational differences (longer latency, decreased amplitude, and increased threshold in preterm infants). Up to 20–25% of NICU infants have abnormal (failed) tests, and most have normal tests at 2–4 months (Stapells & Kurtzberg, 1991). In asphyxiated infants abnormal brainstem auditory evoked potentials are associated with neuromotor impairments. Because infants with congenital infection and persistent pulmonary hypertension may experience progressive hearing loss, they require serial hearing evaluations even if initial auditory evoked responses are normal.

2. **Visual evoked potential**
   a. **Definition.** A visual evoked potential is an electrical response by the CNS to a visual stimulus.
   b. **Indication.** Visual evoked potential may provide information on disorders of the visual pathway and has been used as an indicator for cerebral malfunctioning (eg, hypoxia) (Woods et al, 1981).
   c. **Method.** An electrical response to a visual stimulus (eg, light flash in neonates or checkerboard pattern reversal in older children) is measured via a surface electrode. The electrical response is complex and undergoes significant developmental changes in the preterm infant.
   d. **Results.** When corrected for conceptual age, visual evoked responses allow the detection of various visual pathway abnormalities. Although generalized insults such as severe hypoxemia may result in temporary loss of visual evoked responses, local abnormalities may have similar results (eg, compression of the pathway in hydrocephalus). Persistent visual evoked response abnormalities in postasphyxiated infants have been strongly correlated with poor neurologic outcomes (Muttitt et al, 1991). Although visual evoked potentials may aid in the prognosis of long-term neurodevelopmental outcomes, they may not be helpful in predicting blindness or loss of vision. Improvements in visual evoked responses have also been applied to determine the success of interventions such as a ventricular-peritoneal shunt.

3. **Somatosensory evoked potential**
   a. **Definition.** A somatosensory evoked potential is an electrical response by the CNS to a peripheral sensory stimulus.
   b. **Indication.** Somatosensory evoked potentials allow insight into disorders of the sensory pathway (peripheral nerve, plexus, dorsal root, posterior column, contralateral nucleus, medial lemniscus, thalamus, and parietal cortex).
   c. **Method.** Somatosensory evoked potentials have been recorded over the contralateral parietal scalp after providing an electric stimulus to the median or the posterior tibial nerve. Somatosensory evoked potentials are technically more difficult to obtain than auditory brainstem evoked potentials and are age dependent, with significant changes occurring in the first months of life.
   d. **Results.** Somatosensory evoked potentials may allow evaluation of peripheral lesions such as spinal cord trauma and myelodysplasia as well as cerebral abnormalities such as hypoxia-ischemia, hemorrhage, hydrocephalus, hypoglycemia, and hypothyroidism. Somatosensory evoked potential abnormalities in term infants have a high positive predictive value for neurologic sequelae (Willis et al, 1989) and abnormal neurodevelopmental outcome (Majnemer et al, 1990). Their significance remains *controversial* in the preterm infant.

III. **Clinical neurodevelopmental examination**
   A. **Definition.** The clinical neurodevelopmental examination combines the assessment of posture, movement, extremity and axial muscle tone, deep tendon reflexes, pathologic reflexes (eg, Babinski's sign), primitive (or primary) reflexes, cranial nerve and oromotor function, sensory responses, and behavior by an experienced clinician.
   B. **Indication.** All infants should undergo a brief neurologic examination, including tone and reflex assessment, as part of their initial physical examination. A more detailed neurodevelopmental examination should be performed on high-risk infants. Important risk factors include prematurity, hypoxic-ischemic encephalopathy (Robertson & Finer, 1993), congenital infection, meningitis, significant abnormalities on neuroimaging studies (eg, intraventricular hemorrhage, ventricular dilatation, intraparenchymal hemorrhage, infarct, or cysts), and feeding difficulties.
   C. **Method.** The experienced clinician should examine the infant when stable, preferably during the recovery phase. However, the exam may also be quite useful when performed serially, as with hypoxic-ischemic encephalopathy. The infant's state of alertness may affect many responses, including sensory response, behavior, tone, and reflexes. Normal findings change according to age (actual and postconceptional) (Allen, 1996a, 1996b).
   1. **The full-term neonate.** The normal full-term neonate has flexor hypertonia, hip adductor tone, hyperreflexia (may have unsustained clonus), symmetric tone and reflexes, good trunk tone on ventral suspension, some degree of head lag on pulling to a sitting from a supine position with modulation of forward head movement, presence of pathologic (eg, Babinski's sign) and primitive reflexes (eg, Moro, grasp, and asymmetric tonic neck reflexes), alerting to sound, visual fixation, and a fixed focal length of 8 in.
   2. **The preterm neonate.** Before 30 weeks' postconceptional age, the infant is markedly hypotonic. Extremity flexor and axial tone and the reflexes emerge in a caudocephalad (ie, lower to upper extremity) and centripetal (ie, distal to proximal) manner. Visual attention and acuity improve with postconceptional age. The extremely preterm infant can suck and swallow, but coordination of suck with swallow occurs at ~32–34 weeks' postconceptional age. Flexor tone peaks at term and then becomes decreased in a caudocephalad manner. In comparison to full-term neonates, preterm infants at term have less flexor hypertonia, more extensor tone, more asymmetries, and mild differences in behavior.

D. Results. Abnormalities on neurodevelopmental examination include asymmetries of posture or reflexes (especially significant if marked or persistent), decreased flexor or extremity tone or axial tone for postconceptional age, cranial nerve or oromotor dysfunction, abnormal sensory responses, abnormal behavior (eg, lethargy, irritability, or jitteriness), and extensor neck, trunk, or extremity tone. A normal neonatal neurodevelopmental examination is reassuring, but an abnormal exam cannot be used to diagnose disability in the neonatal period (Allen & Capute, 1989). The more abnormalities are found on examination and the greater the degree of abnormality (eg, marked neck extensor hypertonia), the higher is the incidence of later disability, including cerebral palsy and mental retardation.

REFERENCES

Allen MC: The neonatal neurodevelopmental examination. In Capute AJ, Accardo PJ (eds): *Developmental Disabilities in Infancy and Childhood,* Vol 1, 2nd ed. Brookes, 1996a.

Allen MC: Preterm development. In Capute AJ, Accardo PJ (eds): *Developmental Disabilities in Infancy and Childhood,* Vol 2, 2nd ed. Brookes, 1996b.

Allen MC, Capute AJ: Neonatal neurodevelopmental examination as a predictor of neuromotor outcome in premature infants. *Pediatrics* 1989;83:498.

Bode H, Wais U: Age dependence of flow velocities in basal cerebral arteries. *Arch Dis Child* 1988;63:606.

Di Salvo DN: A new view of the neonatal brain: clinical utility of supplemental neurologic US imaging windows. *Radiographics* 2001;21:943.

Huppi PS, Inder TE: Magnetic resonance techniques in the evaluation of the perinatal brain: recent advances and future directions. *Semin Neonatol* 2001;6:195.

Majnemer A et al: Prognostic significance of multimodality response testing in high-risk newborns. *Pediatr Neurol* 1990;6:367.

Muttitt SC et al: Serial visual evoked potentials and outcome in term birth asphyxia. *Pediatr Neurol* 1991;7:86.

Robertson CM, Finer NN: Long-term follow-up of term infants with perinatal asphyxia. *Clin Perinatol* 1993;20:483.

Stapells DR, Kurtzberg D: Evoked potential assessment of auditory system integrity in infants. *Clin Perinatol* 1991;18:497.

Volpe JJ: *Neurology of the Newborn,* 4th ed. Saunders, 2001.

Willis J et al: Somatosensory evoked potentials predict neuromotor outcome after periventricular hemorrhage. *Dev Med Child Neurol* 1989;31:435.

Woods JR Jr et al: Birth asphyxia: I. Measurement of visual evoked potential (VEP) in the healthy fetus and newborn lamb. *Pediatr Res* 1981;15:1429.

15 Neonatal Bioethics

I. **Introduction.** *Ethics* is a term to describe "doing good." The study of bioethics as a field separate from medicine itself is a recent phenomenon. Physicians historically set and maintained policies concerning ethical behavior in medical practice. During the last 20 years, the distinct study of bioethics has been mostly populated with philosophers and sociologists as opposed to medical doctors. In many ways, this insurgence of different perspectives has been very good for the field of bioethics. However, the *practice* of bioethics is inherently a physician's task. The obligation to act in an ethical manner in medical practice requires that we know something about how we should act and what internal and external guidelines should be followed to accomplish that end. Although we can look at bioethical problems from several perspectives, we focus on virtue ethics in this chapter. Virtue ethics deals with the internal virtues of the physician as a starting point to resolving ethical conflicts. From this framework, we will study specific conflicts in bioethics and possible solutions.

II. **Virtue and the physician.** Despite an increasing public distrust of physicians' motives, the practice of medicine requires physicians to perform in an exceptionally professional manner. Indeed, the very idea of "professional" is closely linked to good conduct and virtuous behavior. Several important virtues make the practice of medicine a profession as opposed to everyday work (Pellegrino & Thomasma, 1993).

   A. **Fidelity to trust.** Trust is an important virtue in any human relationship. This involves not only truth telling but also aspects of consistency, integrity, and confidence. The medical relationship between physician and patient extends even further into this idea of trust. The relationship between professionals such as physicians, lawyers, and ministers is termed a fiduciary relationship (Barber, 1983). In such a relationship, the patient trusts the physician to help the patient, and the physician is expected to provide this help to the best of his or her ability. The patient's trust in a physician is multifactorial; the patient trusts not only that a physician is, in fact, properly trained and competent, but that he or she will also use that training in an unbiased and selfless manner for the patient's welfare. Because of this special trust relationship, physicians should have the fidelity to trust. In other words, as physicians, we should always be found trustworthy.

   B. **Compassion.** If there is one aspect of a physician's character that is most scrutinized by patients, it is compassion. Compassion, although difficult to precisely define, is the quality most associated with ethical behavior. The word *compassion* (*com* meaning "with" and *passion* meaning "suffering") literally means to "suffer with" your patient. This goes beyond *pity* (to feel sorry for the patient's condition) or *empathy* (understanding the cause of the patient's suffering). To express compassion is to abide with the patient during suffering. In today's world of health maintenance organizations (HMOs) and managed care, time for this virtue of compassion is shrinking, but this remains as a quality that sets us apart from those with mere technical knowledge and application.

   C. **Phronesis.** The term *phronesis* was used by Aristotle for the virtue of practical wisdom, the capacity for moral insight, the capacity, in a given set of circumstances, to discern what moral choice or course of action is most conducive to the good of the agent or the activity in which the agent is engaged (Pellegrino, 1983).

   In short, *phronesis* can be defined as "common sense." This ability to examine options and sensibly decide a course of action will always be a physician-centered activity. Phronesis is closely linked to the ability to reason and to do so in an unbiased manner. Its application in medical practice relies heavily on the other virtues, such as trust and compassion.

D. **Justice.** *Justice* is defined as "the rendering to one what is due." As physicians, we have a specific obligation to render to our patients what is due: the patient's healing. The virtue of justice also indicates an unfailing quality. This quality is linked to the rule of nonmaleficence or the avoidance of doing harm to the patient. Physicians owe justice not only to their patients but also to the community and society in general. The physician is influenced in the quality of justice by patient autonomy, economic pressures, and personal beliefs. All of these factors may clarify or contrast issues involving justice.

E. **Fortitude.** *Fortitude* describes not only physical but also mental and emotional courage. We tend to think of courage in terms of a soldier in battle, but physicians display courage in a variety of ways: caring for patients with HIV infection, continuing in our care long past any hour that reasonable jobs would require, and facing the emotional wear and tear of dealing with families in crisis situations.

F. **Temperance.** *Temperance,* or *prudence,* is usually thought of in terms of social activities or moral life. The physician also would be wise to consider this; however, temperance in medicine deals with our use of technology. As new procedures and tests become available, physicians have a tendency to use them regardless of any true advantage they might have over tests that are more standard. We should think twice before ordering the newest and latest test.

G. **Integrity.** To *integrate* is to "bring all parts together." In the same sense, physicians need to have all the parts together. Our outward presentation to patients and families should be that of consistency and predictability. This virtue is important in developing trust in our physician–patient relationships. True integrity, as opposed to a facade of self-confidence, requires self-examination and reflection on an ongoing basis.

H. **Self-effacement.** *Self-effacement* is not "the elevation of oneself above another." This virtue is usually well understood by residents, especially in the relationship between attending and resident. Although physicians are highly trained and skilled in the art of medicine, it is important to remember our place; we are to help the parents (or guardians) in caring for the patient. To presuppose that lengthy schooling gives us some higher authority is faulty. Self-effacement also involves attitudes toward patients in research studies and protocols.

III. **Pediatric issues**
A. **The best-interest standard.** When physicians work with patients who cannot talk, either because of age or because of mental incapacity, we cannot obtain direct consent for treatment and procedures. In these cases, we must decide which treatment options the patient would choose. This is called the "best interest standard," which describes what we should do as physicians: Provide care that is in the patient's best interest. In the case of young children, we normally assume that the parents have the best idea of what constitutes the child's best interest. In other cases, the patient's best interests are decided by a spouse, guardian, or legal appointee. Physicians sometimes assume this role in emergencies when there is not enough time to contact other responsible family members.

B. **Parents as patient advocates**
1. **Parental rights.** In the care of infants and children, the parents are uniformly thought to represent the patient's best interests. They are intimately involved in the child's situation and will be long after the physician is out of the picture. Because of this, the parents should be given great authority in the decision-making process. Unless imminent harm will come to the child, the parents should be permitted to make all decisions concerning the welfare of their child.

2. **Exception cases.** There are a few cases in which parental rights are not maintained. The widest known of these concerns blood transfusions in children of families believing in the Jehovah's Witness sect. Because of religious reasons, the parents refuse all blood transfusions or blood products. Their right to refuse potentially lifesaving therapy, however, commonly does not extend to the children. The reasoning is that this particular request is outside of what is "normal and usual" in American society, and thus the parental right to refuse this therapy is challenged. Normally, a physician can seek a court order that will place the child in the custody of the state, which then consents to blood transfusion. This same standard has been applied to other parental requests that are outside what would be reasonably expected. Refusal of surgery for a correctable anomaly or demand for treatments that have no effectiveness are cases in which parental rights may be refused.

C. **Minors as parents.** Increasingly, we see teenagers—minors themselves—now giving birth to children. This places the parent in a paradoxical role: the teenager who is unable to give consent for herself because she is a minor but holds great authority over her child. In most circumstances, the minor parent is treated with adult status. From this point on, she manages her individual health care issues as well as those of her child. In many cases, there may be an overseer figure, such as a grandparent, who helps in this decision process. It is important to note, however, that the parent does have final say in issues of consent and treatment unless that minor parent is otherwise incapacitated.

D. **Child abuse.** Normally, we think of child abuse as occurring after birth, when we see a number of injuries and problems associated with this, such as physical and emotional abuse, neglect, or sexual abuse. Several states, however, have made proposals to prosecute prenatal child abuse by mothers who act in a harmful or neglectful manner toward their unborn infants. Continued intravenous or cocaine drug abuse is thought of as directly harmful to the fetus and, in some instances, has been prosecuted. In these cases, the child becomes a ward of the state after birth.

IV. **Specific issues in neonatology**

A. **Informed consent.** *Informed consent* is a recent term. It implies the two components required for proper treatment of patients. First, they must be informed completely of the disease and its short- and long-term ramifications. Additionally, the treatment or procedures should be performed in a like manner. Potential major complications, long-term side effects, and indications and benefits of the treatment or procedure must be explained to the understanding of the parents. Possible alternative treatment should also be presented. As physicians, we also need to evaluate the consent that is given. Do the parents have a good understanding of the child's disease, prognosis, and therapeutic options? Are the parents capable of acting in the child's best interest and thus capable of giving consent? Obviously, it is impossible to discuss every complication or ramification of the operation; however, some mention should be made that other complications exist, and the major complications should be listed. These should be explained more fully if the parent desires. The consent obtained should always be durable and written, not assumed merely because the parent voices no dissenting opinion. Emergency and life-threatening situations complicate our ability to obtain informed consent. It is prudent, therefore, to try to discuss potential problems before they develop.

B. **Withholding care.** There is sometimes a feeling among physicians that, in order to provide optimal care, patients should be offered every technologic treatment or procedure possible. In many cases, however, the application of highly technical procedures is not in the best interest of the patient. Frequently, critically ill infants who are not responding to present therapy should have further or more advanced therapy withheld. The decision in these cases rests on whether further therapy will:

- Have its intended effect.
- Reverse the process.
- Restore the quality of life that is acceptable to the patient or the caregivers.

With these goals in mind, one can see that it is as important to obtain informed consent for withholding care as it is for the application of procedures. The physician should not withhold care without discussing this course of action with the parents. Likewise, the decision to withhold care should be discussed with the other physicians and nursing staff involved. The indications for and benefits of withholding care should be clearly defined.

C. **Withdrawing care.** In some cases, care can and should be withdrawn for a number of reasons.
  1. **The care or treatment** rendered no longer accomplishes its intended purpose (ie, futility of care).
  2. **Ongoing evaluations or tests** reveal information changing the diagnosis or prognosis of the patient. In these cases, reevaluation and discussion with the patient's parents are required to provide for the patient's best interest with this new information.
  3. **Care given in an emergency** should be withdrawn if it is contrary to the parents' wishes when they are informed.
     As noted, there are a few legal exceptions to this rule. Overall, the withdrawal of care hinges on the idea of futility. Does the patient benefit from such care? Can we expect the therapy to accomplish both short- and long-term goals? As an example, the use of pressor agents in a moribund infant may reach the point of futility. If the short-term goal (ie, raising the blood pressure) is not accomplished and neither is the long-term goal (ie, restoring health), then therapy is no longer useful and should be withdrawn. The difficulty with withdrawing care rests on the definition of *futility.* This may depend on the health care worker's perspective. The ability of a physician to use the virtues of compassion, phronesis, and temperance come into play when discussing these issues. At every step, the patient's parents should be clearly informed of the decisions and possible outcomes.

D. **Nutrition and patient comfort.** *Nutrition* has been classified as a therapy, that is, as a medicine that could potentially be withdrawn or, in other instances, as one of the basic patient's rights for comfort. In any discussion of ethics and patient care, there is consensus that the patient should be provided some basic comforts despite what other circumstance may be in question. The comfort of nursing care, cleanliness, pain relief, and mere presence are factors considered to be basic to human life and not subject to diminution or withdrawal, secondary to end-of-life issues. In most cases, nutrition (ie, food and water) is classified as one of these basic comfort cares. This has been contested in the legal system in a variety of cases, with a broad spectrum of varying opinions. With this in mind, it is probably wise to assume nutrition and feeding to be basic rights for patient care and to challenge this position only in extreme circumstances. The parents' understanding of nutrition as therapy or as a basic right is important. Agreement among the parents, caregivers, administration, and legal authorities must be obtained if the withdrawal of nutrition is contemplated. The activation and opinion of the institution's bioethics committee may be very helpful in resolving these issues.

E. **Delivery room issues.** Neonatal care in the delivery room requires rapid assessment and quick decision making. In infants with severe congenital anomalies or extreme prematurity, these first few moments of life are critical. In these instances, the pediatrician is called on to make critical decisions within seconds concerning viability, quality of life, and prognosis. Care during this period should be guided by the following general principles.

1. **Discuss as fully as possible** with the parents their wishes and expectations before actual delivery of the child. Coordination between the pediatricians and obstetricians can facilitate this dialogue.
2. **Err on the side of life.** If the mother is unable to express her wishes, then emergency therapy must be performed. It is much better to err on the side of life-sustaining therapy than to withhold such therapy. If in the aftermath of this crisis it is discovered that the parents wish no such therapy, then it is appropriate to withdraw therapy. This, however, gives the parents the opportunity to form their own opinion and exercise their right in protecting the child's best interest.
3. **Noninitiation of resuscitation** in the extremely immature infant or in cases of severe congential anomaly is a challenging problem in neonatology. According to guidelines from the American Heart Association and American Academy of Pediatrics, noninitiation of resuscitation appears appropriate in confirmed gestation of <23 weeks or birth weight <400 g, anencephaly, or confirmed trisomy 13 or 18 (Kattwinkel, 2000) In these cases, all data suggest that resuscitation of these infants is highly unlikely to result in survival or survival without severe disability. In cases in which the antenatal information may be unreliable or with uncertain prognosis, options include a period of resuscitation with the option of discontinuation of the resuscitation if assessment of the infant after delivery does not support the continued efforts. Initial resuscitation and subsequent withdrawal of support may allow time to gather key clinical information and to counsel the family appropriately.
4. **Discontinuation of resuscitation may be appropriate** if the infant fails to have return of spontaneous circulation within 15 min. This is based on strong data suggesting that after a period of 10 min of asystole survival or survival without severe disability is highly unlikely (Kattwinkel, 2000) The Guideline Committee of the American Academy of Pediatrics and American Heart Association recommends that each institution develop local discussions of these issues based on the availability of resources and outcome data.

V. **Conflict resolution**
  A. **Identifying conflict.** *Conflict* is any dispute or disagreement of opinion. This may occur between the physician and the patient or the patient's guardian. Alternatively, conflicts can arise between the physician and the nursing staff, health care workers, and administrative staff or any combination of these. Most ethical issues arise as conflict between differing values or moral ideals. Therefore, the identification of conflict is a key or essential ingredient in bioethical decisions. Conflict is best identified by ongoing communication. Normally, we think of this as communication between physician and patient. However, this is just the first step. Continued communication among members of the health care team, parents, family members, and others involved in the case will uncover unvoiced concerns and opinions. These should be dealt with in an open and honest fashion to obtain consensus about ethical issues.
  B. **Putting virtue into practice.** Section II of this chapter describes various virtues or attributes that will assist a physician in making ethical decisions. Many of these virtues are common for all humans. Others, however, apply specifically to the obligations and responsibilities of a physician. If used, many of these virtues will help the physician defuse or avoid completely many issues of an ethical nature. This is because careful attention to the physician's responsibility and behavior creates an environment in which open dialogue and an exchange of ideas and values can occur between the patient and the physician. This ongoing dialogue automatically corrects many of the miscommunications or conflicts that lead to ethical crises.
  C. **The bioethics consult: obtaining an outside perspective.** Many institutions have standing bioethics committees or departments that can aid in re-

solving bioethical conflicts. Despite our best intentions, we are sometimes unable to resolve conflict with patients or cannot fully explain the necessity of action to patients, causing confusion. In these instances, an outside perspective may be of value. A consultation from the bioethics committee is simply an outside review of the facts and values associated with a particular crisis. This outside observer may be a physician, another health care worker, or a member of the clergy. The purpose of the consult is not to render a "more expert" opinion but to uncover differing moral values and miscommunication that lead to conflict. In many instances, this is all that is needed to resolve these problems. If consensus cannot be obtained in this manner, further interventions are warranted.

D. **The bioethics committee.** A bioethics committee is usually multidisciplinary in membership. Composed of administrators, lawyers, physicians, nursing staff, and clergy, the committee reviews ethical dilemmas put before it. Many bioethics committees also have a standing role in monitoring the ethical behavior of physicians and health care workers at their institution. Activation of the bioethics committee, as opposed to a consult, is a more involved process. The committee's purpose is to not only resolve conflict in particular instances but also provide policy and general guidelines for ethical behavior at that institution. Because of the potential legal ramifications, this body may routinely consult the judiciary system for further advice. It is the usual policy of most committees that the body may be queried by physicians or other health care workers, family members, clergy, or other interested parties. These queries can be put forth without fear of retribution or chastisement from other staff members. The procedure for activating the bioethics committee should be posted in the residents' or physicians' handbook or nursing manual for that patient unit.

E. **The legal system.** On occasion, conflict arises that cannot be resolved by the physician, bioethics consult, or committee opinion. In these instances, outside judiciary opinions should be sought. The bioethics committee can usually be helpful in obtaining this legal opinion. Not only does the committee have familiarity with accessing the judiciary system, but they should also be able to frame the question in such a way to provide the most concise legal response. Activation of the legal system in this way also protects the physician from direct consequence from legal action.

REFERENCES

Barber B: *The Logic and Limits of Trust.* Rutgers University Press, 1983.
Kattwinkel J: *Textbook of Neonatal Resuscitation,* 4th ed. American Heart Association/American Academy of Pediatrics, 2000.
Pellegrino ED: *Pharos Alpha Omega Alpha Honor Medical Society* 1983;46:38.
Pellegrino ED, Thomasma DC: *The Virtues in Medical Practice.* Oxford University Press, 1993.

Universal precautions are indicated on all procedures that involve potentially infectious body fluids.

16 Arterial Access

ARTERIAL PUNCTURE (RADIAL ARTERY PUNCTURE)

 I. **Indications.** Arterial puncture is performed (1) to obtain blood for blood gas measurements and (2) when blood is needed and venous or capillary blood samples cannot be obtained.
 II. **Equipment.** Equipment includes a 23- to 27-gauge scalp vein needle or a 23- to 25-gauge venipuncture needle, a 1- or 3-mL syringe, povidone-iodine and alcohol swabs, a 4 × 4 gauze pad, gloves, and 1:1000 heparin.
III. **Procedure**
  A. For submitting a blood gas sample, most hospitals already have 1-mL syringes coated with heparin. If this is not available, draw a small amount of heparin (concentration 1:1000) into the syringe to be used for submitting the blood gas sample and then discard the excess heparin from the syringe. The small amount of heparin coating the syringe is sufficient to prevent coagulation of the sample. Excessive amounts of heparin may interfere with laboratory results, causing a falsely low pH and $Paco_2$. If any other laboratory test is to be performed, do not use heparin.
  B. The radial artery is the most frequently used puncture site and is described here. Alternative sites are the posterior tibial artery or the dorsalis pedis. Use of femoral arteries should be reserved for emergency situations. Brachial arteries should not be used because there is minimal collateral circulation and a risk of median nerve damage. Temporal arteries should not be used because of the high risk of neurologic complications.
  C. Check for collateral circulation and patency of the ulnar artery by means of the **Allen test.** First, elevate the arm and simultaneously occlude the radial and ulnar arteries at the wrist; then rub the palm to cause blanching. Release pressure on the ulnar artery. If normal color returns in the palm in <10 s, adequate collateral circulation from the ulnar artery is present. If normal color does not return for 15 s or longer or does not return at all, the collateral circulation is poor and it is best not to use the radial artery in this arm. The radial and ulnar arteries in the other arm should then be tested for collateral circulation.
  D. To obtain the blood sample, take the patient's hand in your left hand (for a right-handed operator) and extend the wrist. Palpate the radial artery with the index finger of your left hand (Figure 16–1). Transillumination may also be helpful. Marking the puncture site with a fingernail imprint may be helpful.
  E. Clean the puncture site first with a povidone-iodine swab (preferred for blood cultures) and then with an alcohol swab.
  F. Puncture the skin at about a 30-degree angle, and slowly advance the needle with the bevel up until blood appears in the tubing (see Figure 16–1). With arterial blood samples, little aspiration is needed to fill the syringe.
  G. Collect the least amount of blood needed for this and any other test in a neonate. The volume of blood taken should not exceed 3–5% of the total blood volume (the total blood volume in a neonate is ~80 mL/kg). As an example, if 4 mL of blood is drawn from an infant weighing 1 kg, this represents 5% of the total blood volume.
  H. Withdraw the needle and apply firm, but not occlusive, pressure to the site for ≥5 min with a 4 × 4 gauze pad to ensure adequate hemostasis.

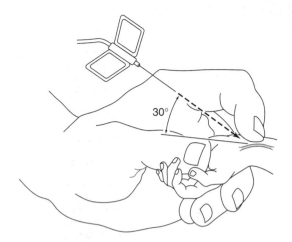

FIGURE 16–1. Technique of arterial puncture in the neonate.

    I. Before submitting an arterial blood gas sample, expel air bubbles from the sample and tightly cap the syringe. Failure to do this can lead to errors in testing. (See the following discussion of inaccuracy of blood gas results.)

    J. Place the syringe in ice, and take it to the laboratory immediately. Note the collection time and the patient's temperature and hemoglobin on the laboratory slip.

IV. Complications

    A. Hematoma. To minimize the risk of hematoma, use the smallest gauge needle possible. Immediately after withdrawing the needle, apply pressure for ~5 min. Hematomas will usually resolve spontaneously.

    B. Arteriospasm, thrombosis, and embolism. These complications can be minimized by using the smallest gauge needle possible. With thrombosis, the vessel will usually recanalize over a period of time. Arteriospasm will usually resolve spontaneously.

    C. Infection. The risk of infection is rare and can be minimized by using strict sterile technique. Infection is commonly caused by gram-positive organisms such as *Staphylococcus epidermidis,* which should be treated with nafcillin or vancomycin and gentamicin (see Chapter 80). Drug sensitivities at the specific hospital should be checked.

    D. Inaccuracy of blood gas results. Excessive heparin in the syringe may result in a falsely low pH and $Paco_2$. Remove excess heparin before obtaining the blood sample. Air bubbles caused by failure to cap the syringe may falsely elevate the Pao_2 and falsely lower the $Paco_2$.

PERCUTANEOUS ARTERIAL CATHETERIZATION

    I. Indications

    A. When frequent arterial blood samples are required and an umbilical arterial catheter cannot be placed or has been removed because of complications, percutaneous arterial catheterization is required.

    B. This procedure is also indicated when intraarterial blood pressure monitoring is required.

    II. Equipment. Use a 22- or 24-gauge needle with a 1-in catheter encasement (Jelco or Angiocath). A 24-gauge needle is recommended for infants weighing <1500 g.

Also needed are an armboard (or two tongue blades taped together), adhesive tape, sterile drapes, povidone-iodine and alcohol swabs, gloves, antiseptic ointment, a needle holder, suture scissors, 4-0 or 5-0 silk sutures, 0.5 normal saline or 0.25 normal saline solution (the latter is preferred in premature infants to decrease the incidence of hypernatremia) in a 1- or 3-mL syringe with heparinized saline solution (1 unit of heparin/mL saline) in a pressure bag, and connecting tubing.

III. **Procedure.** Two methods are described here; both use the radial artery, which is the most common site. An alternative site is the posterior tibial artery. The temporal artery is not recommended because of the risk of central nervous system (CNS) complications. Transillumination may be helpful in locating the artery in premature infants. Arterial catheterization requires a great deal of patience.

A. **Method 1**

   1. Verify adequate collateral circulation using the Allen test (see prior discussion of arterial puncture procedure).

   2. Place the infant's wrist on an armboard (some physicians prefer to use an intravenous bag), and hyperextend the wrist by placing gauze underneath it. Tape the arm and hand securely to the board (Figure 16–2). Put on gloves, and place sterile drapes around the puncture site. Cleanse the site, first with povidone-iodine swabs and then with alcohol swabs.

   3. Puncture both the anterior and posterior walls of the artery at a 30- to 45-degree angle. Remove the stylet. There should be little or no backflow of blood.

   4. Pull the catheter back slowly until blood is seen; this signifies that the arterial lumen has been entered.

   5. Advance the catheter after attaching the syringe and flush the catheter. Never use hypertonic solutions to flush an arterial catheter.

   6. Secure the catheter with 4-0 or 5-0 silk sutures in two or three places. Occasionally, it is not possible to suture the catheter, and it should be securely taped instead.

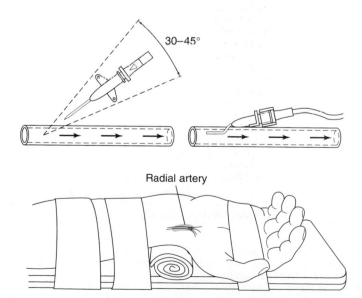

FIGURE 16–2. When placing an indwelling arterial catheter, the wrist should be secured as shown. The catheter assembly is introduced at a 30- to 45-degree angle.

7. Connect the tubing from the heparinized saline pressure bag to the catheter.
8. Place povidone-iodine ointment on the area where the catheter enters the skin and cover the area with gauze taped securely in place.
B. **Method 2 (alternative method)**
   1. Perform steps 1 and 2 as just discussed.
   2. Puncture the anterior wall of the artery until blood return is seen. At this point, the catheter should be in the lumen of the artery.
   3. Advance the catheter into the artery while simultaneously withdrawing the needle. The blood should be flowing freely from the catheter if the catheter is properly positioned.
   4. Attach the syringe and flush the catheter.
   5. Secure the line as in method 1.
IV. **Complications**
   A. **Arteriospasm.** The risk of arteriospasm can be minimized by using the smallest gauge catheter possible and performing as few punctures as possible. If arteriospasm occurs, the catheter must be removed until the spasm resolves.
   B. **Embolism or thrombosis.** To prevent these complications, make certain that air is not introduced into the catheter and that the catheter is flushed with heparinized saline.
   C. **Skin ischemia/necrosis or gangrene.** Adequate collateral circulation decreases the risk of this complication. Always perform the Allen test to verify collateral flow (see prior discussion of arterial puncture procedure).
   D. **Hematoma.** See prior discussion under Arterial Puncture, Procedure.
   E. **Blood loss.** Accidental loss of catheter position, resulting in hemorrhage, can occur.
   F. **Infection.**
   G. **Infiltration of solution.**

UMBILICAL ARTERY CATHETERIZATION

I. **Indications**
   A. When frequent or continuous measurements of arterial blood gases are required.
   B. For continuous arterial blood pressure monitoring.
   C. To provide exchange transfusion.
   D. For angiography.
   E. For resuscitation (umbilical vein [UV] preferred).
II. **Equipment.** Prepackaged umbilical artery catheterization trays usually include sterile drapes, a tape measure, a needle holder, suture scissors, a hemostat, a forceps, a scalpel, and a blunt needle. Also needed are a 3-way stopcock, an umbilical artery catheter (No. 3.5 French for an infant weighing <1.2 kg, No. 5 French for an infant weighing >1.2 kg; newer double-lumen catheters are also available to provide an additional access), umbilical tape, silk tape (eg, Dermicel), 3.0 silk suture, gauze pads, antiseptic solution, gloves, a mask and a hat, a 10-mL syringe, 0.5 normal or 0.25 normal saline flush solution (saline with heparin 1–2 U/mL; to decrease thrombotic complications, it is recommended to use a continuous infusion with heparin), and a 22-gauge needle.
III. **Procedure**
   A. Place the patient supine. Wrap a diaper around both legs and tape the diaper to the bed. This stabilizes the patient for the procedure and allows observation of the feet for vasospasm.
   B. Put on sterile gloves, a mask, a hat, and a sterile gown.
   C. Prepare the umbilical catheter tray by attaching the stopcock to the blunt needle and then attaching the catheter to the blunt needle. Fill the 10-mL syringe with flush solution, and inject it through the catheter.

D. Clean the umbilical cord area with antiseptic solution. Place sterile drapes around the umbilicus, leaving the feet and head exposed. Observe the infant closely during the procedure for vasospasm in the legs or signs of distress.

E. Tie a piece of umbilical tape around the base of the umbilical cord tightly enough to minimize blood loss but loosely enough so that the catheter can be passed easily through the vessel (ie, snug but not tight). Cut off the excess umbilical cord with scissors or a scalpel, leaving a 1-cm stump. A scalpel usually makes a cleaner cut, so that the vessels are more easily seen. There are *usually* two umbilical arteries and one umbilical vein. The arteries are smaller and are usually located at the 4- and 7-o'clock positions. The vein usually has a floppy wall (Figure 16–3A and B).

F. Using the curved hemostat, grasp the end of the umbilicus to hold it upright and steady

G. Use the forceps to open and dilate the umbilical artery. First, place one arm of the forceps in the artery, and then use both arms to gently dilate the vessel (see Figure 16–3C and D).

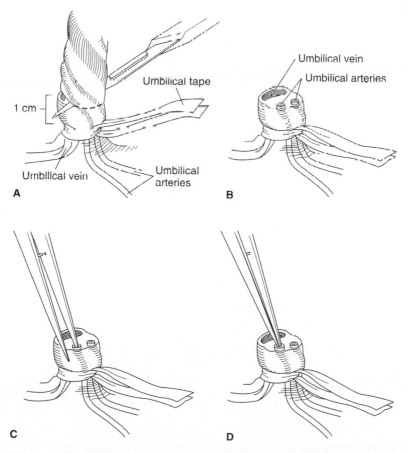

FIGURE 16–3. (A) The umbilical cord should be amputated, leaving a 1-cm stump. **(B)** Identification of the umbilical cord vessels. **(C and D)** A forceps is used to gently dilate the umbilical artery.

H. Once the artery is sufficiently dilated, insert the catheter.
I. Be certain you know the correct length of catheter to be inserted. The catheter is positioned in one of two ways. In **"low catheterization,"** the tip of the catheter lies below the level of L3 or L4. In **"high catheterization,"** the tip lies above the diaphragm at the level of T6–T9. Positioning is usually determined by the routine at a given institution. High positioning is associated with hypertension and an increased risk of intraventricular hemorrhage. High positioning is also associated with a lower incidence of blanching and cyanosis of the extremities. Low positioning has been associated with more episodes of vasospasm of the lower extremities. The length of catheter needed can be obtained from the **umbilical catheter measurements** (Figure 16–4). A rapid method for determining the length needed for low catheterization is to measure two thirds of the distance from the umbilicus to the midportion of the clavicle.

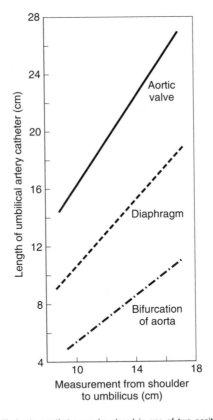

FIGURE 16–4. The umbilical artery catheter can be placed in one of two positions. The low catheter is placed below the level of L3 to avoid the renal and mesenteric vessels. The high catheter is placed between the thoracic vertebrae from T6 to T9. The graph is used as a guide to help determine the catheter length for each position. The low line corresponds to the aortic bifurcation in the graph, whereas a high line corresponds to the diaphragm. To determine catheter length, measure (in centimeters) a perpendicular line from the top of the shoulder to the umbilicus. This determines the shoulder-umbilical length. Plot this number on the graph to determine the proper catheter length for the umbilical artery catheter. It is helpful to add the length of the umbilical stump to the catheter length. *(Based on data from Dunn PM: Localization of the umbilical catheter by postmortem measurement. Arch Dis Child 1966;41:69.)*

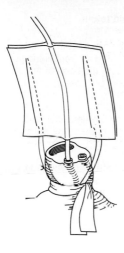

FIGURE 16-5. The umbilical artery catheter is secured with silk tape, which is attached to the base of the cord (through the Wharton's jelly, not the skin or vessels).

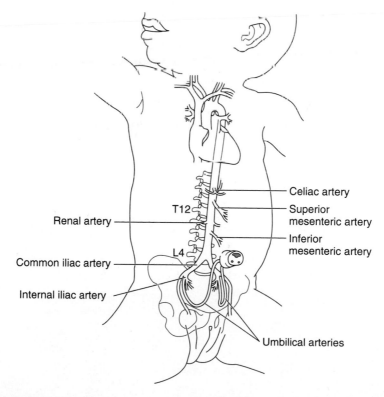

Celiac artery

Superior
mesenteric artery

Inferior
mesenteric artery

T12

Renal artery

L4

Common iliac artery

Internal iliac artery

Umbilical arteries

FIGURE 16-6. Important landmarks, related vessels, and the path of the umbilical artery. The internal iliac artery is also called the hypogastric artery.

J. Once the catheter is in position, aspirate to verify blood return.
K. There are multiple ways to secure the catheter.
   • **Method 1.** Secure the catheter as shown in Figure 16–5. The silk tape is folded over part of the way, the catheter is placed, and the remaining portion of the tape is folded over. Suture the silk tape to the base of the umbilical cord (through the Wharton jelly, not the skin or vessels) using 3.0 silk sutures. Connect the tubing to the monitor and flush it. No special dressing is needed. The umbilical stump with the catheter in place is left open to the air. Once the catheter is secure, loosen the umbilical tape.
   • **Method 2.** Place a purse string suture around the base of the cord (not the skin or vessels). Lightly tighten the suture, and then you can sew the ends through a piece of tape (as in Method 1).
   • **Method 3.** Place a pursestring around the base of the cord, and then you can wrap the ends of the suture around the catheter and tie.
   • **Method 4.** Secure the catheter with a tape bridge.

L. Obtain an abdominal x-ray film to verify the position of a low catheter or a chest x-ray film to check the position of a high catheter. Figure 16–6 shows landmarks and the relationship of umbilical arteries to the other major abdominal arteries. X-ray films showing positioning can be found in Chapter 9.

IV. **Complications**
   A. **Infection.** Infection can be minimized by using strict sterile technique. No attempt should be made to advance a catheter once it has been placed and sutured into position; instead, the catheter should be replaced.
   B. **Vascular accidents.** Thrombosis or infarction may occur. Vasospasm may lead to loss of an extremity. Hypertension is a long-term complication caused by stenosis of the renal artery as a result of improper catheter placement near the renal arteries.
   C. **Hemorrhage.** Hemorrhage may occur if the catheter or tubing becomes disconnected. The tubing stopcocks must be securely fastened. If hemorrhage occurs, blood volume replacement may be necessary.
   D. **Vessel perforation.** The catheter should never be forced into position. If the catheter cannot be easily advanced, use of another vessel should be attempted. If perforation occurs, surgical intervention may be necessary.

17 Bladder Aspiration (Suprapubic Urine Collection)

I. Indications. Bladder aspiration is performed to obtain urine for culture when a less invasive technique is not possible.

II. Equipment. Equipment includes sterile gloves, povidone-iodine solution, a 23- or 25-gauge 1-in needle (a 21- to 22-gauge 1½-in needle can also be used in a larger infant) with a 3-mL syringe attached, 4 × 4 gauze pads, gloves, and a sterile container.

III. Procedure

   A. Be certain that voiding has not occurred within the previous hour so that there will be enough urine in the bladder to make collection worthwhile.

   B. An assistant should hold the infant's legs in the frog-leg position.

   C. Locate the site of bladder puncture, which is ~1–2 cm above the pubic symphysis, in the midline position of the lower abdomen.

   D. Put on sterile gloves, and clean the skin at the puncture site with antiseptic solution three times.

   E. Palpate the pubic symphysis. Insert the needle 1–2 cm above the pubic symphysis at a 90-degree angle (Figure 17–1).

   F. Advance the needle while aspirating at the same time. Do not advance the needle once urine is seen in the syringe. Do not advance the needle more

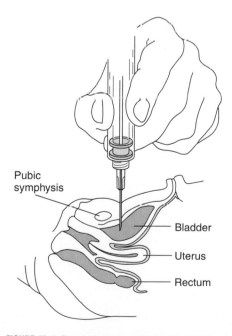

Pubic symphysis

Bladder

Uterus

Rectum

FIGURE 17–1. Technique of suprapubic bladder aspiration.

than 1 in. This precaution helps prevent perforation of the posterior wall of the bladder.

G. Withdraw the needle, and maintain pressure over the site of puncture.

H. Place a sterile cap on the syringe or transfer the specimen to a sterile urine cup, and submit the specimen to the laboratory.

IV. Complications

A. Bleeding. Microscopic hematuria may occur after bladder aspiration but is usually transient and rarely causes concern. Hemorrhage may occur if there is a bleeding disorder. The platelet count should be checked before aspiration is performed; if low, the procedure should not be performed.

B. Infection. Infection is not likely to occur if strict sterile technique is used.

C. Perforation of the bowel. With careful identification of the landmarks described previously, this complication is rare. If the bowel is perforated (indicated by the aspiration of bowel contents), close observation is recommended, and intravenous antibiotics should be considered.

18 Bladder Catheterization

I. Indications

A. Bladder catheterization is performed when a urine specimen is needed and a clean-catch specimen cannot be obtained or suprapubic aspiration cannot be performed.

B. The procedure is performed to monitor urinary output, relieve urinary retention, or obtain a cystogram or voiding cystourethrogram.

C. Bladder catheterization is also done to obtain a bladder residual.

II. Equipment.
Equipment includes sterile gloves, cotton balls, povidone-iodine solution, sterile drapes, lubricant, a sterile collection bottle, and urethral catheters (No. 3.5 French umbilical artery catheter for infants weighing <1000 g; No. 5 French feeding tube for infants weighing 1000–1800 g; No. 8 French feeding tube for infants weighing >1800 g).

III. Procedure

A. Males

1. Place the infant supine, with the thighs abducted (frog-leg position).

2. Cleanse the penis with povidone-iodine solution, starting with the meatus and moving in a proximal direction.

3. Put on sterile gloves, and drape the area with sterile towels.

4. Place the tip of the catheter in sterile lubricant.

5. Hold the penis approximately perpendicular to the body to straighten the penile urethra and help prevent false passage. Advance the catheter until urine appears. A slight resistance may be felt as the catheter passes the external sphincter, and steady, gentle pressure is usually needed to advance past this area. Never force the catheter (Figure 18–1).

6. Collect the urine specimen. If the catheter is to remain in place, some physicians believe that it should be taped to the lower abdomen rather than to the leg in males to help decrease stricture formation caused by pressure on the posterior urethra.

B. Females

1. Place the infant supine, with the thighs abducted (frog-leg position).

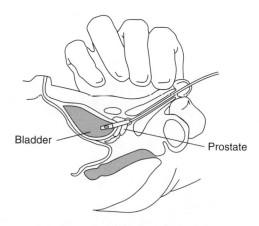

FIGURE 18–1. Bladder catheterization in the male.

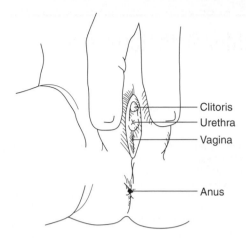

FIGURE 18–2. Landmarks used in catheterization of the bladder in females.

    2. Separate the labia, and cleanse the area around the meatus with povidone-iodine solution. Use anterior-to-posterior strokes to prevent fecal contamination.
    3. Put on sterile gloves, and drape sterile towels around the labia.
    4. Spread the labia with two fingers. See Figure 18–2 for landmarks used in the catheterization of the bladder in females. Lubricate the catheter, and advance it in the urethra until urine appears. Tape the catheter to the leg if it is to remain in position.
IV. Complications
    A. Infection. The risk of introducing bacteria into the urinary tact and then the bloodstream is common. Strict sterile technique is necessary to help prevent infection. "In-and-out" catheterization carries a small risk of urinary tract infection. The longer a catheter is left in place, the greater is the chance of infection. Infections that can occur include sepsis, cystitis, pyelonephritis, urethritis, and epididymitis.
    B. Trauma to the urethra ("false passage") or the bladder. Trauma to the urethra or the bladder is more common in males. It can be prevented by adequately lubricating the catheter and stretching the penis to straighten the urethra. The catheter should never be forced if resistance is felt. Perforation of the bladder or urethra can occur.
    C. Hematuria. Hematuria is usually transient but may require irrigation with normal saline solution.
    D. Urethral stricture. Stricture is more common in males. It is usually caused by a catheter that is too large or by prolonged or traumatic catheterization. In males, taping the catheter to the anterior abdominal wall will help decrease the pressure on the posterior urethra.

19 Chest Tube Placement

I. Indications

A. Tension pneumothorax causing respiratory compromise and decreased venous return to the heart, resulting in decreased cardiac output and hypotension.

B. Pneumothorax compromising ventilation and causing increased work of breathing, hypoxia, and increased $Paco_2$.

C. Drainage of a pleural effusion or to obtain fluid for diagnosis.

II. Equipment.

Prepackaged chest tube trays typically consist of sterile towels, 4 × 4 gauze pads, 3-0 silk suture, curved hemostats, a No. 15 or No. 11 scalpel, scissors, a needle holder, antiseptic solution, antibiotic ointment, 1% lidocaine, a 3-mL syringe, and a 25-gauge needle. The chest tube should be a No. 10 French catheter for infants weighing <2000 g and a No. 12 French catheter for infants weighing >2000 g. Sterile gloves, a mask, hat, and gown, and a suction-drainage system (eg, the Pleur-Evac system) are also needed.

III. Procedure

A. The site of chest tube insertion is determined by examining the anteroposterior and cross-table lateral or lateral decubitus chest films. Air collects in the uppermost areas of the chest, and fluid in the most dependent areas. For air collections, place the tube anteriorly. For fluid collections, place the tube posteriorly and laterally. **Transillumination** of the chest may help detect pneumothorax. With the lights in the room turned down, a strong light source is placed on the anterior chest wall above the nipple and in the axilla. The affected side will usually appear hyperlucent and will "light up" compared with the unaffected side. Transillumination may not reveal a small pneumothorax. Unless the infant's status is rapidly deteriorating, a chest x-ray film should be obtained to confirm pneumothorax before the chest tube is inserted.

B. Position the patient so that the site of insertion is accessible. The most common position is supine, with the arm at a 90° angle on the affected side.

C. Select the appropriate site (Figure 19–1). For anterior placement, the site should be the second or third intercostal space at the midclavicular line. For posterior placement, use the fourth, fifth, or sixth intercostal space at the anterior axillary line. The nipple is a landmark for the fourth intercostal space.

D. Put on a sterile gown, mask, hat, and gloves. Cleanse the area of insertion with povidone-iodine solution, and drape.

E. Infiltrate the area superficially with 0.125–0.25 mL of 1.0% lidocaine and then down to the rib. Infiltrate into the intercostal muscles and along the parietal pleura. Make a small incision (approximately the width of the tube, usually ≤0.75 cm) in the skin over the rib just below the intercostal space where the tube is to be inserted (Figure 19–2A).

F. Insert a closed, curved hemostat into the incision, and spread the tissues down to the rib. Using the tip of the hemostat, puncture the pleura just above the rib and spread gently. Remember that the intercostal nerves, arteries, and veins lie below the ribs (see Figure 19–2A). This maneuver helps create a subcutaneous tunnel that aids in closing the tract when the tube is removed.

G. When the pleura has been penetrated, a rush of air will often be heard.

H. Insert the chest tube through the opened hemostat (see Figure 19–2B). Be certain that the side holes of the tube are within the pleural cavity. The presence of moisture in the tube usually confirms proper placement in the intrapleural cavity. Use of a trocar guide is usually unnecessary and may increase the risk of complications (such as lung perforation). The chest tube should be inserted 2–3 cm for a small preterm infant and 3–4 cm for a term in-

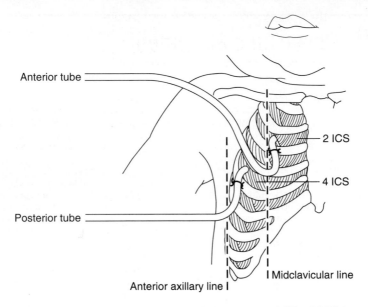

FIGURE 19–1. Recommended sites for chest tube insertion in the neonate. 2 ICS and 4 ICS (second and fourth intercostal space.)

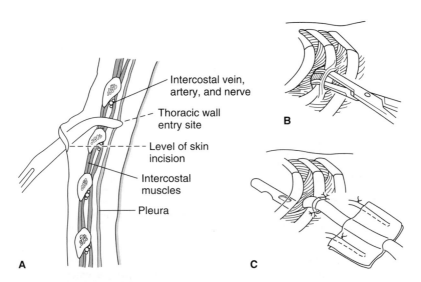

FIGURE 19–2. Procedures of chest tube insertion. **(A)** Level of skin incision and thoracic wall entry site in relation to the rib and the neurovascular bundle. **(B)** Opened hemostat, through which the chest tube is inserted. **(C)** The chest tube is then secured to the skin with silk sutures.

fant. (These are guidelines only; the length of tube to be inserted will vary based on the size of the infant.) An alternative approach to tube insertion is to measure the length from the insertion site to the apex of the lung (approximately the midclavicle) and tie a silk suture around the tube the same distance from the tip. Position the tube until the silk suture is just outside the skin.

I. Hold the tube steady first and then allow an assistant to connect the tube to a water-seal vacuum drainage system (eg, the Pleur-Evac system). Five to 10 cm of suction pressure is usually used. Start at the lower level of suction and increase as needed if the pneumothorax or effusion does not resolve. Systems such as the Pleur-Evac provide continuous suction and water seal. Water seal prevents air from being drawn back into the pleural space.

J. Secure the chest tube with 3.0 silk sutures and silk tape (see Figure 19–2C). Close the skin opening with sutures if necessary. Obtain a chest x-ray film to verify placement and check for residual fluid or pneumothorax. Positioning of the tube must always be verified by a chest x-ray film.

IV. **Complications**
   A. **Infection.** Strict sterile technique will help minimize the risk of infection. Cellulitis is common. Many institutions recommend prophylactic antibiotics (eg, nafcillin [see Chapter 80]) when a chest tube is placed (*controversial*).
   B. **Bleeding.** Bleeding may occur if one of the major vessels (intercostal, axillary, pulmonary, or internal mammary) is perforated or if the lung is damaged during the procedure. This complication can be avoided if landmarks are properly identified. Bleeding is less likely if a trocar is not used. Bleeding may stop during suctioning; however, if significant bleeding continues, immediate surgical consultation is usually necessary.
   C. **Nerve damage.** Passing the tube over the top of the rib will help avoid injury to the intercostal nerve running under the rib.
   D. **Trauma.** Lung trauma can be minimized by never forcing the tube into position.
   E. **Diaphragmatic paralysis.**
   F. **Subcutaneous emphysema.**

20 Endotracheal Intubation

I. **Indications**
   A. To provide mechanical respiratory support.
   B. To obtain aspirates for culture.
   C. To assist in bronchopulmonary hygiene ("pulmonary toilet").
   D. To alleviate subglottic stenosis.
   E. To clear the trachea of meconium.

II. **Equipment.** Equipment includes a correct endotracheal tube (using the guidelines in Table 20–1), a pediatric laryngoscope handle with a blade (No. 00 blade for infants weighing <1000 g, No. 0 blade for infants weighing 1000–3000 g, No. 1 Miller blade for infants weighing >3000 g; straight blades are preferred over curved blades), a bag-and-mask apparatus, an endotracheal tube adapter, an oxygen source with tubing, a suction apparatus, tape, scissors, a stylet (*optional*), gloves, and tincture of benzoin.

III. **Procedure**
   A. The endotracheal tube should be precut to eliminate dead space (cut to 15 cm). Some newer tubes are marked "oral" or "nasal" and should be cut appropriately.
   B. Be certain that the light source on the laryngoscope is working before beginning the procedure. A bag-and-mask apparatus with 100% oxygen should be available at the bedside. Place the stylet (if used) in the endotracheal tube. Flexible stylets are optional but may help guide the tube into position more efficiently. Be sure the tip of the stylet does not protrude out of the end of the endotracheal tube.
   C. Place the infant in the "sniffing position" (with the neck slightly extended). Hyperextension of the neck in infants may cause the trachea to collapse.
   D. Cautiously suction the oropharynx as needed to make the landmarks clearly visible.
   E. Monitor the infant's heart rate and color.
   F. Hold the laryngoscope with your left hand. Insert the scope into the right side of the mouth, and sweep the tongue to the left side.
   G. Advance the blade a few millimeters, passing it beneath the epiglottis.
   H. Lift the blade vertically to elevate the epiglottis and visualize the glottis (Figure 20–1). *Note:* The purpose of the laryngoscope is to vertically lift the epiglottis, not to pry it open.
   I. To better visualize the vocal cords, an assistant may place gentle external pressure on the thyroid cartilage.
   J. Pass the endotracheal tube along the right side of the mouth and down past the vocal cords during inspiration. It is best to advance the tube *only* 2–2.5 cm into the trachea to avoid placement in the right main stem bronchus. It may be helpful to tape the tube at the lip when the tube has been advanced 7 cm in a 1-kg infant, 8 cm in a 2-kg infant, 9 cm in a 3-kg infant, or 10 cm in a 4-kg infant (the rule of "1, 2, 3, 4, 7, 8, 9, 10"). Infants weighing <750 g may only require 6.5-cm insertion. Another way to remember suggested depth is 6 plus the patient's weight in kilograms. The stylet should be removed gently while the tube is held in position.
   K. Confirm the position of the tube. The resuscitation bag is attached to the tube, and an assistant provides mechanical breaths while the physician listens for equal breath sounds on both sides of the chest. Auscultate the stomach to be certain that the esophagus was not inadvertently entered.
   L. Paint the skin with tincture of benzoin. Tape the tube securely in place.
   M. Obtain a chest x-ray film to confirm proper placement of the tube.

TABLE 20–1. GUIDELINES FOR ENDOTRACHEAL TUBE SIZE AND DEPTH OF INSERTION BASED ON WEIGHT AND GESTATIONAL AGE

Weight (g)	Gestational age (weeks)	Endotracheal tube size, inside diameter (mm)	Depth of insertion (cm from upper lip)
<1000	<28	2.5	6.5–7
1000–2000	28–34	3.0	7–8
2000–3000	34–38	3.5	8–9
>3000	>38	3.5–4.0	>9

Based on guidelines from Kattwinkel J: *Textbook of Neonatal Resuscitation,* 4th edition. American Heart Association/American Academy of Pediatrics, 2000.

N. Certain medications can be given through the endotracheal tube. These medications are lidocaine, atropine, naloxone, and epinephrine. These can be remembered by the mnemonic LANE or NEAL.

IV. Complications

A. Tracheal perforation. Tracheal perforation is a rare complication requiring surgical intervention. It can be prevented by careful use of the laryngoscope and the endotracheal tube.

B. Esophageal perforation. Esophageal perforation is usually caused by traumatic intubation. Treatment depends on the degree of perforation. Most injuries can be managed by use of parenteral nutrition until the leak seals, use of broad-spectrum antibiotics, and observation for signs of infection. A barium swallow contrast study may be necessary after several weeks to evaluate healing or rule out stricture formation.

C. Laryngeal edema. Laryngeal edema is usually seen after extubation and may cause respiratory distress. A short course of steroids (eg, dexamethasone) can be given intravenously before and just after extubation. However, systemic dexamethasone has no effect in reducing acute postextubation stridor in neonates.

D. Improper tube positioning (esophageal intubation, right main stem bronchus).

E. Tube obstruction or kinking.

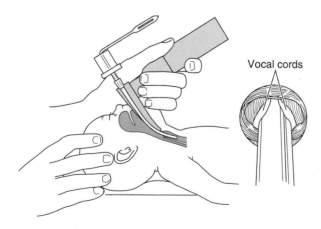

Vocal cords

FIGURE 20–1. Endotracheal intubation in the neonate.

F. **Palatal grooves.** Palatal grooves are usually seen in cases of long-term intubation and typically resolve with time.
G. **Subglottic stenosis.** Subglottic stenosis is most often associated with long-term (>3–4 weeks) endotracheal intubation. Surgical correction is usually necessary. With prolonged intubation, consideration may be given to surgical tracheostomy to help prevent stenosis.

21 Exchange Transfusion

Exchange transfusions are a technique used most often to maintain serum bilirubin at levels below neurotoxicity. The level of bilirubin at which to begin an exchange transfusion is currently under considerable debate (for more details, see Chapter 64). Exchange transfusions are also used to control other conditions, such as polycythemia or anemia. Three types of exchange transfusion are commonly used: (1) 2-volume exchange, (2) isovolumetric 2-volume exchange, and (3) partial exchange (<2 volumes) with normal saline, 5% albumin in saline, or plasma protein fraction (Plasmanate). These procedures are used primarily in sick newborn infants but may also be used for intrauterine exchanges in fetuses at high risk for central nervous system toxicity (eg, erythroblastosis fetalis) by percutaneous umbilical blood sampling and umbilical vein catheterization under ultrasound guidance.

I. **Indications**

A. **Hyperbilirubinemia.** Exchange transfusions are used in infants with hyperbilirubinemia of any origin when the serum bilirubin level reaches or exceeds a level that puts the infant at risk for central nervous system toxicity (eg, kernicterus) if left untreated (see Chapter 39, page 249). Two-volume exchange transfusions over 50–70 min are usually recommended for removal and reduction of serum bilirubin. Efficiency of bilirubin removal is increased in slower exchanges because of extravascular and intravascular bilirubin equilibration.

B. **Hemolytic disease of the newborn.** This results from destruction of fetal red blood cells (RBCs) by passively acquired maternal antibodies. Exchange transfusion aids in removing antibody-coated RBCs, thereby prolonging intravascular RBC survival. It also removes potentially toxic bilirubin from an increased bilirubin load resulting from RBC breakdown and provides plasma volume and albumin for bilirubin binding. Repeated 2-volume exchange transfusions may be needed when RBC destruction is rapid.

C. **Sepsis.** Neonatal sepsis may be associated with shock caused by bacterial endotoxins. A 2-volume exchange may help remove bacteria, toxins, fibrin split products, and accumulated lactic acid. It may also provide immunoglobulins, complement, and coagulating factors.

D. **Disseminated intravascular coagulation (DIC) from multiple causes.** A 2-volume exchange transfusion is preferred; however, depending on the sick infant's condition, any one of the exchange methods may help provide necessary coagulation factors and help reduce the underlying cause of the abnormal coagulation. Repletion of clotting factors by transfusion of fresh-frozen plasma (10–15 mL/kg) may be all that is necessary in less severe cases of DIC.

E. **Metabolic disorders causing severe acidosis (eg, aminoaciduria with associated hyperammonemia).** Partial exchanges are usually acceptable. Peritoneal dialysis may also be useful for treating some progressive metabolic disorders.

F. **Severe fluid or electrolyte imbalance (eg, hyperkalemia, hypernatremia, or fluid overload).** Isovolumetric partial exchanges are recommended to prevent large electrolyte fluctuations with each aliquot of blood exchanged. Transfusions with blood products may bind calcium; therefore, calcium gluconate should be available. Fresh blood products should be used to prevent contribution of the by-products of older blood, such as excess potassium.

G. **Polycythemia.** It is usually best to give a partial exchange transfusion using normal saline. Plasma protein fraction (eg, Plasmanate) or 5% albumin in saline may also be used; however, normal saline is preferred because it reduces both the polycythemia and the hyperviscosity of the infant's circulating blood volume. Either plasma protein fraction or 5% albumin may leave viscosity unchanged despite reductions in circulating red cell mass.

   H. Severe anemia (normovolemic or hypervolemic) causing cardiac failure, as in hydrops fetalis, is best treated with a partial exchange transfusion using packed RBCs.

   I. Any disorder requiring complement, opsonins, or gamma globulin. Infants with these conditions may require frequent exchanges, and their fluid status must be carefully managed. Partial exchanges are recommended.

II. Equipment

   A. Radiant warmer.

   B. Equipment for respiratory support and resuscitation (eg, oxygen or a suctioning device). This equipment and medications used in resuscitation should be immediately available.

   C. Equipment for monitoring the heart rate, blood pressure, respiratory rate, temperature, Pao_2, $Paco_2$, and Sao_2.

   D. Equipment for umbilical artery and umbilical vein catheterization (see Chapters 16 and 27).

   E. Disposable exchange transfusion tray.

   F. Nasogastric tube for evacuating the stomach before beginning the transfusion.

   G. A temperature-controlled device must be used for warming of the blood before and during the transfusion. The device should have an internal disposable coil and connectors to the donor blood bag and the exchange transfusion circuit. The blood should be warmed to a temperature of 37 °C. Use of makeshift water baths or heaters is not advised because blood that is too warm may hemolyze.

   H. An assistant to help maintain a sterile field, monitor and assess the infant, and record the procedure and exchanged volumes.

III. Blood transfusion

   A. Blood collection

   1. Homologous blood. Blood donated by an anonymous donor with a compatible blood type is most commonly used. Donor-directed blood (blood donated by a selected blood type–compatible person) is another option.

   2. Cytomegalovirus (CMV). Seronegative donor blood is preferred. White blood cells harboring CMV can be removed using leukodepletion filters during blood preparation. The use of frozen deglycerolized RBCs, reconstituted with fresh-frozen plasma, is another means of using seropositive blood free of viable CMV.

   3. Hemoglobin S (sickle cell trait). Precautions should be taken to avoid exchange transfusion with donor blood from a carrier. If the donor blood with sickle trait becomes acidic, sickling can occur with expected complications to the patient.

   4. Graft-vs.-host disease. Consideration should be given for using irradiated donor blood to avoid graft-vs.-host disease in known immune-compromised infants and low birth weight infants. Preterm infants who have been transfused in utero or who have received more than 50 mL of transfused blood are candidates for irradiated blood.

   B. Blood typing and cross-matching

   1. Infants with Rh incompatibility. The blood must be type O, Rh-negative, low-titer anti-A, anti-B blood. It must be cross-matched with the mother's plasma and RBCs.

   2. Infants with ABO incompatibility. The blood must be type O, Rh-compatible (with the mother and the infant) or Rh-negative, low-titer anti-A, anti-B blood. It must be cross-matched with both the infant's and mother's blood.

   3. Other blood group incompatibilities. For other hemolytic diseases (eg, anti-Rh-c, anti-Kell, anti-Duffy), blood must be cross-matched to the mother's blood to avoid offending antigens.

4. **Hyperbilirubinemia, metabolic imbalance, or hemolysis not caused by isoimmune disorders.** The blood must be cross-matched against the infant's plasma and RBCs.
C. **Freshness and preservation of blood.** In newborn infants, it is preferable to use blood or plasma that has been collected in citrate phosphate dextrose (CPD). The blood should be <72 h old. These two factors will ensure that the blood pH is >7.0. For disorders associated with hydrops fetalis or fetal asphyxia, it is best to use blood that is <24 h old.
D. **Hematocrit (Hct).** Most blood banks can reconstitute a unit of blood to a desired Hct of 50–70%. The blood should be agitated periodically during the transfusion to maintain a constant Hct.
E. **Potassium levels in donor blood.** Potassium levels in the donor blood should be determined if the infant is asphyxiated or in shock and renal impairment is suspected. If potassium levels are >7 mEq/L, consider using a unit of blood that has been collected more recently or a unit of washed RBCs.
F. **Temperature of the blood.** Warming of blood is especially important in low birth weight and sick newborn infants.

IV. **Procedure**
A. Simple 2-volume exchange transfusion is used for uncomplicated hyperbilirubinemia.
1. **The normal blood volume in a full-term newborn infant is 80 mL/kg.** In an infant weighing 2 kg, the volume would be 160 mL. Twice this volume of blood is exchanged in a 2-volume transfusion. Therefore, the amount of blood needed for a 2-kg infant would be 320 mL. Low birth weight and the blood volume of extremely premature newborns (which may be up to 95 mL/kg) should be taken into account when calculating exchange volumes.
2. **Allow adequate time for blood typing and cross-matching** at the blood bank. The infant's bilirubin level will increase during this time, and this increase must be taken into account when ordering the blood.
3. **Perform the transfusion in an intensive care setting.** Place the infant in the supine position. Restraints must be snug but not tight. A nasogastric tube should be passed to **evacuate the stomach** and should be left in place to maintain gastric decompression and prevent regurgitation and aspiration of gastric juices.
4. **Scrub and put on a sterile gown and gloves.**
5. **Perform umbilical vein catheterization** and confirm the position by x-ray film (see Figure 9–6). If an isovolumetric exchange is to be performed, then an umbilical artery catheter must also be placed and confirmed by x-ray film (see Figure 9–7).
6. **Have the unit of blood prepared.**
   a. **Check the blood types** of the donor and the infant.
   b. **Check the temperature** of the blood and warming procedures.
   c. **Check the Hct.** The blood should be agitated regularly to maintain a constant Hct.
7. **Attach the bag of blood to the tubing and stopcocks according to the directions on the transfusion tray.** The orientation of the stopcocks for infusion and withdrawal must be double-checked by the assistant.
8. **Establish the volume of each aliquot** (Table 21–1).
B. **Isovolumetric 2-volume exchange transfusion.** Isovolumetric 2-volume exchange transfusion is performed using a double setup, with infusion via the umbilical vein and withdrawal via the umbilical artery. This method is preferred when volume shifts during simple exchange might cause or aggravate myocardial insufficiency (eg, hydrops fetalis). Two operators are usually needed: one to perform the infusion and the other to handle the withdrawal.
1. **Perform steps 1–6** as in simple 2-volume exchange transfusion. In addition, perform umbilical artery catheterization.
2. **Attach the unit of blood to the tubing and stopcocks attached to the umbilical vein catheter.** If the catheter is to be left in place after the ex-

TABLE 21-1. ALIQUOTS USUALLY USED IN NEONATAL EXCHANGE TRANSFUSION

Infant weight	Aliquot (mL)
>3 kg	20
2–3 kg	15
1–2 kg	10
850 g–1 kg	5
<850 g	1–3

change transfusion (usually to monitor central venous pressure), it should be placed above the diaphragm, with placement confirmed by chest x-ray film.

3. **The tubing and the stopcocks of the second setup** are attached to the umbilical artery catheter and to a sterile plastic bag for discarding the exchanged blood.

4. **If isovolumetric exchange is being performed because of cardiac failure,** the central venous pressure can be determined via the umbilical vein catheter; it should be placed above the diaphragm in the inferior vena cava.

C. **Partial exchange transfusion.** A partial exchange transfusion is performed in the same manner as 2-volume exchange transfusion. If a partial exchange is for polycythemia (using normal saline or another blood product) or for anemia (packed RBCs), the following formula can be used to determine the volume of the transfusion.

Volume of exchange (mL) =

$$\frac{\text{Estimated blood volume (mL)} \times \text{Weight (kg)} \times (\text{Observed Hct} - \text{Desired Hct})}{\text{Observed Hct}}$$

D. **Isovolumetric partial exchange transfusion** with packed RBCs is the best procedure in cases of severe hydrops fetalis.

E. **Ancillary procedures**

1. **Laboratory studies.** Blood should be obtained for laboratory studies before and after exchange transfusion.

   a. **Blood chemistry studies** include total calcium, sodium, potassium, chloride, pH, $Paco_2$, acid-base status, bicarbonate, and serum glucose.

   b. **Hematologic studies** include hemoglobin, Hct, platelet count, white blood cell count, and differential count. Blood for retyping and cross-matching after exchange is often requested by the blood bank to verify typing and re-cross-matching and for study of transfusion reaction, if needed.

   c. **Blood culture** is recommended after exchange transfusion (*controversial*).

2. **Administration of calcium gluconate.** The citrate buffer binds calcium and transiently lowers ionized calcium levels. Treatment of suspected hypocalcemia in patients receiving transfusions is *controversial.* Some physicians routinely administer 1–2 mL of 10% calcium gluconate by slow infusion after 100–200 mL of exchange donor blood. Others maintain that this treatment has no therapeutic effect unless hypocalcemia is documented by electrocardiogram showing a change in the QT interval.

3. **Phototherapy.** Begin or resume phototherapy after exchange transfusion for disorders involving a high bilirubin level.

4. **Monitoring of serum bilirubin levels.** Continue to monitor serum bilirubin levels after transfusion at 2, 4, and 6 h and then at 6-h intervals. A rebound of bilirubin levels is to be expected 2–4 h after the transfusion.

5. **Remedication.** Patients receiving antibiotics or anticonvulsants will need to be remedicated. Unless the cardiac status is deteriorating or serum digoxin levels are too low, patients receiving digoxin should not be remedicated. The percentage of lost medications is extremely variable. As little as 2.4% of digoxin is lost, but up to 32.4% of theophylline may be lost during a 2-volume exchange transfusion. Determination of drug levels after exchange transfusion is advisable.

6. **Antibiotic prophylaxis** after the transfusion should be considered on an individual basis. Infection is uncommon but is the most frequent complication.

V. **Complications**

A. **Infection.** Bacteremia (usually caused by a *Staphylococcus* organism), hepatitis, CMV infection, malaria, and AIDS have been reported.

B. **Vascular complications.** Clot or air embolism, arteriospasm of the lower limbs, thrombosis, and infarction of major organs may occur.

C. **Coagulopathies.** Coagulopathies may result from thrombocytopenia or diminished coagulation factors. Platelets may decrease by >50% after a 2-volume exchange transfusion.

D. **Electrolyte abnormalities.** Hyperkalemia and hypocalcemia can occur.

E. **Hypoglycemia.** Hypoglycemia is especially likely in infants of diabetic mothers and in those with erythroblastosis fetalis. Because of islet cell hyperplasia and hyperinsulinism, rebound hypoglycemia may result in these infants in response to the concentrated glucose (300 mg/dL) contained in CPD donor blood.

F. **Metabolic acidosis.** Metabolic acidosis from stored donor blood (secondary to the acid load) occurs less often in CPD blood.

G. **Metabolic alkalosis.** Metabolic alkalosis may occur as a result of delayed clearing of citrate preservative from the donated blood by the liver.

H. **Necrotizing enterocolitis.** An increased incidence of necrotizing enterocolitis after exchange transfusion has been suggested. For this reason, the umbilical vein catheter should be removed after the procedure unless central venous pressure monitoring is required. Also, we recommend that feedings be delayed for at least 24 h to observe the infant for the possibility of postexchange **ileus.**

REFERENCES

Edwards M, Fletcher M: Exchange transfusion. In Fletcher MA, MacDonald MG (eds): *Atlas of Procedures in Neonatology,* 2nd ed. Lippincott, 1993.

Lackner TE: Drug replacement following exchange transfusion. *J Pediatr* 1982;100:811.

Luchtman-Jones L et al: The blood and hematopoietic system. In Fanaroff AA, Martin RJ (eds): *Neonatal-Perinatal Medicine—Diseases of the Fetus and Infant,* Vol 2, 6th ed. Mosby-Year Book, 1997.

22 Gastric Intubation

I. **Indications**
   A. **Enteric feeding.** Gastric intubation is needed for enteric feeding in the following situations:
      1. **High respiratory rate.** At some institutions, the infant is given enteric feedings if the respiratory rate is >60 breaths/min to decrease the risk of aspiration pneumonia (*controversial*).
      2. **Neurologic disease.** If neurologic disease impairs the sucking reflex or the infant's ability to feed, enteric feeding is needed.
      3. **Premature infants.** Many premature infants with immature sucking and swallow mechanisms tire before they can take in enough calories with normal feeding to maintain growth.
   B. **Gastric decompression.** Gastric decompression may be required in infants with necrotizing enterocolitis, bowel obstruction, or ileus.
   C. **Administration of medications.**
   D. **Analysis of gastric contents.**
II. **Equipment.** Equipment includes an infant feeding tube (No. 5 for those weighing <1000 g or No. 8 for those weighing ≥1000 g), a stethoscope, sterile water (to lubricate the tube), a syringe (5–10 mL), 2-in adhesive tape, gloves, and suctioning equipment.
III. **Procedure**
   A. Monitor the patient's heart rate and respiratory function throughout this procedure.
   B. Place the infant in the supine position, with the head of the bed elevated.
   C. The length of tubing needed is determined by measuring the distance from the nose to the xiphoid process. Mark the length on the tube. See Table 22–1 for guidelines on insertion length in infants weighing less than 1500 g.
   D. Moisten the end of the tube with sterile water.
   E. The tube can be placed in one of two positions.
      1. **Nasal insertion.** Flex the neck, push the nose up, and insert the tube, directing it straight back. Advance the tube the desired distance.
      2. **Oral insertion.** Push the tongue down with a tongue depressor and pass the tube into the oropharynx. Slowly advance the tube the desired distance.
   F. Continue to observe the infant for respiratory distress or bradycardia.
   G. Determine the location of the tube. One method is to inject air into the tube with a syringe and listen for a rush of air in the stomach. One study found this method unreliable because a rush of air can occur when the tip is in the distal esophagus. Some clinicians recommended either palpating the tube in the abdomen or aspirating the contents to determine the acidity by pH tape. If the location is still uncertain, obtain an x-ray film. If feedings are to be initiated, the position should also be verified by plain x-ray.
   H. Aspirate the gastric contents.
   I. Secure the tube to the face with benzoin and 2-in tape.
IV. **Complications**
   A. **Apnea and bradycardia.** Apnea and bradycardia are usually mediated by a vagal response and will usually resolve without specific treatment.
   B. **Perforation of the esophagus, posterior pharynx, stomach, or duodenum.** The tube should never be forced during insertion.
   C. **Hypoxia.** Always have bag-and-mask ventilation with 100% oxygen available to treat this problem.

TABLE 22-1. GUIDELINES FOR MINIMUM OROGASTRIC TUBE INSERTION LENGTH TO PROVIDE ADEQUATE INTRAGASTRIC POSITIONING IN VERY LOW BIRTH WEIGHT INFANTS

Weight (g)	Insertion length (cm)
< 750	13
750–999	15
1000–1249	16
1250–1500	17

Data from Gallaher KJ et al: Orogastric tube insertion length in very low birth weight infants. J Perinatol 1993; 13:128.

D. **Aspiration.** Aspiration can occur if feeding has been initiated in a tube that is accidentally inserted into the lung or if the gastrointestinal tract is not passing the feedings out of the stomach. Periodically check the residual volumes in the stomach to prevent overdistention and aspiration.

23 Heelstick (Capillary Blood Sampling)

I. **Indications.** This is the most common procedure done in neonatal intensive care nurseries.
   A. Collection of blood samples when only a small amount of blood is needed or when there is difficulty obtaining samples by venipuncture.
   B. Capillary blood gas sampling.
   C. Blood cultures when venous access is not possible.
   D. Newborn metabolic screen
II. **Equipment.** Equipment includes a sterile lancet (a 2-mm lancet if the infant weighs <1500 g or if only a small amount of blood is needed, a 4-mm lancet in larger infants or if more blood is required). Automated lancets are now available ("Tenderfoot" and "Tenderfoot Preemie"). These devices are associated with fewer complications and decreased pain. Also needed are alcohol swabs, 4 × 4 sterile gauze pads, a capillary tube (for hematocrit and bilirubin tests) or a car-away tube (if more blood is needed [eg, for blood chemistry determinations]), clay to seal the end of the tube, a warm washcloth, gloves, and a diaper.
III. **Procedure**
   A. Wrap the foot in a warm washcloth and then in a diaper for 5 min. Although this is not mandatory, it will produce hyperemia, which increases vascularity, making blood collection easier. A warming pad may be used, but its temperature should not exceed >40 °C.
   B. Choose the area of puncture (Figure 23–1). Do not use the center of the heel because this area is associated with an increased incidence of osteomyelitis.
   C. Wipe the area with an alcohol swab, and let it dry. If the area is wet with alcohol, hemolysis may occur, altering the results of blood testing.
   D. Encircle the heel with the palm of your hand and index finger (see Figure 23–1).
   E. Make a quick, deep (≤2.5-mm) puncture with a lancet. Wipe off the first drop of blood. Gently squeeze the heel, and place the collection tube at the site of the puncture. The tube should automatically fill by capillary action. It may be necessary to gently "pump" the heel to continue the blood flow. Allow enough time for capillary refill of the heel. Avoid excessive squeezing, which may cause hemolysis and give inaccurate results. Seal the end of the tube with clay.
   F. Maintain pressure on the puncture site with a dry sterile gauze pad until the bleeding stops. A 4 × 4 gauze pad can be wrapped around the heel and left on to provide hemostasis.
IV. **Complications**
   A. **Cellulitis.** Cellulitis risk can be minimized with the proper use of sterile technique. A culture of tissue from the affected area should be obtained and the use of broad-spectrum antibiotics considered.
   B. **Osteomyelitis.** This complication usually occurs in the calcaneus bone. Avoid the center area of the heel, and do not make the puncture opening too deep. If osteomyelitis occurs, tissue should be obtained for culture, and broad-spectrum antibiotics should be started until a specific organism is identified. Consultation with specialists in infectious disease and orthopedics is usually obtained.
   C. **Scarring of the heel.** Scarring occurs when there have been multiple punctures in the same area. If extensive scarring is present, consider another technique of blood collection, such as central venous sampling.
   D. **Pain.** Pain caused by routine heelsticks in premature infants can cause marked declines in hemoglobin oxygen saturation as measured by pulse

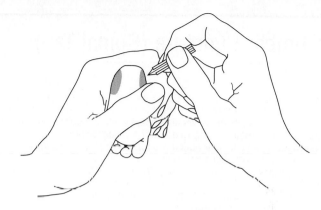

FIGURE 23–1. Use the shaded area when performing a heelstick in an infant.

oximetry. Some institutions advocate topical lidocaine (0.5–1.0%) before the procedure. Automated devices cause less pain. Oral sucrose can also be used for pain reduction.

E. Calcified nodules. These usually disappear by 30 months of age.

F. Inaccurate results. Falsely elevated Dextrostix, potassium, hematocrit, and inaccurate blood gas values can occur with heelstick sampling.

24 Lumbar Puncture (Spinal Tap)

I. **Indications**
   A. Obtain cerebrospinal fluid (CSF) for the diagnosis of central nervous system (CNS) disorders such as meningitis/encephalitis or intracranial hemorrhage.
   B. Drain CSF in communicating hydrocephalus associated with intraventricular hemorrhage. (Serial lumbar punctures for this are *controversial*.)
   C. Administration of intrathecal medications.
   D. Monitor efficacy of antibiotics used to treat CNS infections by examining CSF fluid.
II. **Materials required.** Lumbar puncture kit (usually contains 3 sterile specimen tubes, sterile drapes, sterile gauze, 20- to 22-gauge 1-in spinal needle with stylet, 1% lidocaine), gloves, povidone-iodine solution, 1-mL syringe.
III. **Procedure.** (Normal CSF values are listed in Appendix D.)
   A. An assistant should restrain the infant in either a sitting or a lateral decubitus position, depending on personal preference. An intubated, critically ill infant must be treated in the lateral decubitus position. Some clinicians believe that if CSF cannot be obtained in the lateral decubitus position the sitting position should be used. In the lateral decubitus position, the head and legs must be flexed (knee-chest position). The neck does not have to be fully flexed. Make sure airway patency is maintained. Supplemental oxygen used before the procedure or increasing oxygen if the infant is already on it can prevent hypoxemia.
   B. Once the infant is in position, check for landmarks (Figure 24–1). Palpate the iliac crest and slide your finger down to the L4 vertebral body. Then use the L4–L5 interspace (preferred) as the site of the lumbar puncture. It is sometimes easier to make a nail imprint at the exact location to mark the site.
   C. Prepare the materials (open sterile containers, pour antiseptic [povidone-iodine] solution into the well located in the plastic lumbar puncture kit).
   D. Put gloves on and clean the lumbar area with antiseptic solution, starting at the interspace selected. Prep in a widening circle from that interspace up and over the iliac crest.
   E. Drape the area with one towel under the infant and one towel covering everything but the selected interspace. Keep the infant's face exposed.
   F. Palpate again to find the selected interspace. At this time, 0.1–0.2 mL of 1% lidocaine can be injected subcutaneously for pain relief (*optional*). **Note:** Physiologic instability is not reduced with lidocaine use during the procedure. EMLA (topical lidocaine) may be used (*controversial*).
   G. Insert the needle in the midline with steady force aimed toward the umbilicus.
   H. Advance the needle slowly and then remove the stylet to check for appearance of fluid. One usually does not feel a "pop" as the ligamentum flavum and dura are penetrated, as is the case with older children and adults. It is, therefore, necessary to remove the stylet frequently to keep from going too far and getting a bloody specimen.
   I. Collect ~1 mL of CSF in each of the four sterile specimen tubes by allowing the fluid to drip into the tubes.
   J. Replace the stylet and withdraw the needle.
   K. Maintain pressure on the area, and clean off the antiseptic solution.
   L. For routine CSF examination, send four tubes of CSF to the laboratory in the following recommended order.
      - **Tube 1:** For Gram's stain, culture, and sensitivity testing.
      - **Tube 2:** For glucose and protein levels.

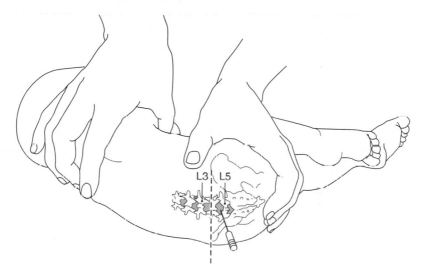

FIGURE 24-1. Positioning and landmarks used for lumbar puncture. The iliac crest (dotted line) marks the approximate level of L4.

- **Tube 3:** For cell count and differential.
- **Tube 4:** Is optional and can be sent for rapid antigen tests for specific pathogens such as group B streptococcus.

M. If a bloody specimen is obtained in the first tube, observe for clearing in the second and third tubes.

1. If bleeding clears, the tap was traumatic.
2. If blood does not clear but forms clots, a blood vessel has probably been punctured. Because CSF has not been obtained, a repeat tap must be done.
3. If blood does not clear and does not clot, the infant probably has had intraventricular bleeding.

IV. Complications

A. Infection. Use of sterile technique will reduce the chance that bacteria may be introduced into the CSF and cause infection. Bacteremia may result if a blood vessel is punctured after the needle has passed through contaminated CSF.

B. Intraspinal epidermoid tumor. This occurs as a result of performing a lumbar puncture with a needle that does not have a stylet. It is caused by the displacement of a "plug" of epithelial tissue into the dura. Note, however, that the incidence of traumatic lumbar puncture is not reduced by the use of a needle without a stylet.

C. Herniation of cerebral tissue through the foramen magnum. This is not a common problem in neonatal intensive care units because of the open fontanelle in infants.

D. Spinal cord and nerve damage. To avoid this complication, use only interspaces below L4.

E. Apnea and bradycardia sometimes occur from respiratory compromise caused by the infant being held too tightly during the procedure.

F. Hypoxia. Increasing the oxygen during the procedure may help to prevent transient hypoxia. Preoxygenation of the patient may also decrease hypoxia.

25 Paracentesis (Abdominal)

I. **Indications**
  A. To obtain peritoneal fluid for diagnostic tests to determine the cause of ascites.
  B. As a therapeutic procedure, such as removal of peritoneal fluid to aid in ventilation.
II. **Equipment.** Equipment includes sterile drapes, sterile gloves, povidone-iodine solution, sterile gauze pads, sterile tubes for fluid, a 10-mL syringe, and a 22- or 24-gauge catheter-over-needle assembly (22-gauge for infants weighing <2000 g, 24-gauge for infants weighing >2000 g).
III. **Procedure**
  A. The infant should be supine with both legs restrained. To restrict all movements of the legs, a diaper can be wrapped around the legs and secured in place.
  B. Choose the site for paracentesis. The area between the umbilicus and the pubic bone is not generally used in neonates because of the danger of perforating the bladder or bowel wall. The sites most frequently used are the right and left flanks. A good rule is to draw a horizontal line passing through the umbilicus and select a site between this line and the inguinal ligament (Figure 25–1).

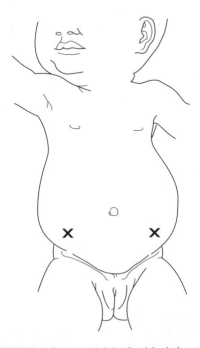

FIGURE 25–1. Recommended sites for abdominal paracentesis.

C. Prepare the area with povidone-iodine in a circular fashion, starting at the puncture site.
D. Put on sterile gloves, and drape the area.
E. Insert the needle at the selected site. A "Z-track" technique is usually used to prevent persistent leakage of fluid after the tap. Insert the needle perpendicular to the skin. When the needle is just under the skin, move it 0.5 cm before puncturing the abdominal wall.
F. Advance the needle, aspirating until fluid appears in the barrel of the syringe. Then remove the needle and aspirate the contents slowly with the catheter. It may be necessary to reposition the catheter to obtain an adequate amount of fluid. Once the necessary amount of fluid is taken (usually 3–5 mL for specific tests or enough to aid ventilation), remove the catheter. If too much fluid is removed or if it is removed too rapidly, hypotension may result.
G. Cover the site with a sterile gauze pad until leakage has stopped.
IV. Complications
A. **Hypotension.** Hypotension is caused by removing too much fluid or removing fluid too rapidly. To minimize this possibility, take only the amount needed for studies or what is needed to improve ventilation. Always remove fluid slowly.
B. **Infection.** The risk of peritonitis is minimized by using strict sterile technique.
C. **Perforation of the intestine.** To help prevent perforation, use the shortest needle possible and take careful note of landmarks (see section III,B). If perforation occurs, broad-spectrum antibiotics may be indicated with close observation for signs of infection.
D. **Perforation of the bladder.** Perforation of the bladder is normally self-limited and requires no specific treatment.
E. **Persistent fluid leak.** The Z-track technique (see section III,E) usually prevents the problem of persistent leakage of fluid. Persistent fluid leaks may have to be bagged to quantify the volume.

26 Pericardiocentesis

I. **Indications**
   A. Treatment of cardiac tamponade caused by pneumopericardium or pericardial effusion.
   B. To obtain pericardial fluid for diagnostic studies in infants with pericardial effusion.
II. **Equipment.** Needed are povidone-iodine solution, sterile gloves and gown, a 22- or 24-gauge 1-in catheter-over-needle assembly, sterile drapes, a 10-mL syringe, a connecting tube, and an underwater seal for use if the catheter is to be left indwelling.
III. **Procedure. It is best if the procedure is done with the help of echocardiography. This will help guide one on insertion and depth of the needle to decrease the incidence of complications.**
   A. Prepare the area (xiphoid and precordium) with antiseptic solution. Put on the sterile gloves and gown.
   B. Drape the area, leaving the xiphoid and a 2-cm circular area around it exposed.
   C. Prepare the needle by attaching the syringe to it. If you want to leave an indwelling catheter, a 3-way stopcock and tubing should be attached to the needle in addition to the syringe.
   D. Identify the area where the needle is to be inserted. The area most commonly used is ~0.5 cm to the left of and just below the infant's xiphoid (Figure 26–1).
   E. Insert the needle at about a 30-degree angle, aiming toward the midclavicular line on the left (see Figure 26–1).
   F. Apply constant suction on the syringe while advancing the needle.
   G. Once air or fluid is obtained (depending on which is to be evacuated), remove the needle from the catheter. Withdraw the necessary amount of air or fluid, that is, enough to relieve symptoms or to obtain sufficient fluid for laboratory studies.

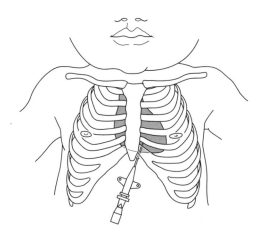

FIGURE 26–1. Recommended sites for pericardiocentesis.

H. If an indwelling catheter is to be left in place, secure it with tape and attach the tubing to continuous suction.

I. Obtain a chest x-ray film to confirm the position of the catheter and the effectiveness of drainage.

IV. **Complications**

A. **Puncturing the heart.** Avoid this complication by advancing the needle only far enough to obtain fluid or air. Another technique to avoid puncturing the heart is to attach the electrocardiogram (ECG) anterior chest lead to the needle with an alligator clip. If changes are seen on the ECG (eg, ectopic beats, changes in the ST segment, or an increase in the QRS voltage), the needle has contacted the myocardium and should be withdrawn. Avoid leaving a metal needle indwelling for continuous drainage. Most needle perforations will heal spontaneously.

B. **Pneumothorax or hemothorax.** This can occur if landmarks are not used and "blind" punctures are done. If this complication has occurred, a chest tube on the affected side is usually needed.

C. **Infection.** Strict sterile technique will minimize the risk of infection.

27 Venous Access

PERCUTANEOUS VENOUS CATHETERIZATION

I. **Indications**
   A. **Administration of intravenous (IV) medications and fluids.**
   B. **Administration of parenteral nutrition.**
II. **Materials required.** An armboard, adhesive tape, a tourniquet, alcohol swabs, normal saline for flush (½ normal saline if there is concern about hypernatremia), povidone-iodine ointment, a needle (a 23- or 25-gauge scalp vein needle or a 22- to 24-gauge catheter-over-needle). Use at least a 24-gauge needle for blood transfusion.
III. **Procedure**
   A. **Scalp vein needle**
      1. **Select the vein to use.** Veins that can be used in the neonate are discussed next (Figure 27–1). It is useful to select the Y region of the vein, where two veins join together. The needle can be inserted in the crotch of the veins.
         a. **Scalp.** Supratrochlear, superficial temporal, or posterior auricular vein.
         b. **Back of the hand.** Dorsal arch vein.
         c. **Forearm.** Median antebrachial or accessory cephalic vein.
         d. **Foot.** Dorsal arch vein.
         e. **Antecubital fossa.** Basilic or cubital vein.
         f. **Ankle.** Greater saphenous vein.
      2. **Shave the area if a scalp vein is to be used.**
      3. **Restrain the extremity** on an armboard, or have an assistant help hold the extremity or the head.
      4. **Apply a tourniquet** proximal to the puncture site. If a scalp vein is to be used, a rubber band can be placed around the head, just above the eyebrows.
      5. **Clean the area with alcohol swabs.**
      6. **Fill the tubing with flush.** Detach the syringe from the needle.
      7. **Grasp the plastic wings** and, using your free index finger, **pull the skin taut** to help stabilize the vein.
      8. **Insert the needle** through the skin and advance ~0.5 cm before entry into the side of the vessel. Alternatively, the vessel can be entered directly after puncture of the skin, but this often results in the vessel's being punctured "through and through" (Figure 27–2).
      9. **Advance the needle** until blood appears in the tubing.
      10. **Gently inject some of the flush** to ensure patency and proper positioning of the needle.
      11. **Connect the IV tubing and fluid, and tape the needle into position.**
   B. **Catheter-over-needle assembly**
      1. **Follow steps 1–5 just presented,** as for the scalp vein needle.
      2. **Fill the needle and the hub with flush** via syringe; then remove the syringe.
      3. **Pull the skin taut** to stabilize the vein.
      4. **Puncture the skin;** then enter the side of the vein in a separate motion. Alternately, the skin and the vein can be entered in one motion.
      5. **Carefully advance the needle** until blood appears in the hub.
      6. **Withdraw the needle** while advancing the catheter.
      7. **Remove the tourniquet,** and gently inject some normal saline into the catheter to verify patency and position.

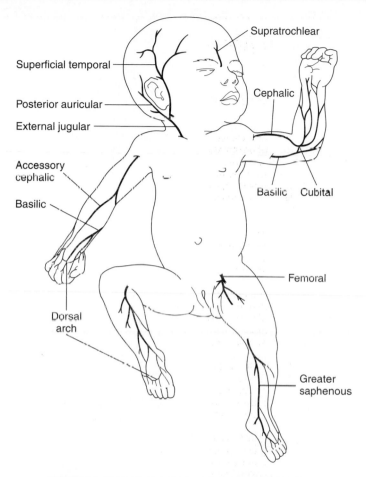

FIGURE 27-1. Frequently used sites for venous access in the neonate.

    8. Connect the IV tubing and fluid, and tape securely in place.
IV. Complications
    A. Infection. The risk of infection can be minimized by using sterile technique, including antiseptic preparation.
    B. Phlebitis. The risk of phlebitis is increased the longer a catheter is left in place, especially if left in >72 h.
    C. Vasospasm. Vasospasm rarely occurs when veins are accessed and usually resolves spontaneously.
    D. Hematoma. Hematoma at the site can often be managed effectively by gentle manual pressure.
    E. Embolus air or clot. Never allow the end of the catheter to be open to the air, and make sure that the IV catheter is flushed free of air bubbles before it is connected.
    F. Infiltration of subcutaneous tissue. IV solution may leak out into the subcutaneous tissue as a result of improper catheter placement or damage to the vessel. To help prevent this, confirm placement of the catheter with the flush solution before the catheter is connected to the IV solution. Infiltration often

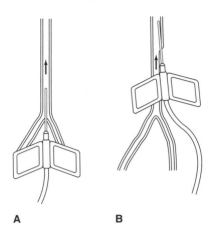

A   **B**

FIGURE 27–2. Two techniques for entering the vein for IV access in the neonate. **(A)** Direct puncture. **(B)** Side entry.

means that the catheter needs to be removed. Avoid hyperosmolar solutions for peripheral infusion.

PERCUTANEOUS CENTRAL VENOUS CATHETERIZATION

I. **Indications.** Insertion of a percutaneous central venous catheter involves inserting a long, small-gauge catheter into a peripheral vein and threading it into a central venous location in the body. The catheter is placed peripherally but is longer than the usual IV device, and hence its tip lies in a more central location. The catheter can be placed in large vessels such as the cephalic and basilic veins in the arm or the saphenous vein in the leg. A percutaneous central venous catheter is helpful especially when it is anticipated that an infant will need IV access for several weeks. This type of device is used commonly with low birth weight infants when it is anticipated that full enteral feedings will not be achieved within a short period. It is used for delivery of fluids, nutritional solutions, and medications.

II. **Equipment.** Cap and mask, sterile gloves, a sterile gown, and a neonatal percutaneous catheter device are needed. Two types of devices are available: **Silastic catheters,** which generally do not have an introducer wire, and **polyurethane catheters,** which contain an introducer wire. Several sizes are available, ranging in diameter from 24 gauge to as small as 28 gauge. (The small catheter is useful in infants weighing <1000 g.) Also required are transparent dressing (for stabilization of the catheter), a sterile tray (any multipurpose tray or tray used for umbilical artery catheter placement may be used), povidone-iodine solution, a tourniquet (or a rubber band), saline flush solution, a T-connector, and sterile tape strips.

III. **Procedure.** For the two commonly used types of catheters (polyurethane catheter with a guide wire and a Silastic catheter without a guide wire), the procedure will vary if a guide wire is or is not present. The placement technique presented next may be used for catheters with a guide wire.
   A. Gather the equipment and assemble the tray with the catheter using sterile technique.
   B. Select a suitable vein in the arm, such as the cephalic or basilic vein, or use the saphenous vein in the leg. Position the infant so that the selected vessel is

accessible. Restrain the infant to prevent contamination of the sterile field with the other extremities.

C. Determine the length of the catheter by measuring the distance between the insertion site and the desired catheter tip location. (For catheters placed in the upper extremities, measure to the level of the superior vena cava or the right atrium; for catheters placed in the lower extremities, measure to the inferior vena cava.) Catheters are typically marked at 5-cm increments to assist with placement.

D. Put on the cap and mask, wash your hands, and then put on the sterile gown and gloves.

E. Prepare the area of insertion with a triple preparation of povidone-iodine solution, and allow the solution to dry.

F. Have an assistant apply the tourniquet.

G. Place sterile drapes around the area of insertion.

H. Remove the plastic protector from the introducer needle, and assess that the catheter is seated inside the introducer needle.

I. Insert the introducer needle into the vein. Confirm entry into the vein by observing for a flashback of blood around the needle at the insertion site. (The blood may not appear *in* the needle, but if the vein had been punctured, blood will appear *at or around* the insertion site.) Do not advance the introducer needle once the flashback (or the blood) has been noted, or you may puncture through the other side of the vessel. (See Figure 27–3.)

J. Release the tourniquet.

K. Hold the introducer needle to maintain the position in the vein, and slowly advance the catheter through the introducer needle with a pair of smooth forceps or fingers into the vein. **(Do not use a hemostat or ridged forceps because it may damage the catheter.)** (See Figure 27–4.)

L. Once the catheter has been advanced to the premeasured location, stabilize the catheter by placing a finger over the vessel where the catheter has been introduced (~1–2 cm above the tip of the introducer needle). Then carefully withdraw the introducer needle completely out of the skin. The area may bleed around the catheter. Hold sterile gauze to the area until the bleeding resolves. (See Figure 27–5.)

M. Separate the introducer needle from the catheter by removing the clip at the top of the needle. Grasp the opposite halves of the introducer needle, and carefully peel each half apart until the needle splits completely. (See Figures 27–6 and 27–7.)

N. While removing the needle, occasionally the catheter will also partially pull out of the vein and will have to be readvanced to the desired location.

O. Remove the stylet wire slowly and steadily from the catheter (do not attempt to reintroduce the stylet once it has been removed from the catheter).

P. As the introducer wire is withdrawn, a blood return may or may not be observed in the catheter, depending on the size of catheter being used. The

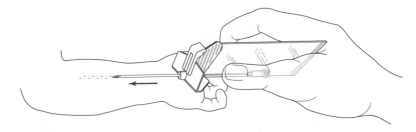

FIGURE 27–3. Technique for insertion of the introducer needle into the vein.

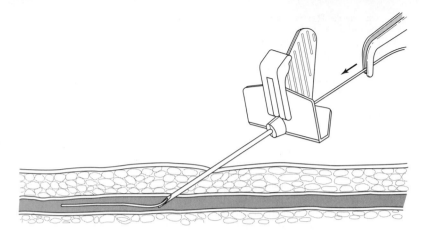

FIGURE 27–4. The catheter is inserted through the introducer needle with forceps.

smaller catheters are less likely to have a blood return. Using a 3-mL syringe, aspirate the blood back through the catheter until the blood reaches the hub. (Slightly more pressure is necessary to withdraw blood through the very small diameter of the catheter; however, if blood is returning, the catheter is patent and in the intravascular system.) Once the blood has been aspirated back to the catheter hub, place a T-connector and flush the catheter with normal saline. (Because of the small diameter of the catheter, it will take slightly more pressure on the syringe to aspirate the blood and to flush solution through the catheter; however, do not use excessive pressure when flushing the catheter because this can cause catheter rupture or fragmentation with possible embolization.)

    Note: It is recommended that the flushing technique be practiced on another catheter before attempting insertion and flushing of a catheter in a patient if the operator is unfamiliar with this type of catheter.

Q. Secure the catheter to the extremity by placing a sterile tape strip over the catheter at the insertion site to anchor the catheter. Curl the remaining external catheter, making sure that there are no kinks, and cover with a sterile transparent dressing. (Do not suture the catheter in place.)

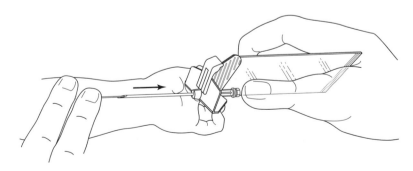

FIGURE 27–5. The catheter is stabilized while withdrawing the needle.

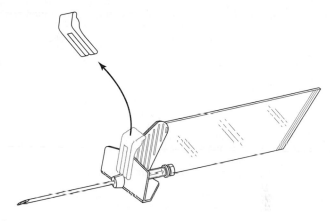

FIGURE 27-6. Technique for separating the introducer needle by removing the needle clip.

R. Connect the IV fluid.

S. Obtain an x-ray film to verify the central catheter tip location. The catheter is radiopaque and can be seen on x-ray film; however, because of its small size, it may be difficult to assess the location of the tip. The manufacturer suggests that it may be necessary to inject a contrast medium (~0.3–1 mL through the catheter just before taking the x-ray film) to assess catheter tip placement.

Note: Ideally, the position of the catheter tip should be in a central location. However, if the catheter has a blood return and is patent but could not be advanced to a central location, it may still be used as a peripheral venous access catheter. Hypertonic solutions should be infused with caution in this case.

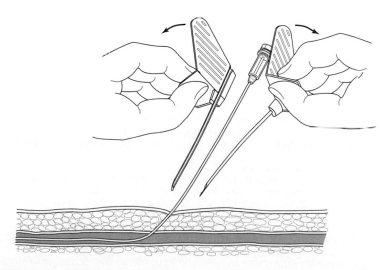

FIGURE 27-7. Technique for removing the needle wing assembly.

  T. Chart the size and the length of catheter that has been inserted and the position of the catheter on x-ray film.

      Note: Catheters that do not contain a guide wire require a different procedure. These catheters will need to be flushed with heparinized saline before being inserted into the vessel. Consult the package insert for instructions specific to the type of catheter.

  U. Precautions

    1. Do not measure the infant's blood pressure on the extremity containing the percutaneous catheter. Doing so could cause occlusion or damage to the catheter.

    2. Do not trim the catheter before placement unless specified by the manufacturer. Doing so may increase the incidence of thrombus formation because of a roughly cut end.

    3. Do not use a hemostat or ribbed forceps to advance the catheter because it could damage the catheter.

    4. When inserting the catheter through the introducer needle, do not pull the catheter back through the introducer needle. Doing so could sever the catheter.

    5. Do not suture the catheter itself. The catheter is very small, and a suture would occlude it.

    6. Do not attempt to infuse blood products or viscous solutions through the catheter; this could cause the catheter to become occluded.

    7. Care should be taken when flushing the catheter. Excessive pressure could rupture it. Do not use a syringe <3 mL to the flush line.

IV. Complications. Only the most common complications have been listed. Refer to the manufacturers' enclosures for a list of further complications.

  A. Infiltration. As with any intravascular device, infiltration is a risk and the area will swell. Because the catheters are longer than peripheral IV catheters, it is necessary to assess for swelling in the area where the tip of the catheter is located, not just at the insertion site.

  B. Catheter occlusion. This catheter is extremely small, fragile, and easily occluded during taping or if the infant bends the extremity containing the catheter. When securing the catheter with the dressing and tape, avoid kinking the catheter; doing so could create an occlusion. If resistance is met when flushing the catheter, do not attempt to flush it any further. Doing so could result in catheter rupture with possible embolization.

  C. Infection or sepsis. Infants requiring this type of catheter are at increased risk for nosocomial infections for many reasons, such as poor skin integrity, an immature immune system, multiple invasive procedures, and exposure to multiple pieces of equipment. Infection specifically related to this type of catheter appears to be related to the length of time the catheter remains in place. Infants who have catheters indwelling for >3 weeks appear to be at greater risk for catheter-related sepsis.

  D. Air embolism. Because these catheters are in a central location, air embolism is a risk. The catheter should be cared for like a central catheter. Special precautions should be taken to avoid air in the line.

  E. Catheter embolus. Do not pull the catheter back through the introducer needle.

V. Maintenance of the catheter

  A. The transparent dressing should remain in place over the catheter. Routine dressing changes are not recommended because of the risk of tearing or dislodging the catheter. The dressing should be changed, using sterile technique, only if the current dressing has drainage under it or is no longer occlusive.

  B. Frequently examine the site and extremity or area in which the catheter is located for inflammation (erythema) or tenderness (as per your neonatal unit's specific IV protocol).

  C. Fluids running through the catheter should be heparinized according to hospital or unit protocol for central catheters.

VI. Removal of the catheter. The catheter can remain in place for several weeks. Several studies have shown an increase in the infection rate after ~2–3 weeks. When ready to remove the catheter, follow the procedure presented next.

A. Gently remove the occlusive dressing from the extremity and the catheter, being careful not to tear the dressing from the catheter.

B. Grasp the catheter tubing near the insertion site, and gently pull the catheter in a continuous movement. If resistance is met, do not apply force and do not stretch the catheter. Doing so could cause the catheter to rupture.

C. Apply a moist, warm compress to the area above the catheter tract for 1 min, and then reattempt removal of the catheter.

D. Once the catheter is removed, inspect and measure it to make sure the entire catheter was removed from the vein. Compare this length with the initial measurement at the time of placement.

E. Cover the area with a sterile dressing.

VENIPUNCTURE (PHLEBOTOMY)

I. Indications

A. To obtain a blood sample for analysis or culture (See also Heelstick, Chapter 23, page 182. Venipuncture typically allows a larger volume of blood to be collected and is the method of choice for obtaining blood cultures.)

B. Administer medications.

II. **Materials required.** A 23- or 25-gauge scalp vein needle, alcohol and povidone-iodine swabs, specimen containers (eg, a red-topped tube), a tourniquet or rubber band (for the scalp), 4 × 4 sterile gauze pads, and a syringe are needed.

III. **Procedure**

A. Have an assistant restrain the infant.

B. Decide which vein to use (to help with vein selection, see Figure 27–1 p 192).

C. If an assistant is not available, restrain the specific area selected for venipuncture. For example, tape the extremity on an armboard.

D. "Tourniquet" the extremity to occlude the vein. Use a rubber band (for the head), a tourniquet, or an assistant's hand to encircle the area proximal to the vein.

E. Prepare the site with antiseptic solution.

F. With the bevel up, puncture the skin, and then direct the needle into the vein at a 45° angle.

G. Once blood enters the tubing, attach the syringe and collect the blood slowly (or administer the medication).

H. Remove the tourniquet.

I. Remove the needle, and apply gentle pressure on the area until hemostasis has occurred. If blood has been collected, distribute it to the appropriate containers to send to the laboratory.

IV. **Complications**

A. **Infection** is a rare complication that can be minimized by using sterile technique.

B. **Venous thrombosis** is often unavoidable, especially when multiple punctures are performed on the same vein.

C. **Hematoma or hemorrhage** is avoided by applying pressure to the site long enough after the needle is removed to ensure hemostasis.

UMBILICAL VEIN CATHETERIZATION

I. Indications

A. Central venous pressure monitoring.

B. Immediate access for IV fluids or emergency medications.

    C. Exchange transfusion or partial exchange transfusion.
    D. Long-term central venous access in extremely low birth weight infants.
II. Materials required. The materials are the same as for umbilical artery catheterization (see p 160), except use a No. 5 French catheter for infants weighing <3.5 kg and a No. 8 French catheter for those weighing >3.5 kg.
III. Procedure
    A. Place the infant supine with a diaper wrapped around both legs to help stabilize the infant.
    B. Prepare the area around the umbilicus with povidone-iodine solution. Put a gown and gloves on.
    C. Prepare the tray as you would for the umbilical artery catheterization procedure (see p 160, Chapter 16: Arterial Access, Umbilical Artery Catheterization, section III,C).
    D. Place sterile drapes, leaving the umbilical area exposed.
    E. Tie a piece of umbilical tape around the base of the umbilicus.
    F. Cut the excess umbilical cord with a scalpel or scissors, leaving a stump of ~0.5–1.0 cm. Identify the umbilical vein. The umbilical vein is thin walled, larger than the two arteries, and close to the periphery of the stump (see Figure 16–3B).
    G. Grasp the end of the umbilicus with the curved hemostat to hold it upright and steady (Figure 27–8A).
    H. Open and dilate the umbilical vein with the forceps.
    I. Once the vein is sufficiently dilated, insert the catheter (Figure 27–8B).
    J. To determine the specific length of catheter needed, see Figure 27–9.
    K. Another method is to measure the length from the xiphoid to the umbilicus and add 0.5–1.0 cm. This number indicates how far the venous catheter should be inserted.
    L. Connect the catheter to the fluid and tubing. Place a piece of silk tape on the catheter, and secure it to the base of the umbilicus with silk sutures (see Figure 16–5, p 163). One can also place a pursestring suture at the base of the cord, not the skin or vessels, and sew it through the tape on two sides. Another way is to place a pursestring suture at the base of the cord and lightly tighten it and then wrap it three times around the cord and tie.

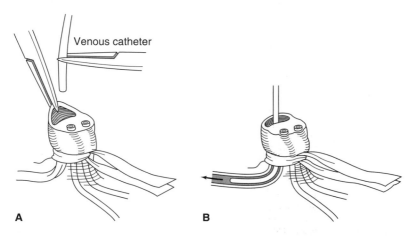

FIGURE 27–8. Umbilical vein catheterization. **(A)** The umbilical stump is held upright before the catheter is inserted. **(B)** The catheter is passed into the umbilical vein.

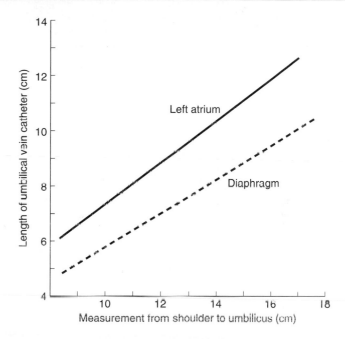

27-9. The umbilical venous catheter is placed above the level of the diaphragm. Determine the shoulder-umbilical length as for the umbilical artery catheter. Use this number and determine the catheter length using the graph. Remember to add the length of the umbilical stump to the length of the catheter. *(Based on data from Dunn PM: Localization of the umbilical catheter by post-mortem measurement. Arch Dis Child 1966;41:69.)*

    M. Obtain an x-ray film to confirm the position (see Figure 9–6, p 108). The correct position for a central venous pressure catheter is with the catheter tip 0.5–1.0 cm above the diaphragm.
    N. Never advance a catheter once it is secured in place.
    O. Occasionally, a catheter will enter the portal vein (Figure 27–10). You should suspect that you have entered the portal vein if you meet resistance and cannot advance the catheter the desired distance or if you detect a "bobbing" motion of the catheter. Several options are available to correct this.
        1. Try injecting flush as you advance the catheter. Sometimes this makes it easier to pass the catheter through the ductus venosus.
        2. Pass another catheter (a smaller size, usually No. 3.5 French) through the same opening. Sometimes this allows one catheter to go through the ductus venosus while the other enters the portal system. The one in the portal system can then be removed.
        3. Apply mild manual pressure in the right upper quadrant over the liver.
IV. Complications
    A. Infection. Minimize the risk of infection through the use of strict sterile technique, and never advance a catheter that has already been positioned.
    B. Thrombolic or embolic phenomenon. Never allow air to enter the end of the catheter. A nonfunctioning catheter should be removed. Never try to flush clots from the end of the catheter.
    C. Hepatic necrosis. Do not allow a catheter to remain in the portal system. In case of emergency placement, the catheter should be advanced only 3 cm (just until blood returns) to avoid hepatic infusion.

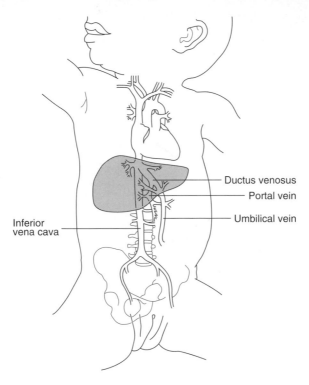

FIGURE 27–10. Anatomic relationships used in the placement of an umbilical venous catheter.

TABLE 27–1. AGENTS ADMINISTERED BY THE INTRAOSSEOUS ROUTE REPORTED IN THE LITERATURE

Fluids	Medications
Crystalloids (normal saline, lactated Ringer's solution, others)	Anesthetic agents
Glucose (dilute if possible when using dextrose 50%)	Antibiotics
Blood and blood products	Atropine
	Calcium gluconate
	Contrast material
	Dexamethasone
	Diazepam
	Diazoxide
	Dobutamine
	Dopamine
	Ephedrine
	Epinephrine
	Heparin
	Insulin
	Isoproterenol
	Lidocaine
	Morphine
	Phenytoin
	Sodium bicarbonate (dilute if possible)

Reproduced with permission from Fletcher MA (ed): *Procedures in Neonatology*, 3rd ed. Lippincott Williams & Wilkins, 2002.

D. **Cardiac arrhythmias.** Arrhythmias are usually caused by a catheter that is inserted too far and is irritating the heart.
E. **Portal hypertension.** Portal hypertension is caused by a catheter that is positioned in the portal system.
F. **Necrotizing enterocolitis (NEC).** NEC is thought to be a complication of umbilical vein catheters, especially if left in place >24 h.

INTRAOSSEOUS INFUSION

I. **Indications.** Intraosseous infusion can be used for emergency vascular access (for administration of fluids and medications) when other methods of vascular access have been attempted and have failed. Many agents have been infused by this technique in the literature, including IV solutions (eg, Ringer's lactate or normal saline), blood and blood products, and a wide variety of medications. See Table 27–1 for a complete list.

II. **Materials required.** Needed are povidone-iodine solution, 4 × 4 sterile gauze pads, a syringe, sterile towels, gloves, an 18-gauge disposable iliac bone marrow aspiration needle (preferred) or an 18- to 20-gauge short spinal needle with a stylet, a short (18–20 gauge) hypodermic needle, or a butterfly (16–19 gauge) needle, a sterile drape, and a syringe with saline flush.

III. **Procedure.** The **proximal tibia** is the preferred site and is described here (Figure 27–11). Other sites are the distal tibia and the distal femur.

A. Restrain the patient's lower leg.
B. Place a small sandbag or IV bag behind the knee for support.
C. Select the area in the midline on the flat surface of the anterior tibia, 1–3 cm below the tibial tuberosity.
D. Clean the area with povidone-iodine solution. Sterile drapes can be placed around the area.
E. Insert the needle at an angle of 10–15 degrees toward the foot to avoid the growth plate.
F. Advance the needle until a lack of resistance is felt (usually no more than 1 cm is necessary), at which point entry into the marrow space should have occurred.
G. Remove the stylet. (*Note:* At this point, aspiration of bone marrow for laboratory studies can be done, if needed. Bone marrow aspirates can be sent for blood chemistry values, carbon dioxide level, pH, hemoglobin level, culture

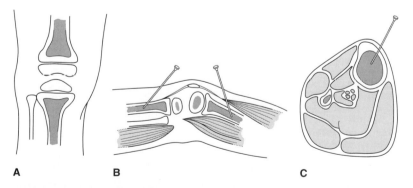

A   B   C

FIGURE 27–11. Technique of intraosseous infusion. **(A)** Anterior view of sites on the tibia and the fibula. **(B)** Sagittal view. **(C)** Cross-section through the tibia. *Reproduced with permission from Hodge D: Intraosseous infusion: a review. Pediatric Emergency Care 1:215, 1985.)*

and sensitivity, and blood type and cross-match.) Secure the needle to the skin with tape to prevent it from dislodging.

H. Attach the needle to IV fluids. Hypertonic and alkaline solutions should be diluted 1:2 with normal saline.

I. Withdraw the needle, and apply pressure over the puncture site.

J. To avoid the risk of infectious complications, this method of vascular access should optimally be used for <2 h.

IV. Complications

A. Fluid infiltration of subcutaneous tissue (most common).

B. Subperiosteal infiltration of fluid.

C. Localized cellulitis.

D. Formation of subcutaneous abscesses.

E. Clotting of bone marrow, resulting in loss of vascular access.

F. Osteomyelitis (rare).

G. Fracture of the bone. X-ray film confirmation of the needle should be done to confirm position and rule out fracture.

H. Compartment syndrome.

I. Blasts in the peripheral blood. Blasts in the peripheral blood have been noted after intraosseous infusions in two patients who have no malignant, infectious, or infiltrative disease of the bone marrow.

J. Sepsis. Minimized by the use of sterile technique.

This section outlines common problems encountered in the neonatal intensive care unit (NICU) or newborn nursery. Guidelines for rapid diagnosis and treatment are given. Clinical situations and institutional guidelines may vary extensively, and recommendations for treatment should be modified based on these factors. If a treatment approach is designated *controversial,* the approach has been useful at some institutions but may not have been confirmed in randomized trials.

28 Abnormal Blood Gas

I. **Problem.** An abnormal blood gas value for a neonate is reported by the laboratory.

II. **Immediate questions**

A. **What component of the blood gas is abnormal?** Accepted normal values for an arterial blood gas sample are pH between 7.35 and 7.45 (pH varies with age, a pH >7.30 is generally considered acceptable), $Paco_2$ between 35 and 45 mm Hg (slightly higher values may be accepted if the blood pH remains normal), and Pao_2 between 55 and 65 mm Hg on room air. Remember that the blood gas measures pH, Pco_2, and O_2, and all the other components (base deficit and bicarbonate) are calculated based on the three levels measured. If one of the components is low (eg, falsely low CO_2), this will falsely elevate the base deficit.

B. **Is this blood gas value very different from the patient's previous blood gas determination?** This is a key question. If the patient has had metabolic acidosis on the last five blood gas measurements and now has metabolic alkalosis, it might be best to repeat the blood gas measurements before initiating treatment. Do not treat the infant on the basis of one abnormal gas value, especially if the infant's clinical status has not changed.

C. **How was the sample collected?** Blood gas measurements can be reported on arterial, venous, or capillary blood samples. Arterial blood samples are the best indicator of pH, $Paco_2$, and Pao_2. Venous blood samples will give a lower pH value and a higher Pco_2 than arterial samples. Capillary samples will give a fair assessment of the infant's pH and Pco_2. Capillary samples give a lower pH value (but not as low as the venous pH) and a slightly higher Pco_2 than arterial samples. An accurate capillary blood gas measurement cannot be obtained on an infant who is hypotensive or in shock.

D. **Is the infant on ventilatory support?** Management of abnormal blood gas levels is approached differently in an intubated infant than in a patient breathing room air.

III. **Differential diagnosis**

A. **Metabolic acidosis.** This is defined as a pH value <7.30–7.35 with a normal CO_2 value and a base deficit >5.

1. **Common causes**

a. Sepsis.

b. Necrotizing enterocolitis.

c. Hypothermia or cold stress.

d. Asphyxia.

e. Periventricular-intraventricular hemorrhage.

f. Patent ductus arteriosus (PDA).

g. Shock.

h. Factitious acidosis (excessive heparin in the syringe). Air contamination can give a large base deficit.

i. Drugs (eg, acetazolamide [Diamox]); for example, benzyl alcohol in doxapram can cause a metabolic acidosis.

2. **Less common causes**
   a. Renal tubular acidosis. This involves a defect in the reabsorption of bicarbonate or the secretion of hydrogen ion and can present in three forms: proximal, distal, or mixed.
   b. Inborn errors of metabolism. See Table 65–1 for those diseases that present with metabolic acidosis.
   c. Maternal use of salicylates and maternal acidosis.
   d. Renal failure.
   e. Congenital lactic acidosis.
   f. Gastrointestinal losses such as frequent loose stools and short bowel syndrome.
B. **Metabolic alkalosis.** This is defined as a pH value >7.45 with a base excess of >5. It is usually iatrogenic and is uncommon.
   1. **Common causes**
      a. Excess alkali administration (eg, sodium bicarbonate, citrate, acetate, or lactate infusion).
      b. Potassium depletion.
      c. Prolonged nasogastric suction.
      d. Diuretic therapy (eg, in patients with bronchopulmonary dysplasia).
   2. **Less common causes**
      a. Pyloric stenosis (vomiting gastric contents that have a high acid concentration).
      b. Bartter's syndrome.
      c. Primary hyperaldosteronism.
C. **Low CO_2, high O_2**
   1. Overventilation.
   2. Air bubble in the syringe.
   3. Hyperventilation therapy, as in persistent pulmonary hypertension.
D. **High CO_2, normal or high O_2**
   1. Obstructed endotracheal tube (eg, mucous plug).
   2. Endotracheal tube down the right main stem bronchus or at the carina.
   3. Pneumothorax.
   4. PDA. Suspect a PDA if the infant has a systolic murmur, active precordium, bounding pulses, and increased pulse pressure. Other clinical signs and symptoms may include congestive heart failure, deteriorating blood gases with an increase in the ventilator settings, and a possible large heart with increased pulmonary vascularity on chest x-ray film.
   5. **Ventilator malfunction.**
   6. **Permissive hypercapnia.** Studies have shown an association between low P_{CO_2} and development of chronic lung disease and cystic periventricular leukomalacia. One study showed decreased risk of chronic lung disease with permissive hypercapnia keeping P_{CO_2} >52 mm Hg. More studies are needed before recommending this practice.
E. **High CO_2, low O_2**
   1. Pneumothorax.
   2. Improper endotracheal tube position. An endotracheal tube positioned in the oropharynx will cause this type of blood gas result.
   3. Increasing respiratory failure.
   4. PDA.
   5. Insufficient respiratory support.
   6. Atelectasis.
   7. Lung disease (intrapulmonary shunt).
F. **Normal CO_2, low O_2**
   1. Agitation.
   2. Pneumothorax.
   3. Improper endotracheal tube position.
   4. Atelectasis.

    5. Pulmonary hypertension.

    6. Pulmonary edema.

IV. Data base

  A. **Physical examination.** Evaluate for signs of sepsis (eg, hypotension or poor perfusion). Check for equal breath sounds; asymmetric breath sounds suggest pneumothorax. Observe for chest wall movement. Listen for breath sounds over the chest versus the epigastric region, which may help determine whether the endotracheal tube is malpositioned. Listen to the heart for any murmur, and palpate for cardiac displacement.

  B. **Laboratory studies**

    1. **Repeat blood gas measurement.** Especially if the result is unexpected or if a major clinical decision is to be made on the basis of venous or capillary blood gas values, an arterial blood sample should be obtained and sent to the laboratory for blood gas values.

    2. **Complete blood cell count with differential** is helpful if sepsis is being considered.

    3. **Serum potassium level.** Severe metabolic alkalosis can cause hypokalemia.

  C. **Radiologic and other studies**

    1. **Pulmonary mechanics.** Many ventilators now provide the tidal volume (TV) delivered. The normal TV is 5–6 mL/kg. If the TV is low, this could mean that not enough pressure is given or there is an obstruction in the endotracheal tube.

    2. **Transillumination of the chest** should be done if pneumothorax is suspected (for details on this procedure, see p 169).

    3. **Chest x-ray study.** A chest x-ray study should be performed if an abnormal blood gas value is reported by the laboratory, unless there is an obvious cause. An anteroposterior view should be obtained to check endotracheal tube placement, rule out air leak (eg, pneumothorax), check heart size and pulmonary vascularity (increased or decreased), and determine whether the infant is being hypoventilated or hyperventilated.

    4. **Abdominal x-ray study.** An abdominal x-ray study should be done if necrotizing enterocolitis is suspected in a patient with **severe metabolic acidosis.**

    5. **Ultrasonography of the head** will allow diagnosis of intraventricular hemorrhage if present.

    6. **Echocardiography.** PDA or other cardiac abnormality may be detected with echocardiography.

V. Plan

  A. **Overall plan.** Verify the blood gas result, find the cause of the problem, and provide appropriate treatment for the specific cause. The first step is to examine the infant. If the infant's clinical status has not changed, repeat blood gas measurements to verify the report. If the clinical status has changed, the abnormal report is probably correct; repeat blood gas measurements can be obtained, but further evaluation of the infant should begin.

  B. **Specific management**

    1. **Metabolic acidosis**

      a. **General measures.** Most institutions treat acidosis with an alkali infusion if the base excess is greater than −5 to −10 or if the pH is ≤7.25. The alkali can be given as one dose over 20–30 min or it can be given as an 8- to 12-h correction. If the acidosis is mild, usually only one dose is given and repeat blood gas measurements are obtained. If the acidosis is severe, a dose is given and correction is started at the same time. One of three medications is used.

        i. **Sodium bicarbonate** can be used if the infant's serum sodium and Pco_2 are not high. If given as a one-time dose, it should be 1–2 mEq/kg diluted 1:1 with sterile water. It should be given over 20–30 min unless the infant is unstable, in which case an intravenous push dose can be given at a rate of 1 mL/min. The total dose required to correct the base deficit is

Bicarbonate dose (mEq) = Base deficit × Body weight (kg) × 0.3

It should be added to the intravenous fluids, and the correction should be given over 8–12 h.

ii. **Tromethamine (THAM)** can be used in infants who have metabolic acidosis but have a high serum sodium (>150 mEq/L) or high P_{CO_2}(>65 mm Hg). *It should be used only in infants who have a good urine output.* (For dosage and other pharmacologic information, see Chapter 80.)

iii. **Polycitrate (Polycitra).** This alkali is especially useful in patients receiving acetazolamide (Diamox). It consists of 1 mEq sodium, 1 mEq potassium, and 2 mEq citrate. Each 1 mEq citrate equals 1 mEq bicarbonate. The dose is 2–3 mEq/kg/day polycitrate in 3 or 4 divided doses. Adjust the dosage to maintain a normal pH.

b. **The underlying cause should be treated** as outlined next.

i. **Sepsis.** Initiate a septic workup and consider broad-spectrum antibiotics. (For specific antibiotic agents, see Chapter 80.)

ii. **Necrotizing enterocolitis.** See Chapter 71.

iii. **Hypothermia or cold stress.** See the section on treatment of hypothermia in Chapter 5.

iv. **Periventricular-intraventricular hemorrhage.** Weekly ultrasonographic examinations of the head and daily head circumferences are indicated. Monitor the infant for signs of increased intracranial pressure (convulsions, vomiting, hypotension).

v. **PDA.** The patient who has a clinically symptomatic PDA should be treated. Treatment includes furosemide, decreased fluid intake, and a course of indomethacin. (For drug dosages, see Chapter 80.)

vi. **Renal tubular acidosis.** Treatment consists of sodium bicarbonate therapy (see section III,A,2,a).

vii. **Inborn errors of metabolism.** See Chapter 65.

viii. **Maternal use of salicylates.** Acidosis usually resolves without treatment.

ix. **Renal failure.** See Chapter 75.

x. **Congenital lactic acidosis.** Correction of the metabolic acidosis (see section III,A) and megavitamin therapy are indicated.

2. **Metabolic alkalosis.** The treatment of metabolic alkalosis depends on the cause.

a. **Excess alkali.** Adjust or discontinue the dose of THAM, sodium bicarbonate, or polycitrate.

b. **Hypokalemia.** If the serum potassium level is low, metabolic alkalosis can occur by a shift of hydrogen ions into cells as potassium is lost. The infant's potassium level should be corrected (see Chapter 44).

c. **Prolonged nasogastric suction** is treated with intravenous fluid replacement, usually with ½ normal saline containing 20 mEq potassium chloride, replaced milliliter for milliliter each shift.

d. **Diuretics.** Mild alkalosis is sometimes seen; no specific treatment is usually necessary.

e. **Bartter's syndrome** is treated with indomethacin and potassium supplements.

f. **Primary hyperaldosteronism** is treated with dexamethasone. (For dosage, see Chapter 80.)

3. **Other causes of abnormal blood gases**

a. **Pneumothorax.** See Chapter 51.

b. **Mucous plug.** If an infant has decreased breath sounds on both sides of the chest and has retractions, a plugged endotracheal tube is proba-

TABLE 28-1. CHANGES IN BLOOD GAS LEVELS CAUSED BY CHANGES IN VENTILATOR SETTINGS

Variable	Rate	PIP	PEEP	IT	F_{IO_2}
To increase Pa_{CO_2}	Decr.	Decr.	NA	NA	NA
To decrease Pa_{CO_2}	Incr.	Incr.	NA[a]	NA[b]	NA
To increase Pa_{O_2}	NA	Incr.	Incr.	Incr.	Incr.
To decrease Pa_{O_2}	NA	Decr.	Decr.	NA	Decr.

PIP, peak inspiratory pressure; PEEP, positive end-expiratory pressure; IT, inspiratory time; F_{IO_2}, fraction of inspired oxygen; Decr., decrease; NA, not applicable; Incr., increase.
[a]In severe pulmonary edema and pulmonary hemorrhage, increased PEEP can decrease Pa_{CO_2}.
[b]Not applicable unless the inspiratory:expiratory ratio is excessive.

bly responsible. The infant can be suctioned, and, if clinically stable, repeat blood gas measurements are obtained. If the infant is in extreme distress, the tube should be replaced.

  c. **Overventilation.** If the blood gas levels reveal overventilation, the ventilation parameters need to be adjusted. If the oxygen level is high, the following parameters can be decreased: oxygen, positive end-expiratory pressure (PEEP), peak inspiratory pressure (PIP), or inspiratory time. If the patient's carbon dioxide level is low, the following parameters can be decreased: rate, PIP, or expiratory time. Deciding which parameter to wean depends on the patient's lung disease and the disease course. See Table 28-1 for changes in blood gas levels caused by changes in ventilator settings.

  d. **Agitation.** An agitated infant may have a drop in oxygenation and may need to be sedated or have ventilator settings changed. One may have to sit by the bedside and try different rates to see whether the infant fights less. If sedation is chosen, phenobarbital, diazepam, lorazepam, midazolam, fentanyl, chloral hydrate, or morphine may be used. (For dosages, see Chapter 80.) Use the agent with which your institution has experience. *Note:* Agitation can be a sign of hypoxia, so a blood gas level should be obtained before ordering sedation. If there is documented hypoxia, attempts to increase oxygenation should be used.

  e. **Problems with endotracheal tube placement.** An infant with a tube placed down the right main stem bronchus will have breath sounds on the right only. An infant with a tube that has dislodged or become plugged will have decreased or no breath sounds on chest auscultation. The patient needs to be reintubated. It is helpful to know and chart the specific mark on the endotracheal tube when it is in correct position so that one will have an idea of whether the tube has been pulled out or pushed in.

  f. **Ventilator malfunction.** The respiratory therapy department should be notified to check the ventilator and replace it if necessary.

  g. **Increasing respiratory failure.** Ventilator settings need to be adjusted.

  h. **Insufficent respiratory support.** If the infant's chest is not moving, the PIP is not high enough and adjustment of the ventilator setting is needed. Also check the TV; if it is low, it could mean not enough pressure is given.

  i. **Atelectasis.** Treatment consists of percussion and postural drainage and possibly increased PIP or PEEP. Percussion should be used with caution in premature infants. A study showed an association with porencephaly in extreme premature infants.

  j. **Pulmonary edema.** Diuretics (eg, furosemide) (see Chapter 80) and mechanical ventilation are indicated.

  k. **Pulmonary hypertension.** See Chapter 62.

29 Apnea and Bradycardia ("A's and B's")

I. **Problem.** An infant has just had an apneic episode with bradycardia. Apnea is the absence of breathing for >20 s or a shorter pause associated with oxygen desaturation or bradycardia (<100 beats/min). Central apnea is the complete absence of respiratory effort. Apnea of prematurity is most prevalent in preemies <36 weeks' gestation and is most commonly central apnea. Obstructive apnea occurs when an infant breathes but no airflow is present because of an obstruction. Mixed apnea is both central and obstructive apnea. Periodic breathing is respiratory pauses <10 s with normal respirations between episodes. This is not associated with bradycardia.

II. **Immediate questions**

A. **What is the gestational age of the infant?** Apnea and bradycardia are common in premature infants. In term infants, they are uncommon and are usually associated with a serious disorder. **Apnea in a term infant is never physiologic;** it usually requires a full workup to determine the cause.

B. **Was significant stimulation needed to return the heart rate to normal?** An infant requiring significant stimulation (eg, oxygen by bag-and-mask ventilation) needs immediate evaluation and treatment. An infant who has had one episode of apnea and bradycardia not requiring oxygen supplementation may not need a full evaluation unless he or she is term.

C. **If the patient is already receiving medication (eg, theophylline) for apnea and bradycardia, is the dosage adequate?** Determining the serum drug level is helpful.

D. **Did the episode occur during or after feeding?** Insertion of a nasogastric tube may cause a vagal reflex, resulting in apnea and bradycardia. Gastroesophageal reflux (GER) may cause apnea and bradycardia generally during or shortly after feeding. Consider aspiration in an infant who has been doing well and feeding.

E. **How old is the infant?** Apnea and bradycardia in the first 24 h are usually pathologic. The peak incidence of apnea of prematurity occurs between 5–7 days postnatal age but can occur earlier.

III. **Differential diagnosis.** Causes of apnea and bradycardia can be classified according to diseases and disorders of various organ systems, gestational age, or postnatal age.

A. **Diseases and disorders of various organ systems**

1. Head and central nervous system
   a. Perinatal asphyxia.
   b. Intraventricular or subarachnoid hemorrhage.
   c. Meningitis.
   d. Hydrocephalus with increased intracranial pressure.
   e. Cerebral infarct with seizures.
   f. Seizures.

2. **Respiratory system**
   a. Hypoxia.
   b. Airway obstruction.
   c. Lung disease.
   d. Inadequate ventilation or performing extubation too early.

3. **Cardiovascular system**
   a. Congestive heart failure.
   b. Patent ductus arteriosus.

    c. Cardiac disorders such as congenital heart block, hypoplastic left heart syndrome, and transposition of the great vessels.
4. **Gastrointestinal tract**
    a. Necrotizing enterocolitis (NEC).
    b. GER.
    c. Feeding intolerance.
5. **Hematologic system**
    a. **Anemia.** There is no specific hematocrit at which apnea and bradycardia will occur. They have been seen in infants with anemia of prematurity. These infants show significant improvement after transfusion.
    b. **Polycythemia.** This disorder is more common in term infants.
6. **Other diseases and disorders**
    a. **Temperature Instability.** Apnea and bradycardia may occur in patients with temperature instability, especially hyperthermia but also hypothermia. Note the incubator temperature. An infant may have a normal body temperature but may have a rise in incubator temperature (meaning that the infant is hypothermic) or may require a lower incubator temperature (meaning that the infant is hyperthermic). Any rapid fluctuation of temperature can cause apnea. Cold stress can occur after birth or during transport or a procedure and may produce apnea.
    b. **Infection (sepsis).**
    c. **Electrolyte imbalance.** Hypoglycemia, hyponatremia, hypernatremia, hypermagnesemia, hyperkalemia, hyperammonemia, and hypocalcemia can cause apnea and bradycardia.
    d. **Vagal reflex.** This may occur secondary to nasogastric tube insertion, feeding, and suctioning.
    e. **Drugs.** High levels of phenobarbital or other sedatives, such as diazepam and chloral hydrate, may cause apnea and bradycardia. Oversedation from maternal drugs such as magnesium sulfate, opiates, and general anesthesia can cause apnea in the newborn.
B. **Gestational age.** See Table 29–1.
    1. **Full-term infants.** In full-term infants of any neonatal age, apnea and bradycardia usually do not result from physiologic causes. The disease or disorder causing apnea and bradycardia must be identified.
    2. **Preterm infants.** More common causes of apnea and bradycardia in preterm infants are listed in Table 29–1. The most common cause is apnea of prematurity. It occurs in infants who are usually <34 weeks' gestation, weigh <1800 g, and have no other identifiable cause of the apnea

TABLE 29–1. MORE COMMON CAUSES OF APNEA AND BRADYCARDIA ACCORDING TO GESTATIONAL AGE

Premature infant	Full-term infant	All ages
Apnea of prematurity	Cerebral infarction	Sepsis
PDA	Polycythemia	NEC
HMD		Meningitis
Respiratory insufficiency of prematurity		Aspiration
PV-IVH		GER
Anemia of prematurity		Pneumonia
Posthemorrhagic hydrocephalus		Cardiac disorder
		Postextubation atelectasis
		Seizures
		Cold stress
		Asphyxia

PDA, patent ductus arteriosus; NEC, necrotizing enterocolitis; HMD, hyaline membrane disease; GER, gastroesophageal reflux; PV-IVH, periventricular-intraventricular hemorrhage.

and bradycardia. Apnea of prematurity usually presents between the second and seventh days of life.

C. **Postnatal age.** Certain types of conditions produce apnea at varying postnatal ages.

1. **Onset within hours after birth:** Oversedation from maternal drugs, asphyxia, seizures, hypermagnesemia, or hyaline membrane disease.
2. **Onset <1 week:** Postextubation atelectasis, patent ductus arteriosus, periventricular-intraventricular hemorrhage, or apnea of prematurity.
3. **Onset >1 week of age:** Posthemorrhagic hydrocephalus with increased intracranial pressure or seizures.
4. **Onset at 6–10 weeks:** Anemia of prematurity.
5. **Variable onset:** Sepsis, NEC, meningitis, aspiration, GER, cardiac disorder, pneumonia, cold stress, or fluctuations in temperatures.

IV. **Data base.** Determine whether there has been any prenatal risk of sepsis. The cord pH should be obtained to rule out birth asphyxia. A history of feeding intolerance will increase the suspicion of NEC.

A. **Physical examination.** Perform a complete physical examination, paying careful attention to the following signs:

1. **Head.** Look for signs of increased intracranial pressure.
2. **Heart.** Listen for a murmur or gallop.
3. **Lungs.** Check for adequate movement of the chest if mechanical ventilation is being used.
4. **Abdomen.** Check for abdominal distention, one of the earliest signs of NEC. Other signs of NEC are decreased bowel sounds and visible bowel loops.
5. **Skin.** An infant with polycythemia has a ruddy appearance. Pallor is associated with anemia.

B. **Laboratory studies**

1. **Complete blood cell count with differential.** Findings may suggest infection, possible anemia, or polycythemia.
2. **Serum electrolyte, calcium, and glucose levels** to rule out metabolic abnormality.
3. **Serum phenobarbital and theophylline levels** are obtained if indicated.
4. **Arterial blood gas levels** should be obtained to rule out hypoxia and acidosis.

C. **Radiologic and other studies**

1. **Chest x-ray study.** A chest x-ray study should be performed immediately if there is any suspicion of heart or lung disease.
2. **Electrocardiography.** If cardiac disease is suspected, electrocardiography should be performed.
3. **Echocardiography.** To evaluate for cardiac disease.
4. **Abdominal x-ray study.** An abdominal x-ray study should be performed immediately if indicated. It may detect signs of NEC (see p 118).
5. **Ultrasonography of the head** is performed to rule out periventricular-intraventricular hemorrhage or hydrocephalus.
6. **Computed tomography (CT) of the head** will detect cerebral infarction and subarachnoid hemorrhage, if present.
7. **Barium swallow** is performed to rule out GER only in cases of apnea and bradycardia associated with feeding.
8. **Lumbar puncture.** Lumbar puncture and a cerebrospinal fluid examination should be performed if meningitis is suspected or if increased intracranial pressure from hydrocephalus is causing apnea and bradycardia.
9. **Esophageal pH probe testing (acid reflux test of Tuttle and Grossman)** is useful in determining whether acidic GER is present. A small-caliber tube (to which a pH electrode is attached) is passed into the distal esophagus. Continuous monitoring can be carried out over 4–24 h. If the pH is acidic, acidic GER is occurring. Most reflux in infants is not acidic.
10. **Electroencephalography.** Because apnea and bradycardia may be a manifestation of seizure activity, an electroencephalogram (EEG) is obtained in any infant who may be having seizures.

11. **Pneumography, thermistor pneumography, and polysomnography.** For a detailed discussion of these procedures, see Chapter 74.

V. **Plan**
  A. **Determine the cause of apnea and bradycardia,** and treat if possible.
  B. **Remember that sepsis is a cause that cannot be overlooked because antibiotics need to be started.** Make sure to rule out sepsis before treating other causes.
  C. **Apnea of prematurity**
   1. **General measures include providing tactile stimulation.**
   2. **Specific treatment**
      a. **Theophylline or caffeine** is used initially. Caffeine seems to have fewer side effects than theophylline, but the choice of drug depends on institutional preference and availability. (For dosages, see Chapter 80.) Therapy can usually be discontinued by postconceptional age (usually 37 weeks), depending on the weight of the infant (usually 1800–2000 g) or if the infant has been free of apnea for 7 days. It is important to remember that the more immature infant will probably require treatment longer. One study found that the incidence of apnea persisting beyond 38 weeks' postconceptional age was significantly higher in the 24- to 27-week infant than in the ≥28-week infant.
      b. **If the just-mentioned drug trial fails, use continuous positive airway pressure (CPAP)** via nasal prongs at a rate of 2–4 cm H_2O and continue administration of the drug. An alternative to nasal CPAP is to use high-flow nasal cannula at 1–2 L/min.
      c. **If apnea persists, begin doxapram.** Doxapram appears to be efficacious when theophylline and caffeine have failed. One concern regarding doxapram is that it contains benzyl alcohol as a preservative. It is important to watch for metabolic acidosis in those infants. If it occurs, consider stopping the medication. (For drug dosage, side effects, and other pharmacologic information, see Chapter 80.) Another risk of doxapram is a possible lengthening of the QTC interval above 440 ms, a life-threatening threshold.
      d. **Mechanical ventilation** should be used if apnea and bradycardia cannot be controlled by drug therapy or nasal CPAP. Low pressures are used at the rate necessary to prevent apnea. (See p 533.)
   3. **Long-term monitoring of respiratory function.** See Chapter 74.
  D. **Anemia.** Most institutions do not treat anemia if the infant is asymptomatic and is feeding and growing and the reticulocyte count indicates that red blood cells are being made (>5–6%). If the hematocrit is low (usually <21–25%, based on the institution), or the infant is symptomatic or not feeding well, and the reticulocyte count is not appropriate for the low hematocrit (ie, the reticulocyte count is <2–3%), transfusion is indicated (*controversial*). If the infant is on oxygen or on respiratory support, transfusion is usually indicated more frequently to maintain a hematocrit at a higher level. Many institutions are now using erythropoietin and iron for anemia of prematurity and decreasing the need for transfusions.
  E. **GER.** Keep the infant in the prone position (head up) as much as possible, and use small-volume, thickened feedings. Prone position has become *controversial* since its association with sudden infant death syndrome (SIDS). *Metoclopramide (Reglan) may also be tried (controversial).* (For dosage and other pharmacologic information, see Chapter 80). GER is very frequent in premature infants. A study measuring esophageal intraluminal impedance (not a routine practice) showed that GER did not play a significant role in the development of apnea of prematurity. There was no temporal relationship between GER and apnea of prematurity. The effectiveness of metoclopramide has not been conclusively proven.

30 Arrhythmia

I. **Problem.** An infant has an abnormal tracing on the heart rate monitor.
II. **Immediate questions**
   A. **What is the heart rate?** Heart rate in newborns varies from 70–190 beats/min. It is normally 120–140 beats/min but may decrease to 70–90 beats/min during sleep and increase to 170–190 beats/min with increased activity such as crying. See Table 30–1 for normal heart rate values.
   B. **Is the abnormality continuous or transient?** Transient episodes of sinus bradycardia, tachycardia, or arrhythmias (usually lasting <15 s) are benign and do not require further workup. Episodes lasting >15 s usually require full electrocardiographic (ECG) assessment.
   C. **Is the infant symptomatic?** A symptomatic infant may need immediate treatment. Signs and symptoms of some pathologic arrhythmias include tachypnea, poor skin perfusion, lethargy, hepatomegaly, and rales on pulmonary examination. All of these signs and symptoms may signify congestive heart failure, which may accompany arrhythmias. Congestive heart failure resulting from rapid cardiac rhythms is unusual with heart rates <240 beats/min.
III. **Differential diagnosis**
   A. **Heart rate abnormalities**
      1. **Tachycardia.** Tachycardia is a heart rate >2 standard deviations above the mean for age (see Table 30–1).
         a. **Benign causes**
            i. Postdelivery.
            ii. Heat or cold stress.
            iii. Painful stimuli.
            iv. Medications (eg, atropine, theophylline [aminophylline], epinephrine, intravenous glucagon, pancuronium bromide [Pavulon], tolazoline, and isoproterenol) can cause tachycardia.
         b. **Pathologic causes**
            i. **More common:** fever, shock, hypoxia, anemia, sepsis, patent ductus arteriosus, and congestive heart failure.
            ii. **Less common:** hyperthyroidism, metabolic disorders, cardiac arrhythmias, and hyperammonemia.
      2. **Bradycardia.** Bradycardia is a heart rate >2 standard deviations below the mean for age (see Table 30–1). Transient bradycardia is fairly common in newborns; rates range from 60–70 beats/min.
         a. **Benign causes**
            i. Defecation.
            ii. Vomiting.
            iii. Micturition.
            iv. Gavage feedings.
            v. Suctioning.
            vi. Medications (eg, propranolol, digitalis, atropine, and infusion of calcium).
         b. **Pathologic causes**
            i. **More common:** hypoxia, apnea, convulsions, airway obstruction, air leak (eg, pneumothorax), congestive heart failure, intracranial bleeding, severe acidosis, and severe hypothermia.
            ii. **Less common:** hyperkalemia, cardiac arrhythmias, pulmonary hemorrhage, diaphragmatic hernia, hypothyroidism, and hydrocephalus.
   B. **Arrhythmias**
      1. **Benign arrhythmias** include any transient episode (<15 s) of sinus bradycardia and tachycardia and any of the benign causes of sinus tachycardia

TABLE 30–1. MINIMUM AND MAXIMUM HEART RATES IN NORMAL NEWBORNS

Age	Minimum	Mean	Maximum	SD
0–24 h	85	119	145	16.1
1–7 days	100	133	175	22.3
8–30 days	115	163	190	19.9

SD, standard deviation.
Reproduced with permission from Hastreiter AR, Abella JE: The electrocardiogram in the newborn period: I. The normal infant. *J Pediatr* 1971;78:146.

and bradycardia noted in sections III,A,1 and 2. Sinus arrhythmia, a phasic variation in the heart rate often associated with respiration, is also benign.
  a. **Premature atrial beats** can occur in the newborn and are usually benign. The QRS is narrow, and the T waves are often discordant. (See the example in Figure 30–1C.) They tend to decrease in number or go away entirely in the first few months of life. A workup is usually not indicated unless the infant has the premature atrial beats in association with structural cardiac disease.
  b. **Unifocal premature ventricular beats** are fairly frequent in the newborn. The QRS is wide, and the T wave is discordant with the sinus T wave. (See Figure 30–1D.) If seen in a newborn, obtain a 12-lead ECG. Do not treat unless the infant is symptomatic. Sometimes premature ventricular contractions (PVCs) become less frequent when the sinus rate increases. PVCs tend to decrease in number or go away entirely in the first few months of life.
  c. **Benign bradycardia** is unusual but not rare.
2. **Pathologic arrhythmias**
  a. **Supraventricular tachycardia (SVT):** the most common type of cardiac arrhythmia seen in the neonate (see Figure 30–1A).
  b. **Atrial flutter:** difficult to distinguish from other SVTs, unless the block is >2:1.
  c. **Atrial fibrillation:** less common than SVT or atrial flutter.
  d. **Wolff-Parkinson-White syndrome** (a short PR interval and delta wave and slow upstroke of the QRS complex): difficult to identify when the rate is fast (see Figure 30–1B).
  e. **Ectopic beats.**
  f. **Ventricular tachycardia.**
  g. **Atrioventricular (AV) block,** with symptoms occurring in newborns with complete AV block and ventricular rates <55 beats/min.
3. **Secondary to extracardiac disease**
  a. **Sepsis (usually tachycardia).**
  b. **Diseases of the central nervous system (usually bradycardia).**
  c. **Hypoglycemia.**
  d. **Drug toxicity.**
      i. **Digoxin.** The effect of this drug is potentiated by hypokalemia, alkalosis, hypercalcemia, and hypomagnesemia.
      ii. **Quinidine.**
      iii. **Theophylline.**
  e. **Adrenal insufficiency.**
  f. **Electrolyte (eg, potassium, sodium, magnesium, or calcium) abnormalities.**
  g. **Metabolic acidosis or alkalosis.**
IV. **Data base**
  A. **Physical examination.** Perform a complete physical examination. Check for signs of congestive heart failure (ie, tachypnea, rales on pulmonary examina-

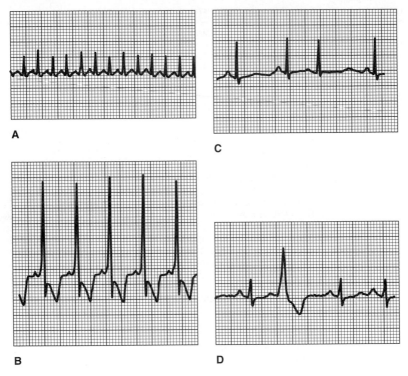

FIGURE 30–1. (A) Supraventricular, narrow QRS tachycardia with a rate of 300 beats per minute. The PR interval is long for this rate. **(B)** Wolff-Parkinson-White syndrome with a short PR interval and a delta upstroke on the QRS complex. The T waves are often discordant. **(C)** A premature atrial beat. The QRS is narrow, and the T wave is concordant with sinus T waves. **(D)** A premature ventricular beat. The QRS is wide, and the T wave is discordant with the sinus T wave.

tion, enlarged liver, and cardiomegaly). Vomiting and lethargy may be seen in patients with digoxin toxicity. Hypokalemia can cause ileus.

B. Laboratory studies
   1. **Electrolyte, calcium, and magnesium levels.**
   2. **Blood gas levels** may reveal acidosis or hypoxia.
   3. **Drug levels** to evaluate for toxicity.
      a. **Digoxin.** Normal serum levels are 0.5–2.0 ng/mL (sometimes up to 4 ng/mL). Elevated levels of digoxin alone are not diagnostic of toxicity; clinical and ECG findings consistent with toxicity are also needed, and many neonates have naturally occurring substances that interfere with the radioimmunoassay test for digoxin.
      b. **Quinidine.** Normal serum levels are 3–7 mg/mL. Toxicity is associated with levels >7 mg/mL.
      c. **Theophylline.** Normal levels are 4–12 μg/mL. Toxicity is associated with levels >15–20 μg/mL.
C. Radiologic and other studies
   1. **ECG.** Full ECG evaluation should be performed in all infants who have an abnormal ECG tracing that lasts >15 s or is not related to a benign condition. Diagnostic features of the common arrhythmias are listed next.

a. **SVT** (see Figure 30–1A)
   i. A ventricular rate of 180–300 beats/min.
   ii. No change in heart rate with activity or crying.
   iii. An abnormal P wave or PR interval.
   iv. A fixed R–R interval.
b. **Atrial flutter**
   i. The atrial rate is 220–400 beats/min.
   ii. A sawtooth configuration seen best in leads V_1–V_3, but often difficult to identify when a 2:1 block or rapid ventricular rate is present.
   iii. The QRS complex is usually normal.
c. **Atrial fibrillation**
   i. Irregular atrial waves that vary in size and shape from beat to beat.
   ii. The atrial rate is 350–600 beats/min.
   iii. The QRS complex is normal, but ventricular response is irregular.
d. **Wolff-Parkinson-White syndrome** (see Figure 30–1B)
   i. A short PR interval.
   ii. A widened QRS complex.
   iii. Presence of a delta wave.
e. **Ventricular tachycardia**
   i. Ventricular premature beats at a rate of 120–200 beats/min.
   ii. A widened QRS complex.
f. **Ectopic beats**
   i. An abnormal P wave.
   ii. A widened QRS complex.
g. **AV block**
   i. **First-degree block**
      (a) A prolonged PR interval (normal range, 0.08–0.12 s)
      (b) Normal sinus rhythm.
      (c) A normal QRS complex.
   ii. **Second-degree block**
      (a) **Mobitz type I**
         • A prolonged PR interval with a dropped ventricular beat.
         • A normal QRS complex.
      (b) **Mobitz type II.** A constant PR interval with dropped ventricular beats.
   iii. **Third-degree block**
      (a) A regular atrial beat.
      (b) A slower ventricular rate.
      (c) Independent atrial and ventricular beats.
      (d) The atrial rate increases with crying and level of activity. The ventricular rate usually stays the same.
h. **Hyperkalemia**
   i. Tall, tented T waves.
   ii. A widened QRS complex.
   iii. A flat and wide P wave.
   iv. Ventricular fibrillation and late asystole.
i. **Hypokalemia**
   i. Prolonged QT and PR intervals.
   ii. A depressed ST segment.
   iii. A flat T wave.
j. **Hypocalcemia.** A prolonged QT interval.
k. **Hypercalcemia.** A shortened QT interval.
l. **Hypomagnesemia.** Same as for hyperkalemia.
m. **Hyponatremia**
   i. A short QT interval.
   ii. Increased duration of the QRS complex.

n. **Hypernatremia**
   i. A prolonged QT interval.
   ii. Decreased duration of the QRS complex.
o. **Metabolic acidosis**
   i. Prolonged PR and QRS intervals.
   ii. Increased amplitude of the P wave.
   iii. Tall, peaked T waves.
p. **Metabolic alkalosis.** An inverted T wave.
q. **Digoxin**
   i. **Therapeutic levels:** A prolonged PR interval and a short QT interval.
   ii. **Toxic levels:** Most common are sinoatrial block, second-degree AV block, and multiple ectopic beats; also seen are AV block and bradycardia.
r. **Quinidine**
   i. **Therapeutic levels:** prolonged PR and QT intervals, a decreased amplitude of P wave, and a widened QRS complex.
   ii. **Toxic levels:** a prolonged PR interval, a prolonged QRS complex, AV block, and multifocal ventricular premature beats.
s. **Theophylline**
   i. **Therapeutic levels:** no effect.
   ii. **Toxic levels:** tachycardia and conduction abnormality.
2. **Chest x-ray studies** should be obtained in all infants with suspected heart failure or air leak.

V. Plan
A. **General management.** First, decide whether the arrhythmia is benign or pathologic, as noted previously. If it is pathologic, full ECG evaluation must be performed. Any acid-base disorder, hypoxia, or electrolyte abnormality needs to be corrected.
B. **Specific management**
   1. **Heart rate abnormalities**
      a. **Tachycardia**
         i. **Benign.** No treatment is necessary because the tachycardia is usually secondary to a self-limited event.
         ii. **Medications.** With certain medications, such as theophylline, you can order a serum drug level to determine whether it is in the toxic range. If it is, lowering the dosage may restore normal rhythm. Otherwise, a decision must be made to accept the tachycardia, if the medication is needed, or to discontinue the drug.
         iii. **Pathologic conditions.** The underlying disease should be treated.
      b. **Bradycardia**
         i. **Benign.** No treatment is usually necessary.
         ii. **Drug-related.** Check the serum drug level if possible, and then consider lowering the dosage or discontinuing the drug unless it is necessary.
         iii. **Pathologic**
            (a) Treat the underlying disease.
            (b) In severe hypotension or cardiac arrest, check the airway and initiate breathing and cardiac compressions.
            (c) Administer atropine, epinephrine, or isoproterenol to restore normal rhythm. (For dosages, see Chapter 80.)
   2. **Arrhythmias.** For dosages of drugs mentioned next and for other pharmacologic information, see Chapter 80; for the technique of cardioversion, see section VI.
      a. **Benign.** Only observation (no other treatment) is indicated.
      b. **Pathologic.** Treat any underlying acid-base disorders, hypoxia, or electrolyte abnormalities.
         i. **SVT**

(a) **If the infant's condition is critical,** electrical cardioversion is indicated, with digoxin started for maintenance therapy.

(b) **If the infant's condition is stable,** vagal stimulation (an ice-cold washcloth applied to the infant's face for a few seconds) can be tried. Adenosine (100 μg/kg), by quick push into a central vein, will convert SVT to sinus rhythm. It may be necessary to double the dose (200 μg/kg). The maximum dose is 300 μg/kg. *Never use* verapamil in infants. Digoxin should be started as a maintenance drug. Another drug that may be used instead of or in addition to digoxin is propranolol. SVT refractory to digoxin and propranolol may be treated with flecainide or amiodarone.

ii. **Atrial flutter**

(a) If the infant's condition is critical (severe congestive heart failure or unstable hemodynamic state), perform electrical cardioversion, with digoxin started for maintenance therapy.

(b) If the infant is stable, start digoxin, which slows the ventricular rate. A combination of digoxin and propranolol may be used instead of digoxin alone.

iii. **Recurrent atrial flutter.** Management is the same as that for atrial flutter.

iv. **Atrial fibrillation.** Management is the same as that for atrial flutter

v. **Wolff-Parkinson-White syndrome.** Treat any symptomatic arrhythmias that may occur. (It is accompanied by a high incidence of SVT.)

vi. **Ventricular tachycardia.** Perform electrical cardioversion (except in digitalis toxicity), with lidocaine started for maintenance therapy. Although lidocaine is the drug of choice, other drugs that may be used are procainamide or phenytoin.

3. **Ectopic beats**
   a. **Asymptomatic.** No treatment is necessary.
   b. **Symptomatic.** With underlying heart disease with ectopic beats that are compromising cardiac output, suppress with phenytoin, propranolol, or quinidine.

4. **AV block**
   a. **First-degree.** No specific treatment is usually necessary.
   b. **Second-degree.** Treat the underlying cause.
   c. **Third-degree (complete).** If the infant is asymptomatic, only observation is necessary. Occasionally, the rate is low enough that transvenous pacing is necessary on an urgent basis, with the need for subsequent permanent pacing. Generally, if the rate is ≥70 beats/min, no problems develop. If the rate is <50 beats/min, the patient usually needs a pacemaker. Between 50 and 70 beats/min is the gray zone. Check the mother for antinuclear antibodies because there is an association with complete heart block.

5. **Arrhythmias secondary to an extracardiac cause**
   a. **Pathologic conditions.** Treat the underlying disease.
   b. **Digoxin toxicity.** Check the PR interval before each dose, obtain a stat serum digoxin level, and hold the dose. Consider digoxin immune Fab (Digibind) (see Chapter 80).
   c. **Quinidine toxicity.** Discontinue medication.
   d. **Theophylline toxicity.** Reduce the dosage or discontinue medication.

6. **Electrolyte abnormalities**
   a. **Check serum electrolyte levels with repeat determinations.**
   b. **Treat electrolyte abnormalities accordingly** (see Chapter 7).

VI. **Technique of cardioversion.** Place the paddles at the apex (left lower chest in the fifth intercostal space in the anterior axillary line) and the base of the heart (right of the midline below the clavicle). Place a saline-soaked gauze pad beneath each paddle to ensure good electrical conduction. The dose is 1–4 J/kg, which should be increased 50–100% each time an electrical charge is delivered. When cardioversion is used for infants with ventricular fibrillation, the synchronization switch should be off.

REFERENCES

Flanagan M et al: Cardiac disease. In Avery GB et al (eds): *Neonatology,* 5th ed. Lippincott, Williams & Wilkins, l999.

Garson A: Medicolegal problems in the management of cardiac arrhythmias in children. *Pediatrics* 1987;79:84.

Lerman B, Belardinelli L: Cardiac electrophysiology of adenosine. *Circulation* 1991;8:1499.

Nagashima M et al: Cardiac arrhythmias in healthy children revealed by 24-hour ambulatory ECG monitoring. *Pediatr Cardiol* 1987;8:103.

Southall R, Johnson B: Frequency and outcome of disorders of cardiac rhythm and conduction in a population of newborn infants. *Pediatrics* 1981;68:58.

31 Bloody Stool

I. **Problem.** A newborn infant has passed a bloody stool.
II. **Immediate questions**
  A. **Is it grossly bloody?** This finding is usually an ominous sign; an exception is bloody stool as a result of swallowed maternal blood, which is a benign condition. A grossly bloody stool usually occurs in infants with a lesion in the ileum or the colon or with massive upper gastrointestinal tract bleeding. Necrotizing enterocolitis (NEC) is the most common cause of bloody stool in premature infants and should be strongly suspected in the differential diagnosis.
  B. **Is the stool otherwise normal in color but with streaks of blood?** This description is more characteristic of a lesion in the anal canal, such as anal fissure. Anal fissure is the most common cause of bleeding in well infants.
  C. **Is the stool positive only for occult blood?** Occult blood often signifies that the blood is from the upper gastrointestinal tract (proximal to the ligament of Treitz). Nasogastric trauma and swallowed maternal blood are common causes. Microscopic blood as an isolated finding is usually not significant. Remember that the Hematest or guaiac tests are very sensitive and can be positive with repeated rectal temperatures.
  D. **Was the infant given vitamin K at birth?** Hemorrhagic disease of the newborn may present with bloody stools, as may any coagulopathy.
III. **Differential diagnosis**
  A. **Occult blood only, no visible blood**
    1. **Swallowing of maternal blood (accounts for 30% of bleeding)** during delivery or breast-feeding (secondary to cracked nipples) may be the cause. Swallowed blood usually appears in the stool on the second or third day of life.
    2. **Nasogastric tube trauma.**
    3. **NEC.**
    4. **Formula intolerance.** Milk protein sensitivity is secondary to cow's milk or soybean formula, and symptoms of blood in the stool usually occur in the second or third week of life.
    5. **Gastritis or stress ulcer (common cause and can be secondary to certain medications).** Stress ulcers may occur in the stomach or the duodenum and are associated with prolonged, severe illness. Steroid therapy, especially prolonged, is associated with ulcers. Hemorrhagic gastritis can occur from tolazoline and theophylline therapy.
    6. **Unknown cause.**
  B. **Streaks of visible blood in the stool**
    1. **Anal fissure.**
    2. **Rectal trauma.** This is often secondary to temperature probes.
  C. **Grossly bloody stool**
    1. **NEC.**
    2. **Disseminated intravascular coagulation.** There is usually bleeding from other sites. This can be secondary from an infection.
    3. **Hemorrhagic disease of the newborn.** This entity occurs from vitamin K deficiency and can be prevented if it is administered at birth. Bloody stools typically appear on the second or third day of life.
    4. **Bleeding diathesis.** Platelet abnormalities and clotting factor deficiencies can cause bloody stools.
    5. **Other surgical diseases,** such as malrotation with midgut volvulus, Meckel's diverticulum, Hirschsprung's enterocolitis, intestinal duplications,

incarcerated inguinal hernia, and intussusception (rare in the neonatal period).
6. **Colitis.** This can be secondary to
   a. **Intestinal infections,** causing colitis with bleeding such as *Shigella, Salmonella, Campylobacter, Yersinia,* and enteropathogenic strains of *Escherichia coli.*
   b. **Dietary/formula intolerance** factors, including allergy and dietary protein-induced colitis.
7. **Severe liver disease.**
8. **Other infections,** such as cytomegalovirus, toxoplasmosis, syphilis, and bacterial sepsis.

IV. **Data base.** The age of the infant is important. If the infant is <7 days old, swallowing of maternal blood is a possible cause; in older infants, this is an unlikely cause.
   A. **Physical examination**
      1. **Examination of peripheral perfusion.** Evaluate the infant's peripheral perfusion. An infant with NEC can be poorly perfused and may appear to be in early or impending shock. Bruising may suggest a coagulopathy.
      2. **Abdominal examination.** Check for bowel sounds and tenderness. If the abdomen is soft and nontender and there is no erythema, a major intra-abdominal process is unlikely. If the abdomen is distended, rigid, or tender, an intra-abdominal pathologic process is likely. Abdominal distention is the most common sign of NEC. Abdominal distention may also suggest intussusception or midgut volvulus. If there are red streaks and erythema on the abdominal wall, suspect NEC with peritonitis.
      3. **Anal examination.** If the infant's condition is stable, perform a visual examination of the anus to check for anal fissure or tear.
   B. **Laboratory studies**
      1. **Fecal occult blood testing (guaiac or Hemoccult test):** to test for the presence of blood.
      2. **Hematocrit and hemoglobin:** to document the amount of blood loss. If a large amount of blood is lost acutely, it takes time for this to be evident on hemoglobin or hematocrit results.
      3. **Apt test:** to differentiate maternal from fetal blood if swallowed maternal blood is suspected. The test is performed as follows: Mix equal parts of the bloody material with water and centrifuge it. Add 1 part of 0.25 mol sodium hydroxide to 5 parts of the pink supernatant. If the fluid remains pink, the blood is fetal in origin because hemoglobin F stays pink. Hemoglobin A from maternal blood is hydrolyzed and changes color from pink to yellow-brown. However, a negative test does not rule out swallowed maternal blood.
      4. **Stool culture.** Certain pathogens cause bloody stools, but they are rare in the neonatal nursery.
      5. **Coagulation studies.** Coagulation studies should be performed to rule out disseminated intravascular coagulation or a bleeding disorder. The usual studies are partial thromboplastin time, prothrombin time, fibrinogen level, and platelet count. Thrombocytopenia can also be seen with cow's milk protein allergy.
      6. **If NEC is suspected, the following studies should be performed:**
         a. **Complete blood cell count with differential.** This test is done to establish an inflammatory response and to check for thrombocytopenia and anemia.
         b. **Serum potassium levels.** Hyperkalemia secondary to hemolysis may occur.
         c. **Serum sodium levels.** Hyponatremia can be seen secondary to third spacing of fluids.
         d. **Blood gas levels.** Blood gases should be measured to rule out metabolic acidosis, which is often associated with sepsis or NEC.

C. **Radiologic and other studies.** A **plain x-ray film of the abdomen** is useful if NEC or a surgical abdomen is suspected. Look for an abnormal gas pattern, a thickened bowel wall, pneumatosis intestinalis, or perforation. Pneumatosis can appear as a "soap bubble" area (see Figure 9–16, p. 118). If a suspicious area appears on the abdominal x-ray film in the right upper quadrant, it is usually not stool. With perforation, one can see the "football sign" on an anteroposterior (AP) film. This is an overall lucency of the abdomen secondary to free intraperitoneal air. Because of the abnormal interface between free air and the peritoneum, the shape resembles a football. A left lateral decubitus view of the abdomen may show free air if perforation has occurred and it cannot be seen on a routine AP film. Surgical conditions usually show signs of intestinal obstruction.

V. **Plan.** The initial plan is to address the loss of volume and give aggressive volume replacement if hypotension is present. Individual plans are as follows:

A. **Swallowed maternal blood.** Observation only is indicated.

B. **Anal fissure and rectal trauma.** Observation is indicated. Petroleum jelly applied to the anus may promote healing.

C. **NEC.** See Chapter 71.

D. **Nasogastric trauma.** In most cases of bloody stool involving nasogastric tubes, trauma is mild and requires only observation. If the tube is too large, replacing it with a smaller one may resolve the problem. If there has been significant bleeding, **gastric lavages** are helpful; it is *controversial* whether tepid water or normal saline is best. Then, if possible, removal of the nasogastric tube is recommended.

E. **Formula intolerance.** This diagnosis is difficult to document, so it is usually made if the patient has remission of symptoms when the formula is eliminated.

F. **Gastritis or ulcers.** Treatment usually consists of ranitidine or cimetidine (for dosages and other pharmacologic information, see Chapter 80). Use of antacids in neonates is *controversial;* some clinicians believe that concretions may result from the use of antacids.

G. **Unknown cause.** If no cause is found, the infant is usually closely monitored. In the majority of the cases, the bleeding will subside.

H. **Intestinal infections.** Antibiotic treatment and isolation are standard treatment. (See Chapter 80 and Appendix G.)

I. **Hemorrhagic disease of the newborn.** Intravenous vitamin K is usually adequate therapy (see Chapter 80).

J. **Surgical conditions (NEC, perforation, volvulus).** These all require immediate surgical evaluation.

32 Counseling Parents Before High-Risk Delivery

I. Problem. The nurse calls to notify you of a pending high-risk delivery. You are on delivery room duty, and you are asked to speak with the parents.

II. Immediate questions

  A. Are both parents and other important family members available? Is a translator needed?

  B. Is the mother too sick or uncomfortable to be able to adequately participate in the discussion? In this situation, other family members are essential to participate in the discussion.

  C. How well do they understand their current situation?

  D. What do they know about neonatal intensive care units (NICUs), pregnancy and neonatal complications, chronic health problems, and neurodevelopmental disability?

III. Differential diagnosis. Although a neonatologist can be called on to counsel expectant parents in a variety of circumstances, the following are common problems that are discussed with parents before delivery.

  A. Preterm delivery.

  B. Intrauterine growth restriction (IUGR).

  C. Maternal drug use.

  D. Fetal distress.

IV. Data base

  A. Maternal/paternal data. Obtain the following information: age of both parents, obstetric history, history of the current pregnancy, medication history, pertinent laboratory and sonographic data, family history, social background and supports, and communication ability.

  B. Fetal. Review current fetal information with the obstetrician: abnormalities of fetal heart rate and fetal tracing, biophysical profile, fetal scalp pH (if done), and any other pertinent tests.

V. Plan

  A. General approach to parent counseling. Parent counseling before delivery is often performed under less than ideal circumstances. Every effort should be made to communicate effectively, explaining all medical terms and avoiding abbreviations and percentages as much as possible. Expectations at delivery, possible complications, and the range of possible outcomes should be covered in addition to the infant's chances of survival. Uncertainties regarding outcome should be acknowledged. Most important, repetition may be necessary in order for parents to comprehend all this information, and an opportunity to review the information should be provided. If NICU admission is anticipated, an opportunity to tour the NICU (and to see other infants hooked up to monitoring and life support equipment) should be offered. Specific and detailed survival and outcome statistics are beyond the scope of this book but are contained in neonatal and obstetric textbooks.

  B. Specific counseling issues

  1. Preterm delivery. The more immature the infant, the greater are the risks of death and all the complications of prematurity, health sequelae, and neurodevelopmental disabilities. Current data, drawn from many published outcome studies, are presented in Table 32–1, although quoting percentages to parents should be avoided.

  a. Immediate questions

TABLE 32–1. ESTIMATES OF MORBIDITY AND MORTALITY USEFUL IN COUNSELING PARENTS

Risk factor	Mortality (%)	Cerebral palsy (%)	Mental retardation (%)	Sensory impairment (%)
None	<1	0.2–0.4	1–3	0.5–2
Prematurity[a]				
GA >30 weeks	<5	—	—	—
GA 27–30 weeks	5–10	—	—	—
GA 25–26 weeks	10–50	14	—	—
GA 23–24 weeks	50–90	12–21	—	—
GA <23 weeks	>>97	50	—	
BW <1500 g	—	5–15	5–17	0.5–6
BW <1000 g	—	7–19	8–25	4–12
BW <750–800 g	—	3–19	3–37	4–15
Severe perinatal depression	35–60	2–30	2–30	Increased
Severe hypoxic-ischemic encephalopathy	60–70	100	100	Increased
Severe persistent pulmonary hypertension	30–80	2–35	2–35	3–20

GA, gestational age; BW, birthweight.
[a]Preterm survival estimates are given in terms of GA for prenatal counseling, but outcome data are published primarily in terms of BW.

i. **What is the infant's gestational age?** This is the most important question because morbidity and mortality are so closely tied to maturity. Both gestational age and birth weight have been used as proxies for maturity in predicting survival and outcome. However, only gestational age is available when counseling parents in labor and delivery.

ii. **Why is preterm delivery threatened?** The very reason for preterm delivery affects infant outcome and the likelihood of delaying delivery (eg, delay is contraindicated with suspected chorioamnionitis).

iii. **Are there signs of fetal distress?** Signs of fetal distress signal either ongoing or impending insult to the fetus.

b. **Specific issues to address with the parents**

i. **Mortality.** The current lower limit of viability is 23–24 weeks' gestation, with occasional survival reported at 21–22 weeks' gestation. Survival at the lower limit of viability requires intubation and mechanical ventilation, but these efforts may merely prolong death. Survival is improved with antenatal steroids but compromised by loss of amniotic fluid before 24 weeks' gestational age.

ii. **Complications of prematurity.** All the complications of prematurity are most common in infants born at the lower limit of viability, and their frequency decreases with increasing gestational age. Complications of prematurity include respiratory distress syndrome, metabolic problems, infection, necrotizing enterocolitis, patent ductus arteriosus, intraventricular hemorrhage, and apnea and bradycardia. Chronic complications include chronic lung disease, periventricular leukomalacia or intraparenchymal cysts, hydrocephalus, poor nutrition, retinopathy of prematurity, and hearing impairment.

iii. **Long-term outcome.** Although the risk of disability is higher in preterm children than in the general population, the majority of preterm children do not develop a major disability (see Table 32–1), such as cerebral palsy or mental retardation. The frequency of neurodevelopmental disability is highest at the lower limit of viability. Learning disability, attention deficit disorder, minor neuromotor dysfunction, and behavior problems are also more frequent in school-age preterm children than in full-term controls.

2. IUGR
   a. Immediate questions. What is the cause of the IUGR? When was it detected? Are there signs of fetal decompensation?
   b. Specific issues to address with parents
      i. IUGR outcome. The most important determinant of IUGR outcome is its cause. Infants with chromosomal disorders and congenital infections (eg, toxoplasmosis or cytomegalovirus) experience early IUGR, often do not tolerate labor and delivery well, and commonly have a disability. The normal fetus initially compensates for fetal deprivation of supply, but when these compensatory mechanisms are overwhelmed, progressive damage to fetal organs occurs, leading to fetal death in utero if there is no intervention.
      ii. Complications of IUGR. IUGR infants are more vulnerable to perinatal complications, including perinatal asphyxia, cold stress, hyperviscosity (polycythemia), and hypoglycemia.
      iii. Long-term outcome. Full-term IUGR infants with fetal deprivation of supply have an increased risk of minor neuromotor dysfunction, learning disability, and behavior problems. Preterm IUGR infants have a risk of major disability (eg, cerebral palsy or mental retardation) that is similar to preterm appropriate for gestational age children **of the same size** (ie, birth weight, not gestational age; see Table 32–1).
3. Maternal use of drugs
   a. Immediate questions. Which drugs did the mother use? When? How much?
   b. Specific issues to address with parents
      i. IUGR. Infants exposed in utero to opiates, cocaine, alcohol, cigarettes, and some prescription drugs can demonstrate IUGR.
      ii. Specific syndromes and risks. Fetal alcohol and fetal hydantoin syndromes are well defined and carry an increased risk of mental retardation but are often difficult to diagnose in the neonatal period.
      iii. Neonatal withdrawal syndrome. Infants exposed in utero to opiates or cocaine may demonstrate neonatal withdrawal syndrome. These infants will have to be closely observed and may require medications to help them through the withdrawal period. Later, these infants have an increased incidence of school and behavior problems.
      iv. Cocaine exposure and risks. Infants with central nervous system infarctions resulting from cocaine exposure are at risk for cerebral palsy, especially hemiplegia.
      v. Sudden infant death syndrome (SIDS). Intrauterine exposure to cigarette smoking increases the risk of SIDS.
4. Signs of fetal distress
   a. Immediate questions. Which signs of fetal distress are evident and for how long? What intervention is planned?
   b. Specific issues to address with parents
      i. Types of fetal distress. There are many different signs of fetal distress, including changes in fetal heart rate patterns, fetal reactivity, meconium staining of amniotic fluid, and decreased fetal movements as well as composite fetal measures (eg, biophysical profile). The type, severity, and duration of insult are important for prognosis, but these cannot be accurately determined.
      ii. Accurate predictors of mortality and morbidity. The only accurate predictors are those related to the infant's response to labor and delivery (eg, low Apgar scores predict mortality; severe perinatal depression or hypoxic-ischemic encephalopathy predicts neurodevelopmental outcome). Infants with chronic intrauterine hypoxia are at increased risk for persistent pulmonary hypertension and

neurodevelopmental disability (whether or not they require extracorporeal membrane oxygenation; see Table 32–1). Infants with severe hypoxic-ischemic encephalopathy who develop a disability tend to have severe multiple disabilities. Nevertheless, the majority of infants who demonstrate signs of fetal distress or acute perinatal depression do not develop hypoxic-ischemic encephalopathy, persistent pulmonary hypertension of the newborn, or neurodevelopmental disability.

REFERENCES

Allen MC: After the intensive care nursery: follow-up and outcome. In Rudolph AM et al (eds): Rudolph's Pediatrics, 21st ed. McGraw-Hill, 2001.

Allen MC: Developmental implication of intrauterine growth retardation. Inf Young Child 1992;5:3.

Allen MC: Outcome and follow-up of high-risk infants. In Taesch W, Ballard RA (eds): Schaeffer and Avery's Diseases of the Newborn, 7th ed. Saunders, 1998.

Aylward GP: Cognitive and neuropsychological outcomes: More than IQ scores. Ment Ret Dev Dis Res Rev 2002;8:234.

Bandstra ES, Bunkett G: Maternal-fetal and neonatal effects of in utero cocaine exposure. Semin Perinatol 1991;15:288.

Bracewell M, Marlow N: Patterns of motor disability in very preterm children. Ment Ret Dev Dis Res Rev 2002;8:241.

Capute AJ, Palmer FB: A pediatric overview of the spectrum of developmental disabilities. J Dev Behav Pediatr 1980;1:66.

Msall ME, Tremont MR: Measuring functional outcomes after prematurity: developmental impact of very low birth weight and extremely low birth weight status on childhood disability. Ment Ret Dev Dis Res Rev 2002;8:258.

Nelson KB, Leviton A: How much of neonatal encephalopathy is due to birth asphyxia? Am J Dis Child 1991;145:1325.

Pena IC et al: The premature small for gestational age infant during the first year of life: comparison by birthweight and gestational age. J Pediatr 1988;113:1106.

Robertson C, Finer N: Term infants with hypoxic-ischemic encephalopathy: outcome at 3–5 years. Dev Med Child Neurol 1985;27:473.

Robertson CMT et al: Eight-year school performance and growth of preterm, small for gestational age infants: a comparative study with subjects matched for birth weight or for gestational age. J Pediatr 1990;93:636.

Sommerfelt K: Long-term outcome for non-handicapped low birth weight infants: is the fog clearing? Eur J Pediatr 1998;157:1.

Wood NS et al: Neurologic and developmental disability after extreme preterm birth. N Engl J Med 2000;343:378.

33 Cyanosis

I. **Problem.** During a physical examination, an infant appears blue. Cyanosis becomes visible when there is more than 3g of desaturated hemoglobin per deciliter. Therefore, the degree of cyanosis will depend on oxygen saturation and hemoglobin concentration. Cyanosis will be visible with much less degree of hypoxemia in the polycythemic compared with the anemic infant. Cyanosis can be a sign of severe cardiac, respiratory, or neurologic compromise.

II. **Immediate questions**

   A. **Does the infant have respiratory distress?** If the infant has increased respiratory effort with increased rate, retractions, and nasal flaring, respiratory disease should be high on the list of differential diagnoses. Cyanotic heart disease usually presents without respiratory symptoms but can have effortless tachypnea (rapid respiratory rate without retractions). Blood disorders usually present without respiratory or cardiac symptoms.

   B. **Does the infant have a murmur?** A murmur usually implies heart disease. Transposition of the great vessels can present without a murmur (approximately 60%).

   C. **Is the cyanosis continuous, intermittent, sudden in onset, or occurring only with feeding or crying?** Intermittent cyanosis is more common with neurologic disorders, because these infants may have apneic spells alternating with periods of normal breathing. Continuous cyanosis is usually associated with intrinsic lung disease or heart disease. Cyanosis with feeding may occur with esophageal atresia and severe esophageal reflux. Sudden onset of cyanosis may occur with an air leak, such as pneumothorax. Cyanosis that disappears with crying may signify choanal atresia. Infants with tetralogy of Fallot may have clinical cyanosis only with crying.

   D. **Is there differential cyanosis?** Cyanosis of the upper or lower part of the body only usually signifies serious heart disease. The more common pattern is cyanosis restricted to the lower half of the body, which is seen in patients with patent ductus arteriosus with a left-to-right shunt. Cyanosis restricted to the upper half of the body is seen occasionally in patients with pulmonary hypertension, patent ductus arteriosus, coarctation of the aorta, and D-transposition of the great arteries.

   E. **What is the prenatal and delivery history?** An infant of a diabetic mother has increased risk of hypoglycemia, polycythemia, respiratory distress syndrome, and heart disease. Infection, such as that which can occur with premature rupture of membranes, may cause shock and hypotension with resultant cyanosis. Amniotic fluid abnormalities, such as oligohydramnios (associated with hypoplastic lungs) or polyhydramnios (associated with esophageal atresia), may suggest a cause for the cyanosis. Cesarean section is associated with increased respiratory distress. Certain perinatal conditions increase the incidence of congenital heart disease. Examples of these include

   - Maternal diabetes or cocaine: D-transposition of the great arteries.
   - Maternal use of lithium: Ebstein's anomaly.
   - Use of phenytoin: atrial septal defect, ventricular septal defect, tetralogy of Fallot.
   - Maternal lupus: atrioventricular block.
   - Maternal congenital heart disease: increased incidence of heart disease in the child.

III. **Differential diagnosis.** The causes of cyanosis can be classified as arising from respiratory, cardiac, central nervous system (CNS), or other disorders.

A. **Respiratory diseases**
   1. **Lung diseases**
      a. **Hyaline membrane disease.**
      b. **Transient tachypnea of the newborn.**
      c. **Pneumonia.**
      d. **Meconium aspiration.**
   2. **Air leak syndrome.**
   3. **Congenital defects** (eg, diaphragmatic hernia, hypoplastic lungs, lobar emphysema, cystic adenomatoid malformation, and diaphragm abnormality).
B. **Cardiac diseases**
   1. **All cyanotic heart diseases,** which include the 5 T's.

      • *Transposition of the great arteries.*
      • *Total anomalous pulmonary venous return.*
      • *Tricuspid atresia.*
      • *Tetralogy of Fallot.*
      • *Truncus arteriosus.*

      Other cyanotic diseases include Ebstein's anomaly, patent ductus arteriosus, ventricular septal defect, hypoplastic left heart syndrome, and pulmonary atresia.
   2. **Persistent pulmonary hypertension of the newborn (PPHN).**
   3. **Severe congestive heart failure.**
C. **CNS diseases.** Periventricular-intraventricular hemorrhage, meningitis, and primary seizure disorder can cause cyanosis. Neuromuscular disorders such as Werdnig-Hoffmann disease and congenital myotonic dystrophy can cause cyanosis.
D. **Other disorders**
   1. **Methemoglobinemia.** May be familial. Pao_2 is within normal limits.
   2. **Polycythemia/hyperviscosity syndrome.** Pao_2 is within normal limits.
   3. **Hypothermia.**
   4. **Hypoglycemia.**
   5. **Sepsis/meningitis.**
   6. **Pseudocyanosis** caused by fluorescent lighting.
   7. **Respiratory depression** secondary to maternal medications (eg, magnesium sulfate and narcotics).
   8. **Shock.**
   9. **Upper airway obstruction.** Choanal atresia is nasal passage obstruction caused most commonly by a bony abnormality. Other causes are laryngeal web, tracheal stenosis, goiter, and Pierre Robin syndrome.
IV. **Data base.** Obtain a prenatal and delivery history (see section II,E).
A. **Physical examination**
   1. **Assess the infant for central versus peripheral cyanosis.** In central cyanosis, the skin, lips, and tongue will appear blue. In central cyanosis, the Pao_2 is <50 mm Hg. In peripheral cyanosis, the skin is bluish but the oral mucous membranes will be pink. Check the nasal passage for choanal atresia.
   2. **Assess the heart.** Check for any murmurs. Assess heart rate and blood pressure.
   3. **Assess the lungs.** Is there retraction, flaring of the nose, or grunting? Retractions are usually minimal in heart disease.
   4. **Assess the abdomen** for an enlarged liver. The liver can be enlarged in congestive heart failure and hyperexpansion of the lungs. A scaphoid abdomen may suggest a diaphragmatic hernia.
   5. **Check the pulses.** In coarctation of the aorta, the femoral pulses will be decreased. In patent ductus arteriosus, the pulses will be bounding.
   6. **Consider neurologic problems.** Check for apnea and periodic breathing, which may be associated with immaturity of the nervous system. Observe

the infant for seizures, which can cause cyanosis if the infant is not breathing during seizures.

B. Laboratory studies

1. **Arterial blood gas measurements on room air.** If the patient is not hypoxic, it suggests methemoglobinemia, polycythemia, or CNS disease. If the patient is hypoxic, perform the 100% hyperoxic test, described next.
2. **Hyperoxic test.** Measure arterial oxygen on room air. Then place the infant on 100% oxygen for 10–20 min. With cyanotic heart disease, the Pao_2 most likely will not increase significantly. If the Pao_2 rises above 150 mm Hg, cardiac disease can generally be excluded but not always. Failure of Pao_2 to rise above 150 mm Hg suggests a cyanotic cardiac malformation, whereas in lung disease the arterial oxygen saturation should improve and go above 150 mm Hg. Remember: In an infant with **severe lung disease** or PPHN the arterial oxygen saturation may not increase significantly. If the Pao_2 increases to <20 mm Hg, PPHN should be considered.
3. **Right-to-left shunt test.** This test should be done to rule out PPHN. Draw a simultaneous sample of blood from the right radial artery (preductal) and the descending aorta or the left radial artery (postductal). If there is a difference of >15% (preductal > postductal), then the shunt is significant. It is sometimes easier to place two pulse oximeters on the infant (one preductal-right hand; one postductal-left hand or either foot). If the simultaneous difference is >10–15%, then the shunt is significant.
4. **Complete blood cell count with differential.** This may reveal an infection process. A central hematocrit of >65% confirms polycythemia.
5. **Serum glucose level.** This will detect hypoglycemia.
6. **Methemoglobin level.** A drop of blood exposed to air has a chocolate hue. To confirm the diagnosis, a spectrophotometric determination should be done by the laboratory.

C. Radiologic and other studies

1. **Transillumination of the chest** (see p 169) should be done on an emergent basis if pneumothorax is suspected.
2. **Chest x-ray** film may be normal, suggesting CNS disease or another cause for the cyanosis (see section III,D). It can verify lung disease, air leak, or diaphragmatic hernia. It can also help diagnose heart disease by evaluating the heart size and pulmonary vascularity. The heart size may be normal or enlarged in hypoglycemia, polycythemia, shock, and sepsis. Decreased pulmonary vascular markings can be seen in tetralogy of Fallot, pulmonary atresia, truncus arteriosus, and Ebstein's anomaly. Increased arterial markings can be seen in truncus arteriosus, single ventricle, and transposition. Increased venous markings can be seen in hypoplastic left heart syndrome and total anomalous pulmonary venous return.
3. **Electrocardiography** (ECG) should be done to help determine the cause of the cyanosis. The ECG is usually normal in patients with methemoglobinemia or hypoglycemia. In those with polycythemia, pulmonary hypertension, or primary lung disease, the ECG is normal but may show right ventricular hypertrophy. It is very helpful in identifying patients with tricuspid atresia; it will show left axis deviation and left ventricular hypertrophy.
4. **Echocardiography** should be performed immediately if cardiac disease is suspected or if the diagnosis is unclear.
5. **Ultrasonography of the head** can be performed to rule out periventricular-intraventricular hemorrhage.

V. Plan

A. General management. Act quickly and accomplish many of the diagnostic tasks at once.

1. **Perform a rapid physical examination.** Transilluminate the chest (see p 169). If a tension pneumothorax is present, rapid needle decompression may be needed (see also p 293).

2. Order stat laboratory tests (eg, blood gas levels, complete blood cell count, and chest x-ray film).
3. Perform the hyperoxic test. See section IV,B,2.
B. Specific management
1. Lung disease. (See Chapter 74.) Respiratory depression caused by narcotics can be treated with naloxone (Narcan) (for dosage, see Chapter 80).
2. Air leak (pneumothorax). (See Chapter 74).
3. Congenital defects. Surgery is indicated for diaphragmatic hernia.
4. Cardiac disease. The use of prostaglandin E$_1$ (PGE$_1$) is indicated for right heart outflow obstruction (tricuspid atresia, pulmonic stenosis, and pulmonary atresia), left heart outflow obstruction (hypoplastic left heart syndrome, critical aortic valve stenosis, preductal coarctation of the aorta, and interrupted aortic arch), and transposition of the great arteries. PGE$_1$ is contraindicated for hyaline membrane disease, PPHN, and dominant left-to-right shunt (patent ductus arteriosus, truncus arteriosus, or ventricular septal defect). If the diagnosis is uncertain, a trial of PGE$_1$ can be given over 30 min in an effort to improve blood gas values.
5. CNS disorders. Treat the underlying disease (see Chapter 72).
6. Methemoglobinemia. Treat the infant with methylene blue only if the methemoglobin level is markedly increased and the infant is in cardiopulmonary distress (tachypnea and tachycardia). Administer intravenously 1 mg/kg of a 1% solution of methylene blue in normal saline. The cyanosis should clear within 1–2 h.
7. Shock. See Chapter 46.
8. Polycythemia. See Chapter 52.
9. Choanal atresia. The infant usually requires surgery.
10. Hypothermia. Rewarming is necessary. The technique is described in Chapter 5.
11. Hypoglycemia. See Chapter 43.

34 Death of an Infant

I. **Problem.** A newborn infant is dying or has just died.
II. **Immediate questions**
  A. **Has the family been prepared for the death, or was it unexpected?** It is important to prepare the family in advance, if possible, for the death of an infant and to be ready to answer questions after the event.
  B. **Was this an early or late neonatal death?** Early neonatal death describes the death of a live-born infant during the first 7 completed days of life. Late neonatal death refers to the death of a live-born infant after 7 but before 28 completed days of life. After 28 days, it is considered an infant death.
  C. **Which family members are present?** Usually several immediate family members in addition to the parents are present at the hospital. This is good for emotional support. Each of the members may adopt a special role. The family should be allowed to go through the immediate process of grieving the way they feel most comfortable (eg, on their own, with the chaplain, with their favorite nurse, or with the physician they trust) and in the location they feel most comfortable (eg, the neonatal intensive care unit [NICU] or family conference room). Attention should be focused on both parents.
  D. **If the family members are not present, is a telephone contact available?** It is good practice to ensure that there is a contact telephone number available for any sick infant. If the family members are not present, telephone contact must be made as soon as possible to alert the family that their infant is dying or has already passed away. In either case, urge the family to come in and be with their infant.
  E. **Are there any religious needs expressed by the family?** The religious needs must be respected and the necessary support provided (eg, priest, rabbi, minister, or pastoral care). Every hospital has pastoral services, and it is useful to inform the minister in advance because some parents may request that their child be baptized before death.
III. **Differential diagnosis.** Not applicable.
IV. **Data base.** It is important to remember that the infant may continue with a gasp reflex for a while even without spontaneous respiration and movement. The heartbeat may be very faint; therefore, auscultation for 2–5 min is advisable. Legal definitions of "death" vary by state.
V. **Plan**
  A. **Preparations**
    1. **The NICU environment.** The noise level should be kept to a minimum. The staff should be sensitive to the emotions of the parents and the family. The infant and family members should be provided privacy in an isolated quiet room or a screened-off area in the NICU. Examination of the infant by the physician to determine death may be done in that same private area, with the family.
    2. **The infant.** Much of the equipment (eg, intravenous catheters and endotracheal tubes) may be removed from the infant unless an autopsy is anticipated. In that case, it is best to leave in place central catheters and possibly the endotracheal tube. The parents should be allowed to hold the infant for as long as they desire. This type of visual and physical contact is important to begin the grieving process in a healthy manner and try to relieve any future guilt.

B. Discussion of death with the family
   1. **Location.** Parents and immediate family members should be in a quiet, private consultation room, and the physician should calmly explain the cause and inevitability of death.
   2. **News of the death.** The physician needs to offer condolences to the family. News of the infant's death can be very difficult for the physician to convey and the family to accept. The physician must be sensitive to the emotional reactions of the family.
C. Effects on the family
   1. **Emotional (grieving).** A brief outline of the normal grieving process may be discussed: shock, denial, sadness, anger, and reorganization.
   2. **Physical. Loss of appetite** and disruption of sleep patterns.
   3. **Other siblings.** It is important to discuss the impact of death on a sibling.
   4. **Surviving twin.** Staff must be aware of the additive stress on the parents looking in on a surviving twin.
D. Practical aspects
   1. **Additional support. Family members should be asked whether they need any support** for transport or funeral arrangements and whether they need a letter to the employer regarding time off from work and so on.
   2. **Written permission** should be obtained for the following: photography, mementos, autopsy, or biopsy.
   3. **Organ donation.** Occasionally, parents and immediate family members may have discussed organ donation before the death of the infant. If not, it can be brought up gently with the family, who will be given adequate time to reflect on it, taking into consideration the requirements for organ donation. Sometimes the parents may want to donate an organ, but this may not be possible because of the presence of infection or inadequate function of the organ before death. This should be explained carefully to the parents. It is best to contact each state organ procurement organization to obtain specific information regarding organ donation.
   4. **Autopsy.** Autopsy can be a vital part of determining the cause of death and may be important in counseling the parents for future pregnancies. It is always a very sensitive issue to discuss with the parents, especially after the loss of their loved one. Parents should always be allowed adequate time to discuss this themselves and with the family if they have not already made up their minds.
   5. **Documentation**
      a. **Neonatal death summary note.** The physician may include a brief synopsis of the infant's history or a problem list. Then the events leading up to the infant's death that day, whether it was sudden or gradual, and the treatment or interventions performed must be noted. It is also important to note conversations with family members while the infant was dying, if not written earlier in separate notes.
      b. **Death certificate. The physician declaring the infant dead initiates the death certificate, following strict guidelines for each county/state.**
E. Follow-up arrangements
   1. **Family contact.** A telephone call from one of the medical team members should be arranged within the first week of death. A letter of sympathy can be sent out along with a brochure (eg, "Hello Means Good-Bye") that will help the family cope with the loss of a loved one. Another contact can be made at the end of the first month to comfort the family, share any further information, and answer questions. Some NICU teams may make contact again at the 1-year anniversary.
   2. **Counseling.** It is extremely important to discuss the arrangements for future counseling and refer the parents to high-risk obstetrics if appropriate. Parents should be allowed to grieve for the death of their child and should

be given the opportunity to contact the physician at a later date, when they are more receptive emotionally.

3. **Autopsy follow-up.** If consent for autopsy has been obtained, an autopsy follow-up conference after ~6–8 weeks is essential. The presence of a geneticist at this follow-up may be appropriate. This autopsy conference not only provides the parents with concrete information but also assists in the process of grieving.

4. **The obstetrician, pediatrician, and family physician** should be notified of the death.

35 Eye Discharge (Conjunctivitis)

I. **Problem.** Eye discharge is noted. Conjunctivitis is the most common neonatal infection.

II. **Immediate questions**

A. **How old is the infant?** Age is an important factor in determining the cause of eye discharge. Within the first 6–24 h of life, the most likely cause is conjunctivitis secondary to the use of ocular silver nitrate drops immediately after birth to prevent gonococcal ophthalmia. At 2–5 days, a bacterial infection is most likely. The organisms that most commonly cause conjunctivitis in the neonatal period are *Neisseria gonorrhoeae* and *Staphylococcus aureus*. *Chlamydia trachomatis* conjunctivitis is usually seen after the first week of life; it often presents as late as the second or third week. *Pseudomonas aeruginosa* infections are typically seen between the 5th and 18th days of life. Herpes conjunctivitis is seen 5–14 days after birth.

B. **Is the discharge unilateral or bilateral?** Bilateral conjunctivitis is seen with infection caused by *C. trachomatis* or *N. gonorrhoeae* or by the use of silver nitrate. Unilateral conjunctivitis is seen with *S. aureus* and *P. aeruginosa*. Herpes simplex keratoconjunctivitis is usually unilateral. Unilateral discharge is seen in lacrimal duct obstruction.

C. **What are the characteristics of the discharge?** It is important to distinguish between purulent and watery discharge. Purulent discharge is more common with bacterial infection. Infection resulting from chlamydia may be watery early in the course and purulent later. A greenish discharge is more characteristic of *P. aeruginosa*.

III. **Differential diagnosis.** Conjunctivitis in the neonate is either infectious (bacterial, viral, or chlamydial) or secondary to a chemical response. One study revealed that 56% of conjunctivitis cases were infectious (the most common being *Chlamydia*) and 44% were of uncertain origin. Other diagnoses that may mimic conjunctivitis and may need to be ruled out include foreign body, lacrimal duct obstruction, trauma to the eye, and glaucoma.

A. **Chemical conjunctivitis** is usually secondary to the use of silver nitrate ocular drops. This is the most common cause of conjunctivitis in underdeveloped countries. It is not seen as frequently as in the past because many nurseries now use erythromycin ophthalmic ointment, which causes less ocular irritation. The recommended topical prophylaxis with erythromycin will not prevent neonatal chlamydial conjunctivitis. Silver nitrate drops are recommended over erythromycin ophthalmic ointment if the patient population has a high number of penicillinase-producing *N. gonorrhoeae*. Povidone-iodine 2.5% is being used in some underdeveloped countries now for ophthalmia neonatorum prophylaxis.

B. **Gonococcal conjunctivitis** is most commonly transmitted from the mother. The incidence is low because of prophylactic treatment immediately after birth. It is considered a medical emergency because, left untreated, it can cause corneal perforation.

C. **Staphylococcal conjunctivitis** is usually a nosocomial infection. It is the most frequent isolate, but it does not always cause conjunctivitis in infants who are colonized.

D. **Chlamydial conjunctivitis** is transmitted from the mother. Conjunctivitis will develop in approximately 25–50% of infants delivered vaginally to mothers with chlamydia. Remember that topical prophylaxis will not prevent neonatal chlamydial conjunctivitis.

E. **Pseudomonal conjunctivitis** is usually a nosocomial infection and is becoming more common in neonatal nurseries. The organism thrives in moisture-filled environments such as respiratory equipment. It occurs most often in hospitalized premature infants or those with depressed immunity. It can be responsible for epidemic conjunctivitis in preemies.

F. **Other bacterial infections** include infections caused by *Haemophilus* spp, *Streptococcus pneumoniae*, and *Enterococcus*.

G. **Herpes simplex keratoconjunctivitis.** Herpes simplex type 2 (HSV-2) can cause unilateral or bilateral conjunctivitis, optic neuritis, and chorioretinitis. It is the most frequent viral cause of conjunctivitis. The conjunctivitis can be superficial or may involve the deeper layers of the cornea. Vesicles may appear on the nearby skin. Most of these infections are secondary to HSV-2 (which occurs through the genital tract or from ascending infection), but some (15–20%) are caused by HSV-1. Herpes should be suspected if the conjunctiva is not responding to antibiotic therapy.

H. **Viral causes (other than herpes).** These are usually associated with other symptoms of respiratory tract disease. The discharge is usually watery or mucopurulent and rarely purulent. Preauricular adenopathy can also be seen. Examples of these are adenovirus and enterovirus.

I. **Lacrimal duct obstruction (dacryostenosis).** In this disorder, the nasolacrimal duct may fail to canalize completely at birth. The obstruction is usually at the nasal end of the duct. The symptoms are persistent tearing and a mucoid discharge in the inner corner of the eye. The disorder is usually unilateral.

IV. **Data base**
A. **Physical examination**
   1. **Ophthalmic examination.** Examine both eyes for swelling and edema of the eyelids, and check the conjunctiva for injection (congestion of blood vessels). A purulent discharge, edema, and erythema of the lids as well as injection of the conjunctiva are suggestive of bacterial conjunctivitis.
   2. **Perform a complete physical examination** to rule out signs of systemic infection.
B. **Laboratory studies**
   1. **Always obtain a Gram's-stained smear of the discharge** to check for white blood cells (a sign of infection) and bacteria (to identify the specific organism). **A sample of the discharge should also be submitted for culture and sensitivity testing.** It will verify the specific organism seen on the Gram's-stained smear and will indicate antibiotic sensitivities.
      a. *N. gonorrhoeae* **conjunctivitis.** Gram-negative intracellular diplococci and white blood cells are seen.
      b. *S. aureus* **conjunctivitis.** Gram-positive cocci in clusters and white blood cells are seen.
      c. *P. aeruginosa* **conjunctivitis.** Gram-negative bacilli and white blood cells are found.
      d. **Chemical conjunctivitis, lacrimal duct obstruction, herpes simplex, and** *C. trachomatis* **conjunctivitis.** The Gram's-stained smear will be negative.
      e. **Conjunctivitis caused by** *Haemophilus* **spp.** Gram-negative coccoid rods are seen.
      f. **Streptococcal or enterococci.** Streptococci are gram-positive spherical cocci, and enterococci are gram-positive lancet-shaped encapsulated diplococci.
   2. **If a chlamydial infection is suspected, material is gathered for Giemsa staining by scraping (*not swabbing*)** the lower palpebral conjunctiva with a wire loop or blunt spatula to obtain epithelial cells. This is a specific (but not sensitive) method for detecting conjunctivitis. Cotton or Calgonite swabs have not proved to be adequate. If chlamydial infection is present, **typical cytoplasmic inclusion bodies** will be seen within the epithelial cells. Rapid antigen detection assays on conjunctival scrapings can

be sent to the laboratory for results. Direct fluorescent antibody (DFA), enzyme immunoassay (EIA), and DNA probes are all diagnostic tests for *Chlamydia*.
3. **If herpes is suspected,** a conjunctival scraping will show multinucleated giant cells with intracytoplasmic inclusions. Also, the conjunctiva should be swabbed and transported on special viral transport media for culture.
C. **Radiologic and other studies.** None are usually needed.
V. **Plan.** Based on the results of the Gram's stain and Giemsa stain, empiric treatment should be started after a specimen of the discharge is sent to the laboratory for culture rather than waiting for the results.
A. **Chemical conjunctivitis.** Observation only is needed. This disorder usually resolves within 48–72 h.
B. **Gonococcal conjunctivitis**
1. Isolate the infant during the first 24 h of parenteral antibiotic therapy.
2. Use strict hand-washing technique because of the highly contagious exudate.
3. Evaluate for disseminated disease. Blood and cerebrospinal cultures must be obtained. Other sites should be cultured if appropriate. Appropriate cultures from the mother should be obtained.
4. Tests for concomitant infection with *C. trachomatis*, congenital syphilis, and HIV infection should also be performed.
5. For gonococcal conjunctivitis without dissemination, administer a single dose of ceftriaxone, 125 mg intravenously (IV) or intramuscularly (IM). For low birth weight infants, the single dose is ceftriaxone sodium, 25–50 mg/kg/day IM or IV (up to a maximum of 125 mg). An alternative therapy is cefotaxime in a single dose (100 mg/kg, given IV or IM).
6. For gonococcal conjunctivitis with dissemination, ceftriaxone, 25–50 mg/kg IV or IM, may be given once every day for 7 days. If meningitis is present, it should be given for a total of 10–14 days. An alternate therapy is cefotaxime (recommended for hyperbilirubinemic infants) at 50–100 mg/kg/day, given IV or IM in 2 divided doses for 7 days or 10–14 days if meningitis is present.
7. In infants born to mothers with gonococcal infection:
   i. Gonococcal conjunctivitis, with routine prophylaxis, is uncommon.
   ii. A very small percentage of infants with gonococcal conjunctivitis are given a single dose of ceftriaxone, 125 mg IV or IM; if premature, give 25–50 mg/kg to a maximum of 125 mg. Cefotaxime is also an alternative.
8. Irrigate the eyes with sterile isotonic saline solution immediately and at frequent intervals (every 1–2 h) until clear. Topical antibiotic therapy is unnecessary when recommended systemic treatment is given.
9. Because gonococcal ophthalmia can lead to corneal perforation and blindness, an ophthalmologic consultation is usually requested.
C. **Staphylococcal conjunctivitis**
1. Isolate the infant to prevent spread of infection.
2. Culture the blood and other areas if appropriate.
3. Systemic therapy with a penicillinase-resistant penicillin (eg, methicillin) should be used for a minimum of 7 days.
4. Topical antibiotics are unnecessary if the patient is on systemic therapy.
D. **Chlamydial conjunctivitis**
1. Topical treatment with erythromycin ophthalmic ointment is ineffective and unnecessary when treating with systemic therapy.
2. Erythromycin suspension, 50 mg/kg/day in 4 divided doses for 14 days orally, is recommended. Oral sulfonamides may be used after the immediate neonatal period for infants who do not tolerate erythromycin. A second course of antibiotics is sometimes required because ~20% of cases will recur after antibiotic therapy.
3. Infantile hypertrophic pyloric stenosis (IHPS) has been seen in infants <6 weeks treated with erythromycin. Counsel patients about the risk and signs

of IHPS. AAP still recommends erythromycin because other treatments have not been well studied.

4. Infants born to mothers with untreated chlamydia are at a high risk for infection. Prophylactic antibiotic treatment is not indicated. Monitor for infection. If adequate fo''ow-up is not possible, some clinicians advocate treatment.

E. **Pseudomonal conjunctivitis**
1. Isolate the patient.
2. Culture blood and other sites if appropriate.
3. Treat the conjunctivitis with gentamicin ophthalmic ointment 4 times/day for 2 weeks.
4. Parenteral therapy for pseudomonas conjunctivitis is recommended because *Pseudomonas* is such a virulent organism. Treatment consists of a β-lactam antibiotic or an appropriate cephalosporin plus an aminoglycoside (gentamicin) for a minimum of 10–14 days. For infections that include meningitis, ampicillin or cephalosporin plus an aminoglycoside is recommended for 21 days.
5. Because this infection may be devastating, an ophthalmologist should be consulted. Infectious disease consult may also be helpful, especially in the management of *Pseudomonas* meningitis.

F. **Other bacterial infections**
1. Local saline irrigation.
2. Topical antibiotics containing a combination of bacitracin, neomycin, and polymyxin can be applied every 6 h for 7–10 days.

G. **Herpes simplex conjunctivitis**
1. Isolate the patient; implement contact precautions.
2. Obtain a complete set of viral cultures (blood, cerebrospinal fluid, eyes, stool or rectum, urine, mouth or nasopharynx, and any lesions).
3. Administer topical ophthalmic therapy with 3% vidarabine ointment, 1% iododeoxyuridine, or 1–2% trifluridine ointment 5 times/day for 10 days.
4. Systemic acyclovir therapy for a minimum of 14 days is indicated. If CNS disease or disseminated disease is present, treat for a minimum of 21 days. (For dosage, see Chapter 80.)
5. Ophthalmologic evaluation and follow-up are necessary because chorioretinitis, cataracts, and retinopathy may develop in these infants.

H. **Lacrimal duct obstruction**
1. Most obstructions clear spontaneously without treatment.
2. Massaging the inside corner of the eye over the lacrimal sac, with expression toward the nose, may help to establish patency.
3. If the problem does not resolve and symptoms persist (usually after 6–7 months), the infant should be evaluated by an ophthalmologist. Probing of the duct is indicated with a success rate of >90%.

36 Gastric Aspirate (Residuals)

I. **Problem.** The nurse alerts you that a gastric aspirate has been obtained in an infant. Gastric aspiration is a procedure by which the stomach is aspirated with an oral or nasogastric tube. The procedure is usually performed before each feeding to determine whether the feedings are being tolerated and digested.

II. **Immediate questions**

A. **What is the volume of the aspirate?** A volume of >30% of the total formula given at the last feeding may be abnormal and requires more extensive evaluation. A gastric aspirate of >10–15 mL is considered excessive.

B. **What is the character of the aspirate (ie, bilious, bloody, undigested, or digested)?** This is important in the differential diagnosis (see section III,A).

C. **Are the vital signs normal?** Abnormal vital signs may indicate a pathologic process, possibly an intra-abdominal process.

D. **Is the abdomen soft, with good bowel sounds, or distended, with visible bowel loops?** Absence of bowel sounds, distention, tenderness, and erythema are signs of peritonitis. Absence of bowel sounds may also indicate ileus.

E. **When was the last stool passed?** Constipation resulting in abdominal distention may cause feeding intolerance and increased gastric aspirates.

III. **Differential diagnosis.** The characteristics of the aspirate can provide important clinical clues to the cause of the problem and are outlined next.

A. **Bilious in color.** Bilious aspirate usually indicates an obstructive lesion distal to the ampulla of Vater. This type of aspirate is usually a serious problem, especially if it occurs in the first 72 h of life.

1. **Bowel obstruction.** One study found that 30% of infants with bilious vomiting in the first 72 h of life had obstruction, of which 20% required surgery.

2. **Necrotizing enterocolitis (NEC).** This occurs mainly in premature infants. Ten percent of the cases involve term infants.

3. **Meconium plug.**

4. **Meconium ileus.**

5. **Hirschsprung's disease.**

6. **Malrotation of the intestine.**

7. **Volvulus.**

8. **Ileus.**

9. **Factitious.** Passage of the feeding tube into the duodenum or the jejunum instead of the stomach can cause a bilious aspirate.

B. **Nonbilious in color**

1. **Problems with the feeding regimen.** Undigested or digested formula may be seen in the aspirate if the feeding regimen is too aggressive. This problem is especially likely in small premature infants who are given a small amount of formula initially and then are given larger volumes too rapidly.

a. **Aspirate containing undigested formula** may be seen if the interval between feedings is too short.

b. **Aspirate containing digested formula** may be a sign of delayed gastric emptying or overfeeding. Also, if the osmolarity of the formula is increased by the addition of vitamins, retained digested formula may be seen.

2. **Other**

a. **NEC.**

b. **Pyloric stenosis.**

c. **Post-NEC stricture.**

    d. Infections.
    e. Inborn errors of metabolism.
    f. Constipation. This is a factor especially if the abdomen is full but soft and no stool has passed in 48–72 h.
    g. Adrenogenital syndrome.
    h. Adrenal hypoplasia.
    i. Formula intolerance. Formula intolerance is an uncommon cause of aspirate but should nonetheless be considered. Some infants do not tolerate the carbohydrate source in some formulas. If the infant is receiving a lactose-containing formula (eg, Similac or Enfamil), a stool pH should be performed to rule out **lactose intolerance.** If the stool pH is acidic (<5.0), lactose intolerance may be present. In these cases, there is usually a strong family history of milk intolerance. It is more common to see diarrhea than gastric aspirates with lactose intolerance.
  C. Bloody in color
    1. Trauma from nasogastric intubation.
    2. Swallowed maternal blood.
    3. Bleeding disorder. Vitamin K deficiency, disseminated intravascular coagulation, and any congenital coagulopathy can cause a bloody aspirate.
    4. Stress ulcer.
    5. Severe fetal asphyxia.
    6. NEC.
    7. Gastric volvulus or duplication. These are rare.
    8. Medications. The following medications can cause a bloody aspirate: tolazoline, theophylline, indomethacin, and corticosteroids. It is important to note that theophylline is a rare cause of bloody gastric aspirate. Tolazoline administration, especially by continuous infusion, can cause a massive gastric hemorrhage.
IV. Data base
  A. Physical examination. Perform a complete physical examination, paying particular attention to the abdomen. Check for bowel sounds (absent bowel sounds may indicate ileus or peritonitis), abdominal distention, tenderness to palpation and erythema of the abdomen (which may signify peritonitis), or visible bowel loops. Check for hernias because they may cause obstruction.
  B. Laboratory studies
    1. A complete blood cell count with differential is performed to evaluate for sepsis, if suspected. The hematocrit and platelet count may be checked if bleeding has occurred.
    2. Blood culture is performed if sepsis is suspected and before antibiotics are started.
    3. Serum potassium level. If ileus is present, a serum potassium level should be obtained to rule out hypokalemia.
    4. Stool pH. If there is a family history of milk intolerance, a stool pH should be obtained to rule out lactose intolerance (the stool pH will usually be <5.0).
    5. Coagulation profile (prothrombin time, partial thromboplastin time, fibrinogen, and platelets). A bloody aspirate may signify the presence of a coagulopathy. In this case, coagulation studies should be obtained.
  C. Radiologic and other studies
    1. Plain x-ray film (flat plate) of the abdomen. A plain x-ray film of the abdomen should be obtained if the aspirate is bilious, if there is any abnormality on physical examination, or if aspirates continue. The x-ray film will show whether the nasogastric tube is in the correct position and will define the bowel gas pattern. Look for an unusual gas pattern, pneumatosis intestinalis, ileus, or evidence of bowel obstruction. It is important to check also a left lateral decubitus film because a perforation can be easily missed on the anteroposterior film.

2. **Upright x-ray film of the abdomen.** If bowel obstruction is suspected on the film, obtain an upright x-ray film of the abdomen and look for air-fluid levels.

3. **Endoscopy** should be considered for ulcer evaluation.

V. **Plan.** The approach to management of the neonate with increased gastric aspirates is usually initially based on the nature of the aspirate.

A. **Bilious aspirate**

1. **Surgical problem (eg, bowel obstruction, malrotation, volvulus, meconium plug).** A nasogastric tube should be placed for decompression of the stomach with continuous suction. Consultation with a pediatric surgeon should be obtained immediately.

2. **NEC.** A nasogastric tube should be placed to rest the gut, and the infant should receive nothing by mouth. (For further management, see Chapter 71.)

3. **Ileus.** If ileus is diagnosed, the patient is fed nothing orally and a nasogastric tube is placed for decompression of the stomach. Ileus in the neonate may be secondary to the following underlying causes, which should be treated if possible.

a. **Sepsis.**

b. **NEC.**

c. **Prematurity.**

d. **Hypokalemia.**

e. **Effects of maternal drugs** (especially magnesium sulfate).

f. **Pneumonia.**

g. **Hypothyroidism.**

4. **Factitious.** An x-ray film will confirm the position of the nasogastric tube distally in the duodenum. Replace or reposition the tube in the stomach.

B. **Nonbilious aspirate**

1. **Aspirate containing undigested formula.** If the volume of undigested formula in the aspirate does not exceed 30% of the previous feeding or 10–15 mL total and the physical examination and vital signs are normal, the volume can be replaced. The time interval between feedings may not be long enough for digestion to take place. If the infant is being fed every 2 h and aspirates continue, the feeding interval may be increased to 3 h. If aspirates still continue, the patient must be reevaluated. An abdominal x-ray film should be obtained. Continuous gavage feedings may be tried; the patient may also have to be fed intravenously to allow the gut to rest.

2. **Aspirate containing digested formula.** The aspirate is usually discarded, especially if it contains a large amount of mucus. If the physical examination and vital signs are normal, continue feedings and aspiration of stomach contents. If reflux continues, the patient must be reassessed. An abdominal film must be taken, and oral feedings should be discontinued for a time to let the gut rest. The number of calories given should be calculated to make certain that overfeeding (usually >130 kcal/kg/day) is not occurring.

3. **Other**

a. **NEC.** See Chapter 71.

b. **Pyloric stenosis.**

c. **Post-NEC stricture.**

d. **Infections.** If sepsis is likely, broad-spectrum antibiotics are started after a laboratory workup is performed. A penicillin (usually ampicillin) and an aminoglycoside (usually gentamicin) are given initially until culture results are obtained (for drug dosages and other pharmacologic information, see Chapter 80). The patient is usually not fed orally if this diagnosis is entertained; an infant with sepsis usually does not tolerate oral feedings.

e. **Inborn errors of metabolism.**

f. Constipation. Anal stimulation can be attempted. If this fails, a glycerin suppository can be given. (See also Chapter 48.)

g. Adrenogenital syndrome.

h. Adrenal hypoplasia.

i. Formula intolerance. A trial of lactose-free formula (eg, ProSobee or Isomil) can be instituted if lactose intolerance is verified.

C. Bloody aspirate

    1. Nasogastric trauma. See Chapter 37.

    2. Gastrointestinal hemorrhage.

        a. Stress ulcer

          i. Stress ulcer is treated with gastric lavages of tepid water, ½ normal saline, or normal saline—5 mL/kg given by nasogastric tube until the bleeding has subsided. (**Note:** There is *controversy* about which fluid to use. Some clinicians believe that hyponatremia may occur if water is used and hypernatremia may occur if normal saline is used. Follow your institution's guidelines. *Never use cold water lavages* because they lower the infant's core temperature too rapidly.)

          ii. If the just-mentioned lavages do not stop the bleeding, a **lavage of 0.1 mL of 1:10,000 epinephrine solution in 10 mL of sterile water** can be used. This recommendation is also *controversial.*

          iii. The infant is usually started on **ranitidine or cimetidine** (for dosages and other pharmacologic information, see Chapter 80). Ranitidine is usually preferred because it has fewer side effects.

          iv. **Antacids** may be used (eg, Maalox, 2–5 mL [depending on the size of the infant], placed in the nasogastric tube every 4 h until bleeding has subsided), but this recommendation is also *controversial;* some clinicians believe that it may cause concretions in the gastrointestinal tract. Another dosage that has been recommended is 0.25 mL/kg of body weight, given 6 times/day.

        b. Disseminated intravascular coagulation. If clotting studies are abnormal and if gastrointestinal hemorrhage and hemorrhage at other sites are occurring, the cause of the coagulopathy must be identified and treated. Immediate transfusion of blood or fresh-frozen plasma, or both, may be needed depending on the amount of blood loss and blood pressure levels. Platelets may be needed depending on the platelet count.

        c. Vitamin K deficiency. Hemorrhage may occur if vitamin K injection was not given at birth or if the infant is receiving an inadequate amount of breast milk. Vitamin K_1 (1 mg subcutaneously or intravenously) should be given.

        d. NEC. See Chapter 71.

37 Gastrointestinal Bleeding from the Upper Tract

I. **Problem.** Vomiting of bright red blood or active bleeding from the nasogastric tube is seen.

II. **Immediate questions**

A. **What are the vital signs?** If the blood pressure is dropping and there is active bleeding from the nasogastric tube, urgent crystalloid replacement is necessary.

B. **What is the hematocrit?** A spun hematocrit should be done as soon as possible. The result is used as a baseline value and to determine whether blood replacement should be performed immediately. Remember: With an acute episode of bleeding, the hematocrit may not reflect the blood loss for several hours.

C. **Is blood available in the blood bank should transfusion be necessary?** Verify that the infant has been typed and cross-matched so that blood will be quickly available if necessary.

D. **Is there bleeding from other sites?** Bleeding from other sites suggests disseminated intravascular coagulation (DIC) or another coagulopathy. If bleeding is coming only from the nasogastric tube, disorders such as stress ulcer, nasogastric trauma, and swallowing of maternal blood are likely causes to consider in the differential diagnosis.

E. **How old is the infant?** During the first day of life, vomiting of bright red blood or the presence of bright red blood in the nasogastric tube is frequently secondary to swallowing of maternal blood during delivery. Infants with this problem are clinically stable, with normal vital signs. Pyloric stenosis in infants is usually present at 3–4 weeks of life.

F. **What medications are being given?** Certain medications are associated with an increased incidence of gastrointestinal (GI) bleeding. The most common of these medications are indomethacin (Indocin), tolazoline (Priscoline), and corticosteroids. A massive gastric hemorrhage may occur during continuous drip infusion of tolazoline. Theophylline is a rare cause of GI bleeding.

G. **Was vitamin K given at birth?** Failure to give vitamin K at birth may result in a bleeding disorder, usually at 3–4 days of life.

III. **Differential diagnosis**

A. **Idiopathic causes.** More than 50% of cases have no clear diagnosis. These usually resolve within several days.

B. **Swallowing of maternal blood.** This accounts for ~10% of cases. Typically, blood is swallowed during cesarean section delivery.

C. **Stress ulcer.**

D. **Nasogastric trauma.**

E. **Necrotizing enterocolitis.** This is a rare cause of upper GI tract bleeding and indicates extensive disease.

F. **Coagulopathy.** Hemorrhagic disease of the newborn and DIC account for ~20% of cases. Also, congenital coagulopathies (most commonly factor VIII deficiency [hemophilia A] and factor IX deficiency [hemophilia B]) can cause GI bleeding from the upper tract. DIC can occur after infection, shock, and severe fetal asphyxia.

G. **Drug-induced bleeding.** Indomethacin, corticosteroids, tolazoline, and other drugs may cause upper GI tract bleeding. Theophylline is a rare cause.

H. **Congenital defects** such as gastric volvulus, malrotation with volvulus, Hirschsprung's disease with enterocolitis, and gastric duplication are rare causes of GI bleeding.

I. **Pyloric stenosis.** Patients present at the 3rd to 4th week of life with nonbilious projectile vomiting (occasionally bloody).

IV. **Data base**

A. **Physical examination.** A complete physical examination should be performed, paying particular attention to the observation of other possible bleeding sites. Palpation of the abdomen may reveal a pyloric olive.

B. **Laboratory studies**

1. **Apt test.** The Apt test should be performed if swallowing of maternal blood is a possible cause (see p 220).

2. **Hematocrit** should be checked as a baseline and serially to gauge the extent of blood loss.

3. **Coagulation studies (prothrombin time, partial thromboplastin time, fibrinogen, and platelets).** These studies should be done to rule out DIC and other coagulopathies.

C. **Radiologic and other studies.** An **abdominal x-ray film** should be obtained to assess the bowel gas pattern and to rule out necrotizing enterocolitis. The x-ray film will also show the position of the nasogastric tube and rule out any surgical problem. Endoscopy should be considered in ulcer diagnosis. Ultrasound scans should be obtained if pyloric stenosis is suspected.

V. **Plan**

A. **General measures.** The most important goal is to stop the bleeding. This measure should be taken in every case except those involving infants who have swallowed maternal blood. (Infants with this problem are usually only a few hours old, are not sick, and have a positive Apt test result. Once stomach aspiration is performed, no more blood is obtained.) To help stop an acute episode of GI bleeding, the following measures can be used:

1. **Gastric lavage.** The technique for gastric lavage is described in Chapter 36.

2. **Epinephrine lavage** (1:10,000 solution), 0.1 mL diluted in 10 mL of sterile water, can be used if tepid water lavages do not stop the bleeding (*controversial*).

3. **Crystalloid replacement.** If the blood pressure is low or dropping, crystalloid (usually normal saline) can be given immediately.

4. **Blood replacement** may be indicated, depending on the result of hematocrit values obtained from the laboratory.

B. **Specific measures**

1. **Idiopathic.** When no cause is determined, the bleeding usually subsides and no other treatment is necessary.

2. **Swallowing of maternal blood.** Perform the Apt test to confirm maternal hemoglobin (see p 220). No treatment is necessary.

3. **Stress ulcer.** Stress ulcer is commonly diagnosed after an episode of GI bleeding. This disorder is difficult to confirm using radiologic studies; thus, they are not often obtained. Remission usually occurs; recurrence is rare. Antacids (eg, Maalox) may be given, but it is considered a *controversial* treatment because of the possibility of concretion formation. If used, the dosage for Maalox is 2–5 mL given by nasogastric tube every 4 h. Ranitidine (now preferred because it results in fewer central nervous system, hepatic, and platelet side effects) or cimetidine is often used during the period of bleeding (for dosages and other pharmacologic information, see Chapter 80).

4. **Nasogastric trauma.** This may occur if the nasogastric tube is too large or insertion is traumatic. Use the smallest nasogastric tube possible. Observation is indicated.

5. **Necrotizing enterocolitis.** Severe cases of necrotizing enterocolitis will cause upper GI bleeding. Treatment is discussed in Chapter 71.

6. **Coagulopathy**
   a. **Hemorrhagic disease of the newborn.** There are three forms of vitamin K deficiency:
      i. **Early form** (first day of life) is related to maternal medications affecting production of vitamin K by the neonate (barbiturates, phenytoin, rifampin, isoniazid, warfarin).
      ii. **Classic form** between day 2 and day 7 of life is more commonly seen in infants with inadequate intake of breast milk and when an infant has not received vitamin K at birth (home delivery).
      iii. **Late form** occurs between 2 weeks and 6 months of age. This is secondary to inadequate vitamin K intake (breast-fed infants) or hepatobiliary disease.

      When vitamin K deficiency is suspected, vitamin K should be administered intravenously or subcutaneously. Intramuscular injection can result in severe hematoma.
   b. **DIC.** If DIC is present, bleeding from other sites is usually seen. Coagulation studies will be abnormal (increased prothrombin time and partial thromboplastin time and decreased fibrinogen levels). Treat the underlying condition and support blood pressure with multiple transfusions of colloid as needed. Platelets may be required. The cause of DIC (eg, hypoxia, acidosis, bacterial or viral disease, toxoplasmosis, necrotizing enterocolitis, shock, or erythroblastosis fetalis) must be investigated. Several obstetric disorders, including abruptio placentae, chorioangioma, eclampsia, and fetal death associated with twin gestation, may give rise to DIC.
   c. **Congenital coagulopathies.** The most common that present with bleeding are secondary to factor VIII deficiency (hemophilia A) and factor IX deficiency (hemophilia B). Specific laboratory testing and appropriate consultation with a pediatric hematologist are appropriate.
7. **Drug-induced bleeding.** The drug responsible for the bleeding should be stopped if possible.
8. **Gastric volvulus and duplication.** Urgent surgical consultation is recommended.
9. **Pyloric stenosis.** Hydration and surgical pyloromyotomy are necessary.

38 Hyperbilirubinemia, Direct (Conjugated Hyperbilirubinemia)

I. **Problem.** An infant's direct (conjugated) serum bilirubin level is 3 mg/dL. (A value >2.0 mg/dL [or a fraction >10–15% of the total serum bilirubin] is abnormal at any age.) A persistent or increasing elevated direct bilirubin is always pathologic and must be evaluated promptly to minimize long-term sequelae. A value >5.0 mg/dL is considered severe.

II. **Immediate questions**

A. **Is the infant receiving total parenteral nutrition (TPN)?** TPN may cause direct hyperbilirubinemia by an unknown mechanism. It usually does not occur until the infant has been on TPN for >2 weeks. It occurs more commonly in sick premature infants.

B. **Is a bacterial or viral infection present?** Infection may cause hepatocellular damage, leading to increased direct bilirubin levels.

C. **Did direct hyperbilirubinemia occur only after feedings had been established?** If this is the case, a metabolic disorder such as galactosemia may be present.

D. **Have any risk factors been identified?** The most important risk factors include low gestational age, early or prolonged exposure to parenteral nutrition, lack of enteral feeding, and sepsis. Episodes of sepsis can be associated with an increase of 30% in the bilirubin level.

III. **Differential diagnosis.** See also Chapter 64.

A. **More common causes of direct hyperbilirubinemia.** Idiopathic neonatal hepatitis and biliary atresia account for ~60–80% of all conjugated hyperbilirubinemia cases.

1. **Idiopathic neonatal hepatitis** is the most common cause. This diagnosis is made after all other known causes have been excluded.

2. **Biliary atresia** is the second most common cause. It is a progressive obliterative process involving the bile ducts. If untreated, the outcome is fatal.

3. **Hyperalimentation.**

4. **Bacterial infection** (sepsis or urinary tract infection).

5. **Intrauterine infection** (TORCH [*t*oxoplasmosis, *o*ther, *r*ubella, *c*ytomegalovirus, and *h*erpes simplex virus], hepatitis B and C, and syphilis).

6. **Inspissated bile (bile plug)** from hemolytic disease.

7. **Choledochal cyst.**

8. **Alpha-antitrypsin deficiency** is the most common genetic cause of cholestasis.

9. **Galactosemia**

B. **Less common causes of direct hyperbilirubinemia**

1. **Bile duct stenosis.**

2. **Neoplasm.**

3. **Cholelithiasis.**

4. **Cystic fibrosis.** Very few of these patients have liver disease in the neonatal period.

5. **Hypothyroidism.**

6. **Rotor's syndrome.**

7. **Dubin-Johnson syndrome,** a genetic defect in the canalicular transport system.

8. **Storage disease (eg, Niemann-Pick disease or Gaucher's disease).**

9. **Metabolic disorders (eg, tyrosinemia, fructosemia).**

10. **Trisomy 21 or 18.**
11. **Other infections, such as varicella, coxsackievirus, echovirus, or *Listeria*.**
12. **Drug induced.**
13. **Shock.**
14. **Alagille syndrome (arteriohepatic dysplasia).**
15. **Zellweger syndrome (cerebrohepatorenal syndrome).**

IV. **Data base.** A detailed history, including prenatal (to evaluate for intrauterine infection or hemolytic disease) and postnatal (feeding history as well as the presence of any acholic stools) histories, should be obtained. The clinical hallmarks of the disease include **icterus, acholic stools, and dark urine.**

A. **Physical examination.** Particular attention should be given to examination of the abdomen. Palpate for an enlarged liver or spleen. Splenomegaly is more common in neonatal hepatitis but can be a late sign in biliary atresia. Check carefully for signs of sepsis. Know the characteristics of the syndromes mentioned previously, and look for any unusual features.

B. **Laboratory studies**
   1. **For the common causes, the workup should be as follows:**
      a. **Liver function tests** should include aspartate aminotransferase (AST [serum glutamic oxaloacetic transaminase, or SGOT]), alanine aminotransferase (ALT [serum glutamic pyruvic transaminase, or SGPT]), alkaline phosphatase, and gamma-glutamyltranspeptidase (GGTP). Elevated levels of AST and ALT signify hepatocellular damage. Elevated alkaline phosphatase levels may signify biliary obstruction. Elevated GGTP is a sensitive but nonspecific indicator of early cholestatic change.
      b. **A complete blood cell count with differential** may help to determine whether infection is present.
      c. **Coombs' test** may indicate the possibility of hemolytic disease.
      d. **Prothrombin time, partial thromboplastin time, and serum albumin level** will help evaluate hepatic function.
      e. **Reticulocyte count** may be elevated (ie, >4–5%) if bleeding has occurred.
      f. **Blood and urine culture.** If sepsis is considered, blood and urine samples must be obtained for culture.
      g. **Testing for viral disease.** Determine the serum total immunoglobulin M (IgM) level. If high, test for TORCH infections (see Chapter 60). Urine is tested for cytomegalovirus, and a serum hepatitis profile is obtained (hepatitis surface antigen and IgM hepatitis A antibody). Hepatitis B markers should be tested in both the mother and the infant.
      h. **Serum alpha₁-antitrypsin levels.** These levels are obtained to rule out alpha₁-antitrypsin deficiency.
      i. **Urine-reducing substance** should be determined if galactosemia is suspected.
   2. **For the less common cause,** perform the following additional studies:
      a. **Serum thyroxine (T₄) and thyroid-stimulating hormone (TSH) levels** should be obtained if hypothyroidism is suspected.
      b. **Sweat chloride test.** A quantitative sweat chloride test should be done to rule out cystic fibrosis.
      c. **Urine metabolic screen.**

C. **Radiologic and other studies**
   1. **Ultrasonography.** Ultrasound examination of the liver and the biliary tract will rule out choledochal cyst, stones, tumor, and masses and will also provide information on the gallbladder. The absence of the gallbladder may suggest biliary atresia.
   2. **Radionuclide scans** allow evaluation of the biliary anatomy.
   3. **Liver biopsy** is usually performed after all other laboratory tests have been performed and a definitive diagnosis is still needed.

4. **Exploratory laparotomy and operative cholangiography** should be done if biliary atresia is suspected or the medical evaluation is inconclusive.

V. **Plan.** The cause of direct hyperbilirubinemia is determined. This section discusses only the treatment plans of the more common causes of cholestatic jaundice. Supportive care is indicated. More detailed management information is presented in Chapter 64.

A. **Biliary atresia.** Exploratory surgery with intraoperative cholangiography is usually the initial step. Hepatic portoenterostomy (the **Kasai procedure**) is currently the initial procedure of choice in infancy; orthotopic liver transplantation is selectively performed for those infants or children with progressive liver failure. Hepatic transplantation offers improved survival and quality of life to those for whom the Kasai operation has not been successful.

B. **Idiopathic neonatal hepatitis.** Supportive care with a fair prognosis exists.

C. **Alpha₁-antitrypsin.** The only curative therapy is liver transplantation.

D. **Hyperalimentation.** Consider stopping TPN completely or using partial parenteral nutrition with some enteral feedings. Most infants recover with clearing of cholestasis in 1–3 months after normal feedings have begun. The use of phenobarbital therapy is *controversial.* Studies have shown that ursodeoxycholic acid is being used in high-risk neonates with TPN-cholestasis with good results. Cholecystokinin as a treatment or prophylactic agent has less conclusively shown a beneficial effect.

E. **Bacterial infection.** If signs of sepsis are present, appropriate cultures should be performed and empiric antibiotic therapy initiated.

F. **Intrauterine infection.** Appropriate antiviral agents or other medications should be started, if indicated.

G. **Inspissated bile** secondary to hemolytic disease is treated with supportive management. The use of phenobarbital is *controversial.*

H. **Choledochal cyst.** The treatment is surgical removal.

I. **Galactosemia.** Immediate elimination of lactose- and galactose-containing products from the diet is required.

39 Hyperbilirubinemia, Indirect (Unconjugated Hyperbilirubinemia)

I. **Problem.** An infant's indirect (unconjugated) serum bilirubin level is 10 mg/dL.
II. **Immediate questions**
   A. **How old is the infant?** *High indirect serum bilirubin levels during the first 24 h of life are never physiologic.* Hemolytic disease (Rh isoimmunization or ABO incompatibility), congenital infection, and polycythemia are likely causes. The age and gestation of the infant help to determine the bilirubin level at which phototherapy should be initiated.
   B. **Is the infant being breast-fed?** Breast milk jaundice is common and may be present; the cause is unknown. There is a familial association. Peak bilirubin levels usually occur 4–10 days after birth.
   C. **What is the family ethnicity?** Glucose-6-phosphate dehydrogenase (G6PD) deficiency occurs more commonly in people of Mediterranean descent. There is a rapid increase in the total serum bilirubin level after 24–48 h of age.
   D. **Is the infant dehydrated?** If the infant is dehydrated, fluid administration may lower the serum bilirubin level. Additional feedings should be given, if tolerated (milk-based formula is recommended in dehydrated breast-fed infants); otherwise, intravenous fluids should be given. For example, a 3-day-old infant is strictly breast-feeding, but his mother's milk has not yet "come in," so he has lost significant weight and becomes dehydrated. Remember that adequate hydration is essential, but excess hydration will not clear the bilirubin any more quickly.
III. **Differential diagnosis.** See also Chapter 64.
   A. **More common causes of indirect hyperbilirubinemia**
      1. **Physiologic hyperbilirubinemia.**
      2. **ABO incompatibility.**
      3. **Breast-feeding or breast milk jaundice.**
      4. **Infection** (eg, congenital syphilis, viral, or protozoal infections). Jaundice as the only sign of underlying sepsis is rare. In one study of 171 newborns readmitted for a mean bilirubin of 18.8 mg/dL, not one case of sepsis was identified.
      5. **Subdural hematoma or cephalhematoma.**
      6. **Excessive bruising.**
      7. **Infant of a diabetic mother.**
      8. **Polycythemia or hyperviscosity.**
   B. **Less common causes of indirect hyperbilirubinemia**
      1. **Rh isoimmunization.** As a result of antenatal treatment of Rh-negative mothers with RhoGAM, this has become a much less frequent cause.
      2. **G6PD deficiency.** With this condition, a late-rising bilirubin will be seen. This is also more common in individuals of certain ethnic backgrounds, such as those from Greece, Turkey, Sardinia, or Nigeria and Sephardic Jews.
      3. **Pyruvate kinase deficiency.**
      4. **Congenital spherocytosis.**
      5. **Lucey-Driscoll syndrome** (familial neonatal jaundice).
      6. **Crigler-Najjar syndrome.**
      7. **Hypothyroidism.**
      8. **Hemoglobinopathy.** α- and β-thalassemias are examples of this.
IV. **Data base**

A. History. It is important to take a complete history. Ask about the infant's feeding regimen and frequency of voiding. Ask about jaundice in previous siblings. Also ask about family ethnicity (if G6PD deficiency is suspected). Is there a familial history of significant hemolytic disease? Is there a history of light-colored stools or dark urine?

B. Physical examination. Pay particular attention to signs of bruising, cephalhematoma, or intracranial bleeding. Check for hepatosplenomegaly.

C. Laboratory studies. Studies have questioned the validity of ordering extensive tests on any infant with possible hyperbilirubinemia. Recommendations suggest that in normal and healthy term infants fewer tests are necessary. It is important to save all cord blood for future testing if necessary.

1. **Normal, otherwise healthy term newborn** (weighing >2500 g and at >37 weeks' gestational age based on recommendations from the American Academy of Pediatrics [AAP]).

    a. **Blood type and ABO and Rh(D) typing** of the mother and a serum screen for isoimmune antibodies.

    b. **Direct Coombs' test, blood type, and Rh(D) type on the infant's cord blood** if the mother has not had prenatal blood grouping or is Rh-negative.

    c. **Total serum bilirubin level** if there is jaundice in the first 24 h or moderate jaundice associated with a positive Coombs' test, parental anxiety, or other signs of illness.

2. **Any other infant**

    a. **Total and direct serum bilirubin levels.** In preterm or ill infants, check levels every 12–24 h depending on the rate of rise and until stable. In term infants, direct bilirubin is indicated only if jaundice is persistent or the infant is ill.

    b. **Complete blood cell count with differential.** This test is indicated if hemolytic disease, anemia, or infection is suspected.

    c. **Mother's blood type with Rh determination.**

    d. **Infant's blood type with Rh determination.**

    e. **Direct and indirect Coombs' tests.**

    f. **Reticulocyte count.** Consider this test if the infant is anemic or hemolytic disease is suspected.

    g. **Red blood cell (RBC) smear.** Fragmented RBCs should be present in hemolysis.

    h. **G6PD screen.** Consider performing a G6PD screen if the infant is of Mediterranean descent, the jaundice is late onset, and there is evidence of hemolysis (low hematocrit, high reticulocyte count, and a peripheral smear showing nucleated RBCs and other fragmented cells).

    i. **Hemoglobin electrophoresis**

    j. **Radiologic and other studies.** None are usually necessary.

V. Plan. See also Chapter 64.

A. Phototherapy. Phototherapy should be initiated according to the guidelines in Tables 39–1 and 39–2. The AAP guidelines (see Table 39–1) are for healthy term infants (>37 weeks) only. Table 39–2 gives recommendations for phototherapy and exchange transfusion in sick and well preterm infants and sick term infants. Remember: These are guidelines only, and each patient must be considered individually. In infants weighing <1000 g, the guidelines may be lowered to 5 mg/dL for phototherapy and 10–12 mg/dL for exchange transfusion. If phototherapy is used, perform the following additional procedures:

1. **Increase the maintenance infusion of intravenous fluids** by 0.5 mL/kg/h if the infant weighs <1500 g and by 1 mL/kg/h if the infant weighs >1500 g. (**Note:** Water supplements to breast-fed infants do not reduce serum bilirubin.) Remember that maintaining adequate hydration and good urine output will help the efficacy of phototherapy because the by-products responsible for the decline in bilirubin are partially excreted in the urine.

TABLE 39–1. AMERICAN ACADEMY OF PEDIATRICS RECOMMENDATIONS FOR THE MANAGEMENT OF HYPERBILIRUBINEMIA IN HEALTHY TERM NEWBORN INFANTS

		Total serum bilirubin, mg/dL		
Age (h)	Consider phototherapy[a]	Exchange transfusion if intensive and intensive Phototherapy	Exchange transfusion and intensive phototherapy fails[b]	phototherapy
≤24[c]				
25–48	≥12 (205)	≥15 (260)	≥20 (340)	≥25 (430)
49–72	≥15 (260)	≥18 (310)	≥25 (430)	≥30 (510)
>72	≥17 (290)	≥20 (340)	≥25 (430)	≥30 (510)

Values in parentheses represent μmol/L.
[a]Phototherapy is an option and depends on clinical judgment.
[b]Intensive phototherapy should result in a total serum bilirubin decline of 1–2 mg/dL within 4–6 h. If this does not occur, it is considered a failure of phototherapy.
[c]Term infants who are clinically jaundiced at <24 h are not considered healthy and require further evaluation.
Modified from American Academy of Pediatrics: Management of hyperbilirubinemia in the healthy term newborn. *Pediatrics* 1994;94:558; American Academy of Pediatrics: Management of hyperbilirubinemia in the healthy term newborn. *Pediatrics* 1995;95:458.

2. **Perform total bilirubin testing** every 6–12 h.
3. **Attempt regular feedings** if possible, and feed frequently. Feeding inhibits the enterohepatic from of bilirubin and helps lower the serum bilirubin level. Studies have revealed that increasing the frequency of breastfeeding will not have a significant effect on the serum bilirubin level in the first 3 days of life.
4. **Phototherapy can be safely discontinued** once serum bilirubin levels have fallen >2 mg/dL below the level at which phototherapy was initiated. Once phototherapy is stopped, the average bilirubin rebound in infants who do not have hemolytic disease is <1 mg/dL.

B. **Drug therapy**
1. **Phenobarbital** has been shown to be effective in reducing the serum bilirubin level by increasing hepatic glucuronosyltransferase activity and conjugation of bilirubin. It is not effective immediately and is usually used in severe cases of prolonged hyperbilirubinemia only. (For dosage and other pharmacologic information, see Chapter 80.)
2. **Studies have revealed that the tin and zinc metalloporphyrins** (SnMP and ZnMP, respectively) are effective and in small trials show a dramatic

TABLE 39–2. RECOMMENDATIONS FOR THE MANAGEMENT OF HYPERBILIRUBINEMIA IN PRETERM INFANTS (SICK AND WELL) AND SICK TERM INFANTS

	Total serum bilirubin level (mg/dL)			
	Well infant		Sick infant	
Weight (g)	Phototherapy	Exchange transfusion	Phototherapy	Exchange transfusion
<1500	5–8	13–16	4–7	10–14
1500–2000	8–12	16–18	7–10	14–16
2000–2500	12–15	18–20	10–12	16–18
>2500	a	a	13–15	17–22

[a]See Table 39–1.

decrease in the need for phototherapy. They work by decreasing the production of bilirubin by competitive inhibition of heme oxygenase.
C. **Exchange transfusion.** (See Tables 39–1 and 39–2.) The procedure for exchange transfusion is discussed in Chapter 21. There is considerable *controversy* concerning the exact level at which to initiate exchange transfusion. The overall status (sick or well), birth weight, gestational age, and age of the infant are important considerations. In many cases, institutional guidelines are established and should be followed. The AAP guidelines for exchange transfusion are for healthy term newborns (>37 weeks) only. Some general guidelines are listed in Table 39–2. Remember: These are guidelines only, and each patient must be considered individually. If the infant is sick (eg, with signs of hemolysis, hypoxemia, acidosis, or sepsis), has a lower gestational age, is on day 1 or 2 of life, or has a low birth weight, this would tend to lower the threshold that is used for exchange transfusion.
D. **Breast-fed infants.** The AAP does not recommend the interruption of breast-feeding in healthy term newborns. The AAP does encourage continued and frequent breast-feeding. Remember that supplementing with water or dextrose water does not lower the bilirubin level. Five treatment options are available. The decision as to which treatment option to use depends on the specific infant, the physician's judgment, and the family circumstances.
   1. Observation and serial bilirubin determinations.
   2. Continue breast-feeding, and administer phototherapy.
   3. Continue breast-feeding but supplement with formula with or without phototherapy.
   4. Interrupt breast-feeding, and substitute formula.
   5. Interrupt breast-feeding, substitute formula, and administer phototherapy. Although phototherapy does not reduce the serum bilirubin concentration in breast-fed infants as quickly as it does in formula-fed infants, it is still effective. Supplemental breast milk rather than formula is advocated by some.
E. **Breast-fed infants with persistent jaundice after 2 weeks.** About 30% of healthy term infants will have persistent jaundice after 2 weeks of age. Treatment is as follows:
   1. If the physical examination is normal and the history of normal urine and stool is obtained, then the infant can be observed. An abnormal history includes pale stools or dark-yellow urine.
   2. Check the newborn screen for hypothyroidism (congenital hypothyroidism is a cause of indirect hyperbilirubinemia).
   3. If jaundice is still present after 3 weeks, a urine bilirubin and total and direct serum bilirubin should be obtained.
F. **Follow-up should be provided for all neonates** discharged <48 h after birth to monitor for bilirubin problems.

40 Hyperglycemia

I. **Problem.** The nurse reports that an infant has a blood glucose level of 240 mg/dL. (Hyperglycemia is defined as a serum blood glucose level >125 mg/dL in term infants and >150 mg/dL in premature infants.) Hyperglycemia in very premature infants has been associated with an increased mortality, increased incidence of intracranial hemorrhage, and developmental delay.

II. **Immediate questions**

A. **What is the serum glucose value on laboratory testing?** Dextrostix values are often inaccurate because the procedure is performed incorrectly or the Dextrostix strips are old and no longer reliable. Chemstrip-bG values are thought to be more reliable by some, but it is best to obtain a serum glucose level from the laboratory before initiating treatment.

B. **Is glucose being spilled in the urine?** A trace amount of glucose in the urine is accepted as normal. If the urinary glucose level is +1, +2, or greater, the renal threshold has been reached and there is an increased chance of osmotic diuresis. Some institutions accept a urinary glucose level of +1 without treating the patient (*controversial*). **Note:** *Each 18-mg/dL rise in blood glucose causes an increase in serum osmolarity of 1 mOsm/L. Normal osmolarity is 280–300 mOsm/L.*

C. **How much glucose is the patient receiving?** Normal initial maintenance glucose therapy in infants not being fed orally is 5–7 mg/kg/min. To determine this, see Chapter 7.

D. **Are there signs of sepsis?** Sepsis may cause hyperglycemia by inducing a stress response (catecholamine mediated).

III. **Differential diagnosis.** Hyperglycemia occurs most often in premature infants. The main concern with hyperglycemia is it can cause hyperosmolarity, osmotic diuresis, and subsequent dehydration. There may be a risk of intracranial hemorrhage with hyperosmolarity.

A. **Excess glucose administration.** Incorrect calculation of glucose levels or errors in the formulation of intravenous fluids may cause hyperglycemia.

B. **Inability to metabolize glucose** may occur with prematurity or secondary to sepsis or stress. Most commonly, a tiny infant on total parenteral nutrition becomes hyperglycemic because he or she does not tolerate the increase in glucose.

C. **Transient neonatal diabetes mellitus** is a rare disorder. The majority of infants are small for gestational age. The disorder may present at any time from 2 days to 6 weeks of age but commonly at 12 days of age. The most common findings are hyperglycemia, dehydration, glycosuria, polyuria, progressive wasting, hypoinsulinism, and acidosis. Ketonuria is absent. The C-peptide levels can be normal or transiently low in the serum or urine.

D. **Medications** such as maternal use of diazoxide can cause hyperglycemia in the infant. Drugs used in infants that have been associated with hyperglycemia include caffeine, theophylline, corticosteroids, and phenytoin.

E. **Insulin-dependent diabetes mellitus.** This is very rare. Insulin is required throughout life. Studies reveal low to absent C-peptide levels.

IV. **Data base**

A. **Physical examination and history.** Perform a complete physical examination. Look for subtle signs of sepsis (eg, temperature instability, changes in peripheral perfusion, or any changes in gastric aspirates if the infant is feeding). Determine maternal and infant medications. Obtain a thorough family history because diabetes can be familial.

B. Laboratory studies
1. **Serum glucose level.** Confirm the rapid paper-strip test result with a serum glucose level.
2. **Urine dipstick testing for glucose level.**
3. **Complete blood cell count with differential** is performed as a screening test for sepsis.
4. **Blood and urine cultures** are indicated if sepsis is suspected and if antibiotics are to be started.
5. **Serum electrolytes.** Hyperglycemia may cause osmotic diuresis, which may lead to electrolyte losses and dehydration. Therefore, it is important to monitor serum electrolyte levels in hyperglycemic patients.
6. **Serum insulin level** is obtained if there is concern about transient neonatal diabetes mellitus. The levels are usually low because of the hyperglycemia.
7. **Serum or urine C-peptide levels.** These levels will be low to absent in insulin-dependent diabetes mellitus.

C. Radiologic and other studies. None are usually required; however, a chest x-ray study may be useful in the evaluation of sepsis.

V. Plan
A. Excess glucose administration
1. **Positive urinary glucose level.** Decrease the amount of glucose being given by decreasing the concentration of dextrose in intravenous fluids or by decreasing the infusion rate. Most infants who are not feeding initially require 5–7 mg/kg/min of glucose to maintain normal glucose levels. Use Dextrostix or Chemstrip-bG testing every 4–6 h, and check for glucose in the urine with each voiding.
2. **Negative urinary glucose level.** If glucose is being given to increase the caloric intake, it is acceptable to have a higher serum glucose level as long as glucose is not being spilled in the urine. Perform Dextrostix and urinary glucose testing every 4–6 h.

B. Inability to metabolize glucose. Sepsis should always be considered in an infant with hyperglycemia. If the blood cell count looks suspicious or there are clinical signs of sepsis, it is acceptable to treat the infant for 3 days with antibiotics and then stop if cultures are negative. Ampicillin and an aminoglycoside are usually given initially (for dosages, see Chapter 80). Treatment of infants unable to metabolize glucose for any reason is described next.
1. **Decrease the concentration of glucose or the rate of infusion until a normal serum glucose level is present.** Do not use a solution that has a dextrose concentration of <4.7%. Such a solution is hypo-osmolar and could cause hemolysis, with resulting hyperkalemia.
2. **Insulin.** Insulin administration has been used in premature infants with success and has allowed more energy intake, promotes glucose tolerance, and promotes weight gain in these infants. Potassium levels need to be monitored when giving insulin therapy. If insulin is used, it can be given in one of two ways:
   a. **An insulin infusion** may be given at a rate of 0.02–0.1 unit/kg/h. Albumin, which used to be added to the bag to prevent insulin from adhering to the plastic tubing, is now considered unnecessary. It is currently thought that, by simply flushing the tubing with an adequate amount of the insulin-containing solution, all binding sites and the tubing will be saturated satisfactorily before beginning the insulin infusion. Dextrostix testing must be performed every 30–60 min until the level of glucose is stable.
   b. **Insulin may be given subcutaneously,** 0.05–0.1 unit/kg every 6 h. Continuous intravenous insulin is preferred. Chemstrip-bG testing (or Dextrostix testing) must be performed every 60 min until the glucose level is stable.

C. Transient neonatal diabetes mellitus
1. **Give intravenous (or oral) fluids,** and monitor the urine output, blood pH, and serum electrolyte levels.

2. **Give insulin** either by constant infusion or subcutaneously (see the dosage just given). Monitor glucose levels with Chemstrip bG testing (or Dextrostix testing) every 4–6 h. This disease usually resolves in days to months.
3. **Consult a pediatric endocrinologist.**
4. **Repeat serum insulin values** to rule out permanent diabetes mellitus.

D. **Medications**
1. **If the infant is receiving theophylline,** the serum theophylline level should be checked to detect possible toxicity, with resulting hyperglycemia. Other signs of **theophylline toxicity** include tachycardia, jitteriness, feeding intolerance, and seizures. If the level is high, the dosage must be altered or the drug discontinued.
2. **With maternal use of diazoxide,** the infant may have tachycardia and hypotension as well as hyperglycemia. Toxicity in the infant is usually self-limited, and only observation is usually necessary.
3. **Caffeine and phenytoin.** If possible, the medication should be discontinued.
4. **Steroids.** Prolonged courses and pharmacologic dosing of corticosteroids are being used much less frequently now for infants with chronic lung disease. When steroid use is deemed necessary, reducing the dose or frequency may limit the hyperglycemia side effect.

41 Hyperkalemia

I. **Problem.** The serum potassium level is >6 mEq/L. Normal potassium levels vary with the technique used by the laboratory. Normal potassium levels are generally between 4 and 6 mEq/L.

II. **Immediate questions**
   A. **How was the specimen collected? What is the central serum potassium level? Is it a true level or factitious?** Blood obtained by heelstick may yield falsely elevated potassium levels secondary to hemolysis. Blood drawn through a tiny needle may cause hemolysis and falsely elevated potassium levels. Clot formation can also cause a falsely elevated potassium. The blood also should not be obtained from a heparin-coated umbilical catheter (release of benzalkonium from a heparin-coated umbilical catheter can elevate results).
   B. **How much potassium is the infant receiving?** Normal amounts of potassium given for maintenance are 1–3 mEq/kg/day.
   C. **Does the electrocardiogram (ECG) show cardiac changes characteristic of hyperkalemia?** Early cardiac changes include tall, "tented" T waves, followed as hyperkalemia worsens by loss of P wave, widening QRS, ST-segment depression, bradycardia, sine wave QRS-T, first-degree atrioventricular (AV) block, ventricular dysrhythmia, and finally cardiac arrest.
   D. **What are the blood urea nitrogen (BUN) and creatinine levels? What is the urine output and weight?** Elevated BUN and creatinine measurements indicate renal insufficiency. Another indication of renal failure is decreasing or inadequate urine output with weight gain.
   E. **Is there associated hyponatremia, hypoglycemia, and hypotension?** If an infant has low sodium and glucose levels, a high potassium level, and hypotension, one needs to rule out adrenal insufficiency.

III. **Differential diagnosis**
   A. **Falsely elevated potassium level.** This is usually caused by hemolysis or clot formation during phlebotomy or heelstick or by drawing of blood proximal to an intravenous site that contains potassium.
   B. **Excess potassium administration.** This can occur from giving too much potassium in the intravenous fluids. Potassium supplements usually are not necessary on the first day of life and often are not necessary until day 3, with the typical requirement of 1–2 mEq/kg/day.
   C. **Pathologic hemolysis of red blood cells.** This may be secondary to intraventricular hemorrhage, use of a hypotonic glucose solution (<4.7% dextrose), sepsis (most commonly, *Pseudomonas*), or Rh incompatibility.
   D. **Renal failure.** Acute renal failure can lead to hyperkalemia.
   E. **Immaturity.** Nonoliguric hyperkalemia occurs in almost half of extremely low birth weight infants. This hyperkalemia occurs without potassium intake or oliguria. This hyperkalemia can result either from a shift of potassium from intracellular to extracellular space associated with decreased sodium- and potassium-activated adenosine triphosphate (Na^+, K^+-ATPase) activity or from immature renal tubular and glomerular functions. Hyperkalemia is very often associated with hyperglycemia as a result of insulin resistance and intracellular energy failure.
   F. **Metabolic or respiratory acidosis.** Systemic acidosis causes potassium to move out of cells, resulting in hyperkalemia. For every 0.1-unit decrease in pH, the serum potassium will increase ~0.3–1.3 mEq/L.
   G. **Tissue necrosis.** In certain disease states, such as necrotizing enterocolitis (NEC), tissue necrosis can occur and hyperkalemia may result.

H. **Medications.** Certain medications contain potassium and will elevate the serum potassium level. Digoxin therapy can lead to hyperkalemia secondary to redistribution of potassium. K^+-sparing diuretics cause decreased potassium losses. Both propranolol and phenylephrine are associated with hyperkalemia. High glucose load can lead to hyperkalemia secondary to increases in plasma osmolality. Hyperkalemia occurs with tromethamine administration. Indomethacin and angiotensin-converting enzyme inhibitors are associated with hyperkalemia.

I. **Adrenal insufficiency.** Adrenal insufficiency can be seen in congenital adrenal hyperplasia and bilateral adrenal hemorrhage. In salt-losing congenital adrenal hyperplasia, the infants will have low serum sodium, chloride, and glucose; elevated levels of potassium; and hypotension. In bilateral adrenal hemorrhage, anemia, thrombocytopenia, and jaundice are seen and bilateral adrenal masses are palpable.

J. **Decreased insulin levels** are associated with hyperkalemia.

IV. **Data base**
A. **Physical examination.** Perform a complete physical examination, paying special attention to the abdomen for signs of NEC (ie, abdominal distention, decreased bowel sounds, and visible bowel loops).

B. **Laboratory studies**
   1. **Serum potassium level.**
   2. **Serum ionized and total calcium levels.** Because hypocalcemia may potentiate the effects of hyperkalemia, maintain normal serum calcium concentrations.
   3. **Serum pH.** The serum pH is obtained to rule out acidosis, which may potentiate hyperkalemia.
   4. **BUN and serum creatinine levels** may reveal renal insufficiency.
   5. **Urine specific gravity** is obtained to assess renal status.

C. **Radiologic studies**
   1. **Abdominal x-ray study.** If NEC is suspected, an abdominal x-ray film should be obtained.
   2. **ECG.** ECG may reveal the cardiac changes characteristic of hyperkalemia and will provide a baseline study (see section II,C).

V. **Plan.** First, document whether there are ECG changes. If there are, **then this is a medical emergency and needs to be treated immediately (see later discussion).** Treat the specific cause. Stop all potassium intake. Check the calculation of potassium in the intravenous fluids, and make sure that excess was not being given. Stop any potassium-containing medications. Correct hypovolemia using the isotonic saline to promote tubular secretion of potassium. Renal failure can be treated with fluid restriction. If adrenal insufficiency exists, hormonal therapy is indicated. With the following plan, it is important to monitor ECG changes during therapy.

A. **Hyperkalemia with ECG changes.** See section II,C.
   1. **Give calcium gluconate (0.5–1 mEq/kg over 5–10 min) or calcium chloride (0.25–0.5 mEq/kg over 5–10 min).** Observe the ECG while infusing the medication. Once the arrhythmia disappears, the bolus can be stopped. This medication will only decrease myocardial excitability. It will not decrease the potassium concentration. Therefore, it is necessary to give the infant a medication immediately that will begin to decrease potassium.
   2. **Several medications can be given** (presented next). More than one medication can be used at a time. Both glucose and insulin and sodium bicarbonate cause cellular intake of potassium. Deciding which one to use depends on your unit's preference: One has not been shown to be superior than the other. Most units choose glucose and insulin, especially in an extremely tiny infant.
      a. **Give sodium bicarbonate.** Correct the base deficit by using the following formula:

$$NaHCO_3 \ (mEq) = 0.3 \times weight \ (kg) \times base \ deficit \ (mEq/L)$$

or give 1–2 mEq/kg over 10–30 min intravenously. Inducing alkalosis will drive potassium ions into the cells. In an extremely tiny infant, it may be better to not give sodium bicarbonate because of the associated risks.

   b. **Glucose and insulin** may be given to drive potassium into the cells. The usual dose is 0.1–0.2 unit/kg/h diluted in 10% dextrose in water. The amount of glucose needed is variable depending on blood glucose levels. Monitor the infant for hypoglycemia.

   c. **Start administration of sodium/calcium polystyrene sulfonate** (see section V,B,4). It will lower the potassium level slowly and is, therefore, of limited value acutely.

B. **Hyperkalemia without ECG changes**

   1. **Stop administration of potassium** in intravenous fluids; also consider stopping any potassium-containing medications or medications known to induce hyperkalemia (indomethacin).

   2. **Check the serum potassium level frequently** (ie, every 1–2 h).

   3. **Furosemide (Lasix)** can be given if renal function is adequate; the usual dose is 1 mg/kg given intravenously (*controversial*). (See Chapter 80.)

   4. **Sodium polystyrene sulfonate (Kayexalate),** or calcium polystyrene sulfonate, a potassium-exchange resin, can be given. One gram of resin removes ~1 mEq of potassium. The usual dose is 1 g/kg/dose orally every 6 h or rectally every 2–6 h. (See Chapter 80.) Oral therapy should not be used in extremely low birth weight infants. This therapy should not be used in extremely low birth weight infants because of risk of irritation, concretions, and necrotizing enterocolitis. This treatment can cause an increase in sodium and calcium. Repetitive rectal use can cause local bleeding.

   5. **Insulin and glucose** can be used (see section V,A,2,b).

   6. **Prevention** of nonoliguric hyperkalemia of extremely low birth weight infants. Potassium should not be administered in the first days of life until good urinary output is established and serum potassium is normal and not rising. Potassium levels should be monitored every 6 h in the first few days of life. Early administration of amino acids (first day of life) may stimulate endogenous insulin secretions and prevent the need for insulin infusion. In one pilot study, albuterol inhalation (400 μg in 2 mL of saline solution repeated every 2 h) until serum potassium less than 5 mEq/L with a maximum of 12 doses) lowered potassium rapidly in premature neonates. No adverse effects related to albuterol were observed. The effect is probably mediated through β-adrenergic receptors on $Na^+ K^+$-ATPase.

C. **Refractory hyperkalemia.** If all of these prior measures fail to lower the potassium level, other measures, such as exchange transfusion with freshly washed packed red blood cells reconstituted with plasma, peritoneal dialysis, or hemofiltration and hemodialysis, must be considered. These methods work immediately and are very effective but are limited by the time involved to prepare for them.

42 Hypertension

I. **Problem.** An infant has a systolic blood pressure (BP) >90 mm Hg. Hypertension is defined as a BP >2 standard deviations above normal values for age and weight, but the definition can vary widely (Table 42–1). Others define neonatal hypertension as a systolic BP >95th percentile for age and sex on three separate occasions. It can also be defined as a systolic BP >90 mm Hg and a diastolic BP >60 mm Hg in full-term infants; for premature infants, the values are systolic >80 mm Hg and diastolic >50 mm Hg. The values for normal BP are given in Appendix C. Hypertension is rare in the newborn infant. The incidence is anywhere from 0.2% (healthy newborn) to 40% (the latter figure reported in infants with chronic lung disease).

II. **Immediate questions**
   A. **How was the BP taken?** Doppler flow ultrasonography is the most reliable noninvasive method of measurement. The size of the cuff is important. The cuff should encircle two thirds of the length of the upper extremity. If the cuff is too narrow, the BP will be falsely elevated. If measurements are taken by means of an umbilical artery catheter, be certain that the catheter is free of bubbles or clots and that the transducer is calibrated; otherwise, erroneous results will occur. Remember that BP rises when the infant is feeding, sucking, or in an upright position.
   B. **Is an umbilical artery catheter in place, or has one been in place in the past?** Umbilical artery catheters are associated with an increased incidence of renovascular hypertension. There is no relation between the duration of catheter placement and the development of hypertension. A catheter-related aortic thrombosis can also produce hypertension. The following conditions are risk factors to thrombus formation in the aorta: bronchopulmonary dysplasia (BPD), patent ductus arteriosus, hypervolemia, and certain central nervous system disorders. Improved catheters and the use of heparin has helped to decrease the incidence of thrombus formation.
   C. **Are symptoms of hypertension present?** Infants with hypertension may be asymptomatic or may have the following symptoms: tachypnea, cyanosis, seizures, lethargy, increased tone, apnea, abdominal distention, fever, and mottling. They may also have congestive heart failure and respiratory distress.
   D. **What is the BP in the extremities?** The BP in a healthy infant should be higher in the legs than in the arms. If the pressure is lower in the legs, coarctation of the aorta may be the cause of the hypertension.
   E. **What is the birth weight and postnatal age of the infant?** Normal BP values increase with increasing birth weight and age. Values rise ~1–2 mm Hg/day during the first week of life and then ~1–2 mm Hg/week over the next 6 weeks.
   F. **Is the infant in pain or agitated?** Pain (such as that from a surgical procedure), crying, agitation, or suctioning can cause a transient rise in BP. The systolic pressure can be 5 mm Hg lower in sleeping infants.
   G. **Does the infant have BPD?** Infants with BPD have a significant problem with hypertension (studies reveal up to 40%). It often occurs after discharge from the nursery.

III. **Differential diagnosis**
   A. **More common causes of hypertension**
      1. **No cause found.**
      2. **Renal artery thrombosis.** Most commonly related to umbilical artery catheterization. This is a very common cause of hypertension.

TABLE 42-1. REPRESENTATIVE 95TH AND 97TH PERCENTILES FOR SYSTOLIC BLOOD PRESSURE IN INFANTS

				Systolic blood pressure (mm Hg)	
Study	Technique	Gestation	Age	95th percentile	97th percentile
American Academy of Pediatrics 2nd Task Force	First auscultation or Doppler ultrasonogram	Term	Day 1 Day 8–30	96 104	
Brompton	Mean of 3 Doppler ultrasonograms	Term	Day 4 6 weeks	95* 113*	
Northern Neonatal Nursing Initiative	Mean of 3 or more Doppler ultra-sonograms	Term	Day 1 Day 10		82 111
Northern Neonatal Nursing Initiative	Mean of 3 or more Doppler ultra-sonograms	24 weeks	Day 1 Day 10		57 71
		28 weeks	Day 1 Day 10		62 83
		32 weeks	Day 1 Day 10		67 94
		36 weeks	Day 1 Day 10		74 104

*Awake.
Adapted from Watkinson M: Hypertension in the newborn baby. *Arch Dis Child Fetal Neonatal Ed* 2002;86:F78.

3. **Aortic thrombosis.**
4. **Obstructive uropathy.**
5. **Infantile polycystic kidneys.**
6. **Renal failure.**
7. **Medications** such as theophylline, pancuronium, doxapram, and corticosteroids.
8. **Fluid overload.**
9. **Pain or agitation.**
10. **BPD.** Approximately 40% of patients with BPD have hypertension. The origin is probably multifactorial (increased renin activity and catecholamine secretion may be associated with chronic lung disease).
11. **Coarctation of the aorta.** There is an increased incidence of coarctation in Turner's syndrome.
12. **Drug withdrawal.**
B. **Less common causes**
1. **Renal artery stenosis.** The infant will be hypertensive from birth. This accounts for 20% of the cases of hypertension in infants.
2. **Renal vein thrombosis.**
3. **Hypoplasia or dysplasia of the kidneys.**
4. **Pyelonephritis.**
5. **Medications** such as ocular phenylephrine, dopamine, vitamin D, and epinephrine.
6. **Primary hyperaldosteronism.**
7. **Neuroblastoma, pheochromocytoma, or Wilms' tumor.**
8. **Hyperthyroidism.**
9. **Adrenogenital syndrome.**
10. **Increased intracranial pressure** secondary to intracranial hemorrhage, hydrocephalus, meningitis, or subdural hemorrhage.
11. **Closure of abdominal wall defects (eg, omphalocele or gastroschisis).**
12. **Seizures.**

13. **Extracorporeal membrane oxygenation (ECMO).** Hypertension is common in infants undergoing ECMO.
14. **Congenital adrenal hyperplasia.** Blood gas studies will reveal a metabolic alkalosis.
15. **Cushing's disease.**

IV. **Data base**
  A. **Physical examination**
    1. **Check the femoral pulse in both legs,** which is absent or decreased in coarctation of the aorta.
    2. **Examine the abdomen** carefully for masses and to determine the size of the kidneys. An enlarged kidney may indicate tumor, polycystic kidneys, obstruction, or renal vein thrombosis.
  B. **Laboratory studies.** Figure 42–1 is an overview of a complete evaluation.
    1. **Assessment of renal function.** To assess renal function, perform the following tests:
       a. **Serum creatinine and blood urea nitrogen (BUN) levels.** Elevated serum creatinine and BUN levels may indicate renal insufficiency, which may be associated with hypertension.
       b. **Urinalysis.** Red blood cells in the urine suggest obstruction, infection, or renal vein thrombosis.
       c. **Urine culture.** To rule out pyelonephritis.
       d. **Serum electrolytes and carbon dioxide.** A low serum potassium level and a high carbon dioxide level will be seen in primary hyperaldosteronism.
    2. **Plasma renin levels** may be elevated in patients with renovascular disease. Levels will be low in those with primary hyperaldosteronism.
  C. **Radiologic and other studies**
    1. **Abdominal ultrasonography.** This is the preferred screening test in neonates to detect abdominal masses as well as kidney obstruction. Doppler flow ultrasonography can be used to screen for arterial or venous problems. Infants who had an umbilical artery catheter should have their aorta and renal arteries studied for thrombi.
    2. **Cranial ultrasonography.** To rule out intraventricular hemorrhage.
    3. **Echocardiography.** Use if a disease such as coarctation is suspected or to evaluate end-organ damage caused by hypertension (eg, left ventricular hypertrophy or decreased contractility).
    4. **Intravenous pyelography.** This is usually of limited value in the newborn because of poor renal concentrating ability.
    5. **Further studies.** The following invasive procedures and laboratory studies are sometimes necessary to further evaluate the infant with hypertension:
       a. **Arteriography** to evaluate renovascular disease **or venacavography** to evaluate renal vein thrombosis.
       b. **Abdominal computed tomography (CT) scan.**
       c. **Renal scan** helps to quantitate the function of each kidney.
       d. **Renal vein renin level** to further evaluate renovascular disease.
       e. **Renal biopsy** to rule out any intrinsic renal disease.
       f. **Twenty-four-hour urinary catecholamines** to evaluate for pheochromocytoma.
       g. **Urinary 17-hydroxysteroid and 17-ketosteroid levels** to evaluate for Cushing's syndrome and congenital adrenal hyperplasia.

V. **Plan**
  A. **General.** Treat any obvious underlying condition. Stop medications if they are causing hypertension. Correct fluid overload by decreasing fluids and administering diuretics. Always check volume status and restrict sodium and fluid intake.
  B. **Drug therapy.** To guide drug therapy, decide whether the hypertension is mild, moderate, or life-threatening. (Dosages are given in Chapter 80.) Remember: Treatment thresholds are unclear, and many of the recommenda-

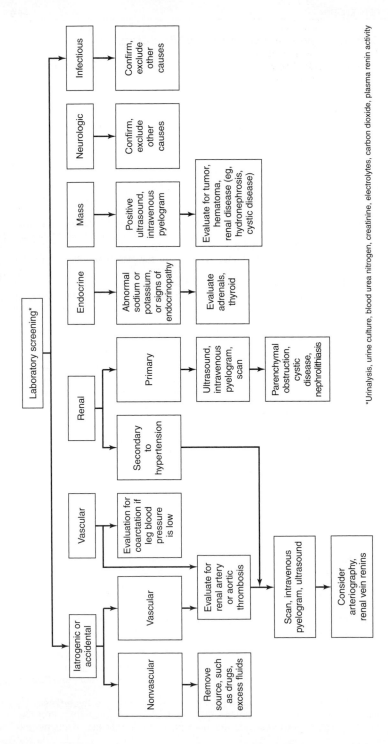

FIGURE 42–1. Evaluation of hypertension in the newborn. (*Modified and reproduced, with permission, from Adelman RD: Hypertension in infants.* Pediatr Ann *[Sept] 1989;18:568.*)

*Urinalysis, urine culture, blood urea nitrogen, creatinine, electrolytes, carbon dioxide, plasma renin activity

tions are *controversial.* More studies are necessary to establish guidelines in preterm infants. Some experts believe that any asymptomatic infant with hypertension with no end-organ involvement should not be treated but observed.

1. **Life-threatening hypertension** (BP extremely high and symptoms present). Labetalol or hydralazine are the intravenous drugs of choice. They may be titrated and the blood pressure will begin to fall within 1 h. Diazoxide (Hyperstat) may cause too rapid and too large a drop in blood pressure, which may cause cerebral underperfusion. Sodium nitroprusside is difficult to use, but it has a very short half-life so its effect can be quickly reversed if the pressure drops too far. See doses in Chapter 80.

2. **Moderate to severe hypertension**
   a. **Begin diuretics first.**
   b. **Add a second-line drug (eg, hydralazine or propranolol).** Begin with a low dose and increase as necessary. Choice of drug depends on your institution. Propranolol is the most extensively used β-blocker and has a low risk of side effects.
   c. **If a third drug is needed with propranolol,** hydralazine can be added.
   d. **Give captopril alone or with a diuretic.** This drug is contraindicated in infants with bilateral renovascular disease. Angiotensin-converting enzyme (ACE) inhibitors also may result in hypotensive events at initiation of therapy and after long-term use. Oliguria and some neurologic complications have been reported after captopril use; therefore, it should be used cautiously.
   e. **Methyldopa** is also used but rarely.

3. **Mild hypertension**
   a. **Simple observation** is required for asymptomatic patients.
   b. **Diuretics** are necessary if nonpharmacologic measures fail. Chlorothiazide or hydrochlorothiazide can be used. These agents are preferred over furosemide because there are fewer electrolyte disturbances. They work well in cases of volume overload but may cause hypotension when used with other agents.
   c. **Propranolol, hydralazine, or captopril may be added** if the previously mentioned measures fail.

REFERENCE

Watkinson M: Hypertension in the newborn baby. *Arch Dis Child Fetal Neonatal Ed* 2002;86:F78.

43 Hypoglycemia

I. **Problem.** An infant has a low blood glucose level on Dextrostix or Chemstrip-bG testing. Hypoglycemia is defined as a plasma glucose <40–45 mg/dL in a term or premature infant (*controversial*)

II. **Immediate questions**

A. **Has the value been repeated, and has a plasma blood sugar sample been sent to the laboratory?** Dextrostix or Chemstrip-bG strips can give incorrect values if the test is not done properly or if the strips used are too old. There can be a wide variation when these results are compared with laboratory-determined plasma levels. Glucose oxidase strips are also quite inaccurate in the low range (<40–50 mg/dL). *Note:* The glucose concentration in whole blood is 10–15% lower than in the plasma. *Never diagnose or treat hypoglycemia based on these screening strips alone.* Always send a serum sample to the laboratory before starting treatment.

B. **Is the infant symptomatic?** Symptoms of hypoglycemia include apnea, hypotonia, inadequate sucking reflex, irritability, irregular respirations, poor sucking or feeding, exaggerated Moro reflex, cyanosis, tremors, pallor, eye rolling, seizures, lethargy, changes in levels of consciousness, temperature instability, and coma. Some infants can have documented hypoglycemia but no symptoms. Rarely, bradycardia, tachycardia, abnormal cry (high pitched), tachypnea, and vomiting present as manifestations of hypoglycemia.

C. **Is the mother a diabetic?** Approximately 40% of infants of diabetic mothers have hypoglycemia. Throughout pregnancy, diabetic mothers have fluctuating hyperglycemia, resulting in fetal hyperglycemia. This fetal hyperglycemia induces pancreatic beta cell hyperplasia, which in turn results in hyperinsulinism. After delivery, hyperinsulinism persists and hypoglycemia results.

D. **How much glucose is the infant receiving?** The normal initial glucose requirement is 5–7 mg/kg/min. If the glucose order was written arbitrarily and not calculated on the basis of body weight, the infant may not be getting enough glucose. (For glucose calculations, see p 73.)

III. **Differential diagnosis**

A. **Causes of transient hypoglycemia**
   1. Perinatal stress.
   2. Sepsis, especially gram-negative.
   3. Asphyxia or hypoxic-ischemic encephalopathy.
   4. Hypothermia.
   5. Polycythemia.
   6. Shock.
   7. Infant of a gestational or insulin-dependent diabetic mother.
   8. Insufficient amount of glucose administered (see section II,D).
   9. Maternal drugs such as β-sympathomimetic agents (eg, terbutaline, ritodrine, chlorpropamide, or propranolol).

B. **Decreased glycogen stores**
   1. Intrauterine growth retardation (IUGR) or small for gestational age.
   2. Premature infants.
   3. Postmature infants.

C. **Causes of recurrent or persistent hypoglycemia**
   1. **Hormone excess hyperinsulinism**
      a. Beckwith-Wiedemann syndrome (visceromegaly, macroglossia, and hypoglycemia).
      b. Islet cell adenoma.
      c. Adenomatosis.

   d. Beta cell hyperplasia or dysplasia.
   e. Nesidioblastosis.
2. **Hormone deficiencies**
   a. Growth hormone deficiency.
   b. Corticotropin (adrenocorticotropic hormone [ACTH]) unresponsiveness.
   c. Thyroid deficiency.
   d. Epinephrine deficiency.
   e. Glucagon deficiency.
   f. Cortisol deficiency, either from hemorrhage or adrenogenital syndrome.
   g. Hypoplastic pituitary or aplasia of the anterior pituitary.
   h. Congenital optic nerve hypoplasia.
   i. Hypothalamic hormone deficiencies.
   j. Midline central nervous system malformations.
3. **Hereditary defects in carbohydrate metabolism**
   a. Glycogen storage disease type I.
   b. Fructose intolerance.
   c. Galactosemia.
   d. Glycogen synthase deficiency.
   e. Fructose-1,6-diphosphatase deficiency.
4. **Hereditary defects in amino acid metabolism**
   a. Maple syrup urine disease.
   b. Propionic acidemia.
   c. Methylmalonic acidemia.
   d. Tyrosinosis.
   e. 3-Hydroxy-3-methylglutaryl-CoA lyase deficiency.
5. **Hereditary defects in fatty acid metabolism.** Medium- and long-chain deficiency.
IV. **Data base**
   A. **History and physical examination.** Evaluate the infant for symptoms of hypoglycemia (see section II,B). Are there signs of sepsis, shock, or dysmorphism suggesting a syndrome?
   B. **Laboratory studies**
      1. **Initial studies for transient hypoglycemia**
         a. **A serum glucose level** should be obtained to confirm the bedside paper-strip determination.
         b. **A complete blood cell count with differential** should be obtained to evaluate for sepsis and to rule out polycythemia.
      2. **Studies for persistent hypoglycemia**
         a. **Initial studies.** One study recommends obtaining only serum glucose, insulin, and ketones. The ratio of insulin to glucose (I/G) is obtained. A level >0.30 indicates a non-hyperinsulinemic cause of hypoglycemia. Serum ketones are low to absent in the presence of hyperinsulinemia.
         b. **Follow-up studies.** If further evaluation is needed, the following tests can be done to help differentiate a metabolic defect, hypopituitarism, and hyperinsulinism:
            i. Insulin.
            ii. Glucose.
            iii. I/G ratio (see section IV,B,2,a).
            iv. Growth hormone.
            v. Cortisol.
            vi. Free fatty acids.
            vii. Thyroxine (T_4), triiodothyronine (T_3), and thyroid-stimulating hormone (TSH).
            viii. Glucagon.
            ix. Uric acid.
            x. Lactate.
            xi. Alanine.
            xii. Ketones.

xiii. Amino acids.
xiv. Somatomedins (insulin-like growth factor [IGF] type I, IGF-II, and IGF-binding proteins).
C. **Radiologic and other studies.** An ultrasonogram or computed tomography (CT) scan of the pancreas is usually done.
V. **Plan**
A. **Overall plan.** Attempt to maintain normoglycemia. Infants at risk for hypoglycemia and those with established hypoglycemia should have glucose screening every 1–2 h until glucose levels are stable and then every 4 h. Once the glucose level is stable, the next step is to determine why the patient is hypoglycemic. Sometimes the cause is obvious, as in the case of an infant of a diabetic mother or one with IUGR. If the cause is not obvious, further workup is necessary.
   1. **Asymptomatic hypoglycemia.** The treatment of asymptomatic hypoglycemia is *controversial*. One method of treatment is presented next. Some clinicians will treat with early feeding if the infant is term, in the first 6–12 h of life, and not high-risk. Others go by a blood level (usually <25 mg/dL), and treat all such infants with parenteral glucose. It is always best to follow your own institution's guidelines.
      a. **Draw a blood sample,** and send it to the laboratory for a stat baseline plasma glucose level.
      b. **For infants with Dextrostix values of <25 mg/dL** or Chemstrip-bG values of <20 mg/dL (confirmed by stat central serum level), **insert an intravenous catheter and start a glucose infusion** of ~6 mg/kg/min (see the calculation on p 73), even if the infant is asymptomatic. (*Controversial:* Some clinicians will treat with early feeding if the infant is term, in the first 6–12 h of life, and not high-risk. They recheck the glucose in 30–60 min and start intravenous treatment only if the repeat blood sugar is still low.) Initially, glucose levels should be checked every 30 min until stable. The infusion should be increased until normoglycemia is achieved. A bolus of glucose in the asymptomatic infant is contraindicated because it is thought to result in hyperglycemia with rebound hypoglycemia (*controversial*).
      c. **For infants with Dextrostix values of 25–45 mg/dL or Chemstrip-bG values of 20–40 mg/dL,** if there are no risk factors for hypoglycemia and the infant is clinically stable, an **early feeding of 5% dextrose in water** or formula can be given. The glucose levels are monitored every 30–60 min until stable and then every 4 h. If the glucose remains low, an intravenous catheter will have to be started with a glucose infusion of 6 mg/kg/min.
   2. **Symptomatic hypoglycemia (transient).** Always treat symptomatic hypoglycemia with parenteral glucose.
      a. **Draw a sample for a stat baseline plasma glucose level.**
      b. **Insert an intravenous catheter, and start a glucose infusion.** Infuse a minibolus (usually not associated with rebound hypoglycemia) of 2 mL/kg of a 10% glucose solution at a rate of 1.0 mL/min. Then give a continuous infusion of glucose at a rate of 6–8 mg/kg/min, and increase the rate as needed to maintain a normal blood glucose (>40–50 mg/dL). The level should be monitored every 30–60 min until stable. Remember: **The highest concentration of glucose that can be infused through a peripheral catheter is 12.5%. If a more concentrated solution is required, a central catheter will have to be placed.** Higher concentrations are hypertonic and may damage the veins. Also, if there is difficulty starting an intravenous catheter, an umbilical venous catheter can be placed emergently.
      c. **If an intravenous catheter cannot be started, glucagon (see Chapter 80) can be given to infants with adequate glycogen stores.** This measure may be particularly effective in infants of diabetic mothers. It

may be less effective in infants who have growth retardation or who are small for gestational age, because of poor muscle mass and glycogen stores. The dose is 300 μg/kg, not to exceed 1.0 mg total dose, and it may be given subcutaneously or intramuscularly while vascular access is being attempted.

3. **Persistent hypoglycemia.** This usually means hypoglycemia persisting or recurring over a period >7 days. Endocrinologic consultation should be obtained.

    a. **Continue administration of intravenous glucose.** Continue to increase the rate of intravenous glucose administration to 16–20 mg/kg/min. Rates higher than 20 mg/kg/min are usually not helpful. If it is evident at this point that the infant still has problems with hypoglycemia, further workup should be initiated as outlined next.

    b. **Perform a definitive workup.** First, obtain blood samples to obtain the I/G ratio and serum ketone level. If the diagnosis is still unclear, the definitive workup of an infant with persistent hypoglycemia consists of obtaining a set of laboratory determinations before and 15 min after the parenteral administration of glucagon (0.3 mg/kg/dose). Laboratory studies include serum glucose, ketones, free fatty acids, lactate, alanine, uric acid, insulin, growth hormone, cortisol, glucagon, T_4, and TSH. The results are interpreted as shown in Table 43–1. Urine collections for catecholamines, organic acids, and specific reducing sugars should be sent to the laboratory. The following methods of treatment can be initiated while waiting for results of the glucagon test:

        i. **Consider a trial of corticosteroids.** The recommended drug is either hydrocortisone sodium succinate (Solu-Cortef), 5 mg/kg/day given intravenously or orally every 12 h, or prednisone, 2 mg/kg/day orally daily.

        ii. **If hypoglycemia persists,** the following medications can be tried. It is not necessary to stop the previous agent when trying a new medication. Often the second drug to use is somatostatin. Other institutions choose glucagon or diazoxide as next-line therapy. Choice of treatment is variable and depends on the institution. If dosages are not given, they can be found in Chapter 80.

           (a) Human growth hormone (somatrem [Protropin]), 0.1 unit/day intramuscularly, is used in infants with growth hormone deficiency.

TABLE 43–1. DIAGNOSIS OF PERSISTENT HYPOGLYCEMIA BEFORE AND AFTER PARENTERAL GLUCAGON ADMINISTRATION

Variable	Hyperinsulinism		Hypopituitarism		Metabolic defect	
	Before	After	Before	After	Before	After
Glucose	↓	↑↑↑	↓	↑/N	↓	↓/N
Ketones	↓	↓	N/↓	N	↑	↑
Free fatty acids	↓	↑	N/↓	N	↑	↑
Lactate	N	N	N	N	↑	↑↑
Alanine	N	?	N	N	↑	↑↑
Uric acid	N	N	N	N	↑	↑↑
Insulin	↑↑	↑↑↑	N/↑	↑	N	↑
Growth hormone	↑	↓	↓	↓	↑	↑
Cortisol	↑	↓	↓[a]	↓[a]	↑	↑
TSH and T_4	N	N	↓[a]	↓[a]	N	N

N, normal or no change; ↑, elevated; ↓, lowered; ?, unknown; TSH, thyroid-stimulating hormone; T_4, thyroxine.
[a]Response may vary depending on the degree of hypopituitarism.
Courtesy of Marvin Cornblath, MD, Baltimore, Maryland.

(b) Diazoxide (for dosage, see Chapter 80).

(c) Somatostatin: Because of its very short half-life, the long-acting analog of somatostatin, octreotide, is actually used. The starting dose is 2–10 μg/kg/day subcutaneously divided every 6–8 h, or by continuous intravenous infusion. Doses up to 40 μg/kg/day have been used.

(d) Glucagon.

(e) Susphrine: The dose is 0.005–0.01 mL/kg/dose subcutaneously, given every 6 h.

(f) Nifedipine.

(g) Surgery to remove most of the pancreas is the treatment of choice in patients with beta cell hyperplasia or nesidioblastosis.

B. Specific treatment plans

1. **Neonatal hyperinsulinism.** Pancreatectomy, removing at least 95% of the organ, is usually necessary. Partial pancreatectomy can be done when hypersecretion is shown to be confined to a small area of the pancreas. Some studies have shown that familial hyperinsulinemic hypoglycemic syndromes of infancy (FHHI) have been managed effectively with diazoxide and long-acting somatostatin preparations.

2. **Congenital hypopituitarism** usually responds to administration of cortisone and intravenous glucose. Administration of human growth hormone may be necessary. (For dosages and other pharmacologic information, see Chapter 80.)

3. **Metabolic defects**
   a. **Type I glycogen storage disease.** Frequent small feedings, avoiding fructose or galactose, may be beneficial.
   b. **Hereditary fructose intolerance.** The infant should begin a fructose-free diet.
   c. **Galactosemia.** The infant should be placed on a galactose-free diet immediately on suspicion of the diagnosis.

44 Hypokalemia

I. **Problem.** A serum potassium value is <4 mEq/L. Normal serum potassium varies with technique used by the laboratory. Normal values are usually between 4 and 6 mEq/L.

II. **Immediate questions**

A. **What is the central serum potassium?** If a low value is obtained by heelstick, central values should be obtained because they may actually be lower than values obtained by heelstick because of the hemolysis of red blood cells.

B. **Are potassium-wasting medications or digitalis being given?** Diuretics may cause hypokalemia. Hypokalemia may cause arrhythmias if digitalis is being administered.

C. **How much potassium is the infant receiving?** Normal maintenance dosages are 1–2 mEq/kg/day.

D. **Is diarrhea occurring, or is a nasogastric tube in place?** Loss of large amounts of gastrointestinal fluids can cause hypokalemia.

III. **Differential diagnosis**

A. **Inadequate maintenance infusion of potassium.** For a further discussion, see Chapter 7.

B. **Abnormal potassium losses**

1. **Medications (most common cause of hypokalemia in the newborn).** Amphotericin B can cause direct renal tubular damage with resulting hypokalemia. Any thiazide diuretic may cause hypokalemia. High and continuous doses of spironolactone with hydrochlorothiazide (Aldactazide) have also resulted in hypokalemia. Gentamicin and carbenicillin are also associated with potassium losses. Corticosteroids also stimulate potassium secretion.

2. **Gastrointestinal tract losses.** Diarrhea, loss of fluid via nasogastric tube, and vomiting may cause hypokalemia. Pyloric stenosis with vomiting can cause hypokalemia.

3. **Primary or secondary hypermineralocorticoidism.** Renal artery stenosis is a cause. In certain forms of congenital adrenal hyperplasia, hypokalemia may occur.

4. **Renal loss of potassium** (other than induced by medications).
   a. **Any cause of polyuria** can be associated with hypokalemia.
   b. **Bartter's syndrome,** a rare form of potassium wasting, secondary to chloride channels anomaly, is characterized by polyuria, hypokalemia, hyponatremia, and hypercalciuria with risk of nephrocalcinosis with elevated levels of aldosterone and renin.
   c. **Proximal renal tubular acidosis type 2**
   d. **Distal renal tubular acidosis type 1.**

C. **Redistribution of potassium by an increase in intracellular uptake**

1. **Alkalosis (metabolic or respiratory).** An increase in pH by 0.1 unit causes a decrease in the potassium level by 0.3–1.3 mEq/L. The decrease is less in respiratory than in metabolic alkalosis.

2. **Insulin.** An increase in insulin causes intracellular uptake in potassium with hypokalemia.

3. **Medications.** Certain medications cause an increase in intracellular uptake of potassium. These include terbutaline, albuterol, isoproterenol, and catecholamines.

IV. **Data base**

A. **Physical examination.** Hypokalemia may cause ileus. Symptoms of hypokalemia include muscle weakness and decreased tendon reflexes, but these are difficult to evaluate in an infant. In pyloric stenosis, a pyloric olive is palpable in 90% of patients.

B. **Laboratory studies**
1. **Repeat measurement of the serum potassium level.**
2. **Spot checks of urinary electrolytes.** Perform periodic spot checks of urinary potassium levels to determine whether urinary losses are high.
3. **Serum electrolytes and creatinine.** This will help to evaluate renal status.
4. **Blood gas levels.** An alkalosis may cause or aggravate hypokalemia (ie, as hydrogen ions leave the cells, potassium ions enter the cells, causing decreased serum potassium levels).

C. **Radiologic and other studies**
1. **Abdominal x-ray study.** If ileus is suspected, an abdominal x-ray film should be obtained. Also, in those infants in whom pyloric stenosis is suspected and an olive cannot be palpated, the diagnostic procedure of choice is abdominal ultrasonography.
2. **Electrocardiography (ECG).** If hypokalemia is present and the infant is unstable, an ECG may show a prominent U wave with prolonged Q–T interval, flattening of the T wave, and a depressed ST segment. Ventricular arrhythmias may also develop. Note that these ECG findings are also seen in hypomagnesemia.

V. **Plan**
A. **General measures.** The problem of hypokalemia is increasing in neonatal intensive care units because of the widespread use of diuretics. The goal of treatment is to increase the potassium intake so that normal blood levels are achieved and maintained. Short-term potassium administration may cause damage to the veins, and sometimes hyperkalemia, because the potassium does not rapidly equilibrate. Therefore, corrections are given slowly, often over 24 h. If too large a bolus is given, cardiac arrest may result. Serum potassium levels should be monitored every 4–6 h until correction is achieved. Once levels reach high normal, decrease the amount of potassium given.

B. **Specific measures.** Any specific defects (ie, renal defects, adrenal disorders, and certain metabolic problems) require specific evaluation and therapy.
1. **Inadequate maintenance infusion of potassium.** Calculate the normal maintenance infusion of potassium that should be given and increase the amount accordingly (normal maintenance infusion is 1–2 mEq/kg/day, usually only necessary after the first day of life).
2. **Abnormal potassium losses**
   a. **Medications.** If the infant is receiving potassium-wasting medications, increase the maintenance dose of potassium. Abnormal potassium loss often occurs in patients with bronchopulmonary dysplasia who are receiving long-term furosemide therapy. Oral supplementation in the form of potassium chloride may be given, 1–2 mEq/kg/day in 3–4 divided doses (with feedings). This amount may be increased or decreased, depending on serum potassium levels. It was once thought that a potassium-sparing diuretic decreased the amount of potassium supplementation; however, a randomized study showed that serum electrolytes sodium and potassium were not affected by the addition of spironolactone.
   b. **Gastrointestinal losses**
      i. **Severe diarrhea** leading to potassium losses in the stool can be corrected by treating the cause of the diarrhea, withholding oral feedings to allow the gut to rest, and giving intravenous fluids. Potassium supplementation may be given intravenously. The initial intravenous dosage of potassium chloride is 1–2 mEq/kg/day. Serum potassium levels are monitored, and the intravenous dosage is increased accordingly.

    ii. Nasogastric drainage. This amount should be measured each shift and replaced milliliter for milliliter with ½ normal saline with 20 mEq of potassium chloride.

    iii. Pyloric stenosis. Correct dehydration if present and if surgery is indicated.

    iv. Bartter's syndrome. Potassium supplementation is given orally, usually at a starting dosage of 2–3 mEq/kg/day, which is increased as necessary to maintain a normal serum potassium level. Certain forms respond to indomethacin.

    v. Hypercalcemia. See Chapter 77.

C. Redistribution

  1. Alkalosis. Determine the cause of metabolic or respiratory alkalosis and treat the underlying disorder.

  2. Medications. The medications should be discontinued if possible.

45 Hyponatremia

I. **Problem.** A 7-day-old infant with an intraventricular bleed has a serum sodium level of 127 meq/L, below the normal accepted value of 135 meq/L.

II. **Immediate questions**

   A. **Is there any seizure activity?** Seizure activity is often seen in patients with extremely low serum sodium levels (usually <120 mEq/L). *This event is a medical emergency, and urgent sodium correction is needed.*

   B. **How much sodium and free water is the patient receiving? Is weight gain or loss occurring?** Be certain that an adequate amount of sodium is being given and that free water intake is not excessive. The normal amount of sodium intake is 2–4 mEq/kg/day. Weight gain with low serum sodium levels is most likely a result of volume overload, especially in the first day or two of life, when weight loss is expected.

   C. **What is the urine output?** With syndrome of inappropriate secretion of anti-diuretic hormone (SIADH), urine output is decreased. If the urine output is in-creased (>4 mL/kg/h), perform a spot check of urine sodium to determine whether sodium losses are high.

   D. **Are renal salt-wasting medications being given?** Diuretics such as furosemide may cause hyponatremia.

III. **Differential diagnosis.** When considering the differential, one needs to ask whether the cause is dilutional (too much volume given), whether it results from a deficiency, or whether there is excessive loss. The most frequent cause of hyponatremia in the neonate is excess fluid administration.

   A. **Volume overload (dilutional hyponatremia).** This can be seen when too much volume is given (a very common cause) and can also be seen in congestive heart failure, renal and liver failure, paralysis with fluid retention, use of diluted formulas, and nephrotic syndrome.

   B. **Inadequate sodium intake.** Maintenance is 2–4 mEq/kg/day.

   C. **Increased sodium loss.** In very low birth weight infants, renal tubular sodium losses are high and an increased amount of sodium is needed (see Chapter 10). Sodium losses can also occur secondary to salt-losing nephropathies, gastrointestinal losses, skin losses with the use of a radiant warmer, third spacing (commonly seen in necrotizing enterocolitis), and adrenal insufficiency.

   D. **Drug-induced hyponatremia.** Diuretics (used frequently with bronchopulmonary dysplasia [BPD]) lead to sodium losses. Indomethacin causes water retention, which causes dilutional hyponatremia. Certain medications, such as opiates, carbamazepine, and barbiturates, can cause SIADH. Infusion of mannitol or hypertonic glucose can cause hyperosmolality with salt wasting.

   E. **SIADH.** SIADH is more commonly seen with central nervous system disorders such as intraventricular hemorrhage, hydrocephalus, birth asphyxia, and meningitis but may also be seen with lung disease. SIADH is often seen in critically ill premature and term neonates.

IV. **Data base**

   A. **Evaluation of the bedside chart.** Evaluate the pertinent information on the bedside chart.

      1. **Check for weight loss or gain.** Weight gain is more likely to be associated with dilutional hyponatremia.

      2. **Check fluid intake and output over a 24-h period.** Normally, infants retain two thirds of the fluid administered, and the rest is lost in the urine or by insensible water loss. If the input is much greater than the output, the patient may be retaining fluid, and dilutional hyponatremia should be considered.

3. **Assess the urine output and specific gravity.** A low urine output with a high specific gravity is more commonly seen with SIADH.

B. **Physical examination.** Perform a complete physical examination. Note signs of seizure activity (eg, abnormal eye movements, jerking of the extremities, and tongue thrusting). Check for edema, which is a sign of volume overload. Look for decreased skin turgor and dry mucous membranes, which are seen in dehydration.

C. **Laboratory studies**
   1. **Specific tests to order**
      a. **Serum sodium and osmolality.**
      b. **Urine spot sodium, osmolality, and specific gravity.**
      c. **Serum electrolytes, creatinine, and total protein** to assess renal function.
   2. **Laboratory results of specific diagnoses**
      a. **Volume overload (dilutional hyponatremia)**
         i. Excess intravenous fluids: increased urine output and decreased urine osmolality and low specific gravity.
         ii. Other (congestive heart failure or paralysis with fluid retention): decreased urine output and increased urine specific gravity.
      b. **Increased sodium losses**
         i. In renal losses, with diuretics and adrenal insufficiency: increased urine output and urine Na⁺ and decreased urine osmolality and specific gravity.
         ii. In skin and gastrointestinal losses and with third spacing: decreased urine output and sodium and increased urine osmolality and specific gravity.
      c. **The diagnosis of SIADH** is made by documenting the following on simultaneous laboratory studies: low urine output, urine osmolality greater than serum osmolality, low serum sodium level and low serum osmolality, and high urinary sodium level and high specific gravity.

D. **Radiologic and other studies.** Usually none are needed. Occasionally, an ultrasonogram of the head may reveal intraventricular hemorrhage as a cause of hyponatremia secondary to SIADH.

V. **Plan**
A. **Emergency measures.** If the infant is having **seizures resulting from hyponatremia** (usually sodium <120 mEq/dL), hypertonic saline solution (3% sodium chloride) should be given. The total body deficit of sodium (see section V,C,3) is calculated, and half of that is given over 12–24 h. Rapid corrections may result in brain damage.

B. **Volume overload (dilutional hyponatremia)** is treated with fluid restriction. The total maintenance fluids can be decreased by 20 mL/kg/day, and serum sodium levels should be monitored every 6–8 h. The underlying cause must be investigated and treated.

C. **Inadequate sodium intake**
   1. **The maintenance sodium requirement for term infants is 2–4 mEq/ kg/day; it is higher in premature infants.** Calculate the amount of sodium the patient is receiving, using the equations in Chapter 7. Readjust the intravenous sodium intake if it is the cause of hyponatremia.
   2. **If the infant is receiving oral formula only, check the formula being used.** Low-sodium formulas such as Similac PM 60/40 may be used. Use of supplemental sodium chloride or a formula with a higher sodium content may be necessary.
   3. **Calculate the total sodium deficit** using the following equation:

Sodium value desired (130–135 mEq/L) −

Infant's sodium value × Weight (kg) × 0.6

The result will be the amount of sodium needed to correct the hyponatremia. Usually, only half of this amount is given over 12–24 h.

D. **Increased sodium losses.** Try to treat the underlying cause and increase the sodium administered to replace the losses.

E. **Drug-induced hyponatremia.** If a renal salt-wasting medication such as furosemide (Lasix) is being given, serum sodium levels will be low even though an adequate amount of sodium is being given in the diet. An increase in sodium intake may be required, often the case in infants with BPD who are receiving diuretics. Most are also receiving oral feedings, so an oral sodium chloride supplement can be used. Start with 1 mEq 3 times/day with feedings and adjust as needed. Some infants may require as much as 12–15 mEq/day. Sodium levels should be kept in the low 130's because higher levels may result in fluid retention when diuretics are used. Indomethacin therapy needs to be treated with fluid restriction.

F. **SIADH.** Restrict fluids, usually to 40–60 mL/kg/day. (This regimen does not allow for fluid loss that accompanies the use of a radiant warmer or phototherapy.) Monitor the serum sodium level and osmolality and the urine output to determine whether the patient is responding. The cause of SIADH is usually obvious; if it is not, further investigation is needed (eg, ultrasonography of the head to diagnose or rule out intraventricular hemorrhage or hydrocephalus or chest x-ray studies to diagnose or rule out lung disease). Use of furosemide can also be tried.

46 Hypotension and Shock

I. **Problem.** The blood pressure (BP) is >2 standard deviations below normal for age. (For normal BP values, see Appendix C; see also Table 42–1.) For infants who are <30 weeks' gestation, a mnemonic that is helpful in remembering BP is that the mean BP should be at least the same number as the gestational age. For example, a 23-week infant should have a mean BP of 23.

II. **Immediate questions**
   A. **What method of measurement was used?** If a cuff was used, be certain that it was the correct width (ie, covering two thirds of the upper arm). A cuff that is too large will give falsely low readings. If measurements were obtained from an indwelling arterial catheter, a "dampened" waveform suggests that there is air in the transducer or tubing or a clot in the system, and the readings thus may be inaccurate.
   B. **Are symptoms of shock present?** Symptoms of shock include tachycardia, poor perfusion, cold extremities with a normal core temperature, lethargy, narrow pulse pressure, apnea and bradycardia, tachypnea, metabolic acidosis, and weak pulse.
   C. **Is the urine output acceptable?** Normal urine output is ~1–2 mL/kg/h. Urine output is decreased in shock because of decreased renal perfusion. If the BP is low but the urine output is adequate, aggressive treatment may not be necessary, because the renal perfusion is adequate. (*Note:* An exception involves the infant with septic shock and hyperglycemia who has osmotic diuresis.)
   D. **Is there a history of birth asphyxia?** Birth asphyxia may be associated with hypotension.
   E. **At the time of delivery, was there maternal bleeding (eg, abruptio placentae or placenta previa) or was clamping of the cord delayed?** These factors may be associated with loss of blood volume in the infant.

III. **Differential diagnosis.** Hypotension (diminished BP) is distinct from shock, which is a clinical syndrome of inadequate tissue perfusion with the clinical signs noted previously.
   A. **Hypovolemic shock** may be secondary to antepartum or postpartum blood loss.
      1. **Antepartum blood loss (associated very often with asphyxia)**
         a. **Abruptio placentae.**
         b. **Placenta previa.**
         c. **Twin-twin transfusion.**
         d. **Fetomaternal hemorrhage.**
      2. **Postpartum blood loss**
         a. **Coagulation disorders.**
         b. **Vitamin K deficiency.**
         c. **Iatrogenic causes** (eg, loss of an arterial catheter).
         d. **Birth trauma** (eg, liver injury, adrenal hemorrhage, intracranial hemorrhage, intraperitoneal hemorrhage).
   B. **Septic shock.** Endotoxemia occurs, with release of vasodilator substances and resulting hypotension. It usually involves gram-negative organisms such as *Escherichia coli* and *Klebsiella* spp but can also occur with gram-positive organisms such as in group B streptococcal and staphylococcal infections.
   C. **Cardiogenic shock**
      1. **Birth asphyxia.**
      2. **Metabolic problems** (eg, hypoglycemia, hyponatremia, hypocalcemia, acidemia) can cause decreased cardiac output with a decrease in BP.
      3. **Congenital heart disease** (eg, hypoplastic left heart or aortic stenosis).

4. **Arrhythmias** can cause a decrease in cardiac output.
5. **Any obstruction of venous return** (eg, tension pneumothorax).
D. **Neurogenic shock.** Birth asphyxia and intracranial hemorrhage can both cause hypotension.
E. **Drug-induced hypotension.** Certain drugs (eg, tolazoline, tubocurarine, nitroprusside, sedatives, magnesium sulfate, digitalis, and barbiturates) will cause vasodilation and a drop in BP. Transient hypotension has been seen after exogenous surfactant administration.
F. **Endocrine disorders.** Complete 21-hydroxylase deficiency and adrenal hemorrhage are the most notable endocrine disorders that can cause hypotension and shock. If there is a low serum sodium, high serum potassium, and hypotension, it is important to rule out adrenogenital syndrome.
G. **Extreme prematurity.** Hypotension is very common in extremely low birth weight (ELBW) infants (40% between 27 and 29 weeks, 60–100% between 24 and 26 weeks). Hypotension in this group is rarely secondary to hypovolemia and more likely due to adrenocortical insufficiency, poor vascular tone, and immature catecholamine responses. Hypotension in ELBW infants has been associated with intraventricular hemorrhage/periventricular leukomalacia (IVH/PVL) and needs to be corrected.
IV. **Data base**
A. **Physical examination.** Particular attention is given to signs of blood loss (eg, intracranial or intra-abdominal bleeding), sepsis, or clinical signs of shock.
B. **Laboratory studies**
1. **Complete blood cell count with differential.** Decreased hematocrit (Hct) will identify blood loss; however, the HCT can be normal in patients with acute blood loss. Elevated/decreased white blood cell count and differential may help identify sepsis as the cause.
2. **Coagulation studies (prothrombin time and partial thromboplastin time) and platelet count,** if disseminated intravascular coagulation is suspected.
3. **Serum glucose, electrolytes, and calcium levels** may reveal a metabolic disorder.
4. **Cultures.** Obtain blood and urine for culture and antibiotic sensitivity testing.
5. **Kleihauer-Betke test** should be performed if fetomaternal transfusion is suspected. The test detects the presence of fetal erythrocytes in the mother's blood by a slide elution technique. A smear of maternal blood is fixed and incubated in an acidic buffer. It causes adult hemoglobin to be eluted from erythrocytes; fetal hemoglobin resists elution. After the slide is stained, fetal hemoglobin cells, if present, appear dark, whereas maternal erythrocytes appear clear.
6. **Arterial blood gases** to assess for hypoxia or acidosis.
C. **Radiologic and other studies**
1. **Chest x-ray study.** An anteroposterior chest x-ray study should be done to assess the heart and lungs and rule out any mechanical cause of shock (eg, pneumothorax).
2. **Ultrasonography of the head is done** in infants in whom intracranial hemorrhage is suspected.
3. **Electrocardiography** should be performed if an arrhythmia is suspected.
4. **Echocardiography** is performed in birth-asphyxiated infants to assess myocardial function. If there is myocardial failure, drug therapy is needed to improve cardiac output. Echocardiography is also useful to rule out a congenital heart lesion.
5. **Central venous pressure measurement.** A venous umbilical catheter can be placed above the diaphragm (at the right atrium) to obtain central venous pressure readings. Normal values are 4–6 mm Hg. If these readings are low, hypovolemia is present and transfusion is usually necessary.

V. Plan

A. General measures

1. **Rapidly assess the infant and determine what is causing the hypotension** in order to direct treatment accordingly. The basic decision is whether the infant requires volume replacement or administration of inotropic agents. The decision is not difficult in the majority of patients. Four parameters are useful in making this decision:

    a. **History.** A history should be obtained to rule out birth asphyxia, blood loss (antepartum or postpartum), drug infusion, and birth trauma (adrenal hemorrhage or liver injury).

    b. **Physical examination.** A careful physical examination will often reveal which organ systems are involved.

    c. **Chest x-ray.** A small heart is seen in volume depletion; a large heart is seen in cardiac disease.

    d. **Central venous pressure.** If it is low (<4 mm Hg), the infant is volume depleted. If it is high (eg, >6 mm Hg), the infant probably has cardiogenic shock.

2. **If you are still unsure of the cause, start empirical volume expansion with crystalloid (eg, normal saline)** (10 mL/kg intravenously over 30 min).

    a. **If there is a response,** continue volume expansion.

    b. **If there is no response,** an inotropic agent (eg, dopamine) should be started (see section V,B,3).

3. **Provide respiratory support as needed.** Blood gas determinations and clinical examinations will dictate whether supplemental oxygen will suffice or whether intubation and mechanical ventilation are necessary.

4. **Correct any metabolic acidosis** with sodium bicarbonate.

B. Specific measures

1. **Hypovolemic shock**

    a. **Volume expansion using intravenous crystalloid** should be given (for dosage, see section V,A,2). Colloids such as albumin or plasma protein fraction (Plasmanate) are to be used with caution. Use of colloids has been associated with increased risk of mortality in critically ill patients. No benefits of use of colloids versus crystalloids (normal saline) has been found in preterm infants. If blood loss has occurred and the patient is severely hypovolemic, immediate volume expansion with a crystalloid is essential. Volume expansion should be continued until adequate tissue perfusion is attained as evidenced by good urinary output and central nervous system function. Meanwhile, a blood sample should be sent to the laboratory for an Hct value, which is used to determine the specific blood products that should be used in blood replacement therapy.

    b. **Blood replacement therapy**

        i. **Hct <40%.** Packed red blood cells should be given, 5–10 mL/kg over 30–40 min. The following formula may also be used to calculate the volume of packed red blood cells needed. This formula assumes that the total blood volume is 80 mL/kg and the Hct of the packed red blood cells is 70%.

$$\text{Volume required} = \frac{(\text{Weight [kg]} \times \text{Total blood volume}) \times (\text{Desired Hct} - \text{Patient's Hct})}{\text{Hct of transfusion product}}$$

        ii. **Hct >50%.** Normal saline, or fresh-frozen plasma (FFP) should be used. FFP is used only if clotting studies are also abnormal.

        iii. **Hct of 40–50%.** Alternating transfusions of packed red blood cells and normal saline should be given.

2. **Septic shock**
   a. **Obtain cultures** (blood and urine [unless in the first 24 h of life, in which case obtain only blood], lumbar puncture for cerebrospinal fluid culture, and other culture studies as clinically indicated).
   b. **Initiate empiric antibiotic therapy** after culture specimens have been obtained. **Intravenous ampicillin and gentamicin** are recommended. **Vancomycin** may be substituted for ampicillin if staphylococcal infection is suspected (usually seen in infants >3 days old who have invasive monitoring catheters or chest tubes in place). Some institutions are advocating the use of **cefotaxime** with vancomycin instead of gentamicin to avoid the nephrotoxicity. (For dosages, see Chapter 80.)
   c. **Use volume expansion and inotropic agents as needed** to maintain adequate tissue and renal perfusion (see sections V,B,1,a and V,B,3,e).
   d. **Use of corticosteroids.** Intravenous corticosteroid therapy for sepsis is *controversial.* Agents such as dexamethasone have been used, however. Studies have shown a single dose or short course of steroids may be beneficial with no associated adverse effects in neonates.
   e. **Use of naloxone.** Naloxone has been used in patients with septic shock and persistent hypotension, but its use is *controversial* (for dosage, see Chapter 80). Studies have shown that the effects of naloxone and methylprednisolone may be synergistic in improving the hemodynamics of these patients. Naloxone is rarely helpful in hypoxic ischemic shock.
   f. **Use of methylene blue.** Methylene blue has been used in septic shock unresponsive to colloid, inotropic agents, and corticosteroids. One study showed that three of five patients had an increase in BP after given a dose of 1 mg/kg over 1 h intravenously. Some required a second infusion. Three of five of these patients were weaned off inotropic agents within 72 h. The mechanism by which this works is that methylene blue is a soluble guanylate cyclase inhibitor. Excess nitric oxide is a mediator of hypotension by dilating vascular smooth muscle through activation of soluble guanylate cyclase.
   g. **Exchange transfusion.** Use of this treatment is *controversial.*
3. **Cardiogenic shock.** First, treat any obvious cause.
   a. **Air leak.** If a tension pneumothorax is causing hypotension by obstructing venous return, immediate evacuation of the air is necessary.
   b. **Arrhythmia.** Recognize the arrhythmia and treat it.
   c. **Metabolic cause.** Metabolic problems need to be corrected.
   d. **Asphyxia.** The hypotension usually responds to inotropic agents. See following discussion.
   e. **In cardiogenic shock,** the goal is to improve cardiac output. Inotropic agents should be used intravenously (for dosages and other pharmacologic information, see Chapter 80).
      i. **Dopamine.** Dopamine is the drug of first choice and has been shown to be superior over dobutamine. Previous studies have suggested that higher than traditionally used dosages (≥30–50 µg/kg/min) may be used without causing α-adrenergic side effects such as decreased renal perfusion and decreased urine output.
      ii. **Dobutamine.** If dopamine fails to improve BP, dobutamine is recommended as a second-line drug. In neonates, it is usually given together with dopamine infusion. Remember: Dobutamine causes peripheral vasodilation.
      iii. **Other agents.** Epinephrine and isoproterenol are sometimes used.
4. **Neurogenic shock.** Neurogenic shock is treated with volume expansion (see section V,B,1,a) and inotropic agents (see section V,B,3,e).
5. **Drug-induced hypotension.** Volume expansion (see section V,B,1,a) will usually maintain the BP in cases of drug-induced vasodilation. If the BP

cannot be maintained, the drug causing hypotension may need to be discontinued.
6. **Endocrine disorders**
   a. **Adrenal hemorrhage** is treated with volume expansion and blood replacement and corticosteroids (see Chapter 80).
   b. **Congenital adrenal hyperplasia** is treated with corticosteroids (see Chapter 80).
7. **Hypotension of ELBW infants.**
   a. **The use of antenatal steroids decreases the risk of hypotension** in ELBW infants.
   b. **Physiologic doses of hydrocortisone** have been used in refractory hypotension with uncertainty of long-term side effects.
   c. **Dopamine** has been shown to be more effective than normal saline in increasing BP in preterm infants. It raised BP in 90% of infants, whereas volume supplementation only was 40% effective.
   d. **More studies** are needed to evaluate safely of use of crystalloids/dopamine to treat low BP in preterm infants.

47 Is the Infant Ready for Discharge?

I. **Problem.** The infant in the neonatal intensive care unit (NICU) or newborn nursery is ready to be discharged home. How can we ensure that this discharge is smooth, safe, and complete?

II. **Immediate questions**

A. **What is the corrected age of the infant?** Most preterm infants are discharged 2–4 weeks before their "due date," but there are variations among hospitals. Infants staying beyond their due date are usually on prolonged assisted ventilation, have severe malformations, or are status post–major surgery. The postconceptual age of 36 weeks is a prime time for consideration for discharge.

B. **Is the infant showing consistent weight gain?** At time of discharge the infant should be gaining weight steadily on breast- or bottle-feeds. Most healthy preterm or term infants with no ongoing problems show an average weight gain of 15–30 g/day. If possible, multiple-gestation infants should be discharged home together, which may necessitate extra allowance on weight criteria. A specific weight requirement at discharge is controversial. Some institutions require that an infant must weigh at least 1800–2000 g at discharge. Others base discharge more on maturity: ability to feed, gain weight, and keep warm.

C. **Is the infant maintaining body temperature in an open crib?** The ability to maintain thermal homeostasis without an external source of heat in an open crib with comfortable clothing is a key determinant of fitness for discharge.

D. **Is the infant feeding satisfactorily? Are any special feeding techniques necessary?** The ability of the infant to breast- or bottle-feed satisfactorily, taking in an adequate number of calories (120 cal/kg/day) in reasonable frequency (every 3–4 h), with each feed not taking more than 30–40 min, is important. If clinical grounds indicate the need for prolonged tube feeding or gastrostomy tube feeding, the parents must be trained to carry out the feedings at home.

E. **Are the vital signs stable? Is there a need for home monitoring? Have arrangements been made for parental training in monitor use and in cardiopulmonary resuscitation?** Episodes of apnea of prematurity along with associated bradycardia and desaturation resolve at about the postconceptional age of 36 weeks. If such episodes persist at 36 weeks of age or at discharge, the infants are usually sent home on varying combinations of cardiopulmonary event monitoring, respiratory stimulants (eg, theophylline or caffeine), and supplemental oxygen. Infant cardiopulmonary resuscitation training is arranged for the parents. If theophylline is still being used, then serum levels should be checked before discharge and monitored during follow-up visits, although this is not usually necessary with caffeine. If home oxygen therapy is needed, pulse oximetry saturations in room air and in oxygen (supine and in a car seat) are recorded before discharge and checked during each follow-up visit.

F. **Are there medications that need to be continued after discharge?** Infants discharged on medications usually have the first prescription filled in the hospital pharmacy. Before the patient's discharge, the parents should be trained in safely administering the medications. Parents are briefed on the duration of administration, importance of the medication, and probable duration of treatment as well as side effects and risks of discontinuing too soon.

G. **Is the audiology screen completed?** A newborn hearing screen (either an otoacoustic emissions [OAE] or an auditory brainstem response [ABR]) is usually performed before discharge. Results are recorded in the patient's record and the discharge summary and are also mailed to each state's Newborn Hearing Screening Program. Any "fail" is usually tested again after clinical inspection of the ear and cleaning of the external auditory meatus, if necessary. "Persistent fail" in a hearing screen warrants Brainstem Auditory Evoked Response (BAER) testing to be arranged within 4 weeks and before 3 months of age. BAER assessment is essential in other clinical conditions in which there is an increased risk for hearing loss and which progressive losses are possible (eg, birth weight <1500 g, family history of deafness, craniofacial anomalies, meningitis, hyperbilirubinemia, inborn errors of metabolism, congenital renal problems, certain genetic syndromes, and prolonged treatment with potentially ototoxic medications).

H. **Is the newborn metabolic screen completed? If so, is it valid and is a repeat test needed?** The content of the newborn metabolic screen varies among states. Screening at birth for phenylketonuria (PKU), hypothyroidism, and galactosemia is almost universal. Other tests, such as sickle cell screen and cystic fibrosis screen, vary regionally based on prevalence. All initial newborn screens should be done per state protocol but essentially at 48 h after birth and preferably after 24 h of protein feeding. The thyroid screen is invalid if done before 48 h because of the surge of thyroid-stimulating hormone (TSH) at birth. The galactosemia test is valid at birth and invalid after blood transfusion for at least 60 days. Any borderline values or abnormal initial metabolic screen results are repeated with more definitive tests (eg, serum thyroxine, TSH, free thyroxine, and thyroxine-binding immunoglobulin).

I. **Are any immunizations due before discharge?** Preterm infants should be immunized at the normal chronologic age with the same vaccine doses as term infants. If the infant is discharged at 2 months of age or older, give DPT (diphtheria-pertussis-tetanus), Hib vaccine (*Haemophilus influenzae* vaccine), and IPV (polio vaccine inactivated) at the appropriate time. Preterm infants usually receive the first hepatitis B vaccine at a weight of 2 kg or before discharge. Infants whose mothers are positive for hepatitis B virus surface antigen or core or "e" antigen (HBsAg, HBcAg, or HBeAg, respectively) need to be given both hepatitis B immunoglobulin and hepatitis B vaccine (high dose) in the first 12 h of life. Preterm infants with chronic lung disease should be considered for respiratory syncytial virus immunoglobulin administration throughout the winter months and influenza vaccination at 6 months of age.

III. **Discharge diagnosis.** A concise list of all the diagnoses for a patient, listed in chronologic order of occurrence, should be generated.

IV. **Data base.** Review the initial history, NICU hospital course, and physical examination at discharge. Compose an organized discharge summary by systems or by problems.

A. **History**
1. **Maternal-fetal conditions** (including prenatal diagnostic tests and medications). Maternal diagnoses need to be reviewed (ie, does the mother have idiopathic thrombocytopenic purpura, systemic lupus erythematosus, and so on?).
2. **Labor and delivery.** Premature rupture of membranes, anesthesia, delivery type, and resuscitation.
3. **Birth history.** Apgar scores, head circumference, length, and weight.

B. **Physical examination.** List any significant abnormal findings noted at birth. Perform a complete physical examination, paying careful attention to the following aspects at discharge:
1. **General.** General disposition, spontaneous activity, phenotypic features of note (if any), weight for gestational or chronologic age, and symmetry. Plot the growth chart and record the percentiles for weight, length, and head circumference.
2. **Skin.** Look for hemangiomas, neurocutaneous markers (eg, café au lait), and scars (eg, surgical, deep-line insertion sites, and chest tube or gas-

trostomy tube sites). Specifically look for erythema, discharge, and unremoved suture threads at incision sites.

3. **Head.** Check for size (occipitofrontal head circumference), shape (dolichocephalic in preemies), rate of growth, state of the fontanelles (including size, if open), sutures, and presence of cephalhematoma or caput. Watch for intravenous infiltrates and necrotic patches in the scalp.

4. **Eyes.** Look specifically for strabismus, red reflex, nystagmus, nasolacrimal duct obstruction, and abnormalities of the sclera and conjunctiva. Elicit the pupillary reflex, and examine the size, color, shape, and symmetry of the pupils.

5. **Ears, nose, and mouth.** Examine the ears at the time of discharge, paying particular attention to patency and any abnormality (eg, preauricular, postauricular sinuses, skin tags, or abnormalities of pinnae), patency of both nostrils (already confirmed with nasogastric tube passage), and examination of the throat to rule out cleft of the soft palate and submucous clefts. Look for natal teeth or prematurely erupted teeth, thrush (*Candida*), and other lesions in the mouth.

6. **Face.** Look for characteristic facies, facial asymmetry (eg, facial nerve paresis or paralysis or torticollis), and hemangiomas in the trigeminal area.

7. **Neck.** The neck should be supple and free of lymphadenopathy and sinuses (eg, branchial). Look for anterior midline masses (eg, ectopic thyroid, thyromegaly, or thyroglossal cyst). Examine the site of deep-line insertions in the neck and upper thorax (eg, extracorporeal membrane oxygenation [ECMO] cannulation or indwelling catheter).

8. **Cardiovascular (eg, murmur or femoral pulse).** Listen for the presence of both normal heart sounds as well as any extraneous clicks or murmurs over the precordium. Assess for murmurs in the neck and interscapular region (eg, peripheral pulmonic stenosis) and axilla. Feel for peripheral pulses on each limb, including femoral pulses. Note the presence of systolic flow murmur secondary to anemia in preemies.

9. **Chest.** Note the shape and symmetry of the chest, abnormalities of the sternum, prominence of the costochondral junctions, significant intercostal and subcostal retractions, abnormalities in the breathing pattern, air entry, and accessory breathing sounds (eg, wheeze or rales). Look specifically at the indwelling catheter site, chest tube insertion site (for infection), and sutures.

10. **Abdomen.** Look for distention, dilated veins, and visible gastric or intestinal peristalsis, and auscultate for bowel sounds. Palpate for visceromegaly or abnormal masses. Check the renal angle for fullness, dullness, or bruit (eg, renal artery stenosis). Note the presence of surgical scars, gastrostomy tube, ventriculoperitoneal catheters, and so on.

11. **Genitalia. In males,** look for the position of the urethral meatus (eg, normal, epispadias, or hypospadias), the stream of urine, and circumcision and for the presence of both testes in the scrotum. **In females,** note the vaginal-anal distance. Examine specifically the hernial orifices for hernia (including umbilical).

12. **Spine.** Specifically look for kyphosis and scoliosis, and record any abnormality already radiologically confirmed (eg, hemivertebrae). Record the presence of cutaneous stigmata such as pigmentation, lipoma, or tuft of hair along the vertebral region.

13. **Presacral area.** Examine the lumbosacral region in detail for spina bifida occulta, any sinus tracts, and cutaneous markers (eg, lipoma or pigmentation). Always perform ultrasound examination of deep pilonidal pits and sinuses to look for cord tethering.

14. **Limbs.** Look for symmetry, palpable peripheral pulses in all four limbs, areas of intravenous infiltrates, erythema or induration in areas of cutdowns, and arterial cannulation. Look for normal passive mobility in all joints and assess muscle tone (eg, hypotonia, hypertonia, and contracture).

15. **Joints.** Look for abnormal shape, limitation of movements, and stability, especially in the hip joint. Assess the hips for congenital hip dysplasia with the Barlow or Ortolani procedure.
16. **Gross neurologic.** Examine for general body tone, posture, spontaneous activity, symmetry of movements, deep tendon reflexes, presence of or abnormal persistence of neonatal reflexes, and involuntary movements.

C. **Laboratory studies (at discharge)**
1. **Hematocrit and reticulocyte count.** Hematocrit at the time of discharge should be >22%, and the reticulocyte count should be >5% (*controversial*) with adequate supplementation of iron and multivitamins as additive to normal dietary intake. Folic acid, B_{12}, and fat-soluble vitamin supplementation may be necessary in infants with short-gut syndrome or loss of distal ileum, including ileocecal valve during surgery.
2. **Serum calcium, phosphorus, and alkaline phosphatase.** Extremely premature infants and low birth weight infants must have these parameters checked during inpatient stay and at discharge along with radiographs of the bones to rule out rickets of prematurity. Vitamin D_3 (1,25-dihydroxy-cholecalciferol) supplementation may be considered in these infants, often as part of a multivitamin (*controversial*).
3. **Repeat newborn metabolic screen.** This is done if necessary for validity, for checking a previously positive screening test, or for a more extensive screen based on clinical suspicion.
4. **Drug levels.** Infants being discharged home on medications such as phenobarbital, theophylline, or caffeine should have levels tested before discharge, and the results should be recorded and the dosage adjusted as necessary.

D. **Radiologic and other studies**
1. **Chest radiograph.** A copy of the most recent radiograph should be sent with the parents to the primary physician for follow-up care of chronic lung disease (eg, bronchopulmonary dysplasia [BPD]).
2. **Head ultrasound scan.** Clearly record the findings of the scans in chronologic order, with emphasis on hemorrhage, ventricular size, and areas of echogenicity suggestive of periventricular leukomalacia and porencephalic cysts.
3. **Electroencephalogram.** Record the results, if done more than once, in chronologic order, indicating assessment of cerebral function in infants with seizures.
4. **Electrocardiogram.** Documentation is useful in cases of congenital heart defect, supraventricular tachycardias, or metabolic problems.
5. **Computed tomography (CT) scan.** If performed to evaluate any area in the infant's body, comment on the findings and interpretation.
6. **Other tests.** Record the findings and recommendations on pneumograms, barium contrast studies, and so on.

V. **Plan.** Once a decision has been made for discharge, compile a checklist of active problems and appointments at discharge.
A. **Ophthalmic check.** An eye examination for evaluation of retinopathy of prematurity is usually recommended for all infants weighing <1200 g and <32 weeks and those ventilated for a prolonged period in high oxygen concentrations. The examination is usually done at 4–6 weeks after birth, and further evaluations are determined by the extent of the disease found on the first exam. Usually, repeat examinations are performed every 1–2 weeks until the retina is normally vascularized. Subsequent examinations periodically over the next months and years are done to detect later-onset problems such as nystagmus, myopia, and astigmatism.
B. **Developmental assessment, including occupational therapy and physiotherapy.** The initial examination and evaluation is done in the NICU before discharge to assess the need for early interventional services.

C. Circumcision. Circumcision is performed at parental request and with their consent before discharge. Remember that the procedure is elective, requires analgesia, and should not be done on small infants, on infants with BPD on oxygen, or on those with ongoing apnea or bradycardia problems. Older infants require anesthesia and analgesia.

D. Social services input. Determine whether this service has been required, including the family's need for housing, financial stability, or other assistance.

E. Follow-up with the primary care physician. Information on the name, location, and choice of follow-up physician should be available at the time of discharge. In any given case, the specialty physician should personally contact the primary care physician by telephone to discuss the patient or to make arrangements for a preliminary discharge summary to be faxed to the primary physician.

F. Follow-up clinical assessment. Parents should be briefed on subspecialty appointments (eg, ophthalmology, pediatric surgery, or neurosurgery) and their importance. Appointments at a neonatal follow-up clinic for monitoring growth and development, with input from a dietitian, social worker, physiotherapist, and developmentalist, are mandatory for very high-risk infants. At the request of the physician, follow-up house visits by a home health nurse to check clinical status, to repeat tests, and to ensure weight gain should be arranged for finite periods, depending on the needs of the individual infant and family. Infants with special needs who require specialized follow-up health surveillance include those with the following conditions:

1. BPD.
2. Neurologic abnormalities.
3. Gastroesophageal reflux.
4. Short gut and the presence of ostomies.
5. Congenital heart disease.
6. Genetic problems.

G. Car seat. Use infant-only car safety seats with 3-point harness systems or convertible car safety seats with 5-point harness systems. Blanket rolls may be placed on both sides of the infant and a rolled diaper or blanket can be used between the crotch strap and the infant to reduce slouching. Parents need to bring the car seat before discharge for training on seating the infant, proper positioning, and support. While the infant is in the car seat, check for oxygen saturation in supine and car seat positions, especially for preemies sent home on oxygen and monitoring for apnea (per the American Academy of Pediatrics' "Safe Transport of the Preemie" policy statement).

H. Brief parents on common issues after discharge. Discuss home temperature and dressing the infant, intercurrent illness and taking temperature, vomiting, bowel movement, diaper rash, sleeping, bathing, stuffy nose and its management, hiccups, crying, breathing pattern, interacting with the infant, going out, visitors and relatives, and a "no smoking" policy inside the house. Review medications, nutrition (type, amount, frequency, and special precautions), and use of supplemental oxygen and the cardiopulmonary monitor as needed.

48 No Stool in 48 Hours

I. **Problem.** No stool has been passed in 48 h. Ninety-nine percent of term infants and 76% of premature infants pass a stool in the first 24 h of life. Ninety-nine percent of premature infants pass a stool by 48 h.

II. **Immediate questions**
  A. **Has a stool been passed since birth?** If a stool has been passed since birth but not in the last 48 h, constipation may be the cause. If a stool has never been passed, imperforate anus or some degree of intestinal obstruction may be present. Table 48–1 shows the time after birth at which the first stool is typically passed.
  B. **What is the gestational age?** Prematurity is associated with delayed passage of stool because of immaturity of the colon and lack of triggering effect of enteral feeds on gut hormones when the patient is maintained on nothing by mouth (NPO) orders.
  C. **Were maternal drugs used that could cause a paralytic ileus with delayed passage of stool?** Magnesium sulfate, which is used to slow the premature onset of labor, may cause paralytic ileus. Narcotics for pain control or use of heroin by the mother may also cause delayed passage of stool in the neonate.

III. **Differential diagnosis**
  A. **Constipation.**
  B. **Anorectal abnormalities** such as imperforate anus
  C. **Bowel obstruction**
    1. **Meconium plug.** A meconium plug is an obstruction in the lower colon and rectum caused by meconium. It is more common in infants of diabetic mothers (as seen in neonatal small left colon syndrome, in which the plug extends to the splenic flexure) and in premature infants. (**Note:** A rectal biopsy should be considered in all these patients because they have an increased incidence [10–15%] of Hirschsprung's disease.)
    2. **Meconium ileus** occurs when meconium becomes obstructed in the terminal ileum. Ninety percent of patients with meconium ileus will have cystic fibrosis and thus should be tested for CF. It is the most common presentation of cystic fibrosis in the neonatal period.
    3. **Hirschsprung's disease** accounts for ~15% of infants who have delayed passage of stool. A functional obstruction is caused by aganglionosis of cells in Meissner's and Auerbach's plexus in the rectum and variable amounts of the distal colon. The affected segment of colon and rectum are aperistaltic.
    4. **Ileal atresia** can occur secondary to meconium ileus, Hirschsprung's disease, incarcerated hernia, or intussusception. Signs include abdominal distention, bilious vomiting, and failure to pass meconium.
    5. **Adhesions.** Postoperatively, such as after surgery for necrotizing enterocolitis, there is a 30% chance of having adhesions.
    6. **Incarcerated hernia.** A hernia is obstructed when its contents cannot be reduced and the bowel is obstructed. Signs include irritability, cramps, bilious vomiting, and abdominal distention. The risk of incarceration for an inguinal hernia in infancy is 20–30%; the risk of bowel obstruction secondary to an inguinal hernia is 9%.
    7. **Malrotation.** Malrotation is the failure of the gastrointestinal tract to properly rotate and adhere. Volvulus is a specific malrotation of the gut and is a **surgical emergency** because it can cause ischemia of the gut, with resulting shock and possibly death. Malrotation without volvulus formation may

283

TABLE 48-1. TIME OF FIRST STOOL BASED ON A STUDY OF 500 TERM AND PRETERM INFANTS

Hours	Full-term infants (%)[a]	Preterm infants (%)[a]
Delivery room (0)	16.7	5.0
1–8	59.5	32.5
9–16	91.1	63.8
17–24	98.5	76.3
24–48	100	98.8
>48	—	100

[a]Percentages are cumulative.
Based on data from Clark DA: Times of first void and stool in 500 newborns. *Pediatrics* 1977;60:457.

present with intermittent episodes of vomiting and abdominal distention. The stooling pattern can be normal.

   D. **Other causes**
      1. **Ileus** can be secondary to the following conditions.
         a. **Sepsis.**
         b. **Necrotizing enterocolitis.**
         c. **Hypokalemia.**
         d. **Pneumonia.**
         e. **Maternal use of magnesium sulfate.**
         f. **Hypothyroidism.**
         g. **Narcotic analgesic therapy.**
      2. **Prematurity** (see section II,B).
IV. **Data base**
   A. **Physical examination.** First, document the patency of the anus. Check for abdominal distention or rigidity, bowel sounds, and evidence of a mass. A rectal examination will determine whether muscle tone is adequate, and it may reveal hardened stool in the colon.
   B. **Laboratory findings**
      1. **A complete blood cell count with differential and blood culture** should be done to rule out sepsis. A sterile urine culture should also be done.
      2. **Urinary drug screening** should be performed on both mother and infant to detect maternal use of narcotics.
      3. **The serum magnesium level** should be determined to detect hypermagnesemia.
      4. **Serum electrolytes** should be measured, especially to rule out hypokalemia.
      5. **Serum thyroxine (T₄) and thyroid-stimulating hormone (TSH) levels** should be determined to detect hypothyroidism.
   C. **Radiologic and other studies**
      1. **Plain film abdominal x-rays.** A flat plate and upright film of the abdomen should be obtained to look for ileus or bowel obstruction in any infant who has not passed stool within 48 h of birth. With Hirschsprung's disease or meconium plug, distention of the colon with multiple air-fluid levels is seen.
      2. **Abdominal x-rays with barium enema** should be obtained in all cases of delayed passage of stool if the patient is symptomatic. These will help to define the disease process and may be therapeutic. Specific findings for each disease are described in section V.
V. **Plan**
   A. **Constipation**
      1. **Digital rectal stimulation** can be tried first.
      2. **Glycerin suppositories** can be used if digital rectal stimulation is unsuccessful.
   B. **Anorectal abnormality:** Imperforate anus
      1. **Obtain pediatric surgical consultation** immediately.

2. **Insert a nasogastric tube** for decompression.
3. **Look for other congenital anomalies.** Genitourinary tract abnormalities are frequently seen with imperforate anus.

C. **Bowel obstruction**
   1. **Meconium plug**
      a. **Barium enema** is performed to verify meconium plug. In infants with this problem, the study usually reveals a normal-sized colon with filling defects.
      b. **If meconium plug is verified** by barium enema, repeated water-soluble enemas are usually given every 4–6 h.
      c. **Acetylcysteine (Mucomyst) enema.** If water-soluble enemas are ineffective, a dilute 4% solution of acetylcysteine and water can be used as an enema to break down the meconium so that it can be passed.
      d. **If normal stooling occurs,** monitor closely.
      e. **If an abnormal pattern of stooling recurs,** further workup (eg, rectal biopsy) is necessary to rule out Hirschsprung's disease, which may be diagnosed in half of these patients.
   2. **Meconium ileus**
      a. **Barium enema** may reveal microcolon. Evidence of perforation, volvulus, or atresia may also be seen.
      b. **Mild obstruction** can be treated with Mucomyst enemas (see section V,C,1,c).
      c. **Complete obstruction** may be relieved by hyperosmolar Gastrografin enema. Adequate fluid and electrolyte replacement must be given.
      d. **Operative management** may be necessary in patients not relieved by enemas with passage of meconium within several hours.
   3. **Hirschsprung's disease**
      a. **Barium enema examination** usually shows a distal narrowed, aganglionic segment leading to a dilated proximal segment.
      b. **Rectal biopsy,** the definitive diagnosis, is performed to confirm aganglionosis.
      c. **Colostomy** is usually indicated once the diagnosis is confirmed.
   4. **Adhesions.** Surgery is usually necessary to lyse the adhesions if a trial of nasogastric decompression fails.
   5. **Incarcerated hernia** is a surgical emergency.
   6. **Malrotation**
      a. **Barium enema** reveals an abnormally placed cecum.
      b. **Surgical correction** is necessary.
   7. **Volvulus**
      a. **Barium enema** reveals obstruction at the midtransverse colon.
      b. **Surgery** should be an immediate intervention.

D. **Ileus**
   1. **Ileus caused by sepsis**
      a. **Broad-spectrum antibiotics** are initiated after a sepsis workup (see Chapter 54) is performed. Intravenous ampicillin and gentamicin are recommended. Vancomycin may be substituted for ampicillin if staphylococcal infection is suspected (for dosages, see Chapter 80).
      b. **A nasogastric tube** should be placed to decompress the bowel. The infant should not be fed enterally.
   2. **Ileus caused by necrotizing enterocolitis.** See Chapter 71.
   3. **Ileus caused by hypokalemia**
      a. **Treat underlying metabolic abnormalities.**
      b. **Place a nasogastric tube to rest the bowel.**

E. **Prematurity.** Conservative treatment is usually recommended in infants who are not vomiting but have progressive abdominal distention, even if microcolon is seen. Treatment consists of a hyperosmolar contrast enema for passage of the stool. (**Note:** Some institutions advocate the use of low-osmolality, water-soluble, iodine-containing contrast enemas because of fewer side effects. Consult a pediatric radiologist for appropriate contrast enema to be used.)

F. Hypothyroidism. If the serum T_4 and TSH levels confirm the presence of hypothyroidism, thyroid replacement therapy is indicated. Consultation with an endocrinologist should be obtained before starting this therapy.

49 No Urine Output in 48 Hours

I. **Problem.** Urine output has been scant or absent for 24 h. Oliguria is defined as urine output <0.5–1 mL/kg/h. One hundred percent of healthy premature, full-term, and postterm infants will void by 24 h of age.

II. **Immediate questions**
   A. **Is the bladder palpable?** If a distended bladder is present, it is usually palpable. A palpable bladder suggests there is urine in the bladder. **Credé's maneuver** (manual compression of the bladder) may initiate voiding, especially in infants receiving medications causing muscle paralysis.
   B. **Has bladder catheterization been performed?** This will determine whether urine is present in the bladder. It is more commonly done in more mature infants.
   C. **What is the blood pressure?** Hypotension can cause decreased renal perfusion and urine output.
   D. **Has the infant ever voided?** If the infant has never voided, consider bilateral renal agenesis, renovascular accident, or obstruction. Table 49–1 shows the time after birth at which the first voiding occurs.

III. **Differential diagnosis.** For a complete discussion of acute renal failure, see Chapter 75.
   A. **Prerenal causes** (inadequate renal perfusion)
      1. **Sepsis.**
      2. **Dehydration.**
      3. **Hemorrhage.**
      4. **Hypotension.**
      5. **Asphyxia.**
      6. **Hypokalemia.**
      7. **Heart failure.**
      8. **Medications.** Certain medications (eg, indomethacin, captopril, and β-agonists), if given to the mother before delivery, can result in renal insufficiency.
   B. **Intrinsic renal failure**
      1. **Renal agenesis.**
      2. **Hypoplastic, dysplastic, or cystic kidneys.**
      3. **Pyelonephritis.**
      4. **Vascular accident** (renal artery and vein thrombosis).
      5. **Nephritis.**
      6. **Infections** such as congenital syphilis, cytomegalovirus, toxoplasmosis, and gram-negative infections.
      7. **Acute tubular necrosis** secondary to shock, dehydration, and asphyxia.
      8. **Medications.** Some nephrotoxic medications include tolazoline, aminoglycosides, indomethacin, amphotericin, α-adrenergic agents, and acyclovir.
   C. **Postrenal causes** (urine is formed but not voided)
      1. **Neurogenic bladder** (from myelomeningocele or medications such as pancuronium or heavy sedation).
      2. **Urethral stricture.**
      3. **Posterior urethral valves** (in males only).
      4. **Extrinsic compression** (eg, sacrococcygeal teratoma)

IV. **Data base**
   A. **Physical examination.** Physical examination may reveal bladder distention, abdominal masses, or ascites. Signs of renal disorders (eg, Potter's facies [low-set ears, inner canthal crease, and so on]) should be noted. Urinary as-

TABLE 49-1. TIME OF FIRST VOID BASED ON A STUDY OF 500 TERM AND PRETERM INFANTS

Hours	Full-term infants (%)[a]	Preterm infants (%)[a]
Delivery room (0)	12.9	21.2
1–8	51.1	83.7
9–16	91.1	98.7
17–24	100	100

[a]Percentages are cumulative.
Based on data from Clark DA: Times of first void and stool in 500 newborns. *Pediatrics* 1977;60:457.

cites may be seen with posterior urethral valves. Oligohydramnios in the mother suggests possible renal problems.
  B. **Laboratory studies.** The following laboratory tests can be obtained to help establish the diagnosis. Interpret the results as outlined in Table 75–1.
    1. **Serum creatinine.**
    2. **Serum electrolytes and blood urea nitrogen will also help to evaluate renal function.**
    3. **Complete blood cell count (CBC) and platelet count.** An abnormal CBC can be seen in sepsis. Thrombocytopenia can be seen in renal vein thrombosis.
    4. **Urinalysis** may reveal white blood cells, suggesting a urinary tract infection.
    5. **Arterial blood pH.** A metabolic acidosis can be seen in anything that causes hypovolemia, hypoperfusion, or hypotension, such as sepsis.
    6. **Urine osmolality.**
    7. **Urine sodium (mEq/L).**
    8. **Urine/plasma creatinine ratio.**
    9. **Fractional excretion of sodium** (see p 554, Chapter 75, section VI,B,2).
    10. **Renal failure index** (see p 554, Chapter 75, section VI,B,2).
  C. **Radiologic and other studies**
    1. **Ultrasonography of the abdomen and kidneys** will rule out urinary tract obstruction and help evaluate for other renal abnormalities.
    2. **Abdominal x-ray studies** may reveal spina bifida or an absent sacrum, suggesting a neurogenic bladder.
V. **Plan.** For management of renal failure, see also Chapter 75.
  A. **Prerenal**
    1. **Treat the specific cause** (eg, sepsis).
    2. **A fluid challenge** can be given (10–20 mL/kg of normal saline).
    3. **Treatment may involve volume therapy or inotropic agents.**
  B. **Renal**
    1. **Supportive measures.**
    2. **Treat the specific cause.**
    3. **Restrict fluid intake, and replace insensible losses.**
  C. **Postrenal**
    1. **If obstruction is distal to the bladder,** perform initial catheterization.
    2. **If obstruction is proximal to the bladder,** urologic surgical intervention should be considered (eg, nephrostomy tubes or cutaneous ureterostomy).
    3. **Neurogenic bladder** is initially managed with catheterization.
    4. **Medications resulting in bladder dysfunction** may be stopped, and bladder function is usually restored.

50 Pneumoperitoneum

I. **Problem.** A pneumoperitoneum (an abnormal collection of air in the peritoneal cavity) is seen on an abdominal x-ray film. The air can be secondary to perforation of the gastrointestinal (GI) tract (most common), it can be from the respiratory tract, or it can be secondary to iatrogenic causes (not very common).

II. **Immediate questions**

A. **Are signs or symptoms of pneumoperitoneum present?** These findings can include abdominal distention, respiratory distress, deteriorating blood gas levels, and a decrease in blood pressure.

B. **Are signs or symptoms of necrotizing enterocolitis (NEC) present?** If so, the pneumoperitoneum is most likely to be associated with GI tract perforation.

C. **Are any signs of air leak present?** If a pneumomediastinum, pulmonary interstitial emphysema, or pneumothorax is present, the peritoneal air collection is more likely to be of respiratory tract origin.

D. **Is mechanical ventilation being given?** High peak inspiratory pressures (PIPs > mean of 34 cm H_2O) can be associated with a pneumoperitoneum.

E. **Did the infant recently undergo abdominal surgery?** Intra-abdominal air is normal in the immediate postoperative period and usually resolves without treatment.

III. **Differential diagnosis.** Pneumoperitoneum develops secondary to perforation of the GI tract, from an air leak from the chest, or iatrogenically. In a neonate, unless the infant is on high ventilator settings and has air leak syndrome, **the cause is GI perforation until proven otherwise.** It is necessary to differentiate the cause so specific treatment can be given.

A. **Pneumoperitoneum associated with GI perforation**

1. **Spontaneous perforation** occurs most commonly in the stomach of a full-term neonate. In a preterm infant, the most common cause of perforation is in the jejunoileal area. However, isolated perforation can also occur in the intestine of a full-term infant. Perforation of the appendix and Meckel's diverticulum has been reported. Isolated rupture at any level of the GI tract has been associated with oral or intravenous indomethacin. A meta-analysis of the effect of early treatment (<96 h) with high doses of steroids for chronic lung disease showed an increased risk of spontaneous GI perforation. An embolic phenomenon secondary to an umbilical artery catheter can also contribute to perforation.

2. **NEC** may also be associated with perforation. A meta-analysis examining the use of indomethacin for intraventricular hemorrhage (IVH) prophylaxis showed a nonsignificant trend toward an increased risk of NEC.

3. **Malrotation with volvulus** has rarely been associated with perforation.

B. **Pneumoperitoneum associated with a respiratory disorder (eg, pneumomediastinum or pneumothorax).**

C. **Iatrogenic pneumoperitoneum** may be caused by improperly performed suprapubic bladder aspiration, by paracentesis, or as a normal transient finding post–exploratory laparotomy.

IV. **Data base**

A. **Physical examination.** Perform a complete physical examination. Clinical evaluation may not help in differentiating whether the pneumoperitoneum is of respiratory or GI tract origin. Clinical signs include abdominal distention and elevation of the diaphragm with increasing respiratory difficulty.

B. **Laboratory studies**
   1. **Preoperative laboratory testing** should be performed, including **serum electrolyte levels and a complete blood cell count.** Elevation of the white blood cell count or a left shift may signify a GI tract perforation. Hyponatremia can be seen with NEC secondary to third spacing of fluid. Thrombocytopenia also can be seen.
   2. **Arterial blood gas levels** should be obtained. They may reveal hypoxemia and increasing P_{CO_2} levels. Metabolic acidosis can be seen with peritonitis.

C. **Radiologic and other studies.** First, confirm the diagnosis of free air by the football sign on anteroposterior (AP) x-ray study, air below the diaphragm on an upright view, or air over the liver on a lateral decubitus view.
   1. **AP x-ray study of the chest and abdomen.** The chest may show signs of air leak syndrome (look for pneumomediastinum or pneumothorax) if suspect air is from the respiratory tract. The abdomen may show signs of NEC or ileus. Air-fluid levels in the peritoneal cavity usually indicate ileus.
   2. **Lateral decubitus x-ray study of the abdomen** with the right side up is the best examination for the detection of free abdominal air. Air rises anteriorly, so that a lucency will be seen over the liver if a perforation has occurred. A lateral decubitus x-ray film should be systematically taken when NEC is suspected, because a pneumoperitoneum can be easily missed on an AP x-ray.
   3. **Paracentesis.** Air obtained by paracentesis (see Chapter 25) may be tested for its oxygen level. If the oxygen level is high, the air is probably from a respiratory tract leak. Fluid may be obtained by paracentesis if the diagnosis is still undetermined. If brownish fluid is obtained, the air is probably of GI tract origin. One can also smear the fluid for white blood cells, which would indicate peritonitis.

V. **Plan**
A. **Emergency measures.** In certain cases, massive accumulation of air in the abdomen causes respiratory compromise from an immobile diaphragm. In these cases, an emergency paracentesis must be done, which diminishes the air under pressure and allows the diaphragm to be mobile, thereby providing relief to the respiratory distress. (For the procedure on abdominal paracentesis, see Chapter 25.)

B. **General measures.** A nasogastric tube with low suction should be placed.

C. **Specific measures**
   1. **Pneumoperitoneum of GI tract origin.** Unless the pneumoperitoneum is of a known iatrogenic origin, **immediate surgical evaluation** is necessary. Exploratory laparotomy is usually the treatment of choice, although in some stable patients only a drain is placed.
      a. **Preoperative laboratory values** should be available.
      b. **The infant should be stabilized** as much as possible before being taken to the operating room.
      c. **The surgical team may request a study with a water-soluble contrast medium given through the nasogastric tube** to try to localize the perforation (see section V,C,4).
   2. **Pneumoperitoneum of respiratory tract origin**
      a. **For asymptomatic patients,** observation is often the treatment of choice, with follow-up x-ray studies usually performed every 8–12 h but more frequently if the patient's clinical course changes.
      b. **For symptomatic patients,** paracentesis can be performed.
   3. **Iatrogenic pneumoperitoneum**
      a. **Pneumoperitoneum caused by suprapubic bladder aspiration or paracentesis** may require surgical exploration.
      b. **Post-exploratory laparotomy** pneumoperitoneum associated with an uncomplicated surgical procedure will resolve spontaneously.

4. **If the cause of the pneumoperitoneum is in doubt, a low-osmolality, water-soluble contrast medium (eg, metrizamide) can be given through a nasogastric tube.** If there is a pneumoperitoneum secondary to a GI perforation, contrast material will pass into the peritoneal cavity and urine.

51 Pneumothorax

I. **Problem.** An infant may have a pneumothorax (an accumulation of air in the pleural space).

II. **Immediate questions**

   A. **Are symptoms of tension pneumothorax present?** *Tension pneumothorax presents as a medical emergency, and the patient's status will deteriorate acutely.* The following signs and symptoms may be seen with tension pneumothorax: cyanosis, hypoxia, tachypnea, a sudden decrease in heart rate with bradycardia, a sudden increase in systolic blood pressure followed by narrowing pulse pressure and hypotension, an asymmetric chest (bulging on the affected side), distention of the abdomen (secondary to downward displacement of the diaphragm), decreased breath sounds on the affected side, and shift of the cardiac apical impulse (most consistent finding) away from the affected side.

   B. **Is the patient asymptomatic?** Asymptomatic pneumothorax is present in 1–2% of neonates. Most of these cases are discovered on chest x-ray film at admission. Up to 15% of these infants were meconium stained at birth.

   C. **Is mechanical ventilation being used?** The incidence of pneumothorax in patients receiving positive-pressure ventilation is 15–30%. A life-threatening tension pneumothorax may result from mechanical ventilation.

III. **Differential diagnosis.** A pneumothorax may be spontaneous, or it may develop secondary to mechanical ventilation, which causes barotrauma.

   A. **Pneumothorax**

      1. **Symptomatic** pneumothorax (includes tension pneumothorax).

      2. **Asymptomatic** pneumothorax.

   B. **Pneumomediastinum.** Air in the mediastinal space that may be confused with a true pneumothorax.

   C. **Congenital lobar emphysema.** Overdistention of one lobe secondary to air trapping occurs most commonly (47%) in the left upper lobe. Other lobe involvement is right upper lobe (20%), right middle lobe (28%), and lower lobes (rare). The causes of congenital lobar emphysema are probably multifactorial.

   D. **Atelectasis with compensatory hyperinflation.** Compensatory hyperinflation may appear as a pneumothorax on a chest x-ray film.

   E. **Pneumopericardium.** In neonates, pneumopericardium and tension pneumothorax can both present as sudden and rapid clinical deterioration. In pneumopericardium, the blood pressure drops, heart sounds are distant or absent, and pulses are muffled or absent. Massive abdominal distention can also be seen. In tension pneumothorax, the blood pressure may initially increase, but then hypotension follows. The chest x-ray film easily differentiates the two. A pneumopericardium has a halo of air around the heart. **The more common event will be a tension pneumothorax.** If one is unsure and time does not permit x-ray verification, it is better to insert a needle in the chest on the suspected side. If no response, then a needle should be inserted on the other side. If there is still no response, then the diagnosis of pneumopericardium should be considered.

IV. **Clinical findings**

   A. **Physical examination.** Perform a thorough examination of the chest. Specific findings are discussed in section II,A. Transillumination is a useful rapid technique in neonates (see section IV,C).

   B. **Laboratory studies.** Blood gas levels may show decreased Pao_2 and increased Pco_2, with resultant respiratory acidosis.

   C. **Radiologic and other studies**

1. **Transillumination.** Transillumination of the chest will define the pneumothorax. The room lights are lowered, and a fiberoptic transilluminator is placed along the posterior axillary line on the side on which pneumothorax is suspected. If pneumothorax is present, the chest will "light up" on that side. The transilluminator may be moved up and down along the posterior axillary line and may also be placed above the nipple. Transilluminate both sides of the chest, and then compare the results. If severe subcutaneous edema is present, transillumination may be falsely positive. Premature infants with pulmonary interstitial emphysema may also have a false-positive transillumination. Large infants with thick chest walls do not transilluminate well. **Always verify the diagnosis of pneumothorax by chest x-ray studies if time permits.**

2. **Chest x-ray studies** are the method of choice for diagnosing pneumothorax. Early pneumothoraces are difficult to diagnose. Early on, one can see separation of lung from the chest wall with no lung markings in that space. The following films will help in making the diagnosis.

   a. **Anteroposterior (AP) view** of the chest will show the following:
      i. **A shift of the mediastinum** away from the side of pneumothorax (with tension pneumothorax).
      ii. **Depression of the diaphragm** on the side of the pneumothorax (with tension pneumothorax).
      iii. **Displacement of the lung** on the affected side away from the chest wall by a radiolucent band of air.

   b. **Cross-table lateral view** will show a rim of air around the lung ("pancaking"). It will *not* help to identify the affected side. This film must be considered together with the AP view to identify the involved side.

   c. **Lateral decubitus view (shot through the AP position)** will detect even a small pneumothorax not seen on a routine chest x-ray film. The infant should be positioned so that the side of the suspected pneumothorax is up (eg, if pneumothorax is suspected on the left side, the film is taken with the left side up).

V. **Plan**

A. **Symptomatic (tension) pneumothorax is an emergency!** A 1- to 2-min delay could be fatal. If a tension pneumothorax is suspected, act immediately. It is better to treat in this setting, even if it turns out that there is no pneumothorax. There is no time for x-ray confirmation. If the patient's status is deteriorating rapidly, a needle or Angiocath can be placed for aspiration, followed by formal chest tube placement. There is no specific sign that distinguishes a tension from a nontension pneumothorax. Signs of a tension pneumothorax from above can also occur in a nontension pneumothorax. Just remember that in a tension pneumothorax there is an ongoing cardiopulmonary deterioration as a result of the progressive increase in intrathoracic pressure.

1. **The site of puncture** should be at the second or third intercostal space along the midclavicular line. Cleanse this area with antibacterial solution (eg, Betadine).

2. **Connect a 21- or 23-gauge scalp vein needle** or a 22- or 24-gauge Angiocath to a 20-mL syringe with a stopcock attached. Have an assistant hold the syringe and withdraw the air.

3. **Palpate the third rib at the midclavicular line.** Insert the needle above the rib, and advance it until air is withdrawn from the syringe. The needle may be removed before the chest tube is placed if the infant is relatively stable, or it may be left in place for continuous aspiration while the chest tube is being placed. If an Angiocath is used, the needle can be removed and the catheter left in place.

4. **Chest tube placement** is discussed in Chapter 19.

B. **Asymptomatic pneumothorax**

1. **If positive-pressure mechanical ventilation is the cause of asymptomatic pneumothorax,** a chest tube will probably need to be inserted be-

cause the pressure being given by the ventilator will prevent resolution of the pneumothorax, and tension pneumothorax may develop. Sometimes needle aspiration is all that is needed. If a pneumothorax develops in a patient who is ready to be extubated, clinical judgment must be used in deciding whether a chest tube should be placed.

2. **If positive-pressure mechanical ventilation is not being administered,** one of two treatments may be used.

   a. **Close observation with follow-up chest x-ray studies** every 8–12 h or sooner if the infant becomes symptomatic. The pneumothorax will probably resolve within 48 h.

   b. **For more rapid resolution of the pneumothorax** in the asymptomatic patient, give the infant 100% oxygen for 8–12 h, a procedure known as *nitrogen washout therapy.* Less nitrogen is able to enter the lungs, and at the same time absorption of nitrogen from the extrapleural space is increased and then exhaled. The total gas tension is decreased, which also facilitates absorption of nitrogen by the blood. *The method should be used only in full-term infants in whom retinopathy of prematurity will not be a problem. Some institutions do not routinely give 100% F_{IO_2}.*

C. **Pneumomediastinum** may progress to a pneumothorax or pneumopericardium. Close observation is required.

D. **Congenital lobar emphysema**

   1. **Asymptomatic.** Conservative management with observation is advocated.

   2. **Symptomatic.** If respiratory failure is occurring, the treatment is usually surgical excision of the affected lobe.

E. **Atelectasis with compensatory hyperinflation**

   1. Chest physiotherapy and postural drainage should be initiated. Chest physiotherapy should be used with caution. A study showed an association with porencephaly in extreme premature infants.

   2. Treatment with bronchodilators is indicated (see p 56, 57).

   3. Positioning the infant with the affected (hyperinflated) side down may speed resolution.

F. **Pneumopericardium** should be treated emergently by pericardiocentesis (see Chapter 26).

52 Polycythemia

I. **Problem.** The hematocrit (Hct) is 68% in a newborn. (The upper limit of normal for a newborn peripheral venous stick is 65%.) Polycythemia occurs in 1.5–4% (higher elevations) of newborn infants. It is rare in premature infants <34 weeks' gestation.

II. **Immediate questions**

A. **What is the central Hct?** In blood obtained by heelstick, the Hct may be falsely elevated by 5–15%. Therefore, treatment should **never** be initiated based on heelstick Hct values alone; a central (peripheral venous stick) Hct is needed. If the sample is from the umbilical vein or radial artery, the upper limit of normal is 63%.

B. **Does the infant have symptoms of polycythemia?** Many infants with polycythemia are asymptomatic. Symptoms and signs of polycythemia include respiratory distress, tachypnea, hypoglycemia, lethargy, irritability, apnea, seizures, jitteriness, vomiting, weak sucking reflex, poor feeding, and cyanosis.

C. **Is the mother diabetic?** Poor control of diabetes during pregnancy leads to chronic fetal hypoxia, which may result in increased neonatal erythropoiesis. Infants of diabetic mothers have a 22–29% incidence of polycythemia.

D. **What is the infant's age?** The Hct reaches a peak at 2–4 h of age. After 18 h of age, hemoconcentration as a result of dehydration may be present.

E. **Is the infant dehydrated?** Dehydration may cause hemoconcentration, resulting in a high Hct. It usually occurs in infants >48 h old.

III. **Differential diagnosis.** See also Chapter 61.

A. **Falsely elevated Hct.** This finding occurs most often when blood is obtained by heelstick.

B. **Dehydration.** Weight loss and decreased urine output are sensitive indicators of dehydration. Hemoconcentration secondary to dehydration is suspected if >8–10% of the birth weight has been lost. It usually occurs on the second or third day of life.

C. **True polycythemia**

1. **Placental transfusion** occurs with delayed cord clamping, twin-twin transfusion, fetomaternal transfusion, or perinatal asphyxia.

2. **Iatrogenic polycythemia.** Too much blood was transfused.

3. **Intrauterine hypoxia** may be caused by placental insufficiency. It may be seen in postmature or small for gestational age infants, preeclampsia/eclampsia, and infants of diabetic mothers as well as with maternal use of the drug propranolol. Maternal smoking and severe maternal heart disease may also cause intrauterine hypoxia.

4. **Other causes**

a. **Chromosomal abnormalities** such as Down syndrome and trisomies 13 and 18.

b. **Beckwith-Wiedemann syndrome.**

c. **Neonatal thyrotoxicosis.**

d. **Congenital adrenal hyperplasia.**

5. **No specific cause found with the polycythemia.**

IV. **Data base**

A. **Physical examination.** Evaluate for possible dehydration. The mucous membranes will be dry. Increased skin turgor is usually not seen. True polycythemia is often, but not always, associated with visible skin changes. Ruddiness, plethora, or "pink-on-blue" or "blue-on-pink" coloration may be evident. In males, priapism may be seen secondary to sludging of red blood cells. Clinical signs are listed in section II,B.

B. Laboratory studies
1. **A central Hct value** must be obtained.
2. **The serum glucose level** should be checked because hypoglycemia is commonly seen with polycythemia.
3. **Serum bilirubin level.** Infants with polycythemia have problems with hyperbilirubinemia because of the increased turnover of red blood cells.
4. **Serum sodium and blood urea nitrogen levels** should be obtained if dehydration is being considered. They are usually high, or higher than baseline values, if dehydration is present.
5. **Urine specific gravity.** A high specific gravity (>1.015) is usually seen with dehydration.
6. **Blood gas levels.** Blood gas levels should be obtained to rule out inadequate oxygenation.
7. **Serum platelet count.** Thrombocytopenia can be seen.
8. **Serum calcium level.** Hypocalcemia can also be seen (less common).
C. Radiologic and other studies. These studies are usually not indicated. One can see cardiomegaly and increased pulmonary vascular markings on a chest-x-ray. An abnormal electrocardiogram and electroencephalogram can be seen, but these tests are not routinely indicated.

V. Plan
A. Falsely elevated Hct (>65%). If the confirmatory central Hct is normal, no further evaluation is needed. If the central Hct is high, either dehydration or true polycythemia is present (for treatment, see sections V,B and V,C).
B. Hemoconcentration secondary to dehydration. If the infant is dehydrated but does not have symptoms or signs of polycythemia, a trial of rehydration over 6–8 h can be attempted. The type of fluid used depends on the infant's age and serum electrolyte status and is discussed in Chapter 7. Usually, 130–150 mL/kg/day is given. The Hct is checked every 6 h and usually decreases with adequate rehydration.
C. True polycythemia. Treatment is usually based on whether or not the infant is symptomatic.
1. **Asymptomatic infants**
   a. **Central Hct of 65–70%.** If the central Hct is 65–70% and the infant is asymptomatic, only observation may be needed. Many of these patients respond to increased fluid therapy; increases of 20–40 mL/kg/day can be attempted. The central Hct must be checked every 6 h. The Hct normally reaches a peak at 2–4 h of age. If the Hct is 70% at birth, it may be 5–10% higher at 2–4 h of age.
   b. **Central Hct of 70–75%.** If the Hct is 70–75% and the infant is asymptomatic, then *controversy* exists as to whether an exchange should be done. It is best to follow your institutional guidelines.
   c. **Central Hct >75%.** Most neonatologists agree that a partial exchange transfusion should be given, although some *controversy* exists. Institutional guidelines should be followed.
2. **Symptomatic infants**
   a. **Central Hct >65%** in the symptomatic infant. Partial exchange transfusion should be given. To calculate the volume of Plasmanate that must be exchanged, use the following formula (blood volume = 80 mL/kg):

$$\text{Volume exchanged} = \frac{(\text{Weight [kg]} \times \text{Blood volume}) \times (\text{Hct of patient} - \text{Desired Hct})}{\text{Hct of patient}}$$

Desired Hct is usually <60, with a goal of bringing it down to 50–55. Partial exchange transfusion may be administered via an umbilical venous catheter. (*Care must be taken not to place it in the liver* [for the technique, see Chapter 21].) A low umbilical artery catheter or a peripheral intravenous catheter can also be used. The fluid that can be used for a partial exchange transfusion is Plasmanate, 5% albumin, normal saline, or fresh-frozen plasma (FFP). FFP is usually not recommended because of the risk of HIV transmission. The decision about which fluid to use depends on a particular institution's preference. Most often, normal saline can be used and is preferred in most institutions. The partial exchange transfusion procedure is discussed in detail in Chapter 21. Serial Hct levels should be obtained after transfusion.

b. **Symptoms with a central Hct of 60–65%.** If all other disease entities are ruled out, these infants may indeed be polycythemic and hyperviscous. In these cases, management is *controversial.* Use clinical judgment and institutional guidelines to decide whether or not this infant should have a partial exchange transfusion.

D. **Observe for complications of polycythemia and disorders that are more common in polycythemic infants.**
   1. **Hyperbilirubinemia.**
   2. **Seizures.**
   3. **Necrotizing enterocolitis (NEC).** There is an increased risk of NEC in neonates with hyperviscosity who received a partial exchange transfusion via an umbilical venous catheter.
   4. **Ileus.**
   5. **Renal failure.**
   6. **Peripheral gangrene.**
   7. **Hypocalcemia.**
   8. **Renal vein thrombosis.**
   9. **Congestive heart failure.**

E. **Note that a partial exchange transfusion decreases viscosity** and ameliorates most symptoms but has not been shown to significantly affect or improve long-term neurologic outcomes.

53 Poor Perfusion

I. **Problem.** You receive a report that an infant "doesn't look good" or looks "mottled." Other descriptions may include "a washed-out appearance" or "poor perfusion."

II. **Immediate questions**
   A. **What is the age of the infant?** Hypoplastic left heart syndrome may cause poor perfusion and a mottled appearance. It may be seen at days 1–21 of life (more commonly at day 2 or 3). In an infant <3 days old, sepsis may be a cause. Associated risk factors for sepsis are premature rupture of membranes or maternal infection and fever.
   B. **What are the vital signs?** If the temperature is lower than normal, cold stress or hypothermia associated with sepsis may be present. Hypotension may cause poor perfusion (see normal blood pressure values in Appendix C). Decreased urine output (<2 mL/kg/h) may indicate depleted intravascular volume or shock.
   C. **Is the liver enlarged and are metabolic acidosis, a poor peripheral pulse rate, and gallop present?** These problems are signs of failure of the left side of the heart (eg, hypoplastic left heart syndrome). Poor perfusion occurs because of reduced blood flow to the skin.
   D. **If mechanical ventilation is being used, are chest movements adequate and are blood gas levels improving?** Inadequate ventilation can result in poor perfusion. Pneumothorax may also be a cause.
   E. **Are congenital anomalies present?** Persistent cutis marmorata may be seen in Cornelia de Lange's syndrome and in trisomies 18 and 21.

III. **Differential diagnosis**
   A. **Sepsis.**
   B. **Cold stress** (in general, a skin temperature <36.5 °C).
   C. **Hypotension, usually with shock.**
   D. **Hypoventilation.**
   E. **Pneumothorax.**
   F. **Necrotizing enterocolitis.**
   G. **Left-sided heart lesions** such as hypoplastic left heart syndrome, coarctation of the aorta, and aortic stenosis.
   H. **Cutis marmorata,** a marbling pattern of the skin (the infant appears poorly perfused), may occur in a healthy infant, especially when exposed to cold stress. Persistent cutis marmorata may be seen in Cornelia de Lange's syndrome and in trisomies 18 (Edwards' syndrome) and 21 (Down syndrome). Persistent mottling can also be seen in hypothyroidism and central nervous system (CNS) dysfunction.

IV. **Data base**
   A. **Physical examination.** Note the temperature and vital signs. Look for signs of sepsis. The cardiovascular and pulmonary examinations are important because they may suggest cardiac problems or pneumothorax. Signs of trisomy 18 include micrognathia and overlapping digits; signs of trisomy 21 include a single palmar transverse crease and epicanthal folds.
   B. **Laboratory studies**
      1. **Complete blood cell count with differential.** These studies suggest the presence of sepsis or a decreased hematocrit.
      2. **Blood gas levels.** These studies reveal inadequate ventilation or the presence of acidosis, which may be seen in sepsis or necrotizing enterocolitis.
      3. **Cultures.** If sepsis is suspected, a complete workup should be considered, especially if antibiotics are to be started. This workup includes cultures of blood, urine, and spinal fluid (if indicated).

C. **Radiologic and other studies**
1. **Transillumination of the chest.** This study can be performed quickly to help determine whether or not a pneumothorax is present (see Chapter 51, Pneumothorax).
2. **Chest x-ray study.** A chest x-ray study should be obtained if pneumonia, pneumothorax, congenital heart lesion, or hypoventilation is suspected. In left-sided heart lesions, the x-ray film shows cardiomegaly with pulmonary venous congestion (except in hypoplastic left heart syndrome, in which the size of the heart may be normal). If a view taken during lung expansion shows that the lungs are down only to the sixth rib or less, hypoventilation should be considered. With hyperventilation, lung expansion will be down to the ninth or tenth rib.
3. **Abdominal x-ray study.** A flat plate x-ray film of the abdomen should be obtained if necrotizing enterocolitis is suspected.
4. **Echocardiography.** Echocardiography should be performed if a congenital heart lesion is suspected. In hypoplastic left heart syndrome, a large right ventricle and a small left ventricle are seen on the echocardiogram, and there is failure to visualize the mitral or aortic valve. In aortic stenosis, the echocardiogram reveals a deformed aortic valve. In coarctation of the aorta, it reveals decreased aortic diameter.
5. **Karyotyping.** Karyotyping is performed if trisomy 18 or 21 is suspected.

V. **Plan**
A. **General plan.** A quick workup should be performed initially. While checking vital signs and quickly examining the patient, order stat blood gas levels and a chest x-ray study. Initiate oxygen supplementation. Transillumination of the chest may need to be done if a pneumothorax is suspected.
B. **Specific plans**
1. **Sepsis.** If sepsis is suspected, a sepsis workup is indicated. Empiric antibiotic therapy may be started at the discretion of the physician.
2. **Cold stress.** Gradual rewarming is necessary, usually at a rate of ≤1 °C/h. It can be accomplished by means of a radiant warmer or incubator or a heating pad. (See also Chapter 5.)
3. **Hypotension or shock.** If the blood pressure is low because of depleted intravascular volume, give crystalloid (normal saline), 10 mL/kg intravenously for 5–10 min. (See Chapter 46.)
4. **Hypoventilation.** If hypoventilation is suspected, it may be necessary to increase the pressure being given by the ventilator. The amount of pressure must be decided on an individual basis. One method is to increase the pressure by 2–4 cm H_2O and then obtain blood gas levels in 20 min. Another method is to use bag-and-mask ventilation, observing the manometer to determine the amount of pressure needed to move the chest.
5. **Pneumothorax.** See Chapter 51.
6. **Necrotizing enterocolitis.** See Chapter 71.
7. **Left-sided heart lesions.** Treat with oxygen, possibly diuretics and digoxin if congestive heart failure is present, and infusion of prostaglandin E_1. Surgery is usually indicated in all these patients, except those with hypoplastic left heart syndrome, for whom it is *controversial*. A full discussion of cardiac abnormalities is located in Chapter 62.
8. **Cutis marmorata.** If this condition is secondary to cold stress, treat the patient as described in section V,B,2. If the condition persists, consider formal karyotyping to rule out trisomies 18 and 21. Thyroid studies will be necessary if hypothyroidism is suspected. If CNS dysfunction is suspected, this should be evaluated further.

54 Postdelivery Antibiotics

I. **Problem.** Two infants are born within the last hour. In one infant, the mother had premature rupture of membranes (ROM) but no antibiotics. In the other infant, the mother was pretreated with antibiotics for a positive group B streptococcus (GBS) culture taken at 36 weeks. Should a sepsis workup be done, and should antibiotics be started in either of these newborns? The incidence of sepsis is 1–10 in 1000 live births and 1 in 250 live premature births.

II. **Immediate questions**

A. **Are there any maternal risk factors for sepsis in the infant?** Risk factors include African race, malnutrition in the mother, maternal colonization of GBS infection, recently acquired sexually transmitted diseases, and maternal age <20 years. Low socioeconomic status and asymptomatic bacteriuria in the mother are associated with increased prematurity and sepsis. Maternal history of a previous infant with GBS infection also increases the risk of sepsis for the unborn infant.

B. **Are there intrapartum risk factors for sepsis in the infant?** These include ROM >18 h, chorioamnionitis (defined as sustained fetal tachycardia, uterine tenderness, purulent amniotic fluid, unexplained maternal temperature >38 °C [>100.4 °F]), any untreated or incompletely treated infection of the mother, and maternal fever without identifiable cause. The use of fetal scalp electrodes in the intrapartum period increases the risk of infection in the infant. Perinatal asphyxia (defined as a 5-min Apgar score <6) with prolonged ROM also increases the risk of infection in the neonate.

C. **Are there any neonatal risk factors involved?** Neonatal risk factors include male sex, twin birth, prematurity, low birth weight, and presence of the metabolic disorder galactosemia (which increases the risk of gram-negative sepsis).

D. **How long before delivery did the membranes rupture?** ROM that occurs >18 h before birth is associated with an increased incidence of infection in the neonate.

E. **Was the infant monitored during labor?** Fetal tachycardia (>160 beats/min), especially sustained, and decelerations (usually late) can be associated with neonatal infection. Prolonged duration of intrauterine monitoring is a risk factor for early-onset group B streptococcal disease.

F. **Did the mother have a cerclage for cervical incompetence?** Presence of a cerclage increases the risk of infection in the infant.

G. **Are signs of sepsis present in the infant?** Signs of sepsis include apnea and bradycardia, temperature instability (hypothermia or hyperthermia), feeding intolerance, tachypnea, jaundice, cyanosis, poor peripheral perfusion, hypoglycemia, lethargy, poor sucking reflex, increased gastric aspirates, and irritability. Other signs include tachycardia, shock, vomiting, seizures, abnormal rash, abdominal distention, and hepatomegaly.

H. **Did the mother have an epidural?** Studies have shown an increase in maternal intrapartum fever with the use of epidural analgesia. Because of this fever, an increase in sepsis evaluations and antibiotic treatment was found. However, the study did not find that epidurals caused infections or even increased the risk of infections.

I. **Was the mother tested for GBS, and did she receive antibiotics if she tested positive?** There are now specific guidelines to follow after delivery if the mother was treated for GBS.

III. **Differential diagnosis**

A. **Infant at increased risk for sepsis.** The factors noted previously can increase the risk of sepsis.

B. **Infant at low risk for sepsis.** Newborns without risk factors noted previously are at low risk of sepsis.

IV. **Data base**

A. **Complete maternal, perinatal, and birth history** should be obtained and reviewed in an attempt to identify risk factors. Maternal history is just as important as the birth history.

B. **Physical examination.** Perform a complete physical examination, searching for signs of sepsis (see section II,G). *Note:* Clinical observation is important. One study found that affect, peripheral perfusion, and respiratory status were key predictors in sepsis compared with feeding patterns, level of activity, and level of alertness. The **maternal clinical examination** should be reviewed with the OB/GYN service.

C. **Laboratory studies**

1. **Complete white blood cell (WBC) count.** An abnormally low or high WBC count is worrisome. Values <6000/mcg or >30,000/mcg in the first 24 h of life are abnormal. A band neutrophil count >20% is abnormal. The total leukocyte count is a very unreliable indicator of infection. A normal WBC count does not rule out sepsis. Only half of infants with WBC <5000 or WBC >20,000 have positive blood cultures. The total neutrophil count can be calculated, and normal reference ranges can be found in Tables 54–1 and 54–2. It is important to remember that **a single WBC count is not very helpful.** It is important to **repeat the WBC count** in 4–6 h. Studies reveal that repeating the WBC count helps to increase the validity of the test when it is used to screen for sepsis.

2. **Peripheral blood cultures.** Antibiotic removal device (ARD) bottles should be used if the mother has been receiving antibiotics.

3. **Suprapubic aspiration of urine for urinalysis and culture** (*controversial*). Many institutions do not perform this procedure in newborn infants with possible sepsis on day 1 of life because newborns rarely present with a urinary tract infection the first day.

4. **Lumbar puncture for cerebrospinal fluid examination** is indicated if a decision is made to give antibiotics. This measure is *controversial;* some institutions perform a lumbar puncture only if the infant has signs of central nervous system infection.

5. **Maternal laboratory tests**
   a. **Maternal endocervical culture for GBS.**
   b. **Endocervical culture for chlamydia and gonorrhea.**
   c. **Urinary analysis and culture.**
   d. **Any other pertinent laboratory values.**

6. **Baseline serum glucose levels.**

7. **Arterial blood gas levels.**

8. **Antigen detection assays.** These include the latex agglutination test for GBS, counterimmunoelectrophoresis (CIE), and bacterial antigens (GBS, *Streptococcus pneumoniae,* and *Escherichia coli* are available). These tests can be done on serum, urine, and cerebrospinal fluid.

9. **Other laboratory tests that are sometimes used to help diagnose sepsis.** None of the following tests should be used alone to diagnose sepsis. If used together, or **repeated values** become more abnormal, they may help in deciding who should receive antibiotics.
   a. **Total neutrophil count** (is more sensitive than the total leukocyte count but too often normal in case of infection). See Tables 54–1 and 54–2.
   b. **Total immature neutrophil count** (is poorly sensitive; could have a better positive predictive value). See Tables 54–1 and 54–2.
   c. **Ratio of immature to total neutrophils (I–T)** (greatest value relies on good negative predictive value; likelihood of infection is minimal if I–T ratio is normal). See Tables 54–1 and 54–2.
   d. **C-reactive protein (CRP).** This is a quantitative test. Normal values are ≤1 mg/dL. An increasing CRP is worrisome. The main interest of

TABLE 54–1. NEONATAL NEUTROPHIL INDICES REFERENCE RANGES (per mm³)

Variable	Birth	12 h	24 h	48 h	72 h	>120 h
Absolute neutrophil count[a]	1800–5400	7800–14,400	7200–12,600	4200–9000	1800–7000	1800–5400
Immature neutrophil count[b]	<1120	<1440	<1280	<800	<500	<500
I:T ratio[c]	<0.16	<0.16	<0.13	<0.13	<0.13	<0.12

[a]Total count includes mature and immature forms.
[b]Includes all neutrophils except segmented ones.
[c]Ratio of absolute neutrophil count divided by immature neutrophil count.
Based on data from Manroe BL et al: The neonatal blood count in health and disease: I. Reference values for neutrophilic cells. *J Pediatr* 1979;95:89.

CRP would be its good negative predictive value if repeated over 1–3 days.
   e. **Erythrocyte sedimentation rates.** These are increased with infection. This has a very limited value in diagnosing or monitoring infection.
   f. **Gastric aspirate stain and culture.**
10. **Laboratory tests that could be helpful in screening for sepsis but are not routinely used because of their lack of availability:**
   a. **Cytokines.** Elevated levels of tumor necrosis factor-alpha (TNF-α) and interleukin-6 (IL-6) may be helpful in diagnosing sepsis.
   b. **Fibrinogen.** Plasma fibrinogen levels increase with infection.
   c. **Fibronectin.** Decreased fibronectin levels may be an early marker for sepsis.
D. **Radiologic studies.** If there are signs of respiratory infection, obtain a chest x-ray to rule out pneumonia.

V. **Plan**
A. **General measures.** For the majority of cases, a decision about whether an infant requires a sepsis workup and antibiotics is usually straightforward. These infants either are clinically sick or have a positive history of an increased risk for sepsis and some clinical signs, thereby making the antibiotic decision easy. However, if an infant does not have a clear-cut history and clinical presentation, the decision is difficult. It is important to remember that one single test is often not helpful and to "repeat, repeat, and repeat" the test. Once the decision is made to treat the infant, treatment usually involves 48 h of antibiotics after obtaining cultures. The following guidelines can be used to help make the decision to treat:
   1. **Use of septic scoring systems.** Some institutions have devised their own septic scoring systems to help decide which infants should be treated. Many studies of scoring systems (that use a varied combination of the laboratory tests mentioned previously) have shown that they all have limited

TABLE 54–2. REFERENCE RANGES FOR NEUTROPHIL COUNTS IN VERY LOW BIRTH WEIGHT INFANTS (<1500 g)

Age	Absolute neutrophil count (mm³)
Birth	500–6000
18 h	2200–14,000
60 h	1100–8800
120 h	1100–5600

Based on data from Mouzinho A et al: Revised reference ranges for circulating neutrophils in very-low-birth-weight neonates. *Pediatrics* 1994;94:76.

value in screening for sepsis. The accuracy of a negative panel was a better predictor than a positive panel.

2. **If no septic scoring system is used,** a few general guidelines can be followed when deciding whether or not to treat the infant.

a. **If the infant is symptomatic regardless of history and laboratory values, send culture specimens and initiate empiric antibiotic therapy.**

b. **In the presence of chorioamnionitis,** the infant should be treated whether or not the mother received antibiotics before delivery.

c. **In the presence of other risk factors,** including previous infant with GBS disease, GBS bacteriuria during pregnancy, delivery <37 weeks, and rupture of membranes >18 h:

   i. **Mother treated with more than 2 doses of antibiotics:** No treatment is recommended if infant is asymptomatic, but the infant should be observed for at least 48 h.

   ii. **Mother inadequately or not treated:**

   - Some centers would elect to observe the infant for at least 48 h. It is debated whether blood cultures and CBC should be obtained, because the CBC is poorly sensitive and the majority of infection occurs before the results of blood cultures are available.
   - Another option is to treat the infant after the blood culture and CBC are obtained. Some centers use selective neonatal chemoprophylaxis (SNC):penicillin G, 50,000 units intramuscularly for more than 2 kg and 25,000 units for <2 kg given within 1 h of birth. Send culture specimens to the laboratory, and initiate empiric antibiotic therapy.

d. **In the absence of risk factors, when GBS screen is obtained at 35–37 weeks' gestation:**

   i. **GBS screen is positive or unknown**

   (a) **If the mother was treated with more than 2 doses of antibiotics,** one option is to observe the infant for at least 48 h.

   (b) **If the mother was treated with less than 2 doses of antibiotics,** one option is to observe the infant for at least 48 h (+/– blood cultures and CBC). The second option is to treat (possibly with SNC) after collection of a blood culture and a CBC.

   ii. **GBS screen is negative.** No treatment is recommended, but it is preferable to observe the infant for 48 h.

B. **Antibiotic therapy**

1. **If the decision is to treat**

a. **Obtain cultures** of the blood, urine, and spinal fluid (cultures of urine and spinal fluid are *controversial*). Any other cultures that seem appropriate should be sent to the laboratory (if there is eye discharge, send a Gram's stain and culture and so on).

b. **Ampicillin and gentamicin** are the antibiotics most commonly used for empiric initial therapy in a newborn. (For specific dosing, see Chapter 80.)

2. **Discontinuing antibiotics** is another *controversial* topic. The following guidelines may be used:

a. **If the cultures are negative and the patient is doing well,** antibiotics may be stopped after 48–72 h. A normal I–T ratio and serial negative CRP might help to determine whether antibiotics can be stopped because of their high negative predictive value.

b. **If the cultures are negative but the infant had signs of sepsis,** some clinicians treat the infant for 7–10 days.

c. **If the cultures are positive,** treat accordingly.

55 Pulmonary Hemorrhage

I. **Problem.** Grossly bloody secretions are seen in the endotracheal tube. Pulmonary hemorrhage occurs in 0.8–1.2 per 1000 live births. It occurs most commonly in acutely ill infants on mechanical ventilation and between 2 and 4 days of age. The mortality rate is higher immediately after pulmonary hemorrhage.

II. **Immediate questions**

   A. **Are any other signs or symptoms abnormal?** Typically, an infant with pulmonary hemorrhage is a ventilated low birth weight infant, 2–4 days old (usually in the first week of life). The infant has a sudden deterioration in respiratory status. The infant suddenly becomes hypoxic, has severe retractions, and may experience associated pallor, shock, apnea, bradycardia, and cyanosis.

   B. **Is the infant hypoxic? Has a blood transfusion recently been given?** Hypoxia or hypervolemia (usually caused by overtransfusion) may cause an acute rise in the pulmonary capillary pressure and lead to pulmonary hemorrhage.

   C. **Is bleeding occurring from other sites?** If there is bleeding from multiple sites, coagulopathy may be present, and coagulation studies should be obtained. Volume replacement with colloid or blood products may be needed.

   D. **What is the hematocrit (Hct) of the tracheal blood?** If the Hct is close to the venous Hct, it represents a true hemorrhage, and the blood is usually from trauma, aspiration of maternal blood, or bleeding diathesis. If the Hct is 15–20 percentage points lower than the venous Hct, the bleeding probably represents hemorrhagic edema fluid. This is seen with the majority of cases of pulmonary hemorrhage (such as those secondary to patent ductus arteriosus [PDA], surfactant therapy, and left-sided heart failure; see others discussed later).

III. **Differential diagnosis**

   A. **Direct trauma.** Trauma to the airway may be a result of nasotracheal or endotracheal intubation. Vigorous suctioning can also cause trauma to tissues and bleeding. Trauma during chest tube insertion can cause hemorrhage.

   B. **Aspiration of gastric or maternal blood** is often seen after cesarean section. The majority of blood is usually obtained from the nasogastric tube, but blood may be seen in the endotracheal tube.

   C. **Coagulopathy** may be related to sepsis or congenital. This is a rare cause of pulmonary hemorrhage but may exacerbate the problem.

   D. **Other disorders associated with pulmonary hemorrhage**
   1. **Hypoxia.**
   2. **Hypervolemia** is often the result of overtransfusion.
   3. **Congestive heart failure** (especially in pulmonary edema caused by PDA).
   4. **Respiratory distress syndrome.**
   5. **Severe Rh incompatibility.**
   6. **Pneumonia** caused by gram-negative organisms is commonly associated with pulmonary hemorrhage.
   7. **Hemorrhagic disease of the newborn** resulting from failure to administer vitamin K.
   8. **Intrauterine growth retardation.**
   9. **Severe hypothermia.**
   10. **Surfactant administration.** Pulmonary hemorrhage has occurred within hours of surfactant therapy. The cause is not definite but may be related to a rapid increase in pulmonary blood flow (PBF) because of improved lung function after surfactant treatment. The marked increase of PBF may cause hemorrhagic pulmonary edema. Reports show a significant relation-

ship between pulmonary hemorrhage and a clinical PDA in surfactant-treated infants.
11. **Mechanical ventilation.**
12. **Infection.**
13. **Oxygen therapy.**

IV. **Data base**
  A. **Physical examination.** Note the presence of other bleeding sites, signs of pneumonia or other infection, or congestive heart failure.
  B. **Laboratory studies**
    1. **Complete blood cell count with differential and platelet count.** With pneumonia or other infection, results of these studies may be abnormal. Thrombocytopenia may be seen. The Hct should be checked to determine whether excessive blood loss has occurred.
    2. **Coagulation profile (prothrombin time, partial thromboplastin time, thrombin time, and fibrinogen level)** may reveal coagulation disorders.
    3. **Arterial blood gas levels** will detect hypoxia.
    4. **Apt test,** if aspiration of maternal blood is suspected (rarely needed) (see Chapter 31, p 220).
  C. **Radiologic and other studies.** A chest x-ray study will rule out pneumonia, respiratory distress syndrome, and congestive heart failure. In a pulmonary hemorrhage, x-ray findings depend on whether the hemorrhage is focal (patchy, linear, or nodular densities) or massive (the film shows a complete white-out). The chest x-ray film can also be clear.

V. **Plan**
  A. **Emergency measures**
    1. **Suction the airway** initially until bleeding subsides.
    2. **Increase the oxygen concentration.**
    3. **Increase the positive end-expiratory pressure (PEEP)** to 0–8 cm H_2O; it may cause tamponade of the capillaries. Sometimes higher levels are required to stop the bleeding.
    4. **Consider increasing the peak inspiratory pressure (PIP)** if bleeding does not subside to improve ventilation and raise the mean airway pressure.
    5. **Consider giving epinephrine** through the endotracheal tube (controversial). This may cause constriction of the pulmonary capillaries.
  B. **If mechanical ventilation is not being used,** consider initiating its use in providing the treatments outlined previously.
  C. **General measures**
    1. **Support and correct the blood pressure** with volume expansion and colloids (see Chapter 46: Hypotension and Shock).
    2. **Correct acidosis.**
    3. **Blood volume and Hct** should be restored with transfusion, if necessary. However, in many cases the infant has not had a large volume loss; thus, administering excessive fluid volume may only worsen the situation (an increased left atrial pressure may increase the pulmonary edema.)
    4. **Treat the underlying disorder.**
  D. **Specific therapy**
    1. **Direct nasotracheal or endotracheal trauma.** If there is significant bleeding immediately after an endotracheal or nasotracheal intubation, trauma is the most likely cause; surgical consultation is indicated.
    2. **Aspiration of maternal blood.** If the infant is stable, no treatment is needed because the condition is typically self-limited.
    3. **Coagulopathy**
      a. **Hemorrhagic disease of the newborn.** Vitamin K, 1 mg intravenously, should be given.
      b. **Other coagulopathies.** Fresh-frozen plasma, 10 mL/kg every 12–24 h, may be given. If the platelet count is low, transfuse 1 unit and monitor closely. Monitor the prothrombin time, partial thromboplastin time, platelet count, and fibrinogen level.

56 Sedation and Analgesia in a Neonate

I. **Problem.** An infant with pulmonary hypertension with extreme lability needs sedation. Should the infant be sedated, and which agent is available to use?

II. **Immediate questions**

A. **What is the indication for the sedation?** Agitation and movement by the infant during procedures such as extracorporeal membrane oxygenation (ECMO) can risk injury. Certain procedures (eg, magnetic resonance imaging [MRI]) mandate that the infant be immobilized, so sedation is required. Infants with extreme lability on mechanical ventilation may benefit from sedation.

B. **Why does the infant need analgesia?** If the newborn is to undergo procedures such as elective circumcision, local analgesia is usually administered. For emergency procedures such as chest tube placement, the need for analgesia must be weighed against the delay of administering the analgesic agent.

C. **If treating for agitation while an infant is on mechanical ventilation, is the infant adequately ventilated?** Hypoxia and inadequate ventilation can result in agitation, and sedation is dangerous in these situations.

D. **Is sedation needed for a short period (ie, for a diagnostic procedure) or long-term?** Certain medications are indicated for short-term sedation (ie, chloral hydrate) and should not be used long-term.

III. **Differential diagnosis and indications**

A. **Indications for analgesia.** Whether a newborn can experience pain remains in the philosophical realm, but they undeniably react to painful stimuli (nociception). Such stimuli elicit both clinical symptoms (eg, tachycardia, hypertension, and decreased oxygenation) and complex behavioral responses in term as well as preterm infants. By 23 weeks' gestation, the nervous system has developed sufficiently to enable the conduction of nociceptive stimuli from peripheral skin receptors up to the cortical regions of the brain. The development of the descending inhibiting pathways occurs at a later stage. Because of this, the more immature infant may have an even lower threshold for noxious stimulus than at a later age. Possibly neonates have an increased sensitivity to pain compared with older age groups. During surgical interventions, the neonate (including the preterm infant), like the adult, mounts a large hormonal response that consists of the release of catecholamines, β-endorphins, corticotropin, growth hormone, and glucagon as well as the suppression of insulin secretion. This hormonal response is reduced by prior administration of appropriate analgesia or anesthesia. Although we do not know whether or not the neonate experiences psychological distress and lasting psychological sequelae, there are enough reasons to attempt to control exposure to pain as well as other unpleasant experiences.

1. **Major surgical procedures** such as ligation of the ductus arteriosus, laparotomy, and placement of a central venous catheter require anesthesia. General anesthesia should be provided by inhalation of anesthetic gases or intravenous (IV) administration of narcotic agents. In all these conditions, **the use of paralytic agents without analgesia is absolutely contraindicated.**

2. **Postoperative management**

a. **Narcotic agents should always be included in the immediate postoperative period.** Supplementary sedation is often provided by benzodiazepines or chloral hydrate, which are useful to combat agitation and potentiate the effect of opiates. It is important to remember that these

sedative agents do not have any analgesic effect and, therefore, cannot be given alone to relieve pain.
   b. **Other pain-relieving agents have, in general, little role in postoperative management.** Acetaminophen has only a weak analgesic effect and should be indicated at this age mostly for its antipyretic action. Aspirin should not be given in neonates for risk of bleeding.
3. **Minor surgical procedures.** Analgesia for "minor" procedures is mostly provided by local anesthesia, at times supplemented by small doses of opiates or sedative agents.
   a. **Unless the child's condition requires extreme urgent action, provide analgesia for procedures** such as chest tube insertion and vascular cutdown.
   b. **The need for analgesia for circumcision** is becoming less controversial and is now widely accepted.
   c. **The effectiveness and need for analgesia for more minor procedures** such as lumbar puncture have not been demonstrated.
4. **"Stressful" conditions.** There is wide controversy with regard to providing analgesia or sedation in "stressful" conditions, akin to "anxiolysis" in the adult and pediatric population. The period during which mechanical ventilation and its related routine procedures are provided has been identified as the most frequent time when infants are being "stressed."
   a. **The arguments to favor analgesia or sedation for these situations are as follows:**
      i. **It reduces the level of various biochemical markers** of stress such as blood levels of catecholamines, cortisol, and β-endorphin.
      ii. **It lessens the duration of hypoxemia** associated with endotracheal suctioning.
      iii. **Additional argument for its use** involves the difficulty in diagnosing discomfort and pain when the infant is under muscle paralysis.
   b. **The arguments against such routine use of analgesia or sedation are as follows:**
      i. **The pharmacokinetic characteristics of narcotic agents** in the preterm infant are variable and not always predictable.
      ii. The same assumed safe dose for some infants can, for others, result in severe hemodynamic and respiratory depression as well as toxic accumulation, leading to a transient comatose state.
      iii. **The prolonged use** (sometimes as little as 4 days) of narcotic and sedative agents has been associated with the rapid development of tolerance, withdrawal, and encephalopathy and the requirement for higher ventilatory support in the early phase of respiratory distress syndrome. Furthermore, it often delays weaning from mechanical ventilation.
      iv. **Treating for "agitation"** by sedation can be dangerous when the former is the result of inadequate ventilation or hypoxemia. Therefore, before treating agitation, one must always ensure, by careful physical examination, that the endotracheal tube is not obstructed or misplaced and that adequate ventilating pressures are being used.
B. **Indications for sedation**
   1. **Extreme respiratory lability.** Infants who have demonstrated extreme respiratory lability develop hypoxemia rapidly with minimal handling. Infants with severe pulmonary hypertension and pulmonary vascular hyperreactivity are often candidates for sedation.
   2. **Therapeutic procedures.** When it is necessary to prevent the child from moving vigorously (eg, during ECMO), sedation may be needed to prevent accidental dislodgment of the vascular cannulas.
   3. **Diagnostic procedures.** Procedures that require the child to be immobilized include imaging procedures such as MRI, cardiac catheterization, and occasionally computed tomography (CT) scan.

IV. Data base

A. Physical examination. Before instituting any type of sedation or analgesia, there must be a clear diagnosis. The physical examination is directed at the underlying condition.

B. Laboratory studies. These are usually not needed, except in the context of the underlying disease.

C. Radiologic and other studies. Such studies are usually not needed, except in the context of the underlying disease.

V. Plan

A. General management. Prevention of distress and pain should be a priority in the neonatal unit and in newborn nurseries. Measures to prevent or minimize stress in the neonate should include the following:

1. **Reduce noise (eg, close the incubator door gently).**
2. **Protect the infant from intense light.**
3. **Cluster blood drawings as much as possible.**
4. **Use a spring-loaded lance for heelstick phlebotomy.**
5. **Replace tape with a self-adhesive bandage.**
6. **Perform intratracheal suctioning only if indicated.**
7. **Use adequate medication before invasive procedures.**

B. Specific agents (see also Chapter 80)

1. **Pharmacologic management provided by systemic analgesia**

   a. **Opiates.** All opiates may lead to respiratory depression and hypotension. Muscular rigidity is seen mostly with the synthetic opiates with rapid IV administration, such as fentanyl (≥10 mcg/kg), sufentanil, or especially alfentanil. Muscular rigidity can be counteracted by use of a muscle-relaxing agent (eg, pancuronium) and acutely reversed by naloxone (0.1 mg/kg).

      i. **Morphine sulfate.** IV bolus: 50–200 mcg/kg; IV infusion: 10–40 mcg/kg/h. The peak action occurs in 20 min and lasts for 2–4 h in full-term infants and 6–8 h in preterm infants.

      ii. **Fentanyl (Sublimaze).** This has a shorter duration of action than morphine and does not compromise myocardial function. The dose for anesthesia is IV bolus, 10–50 mcg/kg, and for analgesia, 1–4 mcg/kg. A continuous IV infusion of 1–3 mcg/kg/h may be used for ongoing sedation.

      iii. **Meperidine (Demerol).** Give 1 mg/kg every 4–6 h IV, intramuscularly, or orally.

      iv. **Alfentanil.** Give 20 mcg/kg or by continuous IV, 3–5 mcg/kg/h. (*Note:* Alfentanil has a higher incidence of chest wall rigidity and hypotension than fentanyl; therefore, its use should be discouraged in neonates.)

      v. **Sufentanil.** Give 0.2 mcg/kg over 20 minutes. By continous IV, 0.05 mcg/kg/h.

   b. **Ketamine** can provide anesthesia for a short duration at 0.5–2 mcg/kg per dose. Often used in association with midazolam. Its utilization in the neonatal intensive care unit has been limited. It may be of value, possibly in combination with atropine sulfate, for sedation before endotracheal intubation. Infants with severe bronchopulmonary dysplasia and refractory bronchospasm may also benefit from the use of ketamine for its additional bronchodilatory effect.

2. **Pharmacologic management provided by local analgesia**

   a. **Subcutaneous infiltration with lidocaine,** 0.5% concentration. Use solution without epinephrine.

   b. **Percutaneous administration of EMLA cream.** This is a eutectic mixture (ie, liquid at room temperature) of 2.5% lidocaine and 2.5% prilocaine. A single dose of 0.5–1.25 g of EMLA cream applied under an occlusive dressing provides adequate local anesthesia 60–80 min later. In the term infant, it may be an alternative to penile dorsal block for anesthesia during circumcision. The risk of methemoglobinemia (from prilocaine) may restrict its use to the full-term infant, and repeated doses should be avoided.

3. **Pharmacologic management provided by sedative-hypnotics**
   a. **Benzodiazepines**
      i. **Midazolam (Versed)** has a rapid onset of action (1–2 min) and can produce apnea if given too rapidly. Its very short half-life (1–2 h) makes it a good choice for brief rapid sedation. Midazolam is given as a single dose, 50–100 mcg/kg, or by continuous infusion at a rate of 0.4–0.6 mcg/kg/min. Withdrawal may occur when given continuously for >48 h.
      ii. **Lorazepam (Ativan)** has a longer duration of action and may require less frequent dosing (50–100 mcg/kg every 8 h).
   b. **Barbiturates.** Phenobarbital has a slow onset and long duration of action. The loading dose is 10–20 mcg/kg.
   c. **Chloral hydrate.** This sedative-hypnotic is used primarily for short-term sedation. It is especially useful during diagnostic procedures such as CT scan and MRI. It can be administered either orally or rectally. The onset of action is usually within 10–15 min. Administer 20–40 mg/kg every 6–8 h for sedation. It should not be used long-term.
   d. **Acetaminophen.** The usual dose is 10 mg/kg every 6–8 h. The jaundiced neonate should receive a reduced dose of 5 mg/kg.
4. **Nonpharmacologic management.** Physical measures such as the use of swaddling, containment, or facilitated tucking as well as skin-to-skin contact with the mother are likely to be efficacious in decreasing the noxious effect of the "routine procedures" (such as heelstick) needed for the management of the sick infant.

   Sucrose reduces procedural pain in the neonate. The effective dose is ~2 ml of a 12% sucrose solution given by syringe or pacifier 2 min before procedures such as heelstick or venipuncture. The potential risk for fluid overload, hyperglycemia, and necrotizing enterocolitis should limit this method to infants >34 weeks' gestation.

REFERENCE

Anand KJS: Consensus statement for the prevention and management of pain in the newborn. *Arch Pediatr Adolesc Med* 2001;155:173.

57 Seizure Activity

I. **Problem.** The nurse reports that an infant is having abnormal movements of the extremities consistent with seizure activity. Neonatal seizures are rarely idiopathic in the newborn and are a common manifestation of a serious central nervous system (CNS) disease. This is why quick intervention is necessary.

II. **Immediate questions**

A. **Is the infant really seizing?** This question is very important and is often initially difficult to answer. **Jitteriness** is sometimes confused with seizures. In a jittery infant, eye movements are normal. The hands will stop moving if they are grasped, and movements are of a fine nature. In an infant who is seizing, eye movements can be abnormal (eg, staring, blinking, nystagmoid jerks, or tonic horizontal eye deviation). The hands continue to move if grasped, and movements are of a coarser nature. The electroencephalogram (EEG) is normal with jitteriness and abnormal with seizure activity.

B. **Is there a history of birth asphyxia or risk factors for sepsis?** Asphyxia and sepsis with meningitis may cause neonatal seizures.

C. **What is the blood glucose level?** Hypoglycemia is an easily treatable cause of seizures in the neonatal period.

D. **How old is the infant?** The age of the infant is often the best clue to the cause of the seizures. Common causes for specific ages are as follows:

1. **At birth.** Maternal anesthetic agents: can see severe tonic seizures typically in the first few hours of life.

2. **Day 1.** Metabolic abnormalities such as hypoglycemia, hypocalcemia, hypoxic-ischemic encephalopathy (presenting at 6–18 h after birth and becoming more severe in the next 24–48 h).

3. **Days 2–3.** Drug withdrawal or meningitis.

4. **Day 5 or greater.** Hypocalcemia, TORCH infections (*t*oxoplasmosis, *o*ther, *r*ubella, *c*ytomegalovirus, and *h*erpes simplex virus), or developmental defects.

5. **More than 1–2 weeks.** Methadone withdrawal.

III. **Differential diagnosis.** See also Chapter 72.

A. **Seizure activity** may be secondary to the following conditions:

1. **Hypoxic-ischemic cerebral injury.**

2. **Intracranial hemorrhage,** including subarachnoid, periventricular-intraventricular, or subdural.

3. **Neonatal cerebral infarction** is a common cause of seizures in **full-term** infants. Its origin remains unclear, but it is found in ~1 in 4000 infants.

4. **Metabolic abnormalities**
   a. **Hypoglycemia.**
   b. **Hypocalcemia.**
   c. **Hypomagnesemia.**
   d. **Hyponatremia or hypernatremia.**
   e. **Pyridoxine dependence.**

5. **Infection**
   a. **Meningitis.**
   b. **Sepsis.**
   c. **TORCH infections.**

6. **Neonatal drug withdrawal** (discussed in Chapter 67). Seizures are an uncommon manifestation of withdrawal. One can see abnormalities on the EEG or seizures in infants exposed to maternal cocaine abuse in utero.

7. **Inborn errors of metabolism** (see also Chapter 65).
   a. **Maple syrup urine disease.**

  b. **Methylmalonic acidemia.**
  c. **Nonketotic hyperglycinemia.**
  8. **Maternal anesthetic agents (rare cause).** If a local anesthetic (eg, mepivacaine) is accidentally injected into the infant's scalp during a pudendal, paracervical, or epidural block, seizures can occur at birth.
  9. **Drug toxicity.** Agents such as theophylline.
  10. **Developmental abnormalities.** Cerebral malformations can cause seizures. Often, the infant will have obvious anomalies of the face or head if developmental abnormalities are present.
  11. **CNS trauma.** Usually, there is a history of a difficult delivery.
  12. **Hydrocephalus.** Twenty percent of infants with periventricular or intraventricular hemorrhage will develop posthemorrhagic hydrocephalus.
  13. **Polycythemia** with hyperviscosity.
  14. **Four epileptic syndromes that present in the newborn period:**
     a. **Benign familial neonatal seizures.** Presents usually on the third day of life.
     b. **Fifth day fits.** Benign syndrome.
     c. **Early myoclonic encephalopathy.** Presents within hours of birth. Infants usually die within the first 2 years of life.
     d. **Early infantile epileptic encephalopathy (Ohtahara's syndrome).** Severe epileptic syndrome.
  B. **Jitteriness.** This benign condition is differentiated from seizures as described in section II,A.
  C. **Benign myoclonic activity.** These isolated jerky, nonrepetitive movements of an extremity or other part of the body occur mainly during sleep and are benign.
IV. **Data base**
  A. **History.** A detailed history will help in diagnosing seizure activity. The nurse or physician observing the activity should record a complete description of the event on the chart.
  B. **Physical examination.** Perform a complete physical examination, with close attention to the neurologic status. Look at the scalp for evidence of injection.
  C. **Laboratory studies**
    1. **Metabolic work-up**
      a. **Serum glucose level.** If the glucose level on paper-strip testing is <40 mg/dL, obtain a serum glucose value from the laboratory.
      b. **Serum sodium level.**
      c. **Serum ionized and total calcium levels.** Only an ionized calcium level is usually necessary, but if this test cannot be done, a total calcium study should be ordered. Ionized calcium is the most accurate measurement of calcium.
      d. **Serum magnesium level.**
    2. **Infection workup**
      a. **Complete blood cell count with differential.** A hematocrit will also rule out polycythemia.
      b. **Blood, urine, and cerebrospinal fluid (CSF) cultures (for bacteria and viruses).**
      c. **Serum immunoglobulin M (IgM)- and IgM-specific TORCH titers.** The serum IgM titer may be elevated in TORCH infections.
    3. **Urine drug screening,** if drug withdrawal is suspected.
    4. **Theophylline level,** if the infant is on this medication and toxicity is suspected.
    5. **Blood gas levels** to rule out hypoxia or acidosis.
    6. **Coagulation studies** (if there is evidence of hemorrhage).
    7. **Studies for inborn errors of metabolism** (serum ammonia, lactate, CSF lactate, urine organic acids/serum amino acids).
  D. **Radiologic and other studies**

1. **Ultrasound examination of the head.** This will confirm periventricular-intraventricular hemorrhage (PV-IVH). (**Note:** The coexistence of IVH and seizures does not necessarily mean the two are related.)
2. **Computed tomography (CT) scan of the head.** A CT scan can be done to diagnose subarachnoid or subdural hemorrhage. It may also reveal a congenital malformation. It is also done if cerebral infarction is suspected.
3. **Lumbar puncture.** The presence of blood in the CSF suggests IVH. Cultures of the fluid should be done to diagnose infection. (See Chapter 24.)
4. **Electroencephalography (EEG).** It is usually not possible to perform an EEG during the episode of seizure activity. The EEG is rarely helpful in making a specific diagnosis. This study should be done at some time after seizure activity has been documented. It may confirm seizure activity and may also be used as a baseline study. It will also show changes consistent with the localization of the lesion in cerebral infarction. The interictal pattern is also helpful in predicting future seizure activity.
5. **Magnetic resonance angiography.** This can be used and is helpful in making the diagnosis of cerebral infarction.

V. Plan
A. **General measures.** Once it is determined that the infant is having seizures, because the other two diagnoses (jitteriness and benign myoclonic activity) are benign conditions, the following measures should be taken. Immediate management is necessary.
   1. **Rule out hypoxia.** Send a blood sample to the laboratory for measurement of blood gases, and start oxygen therapy. Assess the infant's airway and breathing. Intubation and mechanical ventilation may be necessary to maintain ventilation and oxygenation. Correct any metabolic acidosis.
   2. **Check the glucose level.** A Dextrostix or Chemstrip-bG paper-strip test should be done to rule out hypoglycemia. Also, send a blood sample to the laboratory for a stat serum glucose level for confirmation of the paper-strip test result. If the paper-strip test shows low blood glucose, it is acceptable to give 10% glucose, 2–4 mL/kg by intravenous push, before obtaining results from the laboratory.
   3. **Obtain stat serum calcium, sodium, and magnesium levels.** If these levels were low on earlier values and a metabolic disorder is strongly suspected as the cause of the seizures, it is acceptable to treat the infant before new laboratory values are available. If serum magnesium levels are low, magnesium can also be given.
   4. **Anticonvulsant therapy.** If hypoxia and all metabolic abnormalities have been treated or if blood gas and metabolic workup values are normal, start anticonvulsant therapy. For detailed pharmacologic information, see Chapter 80.
      a. **Give phenobarbital as the first-line drug.** Initially, 20 mg/kg is given as the loading dose, but additional doses of 5mg/kg up to 40 mg/kg can be given if the seizures have not stopped.
      b. **If seizures persist,** give phenytoin (Dilantin), 20 mg/kg/dose, at a rate of 1 mg/kg/min or less. Fosphenytoin may be preferred (see dosage in Chapter 80). It has been associated with fewer side effects than phenytoin, but experience in neonates has been limited.
      c. **A trial of pyridoxine** with EEG monitoring is now recommended.
      d. **If seizures still persist,** the following drugs may be used (depending on institutional preference). If a benzodiazepine is used, respiratory depression is more likely to occur, but this is usually not a problem because most infants are already on mechanical ventilation.
         i. **Diazepam** is effective if given by a continuous infusion of 0.3 mg/kg/h.
         ii. **Lorazepam,** given intravenously, can be repeated 4–6 times in a 24-h period.
         iii. **Intravenous midazolam** has been found to be effective.

    iv. Oral carbamazepine has been found to be effective.

    v. Paraldehyde, given rectally, has usually been used as a last effort.

B. Specific measures

  1. **Hypoxic-ischemic injury.** Seizures secondary to birth asphyxia usually present at anywhere from 6–18 h of age.

    a. **Careful observation** by the physician and nursing staff is required to detect seizure activity.

    b. **Prophylactic phenobarbital** is used at some institutions (*controversial*).

    c. **Restrict fluids to ~60 mL/kg/day.** Monitor serum electrolytes and urine output.

    d. **If seizures begin,** follow the guidelines given in section V,A,4.

  2. **Hypoglycemia.** Treat and determine the cause, as outlined in Chapter 43.

  3. **Hypocalcemia.** Slowly give 100–200 mg/kg calcium gluconate intravenously. Make certain that the infant is receiving maintenance calcium therapy (usually 50 mg/kg every 6 h). Monitor the heart rate continuously, and make sure that the intravenous line is correctly positioned.

  4. **Hypomagnesemia.** Give 0.2 mEq/kg magnesium sulfate intravenously every 6 h until magnesium levels are normal or symptoms resolve.

  5. **Hyponatremia.** See Chapter 45.

  6. **Hypernatremia.** Treat the seizure activity as described in section V,A,4. If hypernatremia is secondary to decreased fluid intake, increase the rate of free water. The amount of sodium needs to be decreased; it should be reduced over 48 h to decrease the possibility of cerebral edema.

  7. **Hypercalcemia.** Usual treatment plans include the following.

    a. **Increase intravenous fluids by 20 mL/kg/day.**

    b. **Administer a diuretic** (eg, furosemide [Lasix], 1–2 mg/kg/dose every 12 h).

    c. **Administer phosphate, 30–40 mg/kg/day** orally or intravenously.

  8. **Pyridoxine dependence.** Pyridoxine, 50–100 mg, is given intravenously with EEG monitoring. Confirmation of pyridoxine dependence is the cessation of seizures on EEG with treatment.

  9. **Infection.** If sepsis is suspected, a complete workup should be performed and empiric broad-spectrum antibiotic therapy initiated. Antiviral therapy (acyclovir) should be considered in infants 2–3 weeks of age (for treatment of herpes simplex virus encephalitis). A complete septic workup includes white blood cell count with differential, blood culture, urine and serum antigen test (Wellcogen), lumbar puncture and culture for bacteria and viruses (if indicated), and urinalysis and urine culture (if indicated).

 10. **Drug withdrawal syndrome.** Supportive therapy and anticonvulsants are used. See Chapter 67.

 11. **Subarachnoid hemorrhage.** Only supportive therapy is necessary.

 12. **Subdural hemorrhage.** Only supportive therapy is necessary, unless the infant has lacerations of the falx and tentorium for which rapid surgical correction is necessary. Hemorrhage over cerebral convexities is treated by subdural taps.

 13. **CNS trauma.** In cases of depressed skull fracture, elevation of the bone may be necessary.

 14. **Hydrocephalus.** Repeated lumbar taps may be necessary, or a shunt may be placed.

 15. **Polycythemia.** Partial plasma exchange is necessary. See Chapter 21.

 16. **Cerebral infarction**

    a. **Supportive therapy.**

    b. **Treat the seizures.** Some resolve and others progress to epilepsy.

    c. **Close follow-up** is necessary because of possible neurologic sequelae (eg, hemiplegia, cognitive difficulties, delays in language acquisition, and developmental delay).

    d. **Most of the cases** have a normal outcome.

 17. **Accidental injection.** Vigorous support and removal of the drug by diuresis is recommended.

58 Traumatic Delivery

I. **Problem.** An infant is noted to have severe bruises after birth, and a nurse observes that the infant is not using his or her right arm. The birth was traumatic, and he or she calls you to evaluate the infant. Birth injuries are injuries that occur during the birth process. The incidence is ~2–7 per 1000 live births.

II. **Immediate questions**
   A. **Is there any reason the infant would have a birth injury?** Certain factors predispose the infant to birth injuries. These include macrosomia, dystocia, prolonged labor, abnormal presentation (especially breech), cephalopelvic disproportion, and prematurity.
   B. **Is the injury so serious that it requires immediate attention?** The majority of birth injuries are not serious and do not require immediate treatment. Significant injuries requiring immediate intervention, such as abdominal organ injuries that present as shock and require surgery, need to be identified early. It is important to distinguish and recognize the different injuries so that appropriate treatment can be given.
   C. **Were forceps or vacuum extraction used during the delivery?** Studies suggest that the use of midforceps and vacuum extraction may increase the infant's risk of fractures and paralysis.

III. **Differential diagnosis**
   A. **Skin**
      1. **Petechiae.** In birth trauma, petechiae are usually localized (eg, on the head, neck, upper chest area, and lower back). There is no associated bleeding, and no new lesions appear. If petechiae are diffuse, suspect systemic disease. If there is associated bleeding, suspect disseminated intravascular coagulation.
      2. **Forceps injury.** Frequently, linear marks are seen across both sides of the face. The area is usually red.
      3. **Subcutaneous fat necrosis.** Typically, this involves the shoulders and the buttocks with a well-circumscribed lesion of the skin and underlying tissue. It usually appears between 6 and 10 days of age. Lesion size is 1–10 cm. It can be irregular and hard, and the overlying skin can be purple or colorless.
      4. **Ecchymoses.** Bruising can occur after a traumatic delivery, especially when labor is rapid or the infant is premature.
      5. **Lacerations.** Lacerations can occur secondary to the use of a scalpel during a cesarean section. They usually occur on the buttocks, scalp, or thigh.
   B. **Head**
      1. **Caput succedaneum.** This is an area of edema over the presenting part of the scalp during a vertex delivery. The area of edema is usually associated with bruising and petechiae. It crosses the midline of the skull and suture lines. The bleeding is external to the periosteum.
      2. **Cephalhematoma.** This is caused by bleeding that occurs below the periosteum overlying one cranial bone (usually the parietal bone). **There is no crossing of the suture lines.** The overlying scalp is not discolored, and the swelling sometimes takes days to become apparent. The incidence of associated skull fracture is 5–10% and is most often a linear fracture.
      3. **Subgaleal hemorrhage.** This is a collection of blood in the soft tissue space under the aponeurosis but above the periosteum of the skull. Diffuse swelling of the soft tissue, often spreading toward the neck and behind the ears, can be seen. Periorbital swelling is also evident. Associated symptoms include anemia, hypotonia, seizures, and pallor.

  4. Intracranial hemorrhage
  a. Subarachnoid. This is usually asymptomatic. Seizures and other complications are rare.
  b. Epidural. This is very rare and also very difficult to diagnose. Clinical symptoms are usually delayed.
  c. Subdural. These infants present shortly after birth with stupor, seizures, a full fontanelle, unresponsive pupils, and coma.
  5. Skull fracture. These are uncommon in neonates; most are linear and are associated with a cephalhematoma. Depressed fractures are often visible. Fractures at the base of the skull may result in shock.
C. Face
  1. Fractures. Fractures of the nose, mandible, maxilla, and septal cartilage can occur. These can often present as respiratory distress or feeding problems.
  2. Dislocations of the facial bones. Nasal septal dislocation (the most common facial injury) can occur and present as stridor and cyanosis.
  3. Facial nerve palsy. This often occurs secondary to forceps compressing the nerve.
  a. Central paralysis involves the lower half or two thirds of the contralateral side of the face. On the paralyzed side, the nasolabial fold is obliterated, the corner of the mouth droops, and the skin is smooth and full. When the infant cries, the wrinkles are deeper on the normal side and the mouth is drawn to the normal side.
  b. Peripheral paralysis involves the entire side of the face. At rest, the infant has an open eye on the affected side. When the infant cries, the findings are similar to those with central paralysis.
D. Eye
  1. Eyelids. Edema and bruising can occur. Swollen eyelids should be forced open to examine the eyeball. Laceration of the eyelid can also occur
  2. Orbit fracture can occur rarely. Immediate ophthalmologic evaluation is necessary if disturbances of the extraocular muscle movements and exophthalmos are evident. Severe injuries may result in death.
  3. Horner's syndrome (miosis, partial ptosis, enophthalmos, and anhidrosis of the ipsilateral side of the face). Delayed pigmentation of the ipsilateral iris can be seen.
  4. Subconjunctival hemorrhage. This is a common finding.
  5. Cornea. Haziness can occur secondary to edema. With persistent haziness, suspect rupture of Descemet's membrane.
  6. Intraocular hemorrhage
  a. Retinal hemorrhage can occur. Most commonly, a flame-shaped or streak hemorrhage is found near the optic disk. A sheet hemorrhage is associated with a subdural bleed.
  b. Hyphemas. Gross blood is seen in the anterior chamber.
  c. Vitreous hemorrhage. Indicated by floaters, absent red reflex, and blood pigment seen on slit-lamp exam by the ophthalmologist.
E. Ear. Ear injuries can occur because of forceps placed near the ears.
  1. Abrasions and bruising.
  2. Hematomas.
  3. Avulsion of the auricle. This can occur because of misplacement of the forceps.
  4. Laceration of the auricle.
F. Vocal cord injuries. Although these are rare, they can occur as a result of excessive traction on the head during delivery.
  1. Unilateral paralysis involves the recurrent laryngeal branch of one of the vagus nerves in the neck. Clinically, hoarseness and mild to moderate stridor with inspiration are seen.
  2. Bilateral paralysis is caused by trauma to both recurrent laryngeal nerves. Symptoms at birth include respiratory distress, stridor, and cyanosis.

G. Neck and shoulder injuries
  1. **Clavicular fracture.** This is the most common bone fracture during delivery. If the fracture is complete, symptoms involve decreased or absent movement of the arm, gross deformity of the clavicle, tenderness on palpation, localized crepitus, and an absent or asymmetric Moro's reflex. Greenstick fracture usually presents with no symptoms, and the diagnosis is made because of callus formation at 7–10 days.
  2. **Brachial palsy.** Trauma to the spinal roots of the fifth cervical through the first thoracic spinal nerves (brachial plexus) during birth. There are three different presentations.
      a. **Duchenne-Erb.** This involves the upper arm and is the most common type. The fifth and sixth cervical roots are affected, and the arm is adducted and internally rotated. Moro's reflex is absent (sometimes it can be asymmetric or weakened), but the grasp reflex is intact.
      b. **Klumpke.** This involves the lower arm, because the seventh and eighth cervical and first thoracic roots are injured, and is rare. The hand is paralyzed, the wrist does not move, and the grasp reflex is absent (ie, dropped hand). Cyanosis and edema of the hand can also occur. An ipsilateral Horner's syndrome (ptosis, miosis, and enophthalmos) can be seen because of injury involving the cervical sympathetic fibers of the first thoracic root. Phrenic nerve paralysis with Klumpke's palsy is evident.
      c. **Entire arm paralysis.** The patient will have a flaccid arm, hanging limply with no reflexes.
  3. **Phrenic nerve paralysis.** Difficult breech delivery can cause diaphragmatic paralysis. This usually occurs with upper brachial nerve palsy. It is associated with cyanosis, tachypnea, irregular respirations, and thoracic breathing with no bulging of the abdomen.
  4. **Sternocleidomastoid muscle (SCM) injury** (muscular or congenital torticollis). A well-circumscribed, immobile mass in the midportion of the SCM that enlarges, regresses, and disappears. This results in a transient torticollis after birth. The head tilts toward the involved side, the chin is elevated and rotated, and the patient cannot move the head into normal position.
H. Spinal cord injuries. These injuries are rare and are caused by stretching of the cord. Symptoms vary, depending on the location of the injury. The higher the injury, the greater is the risk of respiratory problems.
  1. **Infants with a high cervical lesion** usually have severe respiratory depression with paralysis at birth. There is a high rate of mortality.
  2. **Upper or midcervical lesions** usually present without symptoms but can have hypotonia. The mortality rate is high.
  3. **Lesions in the seventh** cervical to first thoracic roots present with paraplegia and urinary and respiratory problems.
  4. **Partial spinal cord injuries.** On neurologic examination, these infants have signs of spasticity.
I. Abdominal organ injuries. These injuries should be suspected with shock, increasing abdomen, anemia, and irritability. These infants can be asymptomatic for hours and then crash.
  1. **Liver rupture.** The liver is the most common organ affected. This presents with sudden circulatory collapse (a hematoma ruptures through the capsule).
  2. **Spleen rupture.** Blood loss and hemoperitoneum.
  3. **Adrenal hemorrhage.** Symptoms include fever, tachypnea, mass in the flank, pallor, cyanosis, poor feeding, shock, vomiting, and diarrhea.
  4. **Kidney damage.** Same as others; presents as ascites, flank mass, and gross hematuria.
J. Extremity injuries
  1. **Fractured humerus.** This is the second most common fracture during birth trauma. The arm is immobile, with tenderness and crepitation on palpation. Moro's reflex is absent on the affected side.

2. **Fractured femur.** This may occur secondary to breech delivery. Deformity is usually obvious. The affected leg does not move, and there is pain with assisted movement.
3. **Dislocation.** Rare, this usually involves the radial head. Examination reveals adduction, internal rotation of the affected arm, and poor Moro's reflex. Palpate lateral and posterior displacement of the radial head.
K. **Genital injuries**
   1. **Edema, bruising, and hematoma of the scrotum and penis** can occur, especially in large infants and breech deliveries. Injury does not affect micturition.
   2. **Testicular injury.** Testicular and epididymal injury can occur. Findings are scrotal swelling, with the infant experiencing vomiting and irritability. A **hematocele** can form if the tunica vaginalis testis is injured; the scrotum will not transilluminate.
IV. **Data base**
   A. **Physical examination**
      1. **Skin.** Look for petechiae, bruising, and any lacerations. Check the side of the face for forceps marks. Look for and palpate any area that looks like fat necrosis.
      2. **Head.** Carefully examine the head for any evidence of a caput succedaneum, cephalhematoma, subgaleal hemorrhage, or fracture. Check to see whether the suture lines are crossed; this helps one to differentiate between the caput succedaneum and cephalhematoma. Depressed skull fractures are obvious; others may require radiologic studies.
      3. **Face.** Examine the face at rest and during crying to look for any facial nerve palsy. Check for any signs of respiratory distress (eg, stridor or cyanosis).
      4. **Eyes.** Carefully examine the eyeball and the eyelid. Make sure that extraocular muscle movements are normal. Check for the red reflex.
      5. **Ears.** Carefully examine the front and back of the ear, looking for lacerations, swelling, and hematomas.
      6. **Vocal cords.** If injury is suspected, examine the vocal cords by direct laryngoscopy or use a flexible fiberoptic laryngoscope.
      7. **Neck and shoulder injuries.** Carefully examine the neck and the shoulder. Check Moro's and grasp reflexes. Examine the arm to see whether movement is normal. Check respirations, and note any thoracic breathing. Make sure that the head rests in a normal position and is not tilted.
      8. **Spinal cord.** A careful and thorough neurologic examination should be done.
      9. **Abdomen.** Examine the abdomen, and check for ascites, masses, and increase in size.
      10. **Extremities.** Observe for movement and deformity.
      11. **Genitalia.** Examine the testes and the penis; transilluminate the scrotum.
   B. **Laboratory studies**
      1. **Skin**
         a. **Platelet count.** A normal platelet count excludes neonatal thrombocytopenia.
         b. **Serum bilirubin test.** Hyperbilirubinemia may result from reabsorption of blood from extensive ecchymoses.
         c. **Serum hematocrit.** Anemia may result from severe ecchymoses.
      2. **Head**
         a. **Hematocrit.** Blood loss can occur, requiring transfusions, especially in subgaleal hemorrhage.
         b. **Serum bilirubin.** Significant hyperbilirubinemia may result.
      3. **Face.** Arterial blood gas may be indicated in those infants with respiratory distress.
      4. **Eyes.** No laboratory tests are usually required.
      5. **Ears.** No laboratory tests are usually required.

6. **Vocal cords.** No laboratory tests are usually required.
7. **Neck and shoulder.** Arterial blood gas will help diagnose hypoxia associated with phrenic nerve paralysis.
8. **Spinal cord.** The usual laboratory tests are required for respiratory depression and shock, if indicated.
9. **Abdomen**
   a. Hematocrit, to rule out anemia and blood loss.
   b. Urine dipstick, to check for hematuria.
   c. Abdominal paracentesis with fluid sent to the laboratory for cell count with differential.
10. **Extremities.** No laboratory tests are usually needed.
11. **Genitalia.** No laboratory tests are usually needed.

C. **Radiologic and other studies**
   1. **Skin.** No studies are usually needed.
   2. **Head.** Skull radiographs should be obtained to rule out the possibility of skull fractures. A computed tomography (CT) scan can also be obtained and can be useful in the diagnosis of an intracranial hemorrhage.
   3. **Face.** Radiographs and a cranial CT scan will help diagnose facial fractures.
   4. **Eyes.** Radiographs, to rule out orbit fracture, may be indicated.
   5. **Ears.** No radiologic studies are necessary.
   6. **Vocal cord injury.** No radiologic studies are necessary.
   7. **Neck and shoulder**
      a. **A radiograph of the clavicle** is necessary for confirmation of the diagnosis.
      b. **An x-ray film of the chest** for phrenic nerve paralysis will show an elevated diaphragm.
      c. **Fluoroscopy** reveals elevation of the affected side and descent of the normal side on inspiration: Opposite movements occur with expiration.
      d. **Ultrasonogram of the diaphragm** will show abnormal motion on the affected side.
   8. **Spinal cord**
      a. Cervical and thoracic spine radiographs should be obtained.
      b. Magnetic resonance imaging (MRI) is the most reliable method for diagnosing spinal cord injuries.
   9. **Abdomen.** Ultrasonogram will diagnose liver and splenic rupture, adrenal hemorrhage, and kidney damage.
   10. **Extremities.** An x-ray film of the extremities confirms the diagnosis.
   11. **Genitalia.** Ultrasonography may be diagnostic.

V. **Plan**
   A. **Skin**
      1. **Petechiae.** No specific treatment is necessary. Traumatic petechiae usually fade in 2–3 days.
      2. **Subcutaneous fat necrosis.** The lesions require minimal pressure at the affected site and observation only. They disappear within a couple of months. Closely monitor the first 6 weeks for symptomatic hypercalcemia (vomiting, fever, and weight loss with high serum calcium), which can occur in these infants. This can usually be treated with intravenous hydration, furosemide, and hydrocortisone therapy.
      3. **Ecchymoses.** No specific treatment is necessary, and they resolve within 1 week. Watch for hyperbilirubinemia (reabsorption of blood from a bruised area), anemia (blood loss from bruising), and hyperkalemia.
      4. **Lacerations.** If superficial, the edges may be held together with butterfly adhesive strips. If deeper, they should be sutured with 7-0 nylon. Healing is usually rapid.
   B. **Head**
      1. **Caput succedaneum.** No specific treatment is necessary. It resolves within several days.

2. **Cephalhematoma.** Usually no treatment is necessary, and it resolves anywhere between 2 weeks and 3 months. In some cases, blood loss and hyperbilirubinemia can occur.
3. **Subgaleal hemorrhage.** If hypovolemic shock develops, it requires immediate treatment. Surgery is done if the bleeding does not subside. Death may occur. Look for coagulopathies and treat as needed.
4. **Skull fracture.** Linear fractures do not require treatment. Depressed skull fractures may require surgery, depending on their size and clinical course.
5. **Intracranial hemorrhage.** Circulatory and ventilatory support are indicated in deteriorating conditions.
   a. **Subarachnoid.** Resolution usually occurs without treatment.
   b. **Epidural.** Prompt surgical evacuation for large bleeds. Prognosis is good with early treatment.
   c. **Subdural.** Subdural taps are indicated to drain a large hematoma.
C. **Face**
1. **Facial nerve injury.** No specific therapy is necessary. Full resolution usually occurs within a couple of months.
   a. **Complete peripheral paralysis.** Cover the exposed eye with an eye patch and instill synthetic tears (1% methylcellulose drops) every 4 h.
   b. **Electrodiagnostic testing** may be beneficial in predicting recovery.
2. **Fractures. Maxilla, lacrimal, and nose fractures** require immediate evaluation. An oral airway is required, and surgical consultation is needed. The fractures must be reduced and fixated.
D. **Eyes**
1. **Eyelids.** Edema and bruising usually resolve within 1 week. Laceration of the eyelid may require microsurgery.
2. **Orbit fracture.** Immediate ophthalmologic consultation is required.
3. **Horner's syndrome.** No treatment is necessary, and resolution usually occurs.
4. **Subconjunctival hemorrhage.** No treatment is necessary because the blood is usually absorbed within 1–2 weeks.
5. **Cornea.** Haziness disappears usually within 2 weeks. If persistent and if rupture of Descemet's membrane has occurred, then a white opacity of the cornea will occur. This is usually permanent.
6. **Intraocular hemorrhage**
   a. **Retinal hemorrhage.** This usually disappears within 1 week. No treatment is necessary.
   b. **Hyphema.** This usually resolves without treatment within 1 week.
   c. **Vitreous hemorrhage.** If resolution does not occur within 1 year, surgery must be considered.
E. **Ears**
1. **Abrasions and ecchymoses.** These injuries are usually mild and require no treatment, except for keeping the area clean. They resolve spontaneously.
2. **Hematomas.** Incision and evacuation may be indicated.
3. **Avulsion of the auricle.** Surgical consultation is required if cartilage is involved.
4. **Laceration of the ear.** Most of these can be sutured with 7-0 nylon sutures.
F. **Vocal cords**
1. **Unilateral paralysis.** Observe these infants closely. Keeping them quiet and giving small, frequent feedings will decrease their risk of aspiration. This condition usually resolves within 4–6 weeks.
2. **Bilateral paralysis.** Intubation is required if there is airway obstruction. Ear-nose-throat consultation and tracheostomy are usually required. The prognosis is variable.
G. **Neck and shoulder**
1. **Clavicular fracture.** Treatment is immobilization, and the prognosis is excellent.

2. **Brachial palsy.** Treatment is immobilization and prevention of contractures, until recovery of the brachial plexus. Recovery is usually good but may take many months.

3. **Phrenic nerve paralysis.** Treatment is usually nonspecific, and the prognosis is good.

4. **SCM.** Most recover spontaneously. Passive exercise may be indicated and appropriate positioning of the infant is recommended. If it is not resolved within 1 year, surgery should be considered.

H. **Spinal cord.** Treatment is supportive. Specific therapy needs to be directed at the bladder, bowel, and skin because these present as ongoing problems. The prognosis depends on the level and severity of the injury.

I. **Abdomen.** The prognosis for all of these depends on early recognition and treatment.

1. **Liver rupture.** Treatment consists of transfusion, laparotomy with evacuation of hematomas, and repair of any laceration.

2. **Splenic rupture.** Treatment consists of transfusion of whole blood and exploratory laparotomy, with preservation of the spleen if possible.

3. **Adrenal hemorrhage.** Treatment is with packed red blood cells and intravenous steroids.

4. **Kidney damage.** Treat with supportive measures or with laparotomy if severe.

J. **Extremities**

1. **Fractured humerus.** Obtain an orthopedic consultation. Immobilize the arm. The prognosis is excellent.

2. **Fractured femur.** Treatment is traction, with an orthopedic consultation. The prognosis is excellent.

3. **Dislocation.** Treatment is immediate reduction with immobilization of the arm.

K. **Genitalia**

1. **Edema and bruising.** These usually resolve within 4–5 days, and no treatment is necessary.

2. **Testicular injury.** Urologic consultation is necessary.

3. **Hematocele.** Elevate the scrotum with cold packs. Resolution occurs without other treatment, unless there is a severe underlying testicular injury.

59 Vasospasms

I. **Problem.** An infant with an indwelling umbilical artery catheter develops vasospasm in one leg. Another infant with a radial artery catheter develops a vasospasm.

II. **Immediate questions**
   A. **Can the catheter be removed?** Evaluate the need for the catheter. If the catheter can be removed, this is the treatment of choice. Vasospasm is most commonly related to the use of umbilical artery catheters, but it can also occur in radial artery catheters.
   B. **Was a medication given recently through the catheter?** The majority of medications, if given too rapidly, can cause vasospasm.
   C. **Is the vasospasm severe?** Deciding whether the vasospasm is severe or less severe may dictate treatment choices.
   D. **Is there a pulse in the affected extremity?** This is very important because if there is a loss of pulse, then a thrombus may be present, which is a medical emergency.

III. **Differential diagnosis**
   A. **Vasospasm.** Vasospasm is a muscular contraction of a vessel, manifested by acute color change (white or blue) in the upper or lower extremity, sometimes only on the toes or fingers and sometimes over the entire extremity. Occasionally, the color change extends to the buttocks and the abdomen. The change in color may be transient or persistent. It may be caused by prior injection of medication or a thromboembolic phenomenon. Arterial blood sampling can also be a predisposing factor.
   B. **Thromboembolic phenomenon.** A **thrombus** is a clot formation at a specific site in a vessel. It can cause complete obstruction, resulting in loss of pulses and an extremity that is white. An **embolus** is a clot that lodges in a blood vessel and may cause obstruction or vasospasm. Approximately 89% of vascular thromboses are associated with intravascular catheters and their use.

IV. **Data base**
   A. **Physical examination.** The severity of the vasospasm must be assessed because it dictates treatment. The areas of involvement, appearance of the skin over the involved areas, and pulses of the affected extremity are measures of severity. Compare the affected extremity with the other extremity.
      1. **Severe vasospasm** involves a large area of one or both legs, the abdomen, or the buttocks. In the upper extremity, a severe vasospasm includes most of the arm and all of the fingers. The skin may be completely white. Pulses of the affected extremity are present.
      2. **Less severe vasospasm** involves a small area of one or both legs (usually some of the toes and part of the foot). In the arm, it can involve part of the extremity and some fingers. The skin has a mottled appearance. Pulses of the affected extremity are present.
      3. **Thrombosis.** If pulses are absent, thrombosis (a **medical emergency**) is likely.
   B. **Laboratory studies.** Laboratory tests are not usually needed. However, the following laboratory tests should be obtained if thrombosis is suspected and streptokinase is to be used:
      1. **Thrombin time.**
      2. **Activated partial thromboplastin time.**
      3. **Prothrombin time.**
      4. **Hematocrit.**
      5. **Platelet count. (Local thrombus can be a cause of thrombocytopenia.)**

C. **Radiologic and other studies**
   1. **Real-time ultrasonography,** with or without color Doppler flow imaging, can be used to diagnose thrombosis. One study showed that this method underestimated the number of thromboses and had significant false-positive results as well.
   2. **Contrast angiography** performed through the umbilical artery catheter can be used to diagnose aortoiliac thrombosis. (In several studies, this procedure was found to be the most effective diagnostic technique.) A contrast study should be considered before administrating a fibrinolytic agent.
   3. **An x-ray study of the abdomen** should be done to determine catheter placement.

V. **Plan**
   A. **Vasospasm.** (*Note:* Treatment is *highly controversial,* and guidelines vary extensively. **Check your institution's guidelines before initiating treatment.**)
      1. **Severe vasospasm of the leg**
         a. **If possible, remove the catheter.** The vasospasm should then resolve spontaneously.
         b. **If it is not possible to remove the catheter (as in a tiny infant) and this is the only catheter, then tolazoline,** 0.02–0.2 mg/kg/h through the catheter as a continuous infusion for 34 h, can be used. If the vasospasm resolves, the infusion may be stopped. If the vasospasm does not resolve, remove the catheter. This treatment is *highly controversial!*
      2. **Less severe vasospasm of the leg**
         a. **Conservative.** Wrap the entire *unaffected* leg in a warm—not hot—washcloth. This measure will cause reflex vasodilation of the vessels in the affected leg, and the vasospasm may resolve. *Treatment should continue for 15–30 min before a beneficial effect will be seen.*
         b. **Papaverine.** If the just [Δ]mentioned treatment does not work, administer papaverine hydrochloride, 1 mg intramuscularly, in the unaffected leg (*controversial*). *Papaverine is a mild vasodilator; if it is going to work, the effect is usually apparent within 30 min.*
         c. **Tolazoline.** If both of the just mentioned treatments fail, tolazoline may be given as described in section V,A,1,b, for severe vasospasm.
         d. **Catheter removal.** If all of the just mentioned treatments fail, it is best to remove the catheter.
      3. **Vasospasm from peripheral artery catheters.** There has been an increase in the use of peripheral arterial catheters, with an associated increase in vasospasms.
         a. **If possible, remove the catheter.**
         b. **When it is not possible to remove the catheter (ie, the catheter is vital for patient care),** tolazoline (0.02–0.2 mg/kg/h) has been given successfully as a continuous infusion and prolonged the life of the catheter between 3 and 168 h. One study reported complete resolution in five of the six patients treated with tolazoline.
         c. **Studies reveal that a papaverine-containing infusion** (60 mg/500 mL) reduces the risk of failure of peripheral arterial catheters (*controversial*).
   B. **Problems after vasospasm with peripheral tissue ischemia.** Ischemia can sometimes occur after a vasospasm. Studies have shown that topical 2% nitroglycerin (*controversial*) ointment (4 mm/kg of body weight) has been applied to the ischemic area with resolution with no adverse effects except mild episodes of decreased blood pressure.
   C. **Thromboembolic phenomenon.** If thrombosis is suspected and there is loss of pulses in the affected extremity, it is a **medical emergency.** Management is *highly controversial.*
      1. **Do not remove the catheter.** Leave the catheter in place to facilitate arteriography and streptokinase infusion, if needed.

2. **Emergency consultation** with a vascular surgeon is recommended.
3. **Infusion of intra-arterial streptokinase** has been successful in some infants. For dosage, see Chapter 80. In one study, lower doses of streptokinase 500 units/kg/h instead of 1000 units/kg/h was shown to be effective and was well tolerated.
4. **Immediate surgery** may be indicated.

60 Ambiguous Genitalia

I. **Definition.** Ambiguous genitalia are present when the sex of an infant is not readily apparent after examination of the external genitalia. If the appearance resembles neither a male with a normal phallus and palpable testes nor a female with an unfused vaginal orifice and absence of an enlarged phallic structure, the genitalia are ambiguous and investigation before gender assignment is indicated.

II. **Embryology.** The early fetus, regardless of the genetic sex (XX or XY), is bipotential and can undergo either male or female differentiation. The innate tendency of the embryo is to differentiate along female lines.

    A. **Development of the gonads.** Gonadal development occurs during the embryonic period (the third through the seventh to eighth weeks of gestation).

        1. **Testicular differentiation.** Gonadal differentiation is determined by the absence or presence of the Y chromosome. If the **Y chromosome** (more specifically, the sex-determining region of the Y or *SRY* gene) is present, the gonads will differentiate as testes. The testes will then produce and release testosterone, which is converted to **dihydrotestosterone (DHT)** in the target organ cells by 5α-reductase. DHT will induce male differentiation of the external genitalia (see section II,B,1). The testes descend behind the peritoneum and normally reach the scrotum by the eighth or ninth month.

        2. **Ovarian differentiation.** In the female fetus, where the Y chromosome/*SRY* gene is absent, the gonads form ovaries (even in 45,X Turner's syndrome, histologically normal ovaries are present at birth). The ovaries do not produce testosterone, and female differentiation proceeds. Two X chromosomes are needed for differentiation of the primordial follicle. If part or all of the second X chromosome is missing, ovarian development fails, resulting in atrophic, whitish, streaky gonads by 1–2 years of age.

    B. **Development of external genitalia.** This part of sexual differentiation occurs in the fetal period, beginning in the seventh week of gestation and proceeds up to the 14th week (about 16 weeks after the last menstrual period).

        1. **Normal male.** At ~9 weeks postconception age, in the presence of systemic androgens (especially DHT), masculinization begins with lengthening of the anogenital distance. The urogenital and labioscrotal folds fuse in the midline (beginning caudally and progressing anteriorly), leading to the formation of the scrotum and the penis.

        2. **Normal female.** In the female fetus, the anogenital distance does not increase. The urogenital and labioscrotal folds do not fuse and instead differentiate into the labia majora and minora. The urogenital sinus divides into the urethra and the vagina.

III. **Pathophysiology**

    A. **Virilization of female infants (female pseudohermaphroditism).** Most neonates with ambiguous genitalia belong to this group. They have a 46,XX karyotype, are *SRY*-negative, and have exclusively ovarian tissue. The degree of masculinization of the female newborn depends on the potency of the androgenic stimulation to which she is exposed, the stage of development at the time of initial exposure, and the duration of exposure.

        1. **The most common cause** of excess fetal androgens is autosomal recessively inherited **enzymatic deficiencies in the cortisol pathway,** leading to excessive corticotropin (adrenocorticotropic hormone [ACTH]) stimulation with **congenital adrenal hyperplasia (CAH)** and excessive production of adrenal androgens (dehydroepiandrosterone and androstenedione) and testosterone (Figure 60–1). Most common is **21-hydroxylase defi-**

ciency, which causes inadequate cortisol levels, leading to excessive ACTH stimulation (lack of negative feedback to the hypothalamus and pituitary), adrenal hyperplasia, and excessive production of adrenal androgens (dehydroepiandrosterone and androstenedione) and testosterone, producing virilization. **Two forms** are seen in neonates, depending on the associated **relative or absolute aldosterone deficiency: a simple virilizing form and a salt-losing form.** In the first form, the salt loss is mild and adrenal insufficiency tends not to occur, except in stressful circumstances. In the second, adrenal insufficiency occurs under basal conditions and tends to manifest in the neonatal period or soon thereafter as an adrenal crisis. The extent of virilization is not a reliable indicator of the degree of adrenal insufficiency, and the electrolyte status of all infants with 21-hydroxylase deficiency should be monitored. **11-Hydroxylase enzyme deficiency** is less common and is associated with salt retention, volume expansion, and hypertension.

  2. **Other, less common causes** are virilizing maternal or fetal tumors or maternal androgen ingestion or topical use.

B. **Inadequate virilization of male infants (male pseudohermaphroditism).** This problem is caused by inadequate androgen production or incomplete end-organ response to androgen. These patients have a 46,XY karyotype and exclusively testicular tissue. All of these abnormalities are uncommon, and most require extensive laboratory investigation before a final diagnosis can be confirmed.

  1. **Decreased androgen production** can be caused by one of five rare enzyme defects, which are inherited in an autosomal recessive manner. Three of these defects also cause cortisol deficiency and **nonvirilizing adrenal hyperplasia,** and two are specific to the testosterone pathway. Other causes of decreased androgen production include **deficiency of müllerian-inhibiting substance** (the most common presentation is a male in-

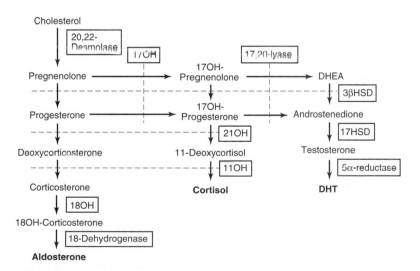

FIGURE 60–1. Adrenal metabolic pathways involved in ambiguous genitalia. 11OH, 11-Hydroxylase; 17OH, 17-hydroxylase; 18OH, 18-hydroxylase; 21OH, 21-hydroxylase; 3βHSD, 3β-hydroxysteroid dehydrogenase; 17HSD, 17-hydroxysteroid dehydrogenase; DHEA, dehydroepiandrosterone; DHT, dihydrotestosterone.

fant with inguinal hernias that contain the uterus or fallopian tubes); **testicular unresponsiveness to human chorionic gonadotropin (hCG) and luteinizing hormone (LH)**; and **anorchia** (absent testes caused by loss of vascular supply to the testis during fetal life). The association of **microphallus** and **hypoglycemia** suggests a **pituitary deficiency** with absence of gonadotropins, ACTH, or growth hormone.

2. **Decreased end-organ response to androgen** is often referred to as **testicular feminization** and can be caused by a defect in the androgen receptor or an unknown defect with normal receptors. It can be total (labial testes with otherwise normal-appearing female genitalia) or, more commonly, partial (incomplete virilization of a male).

3. **5α-Reductase deficiency** results in failure of the external genitalia to undergo male differentiation. The outcome is a neonate with female or ambiguous external genitalia but with a 46,XY karyotype, normally developed testes, and male internal ducts.

C. **Disorders of gonadal differentiation**

1. **True hermaphroditism.** The presence of both a testis and an ovary (or ovotestes) in the same individual is a rare cause of ambiguous genitalia. Most individuals with true hermaphroditism have a 46,XX karyotype, but mosaics of 46,XX, 45,X, 46,XY, and multiple X/multiple Y have all been reported. The appearance of the genitalia is variable, but about three fourths of these infants have adequate phallus size to be raised as males. The chances of fertility are extremely poor.

2. **Gonadal dysgenesis**

   a. **Pure gonadal dysgenesis** is characterized by the presence of a streak gonad bilaterally (complete gonadal dysgenesis) or unilaterally (partial gonadal dysgenesis). It is important to distinguish the X-chromosomal from the Y-chromosomal form because the streak gonads in the Y-positive patients carry a significant **risk for tumor development.**

   b. **Mixed gonadal dysgenesis** is characterized by the presence of a unilateral functioning testis and a contralateral streak gonad. All patients have a Y chromosome and some degree of virilization of the external genitalia. Mixed gonadal dysgenesis is associated with a high incidence of gonadal malignancy in mid to late childhood, and the gonads should, therefore, be removed.

D. **Chromosome abnormalities, syndromes, and associations.** Chromosomal abnormalities do not usually lead to ambiguous genitalia. Examples are **Turner's syndrome** (45,X) and **Klinefelter's syndrome** (47,XXY). However, ambiguous genitalia have been reported occasionally in **trisomies 13 and 18, 4p− syndrome, and triploidy.** Single-gene disorders and syndromes such as **Smith-Lemli-Opitz syndrome, Rieger's syndrome, and camptomelic dysplasia** can also be associated with external sexual ambiguity. **CHARGE and VACTERL associations** can include ambiguous genitalia.

IV. **Diagnostic evaluation.** Please note that the American Academy of Pediatrics has issued a policy statement on the evaluation of the newborn with developmental anomalies of the external genitalia.

A. **History.** A careful history should be obtained from the parents. **Family history** of early neonatal deaths (a death in early infancy accompanied by vomiting and dehydration may be secondary to CAH), consanguinity of the parents (increased risk for autosomal recessive disorders), and female relatives with amenorrhea and infertility (male pseudohermaphroditism) are significant, as are a **maternal history** of virilization or CAH and ingestion or topical use of drugs during pregnancy (particularly androgens or progestational agents).

B. **Physical examination**

1. A **general** examination should address the presence of any of the following: dysmorphic features (syndromes and chromosomal abnormalities), hypertension or hypotension, areolar hyperpigmentation, and signs of dehydration (as signs of CAH).

2. **Genitalia.** Gonads: The number, size, and symmetry of gonads should be evaluated. Palpable gonads below the inguinal canal are almost certainly testes. Ovaries are not found in scrotal folds or in the inguinal region. However, the testes may be intra-abdominal. Phallus length: Measured from the pubic ramus to the tip of the glands, a stretched penile length in a full-term infant should be ≥2.0 cm. Urethral meatus: Look for hypospadias (usually accompanied by chordee). Labioscrotal folds: Findings can range from unfused labia majora, variable degrees of posterior fusion, and bifid scrotum to fully fused, normal-appearing scrotum. The presence of a vaginal opening or urogenital sinus should be determined. A rectal examination, to determine presence of a uterus, should always be performed.

C. **Radiographic studies**
1. **Ultrasonography** to evaluate adrenal and pelvic structures: Although a uterus is sometimes palpable on rectal examination shortly after birth (because of enlargement in response to maternal estrogen), ultrasonography seems less invasive. The presence and localization of gonads may also be clarified by ultrasonography. Adrenal ultrasonography has been shown to be sufficiently sensitive to determine adrenal abnormalities in the majority of patients with untreated adrenal hyperplasia.
2. **Contrast studies** to outline the internal anatomy (sinography, urethrography, vesiculocystoureterography, and intravenous urography) may be indicated before reconstructive surgery.

D. **Laboratory studies**
1. **Initial evaluation.** An important test in the initial evaluation is the **chromosome analysis.** Most cytogenetic laboratories can provide some results of a karyotype within 2–3 days. In situ hybridization techniques (**fluorescent in situ hybridization [FISH]**) may allow even faster determination of the sex chromosome status. Buccal smears provide a quick answer but are notoriously unreliable. The remainder of the diagnostic evaluation depends on the sex chromosome status; accuracy is paramount. Blood for **basic biochemical studies** can be obtained at the same time as the karyotype, including 17-hydroxyprogesterone (17-OHP), testosterone, dihydrotestosterone, sodium, and potassium levels. Other tests may be necessary, depending on the results of the karyotype. Biochemical tests will, therefore, be discussed in the context of the different chromosomal constellations.
2. **Normal 46,XX karyotype.** This finding implies virilization of a genetic female and is caused by excessive maternal or fetal androgen. If the mother is not virilized, the infant almost always has **virilizing adrenal hyperplasia.** To confirm the diagnosis, measure the following:
   a. **17-OHP.** This is the immediate precursor to the enzyme defect in 21-hydroxylase enzyme deficiency and one step before that in 11-hydroxylase enzyme deficiency. In infants with either defect, the serum or plasma level of 17-OHP will be 100–1000 times the normal infant level. Note that the 17-OHP level may be somewhat elevated in normal infants within the first 24 h of life; a repeat level several days later may be indicated while fluid and electrolyte balance is monitored.
   b. **Daily serum measurements of sodium and potassium.** Infants with 21-hydroxylase enzyme deficiency will usually have relative or absolute aldosterone deficiency and will begin to demonstrate hyperkalemia at days 3–5 and hyponatremia 1–2 days later. If hyperkalemia becomes clinically significant before the 17-OHP result is available, begin treatment empirically with intravenous saline, cortisol, and Florinef because the diagnosis is virtually certain (for dosages, see sections V,C,1,a and b).
   c. **Serum testosterone.** About 3% of infants with ambiguous genitalia will be true hermaphrodites, and most will have 46,XX chromosomes. If the 17-OHP is not elevated and there is no maternal virilization, elevated testosterone suggests hermaphroditism or fetal testosterone-producing tumor.

3. **Normal 46,XY karyotype.** The differential diagnosis of an **incompletely virilized genetic male** is extremely complex and includes in utero testicular damage, defects of testosterone synthesis, end-organ resistance, and an enzymatic defect in the conversion of testosterone to dihydrotestosterone. The laboratory evaluation is correspondingly complex and usually proceeds through a number of steps before the results of the preceding step become available.

   a. **Testosterone (T) and dihydrotestosterone (DHT).** These hormone levels should be measurable and are higher in newborns than later in childhood. In the male pseudohermaphrodite, testosterone is low in any defect in testosterone production. The T–DHT ratio should be between 5:1 and 20:1 when expressed in similar units. A high T–DHT ratio suggests 5α-reductase deficiency (see also section IV,D,3,c: the hCG stimulation test). **Androstenedione** levels are measured to diagnose **17-ketosteroid reductase deficiency.**

   b. **LH and follicle-stimulating hormone (FSH).** These hormones are also higher in infancy than they are in childhood. A diagnosis of gonadotropin deficiency is suspected if these values are low in a reliable assay but can be confirmed in infancy only if there are other pituitary hormone deficits. Remember: Growth hormone and ACTH deficiency are manifested in the newborn period as hypoglycemia. In primary gonadal defects and some androgen-resistant states, LH and FSH are elevated.

   c. **hCG stimulation test.** hCG is administered to stimulate gonadal steroid production when testosterone values are low (as in gonadotropin deficiency or a defect in testosterone synthesis). Recommendations vary, but a dose of 500–1000 units every day or every other day for 3 doses is most common. Then testosterone and DHT are measured again to evaluate the gonadal response. A rise in the testosterone level confirms the presence of Leydig cells and, by implication, testicular tissue. In patients with 5α-reductase deficiency, the basal T–DHT ratio may be normal but elevated after hCG stimulation. It is wise to obtain enough blood after hCG injection to measure other steroid intermediates if the testosterone is low. Considering the complexity of male pseudohermaphroditism, the restrictions in drawing blood from newborns, and the fact that many specific tests can be performed only in special laboratories, involvement of a pediatric endocrinologist in the planning and interpretation of these tests seems indicated. In any case, it is always advisable to ask the initial processing laboratory to freeze any remaining serum or plasma.

4. **Abnormal karyotype.** Mixed gonadal dysgenesis with a dysplastic gonad is the great risk for infants with abnormal karyotype and ambiguous genitalia. **Hormone studies** are unlikely to be revealing in this circumstance. Note that a normal karyotype from peripheral white blood cells does not exclude mosaic chromosomal abnormalities and that there is a limit in the resolution of conventional karyotypes. **DNA analysis** (FISH probes or Southern analysis) may contribute in some situations. These techniques may allow detection of *SRY* gene material in 46,XX phenotypic males and be useful in determining whether Y material is present in a 45,X individual, placing the patient at risk for gonadoblastoma.

V. **Management**

  A. **General considerations.** An important aspect of the treatment of ambiguous genitalia in an infant is to protect the privacy of the parents and the child while diagnostic studies are in progress. Once a diagnosis has been established, gender may be assigned (see section V,D) and steroid replacement, gonadal removal, and reconstructive surgery can be considered or, if indicated, initiated.

  B. **Initial measures**

1. **Early instructions for the parents.** As soon as the abnormality is noted, a physician responsible for the infant should be identified and the parents should be informed. The family should be told that their infant is generally healthy (if this is true) but that the genitalia are "incompletely developed" and that it is not possible, at present, to identify the sex of their child. It is best to use gender-nonspecific nouns such as baby, infant, or child rather than gender-specific pronouns at this point to avoid showing a bias to the parents. Meet with the parents as soon as possible to discuss the situation (the delivery room is usually not appropriate for an in-depth discussion). Parents frequently imagine grotesque findings, and examining the infant with them will provide reassurance and facilitate bonding with their child. All attempts to identify the sex of the child on the basis of appearance should be resisted, although there is likely to be great pressure to do so from parents, relatives, and professional personnel. It is important not to complete the birth certificate or make any reference to gender in any of the permanent medical records of the mother or the child. *It is advisable to isolate the child and parents from the inquiries of the community.* Parents may want to delay sending out birth announcements and telling anyone outside the immediate family that the infant has been born until a gender assignment has been made. Whatever the final gender assignment, many children will live the majority of their lives in the community of birth, and confusion about gender assignment because of premature release of information will never be completely forgotten. Parents should be reassured that in most cases the gender will be determined as soon as test results are available, and some specialists discourage the use of unigender names in the early neonatal period. There have been discussions as to whether it is advisable in more complicated cases to delay the gender assignment until the child gets older (see section V,D). In this scenario, a name that is appropriate for either males or females may be used.
2. **Early referral.** It is advisable to seek consultation from a specialist in the evaluation of children with ambiguous genitalia (usually an endocrinologist or geneticist) as soon as feasible. It is never acceptable to discharge a child from the nursery before detailed evaluation of the cause of ambiguous genitalia. In most cases, a complete diagnosis, assignment of the sex of rearing, and a plan for future treatment are accomplished before discharge.
C. **Medical management**
   1. **Congenital adrenal hyperplasia.** The most immediate concern in a neonate with abnormal genitalia is whether CAH is present. The onset of adrenal insufficiency occurs between days 3 and 14 in 50% of affected patients. All forms of adrenal hyperplasia have absolute or relative cortisol deficiency and require early diagnosis and replacement therapy to prevent vascular collapse.
      a. **Glucocorticoid therapy** should be instituted as soon as possible. Maintenance cortisol replacement therapy is usually given orally, but some endocrinologists give intramuscular **cortisone acetate** (10–25 mg/day intramuscularly [IM] for 2–3 days followed by 37.5 mg/m^2 IM every 3 days) in children <6 months because of concerns that oral hydrocortisone is absorbed erratically in these infants. **Hydrocortisone** is the oral preparation of choice. Doses usually range from 10–20 mg/ m^2/day given in 3 divided doses. The dose requires adjustments for growth and during periods of stress, and follow-up with a pediatric endocrinologist is advised.
      b. **Mineralocorticoid therapy.** Fludrocortisone acetate (Florinef) is the drug of choice. The usual dose is 0.05–0.1 mg orally daily. Unlike hydrocortisone, the dose of Florinef does not change with increase of body size or during stress. Many endocrinologists also recommend sodium supplementation (1–5 mEq/kg/day).

2. **Incompletely virilized genetic male.** Treatment with **Depo-Testosterone** might be considered by a pediatric endocrinologist. The usual dose is 25 mg IM at 3- to 4-week intervals for 3 doses. This regimen is followed to evaluate whether adequate growth of the phallus occurs, and this therapy may be attempted before a final decision is made to raise a child with ambiguous genitalia as a male.

D. **Gender assignment.** Gender assignment is beyond the scope of this brief discussion. In general, however, the sex of rearing should be determined only when the final diagnosis is secure. Gender assignment has been traditionally approached as though individuals are psychosexually neutral at birth and as though healthy psychosexual development is intimately related to the appearance of the external genitals. One focus had been to ensure appropriate sexual function as adults. Responses to testosterone therapy and surgical issues such as the question of whether it is simpler to construct a vagina than a satisfactory and functional penis are also of foremost importance for the decision. However, these relatively established beliefs have been challenged: It is now believed that prenatal and early exposure of the brain to androgens, if present, may influence gender-specific behavioral patterns and sexual identity in addition to the external appearance of the genitalia or their future function. Another newly argued point is time of gender assignment. Traditionally, the approach has been to assign gender as soon as possible after birth and to try to then reconstruct or correct the external genitalia to fit the gender assigned. It has been suggested that it may be beneficial to wait in the more complex cases and involve the child in the final decision. There is evidence that some patients who are genetically 46,XY but had been raised as females because of inadequate phalluses at birth do identify themselves with the male role and have expressed dissatisfaction with the initial gender assignment. Some have even switched sex back to males. In view of this new information, it is advisable to counsel the parents of the infant with ambiguous genitalia to wait until all facts have been presented and discussed. A multidisciplinary team of pediatricians, urologists, endocrinologists, geneticists, and psychiatrists should be involved in counseling the parents and, later, the child, and each case must be approached based on its uniqueness.

VI. **Prognosis.** To ensure the best social and psychological outcome possible, continuous psychological support may be indicated. Referral to support groups should be considered; if indicated, genetic counseling can be offered. Other morbidity and mortality are largely dependent on associated anomalies, the presence or absence of adrenal dysfunction, and the need and extent of surgical interventions. Many patients with ambiguous genitalia are fertile as adults. This is in part because of the advances and options of modern reproductive technologies.

REFERENCES

Al-Agha AE et al: The child of uncertain sex: 17 years of experience. *J Paediatr Child Health* 2001;37:348.

Al-Alwan I et al: Clinical utility of adrenal ultrasonography in the diagnosis of congenital hyperplasia. *J Pediatr* 1999;135:71.

American Academy of Pediatrics Committee on Genetics: Evaluation of the newborn with developmental anomalies of the external genitalia. *Pediatrics* 2000;106:138.

Anhalt H et al: Ambiguous genitalia. *Pediatr Rev* 1996;17:213.

Charest NJ (ed): Sexual differentiation and evaluation of ambiguous genitalia (special issue). *Semin Perinatol* 1992;5.

Diamond M, Sigmundson HK: Management of intersexuality. *Arch Pediatr Adolesc Med* 1997a; 151:1046.

Diamond M, Sigmundson HK: Sex reassignment at birth: long-term review and clinical implications. *Arch Pediatr Adolesc Med* 1997b;151:298.

Donahoe PK, Schnitzer JJ: Evaluation of the infant who has ambiguous genitalia, and principles of operative management. *Semin Pediatr Surg* 1996;5:30.

Gooren LJ: Androgen-resistance syndromes: considerations of gender assignment. Curr Ther Endocrinol Metab 1997;6:380.

Griffin JE: Androgen resistance: the clinical and molecular spectrum. N Engl J Med 1992; 326:611.

Grumbach MM, Conte FA: Disorders of sexual differentiation. In Wilson JD, Foster DW (eds): Williams' Textbook of Endocrinology, 8th ed. Saunders, 1992.

Hernanz-Schulman M et al: Sonographic findings in infants with congenital adrenal hyperplasia. Pediatr Radiol 2002;32:130.

Holm IA: Ambiguous genitalia in the newborn. In Herriot SJ et al (eds): Pediatric and Adolescent Gynecology, 4th ed. Lippincott-Raven, 1997.

Izquierdo G, Glassberg K: Gender assignment and gender identity in patients with ambiguous genitalia. Urology 1993;42:232.

Lee MM, Donahoe PK: The infant with ambiguous genitalia. Curr Ther Endocrinol Metab 1997; 6:216.

Malasanos TH: Sexual development of the fetus and pubertal child. Clin Obstet Gynecol 1997; 40:153.

Mandel J: Sexual differentiation: normal and abnormal. In Walsh PC et al (eds): Campbell's Urology, 7th ed. Saunders, 1997.

McGillivray BC: Genetic aspects of ambiguous genitalia. Pediatr Clin North Am 1992;39:307.

Migeon CJ, Berkovitz GD: Congenital defects of the external genitalia in the newborn and prepubertal child. In Koehler SE, Rock JA (eds): Pediatric and Adolescent Gynecology. Raven, 1992.

Reiner WG: Assignment of sex in neonates with ambiguous genitalia. Current Opin Pediatr 1999; 11:363.

Schober JM: Quality-of-life studies in patients with ambiguous genitalia. World J Urol 1999; 17:249.

Slaughenhoupt BL: Diagnostic evaluation and management of the child with ambiguous genitalia. J Kentucky Med Assoc 1997;95:134.

Stradtman EW Jr: Female gender reconstruction surgery for ambiguous genitalia in children and adolescents. Curr Opin Obstet Gynecol 1991;3:805.

Zaontz MR, Packer MG: Abnormalities of the external genitalia. Pediatr Clin North Am 1997;44:1267.

61 Blood Abnormalities

ABO INCOMPATIBILITY

I. **Definition.** Isoimmune hemolytic anemia may result when ABO incompatibility occurs between the mother and the newborn infant. This disorder is most common with blood type A or B infants born to type O mothers. The hemolytic process begins in utero and is the result of active placental transport of maternal isoantibody. In type O mothers, isoantibody is predominantly 7S-IgG (immunoglobulin G) and is capable of crossing the placental membranes. Because of its larger size, the mostly 19S-IgM (immunoglobulin M) isoantibody found in type A or type B mothers cannot cross. Symptomatic clinical disease, which usually does not present until after birth, is a compensated mild hemolytic anemia with reticulocytosis, microspherocytosis, and early-onset unconjugated hyperbilirubinemia.

II. **Incidence.** Risk factors for ABO incompatibility are present in 12–15% of pregnancies, but evidence of fetal sensitization (positive direct Coombs' test) occurs in only 3–4%. Symptomatic ABO hemolytic disease occurs in <1% of all newborn infants but accounts for approximately two thirds of observed cases of hemolytic disease in the newborn.

III. **Pathophysiology.** Transplacental transport of maternal isoantibody results in an immune reaction with the A or B antigen on fetal erythrocytes, which produces characteristic **microspherocytes.** This process eventually results in complete extravascular hemolysis of the end-stage spherocyte. The ongoing hemolysis is balanced by compensatory reticulocytosis and shortening of the cell cycle time, so that there is overall maintenance of the erythrocyte indices within physiologic limits. A paucity of A or B antigenic sites on the fetal (in contrast to the adult) erythrocytes and competitive binding of isoantibody to myriad other antigenic sites in other tissues may explain the often mild hemolytic process that occurs and the usual absence of progressive disease with subsequent pregnancies.

IV. **Risk factors**
   A. **A_1 antigen in the infant.** Of the major blood group antigens, the A_1 antigen has the greatest antigenicity and is associated with a greater risk of symptomatic disease.
   B. **Elevated isohemagglutinins.** Antepartum intestinal parasitism or third-trimester immunization with tetanus toxoid or pneumococcal vaccine may stimulate isoantibody titer to A or B antigens.
   C. **Birth order.** Birth order is not considered a risk factor. Maternal isoantibody exists naturally and is independent of prior exposure to incompatible fetal blood group antigens. First-born infants have a 40–50% risk for symptomatic disease. Progressive severity of the hemolytic process in succeeding pregnancies is a rare phenomenon.

V. **Clinical presentation: symptoms and signs**
   A. **Jaundice.** Icterus is often the sole physical manifestation of ABO incompatibility with a clinically significant level of hemolysis. The onset is usually within the first 24 h of life. The jaundice evolves at a faster rate over the early neonatal period than nonhemolytic physiologic pattern jaundice.
   B. **Anemia.** Because of the effectiveness of compensation by reticulocytosis in response to the ongoing mild hemolytic process, erythrocyte indices are maintained within a physiologic range that is normal for asymptomatic infants of the same gestational age. Additional signs of clinical disease (eg, hepatosplenomegaly or hydrops fetalis) are extremely unusual but may be

seen with a more progressive hemolytic process (see Rh Incompatibility, pp 344–349). Exaggerated physiologic anemia may occur at 8–12 weeks of age, particularly when treatment during the neonatal period required phototherapy or exchange transfusion.

VI. Diagnosis. Obligatory screening for infants with unconjugated hyperbilirubinemia includes the following studies:

A. Blood type and Rh factor in the mother and the infant. These studies establish risk factors for ABO incompatibility.

B. Reticulocyte count. Elevated values after adjustment for gestational age and degree of anemia, if any, will support the diagnosis of hemolytic anemia. For term infants, normal values are 4–5%; for preterm infants of 30–36 weeks' gestational age, 6–10%. In ABO hemolytic disease of the newborn, values range from 10–30%.

C. Direct Coombs' test (direct antiglobulin test). Because there is very little antibody on the red blood cell (RBC), the direct Coomb's test is often only weakly positive at birth and may become negative by 2–3 days of age. A strongly positive test is distinctly unusual and would direct attention to other isoimmune or autoimmune hemolytic processes.

D. Blood smear. The blood smear typically demonstrates **microspherocytes, polychromasia** proportionate to the reticulocyte response, and **normoblastosis** above the normal values for gestational age.

E. Bilirubin levels (fractionated or total and direct). Indirect hyperbilirubinemia is mainly present and provides an index of the severity of disease. The rate at which unconjugated bilirubin levels are increasing suggests the required frequency of testing, usually every 4–8 h until values plateau.

F. Additional laboratory studies. Supportive diagnostic studies may be indicated on an individual basis if the nature of the hemolytic process remains unclear.

  1. Antibody identification (indirect Coombs' test). The indirect Coombs' test is more sensitive than the direct Coombs' test in detecting the presence of maternal isoantibody and will identify antibody specificity. The test is performed on an eluate of neonatal erythrocytes, which is then tested against a panel of type-specific adult cells.

  2. Maternal IgG titer. The absence in the mother of elevated IgG titers against the infant's blood group will tend to exclude a diagnosis of ABO incompatibility.

VII. Management

A. Antepartum treatment. Because of the low incidence of moderate to severe ABO hemolytic disease, invasive maneuvers before term is reached (eg, amniocentesis or early delivery) are usually not indicated.

B. Postpartum treatment

  1. General measures. The maintenance of adequate hydration (see Chapter 7) and evaluation for potentially aggravating factors (eg, sepsis, drug exposure, or metabolic disturbance) should be considered.

  2. Phototherapy. Once a diagnosis of ABO incompatibility is established, phototherapy may be initiated before exchange transfusion is given. Because of the usual mild to moderate hemolysis, phototherapy may entirely obviate the need for exchange transfusion or may reduce the number of transfusions required. For guidelines on phototherapy, see Chapter 39.

  3. Exchange transfusion. See Chapters 21 and 39.

  4. Intravenous immunoglobulin (IVIG). By blocking neonatal reticuloendothelial Fc receptors, and thus decrease hemolysis of the antibody-coated RBCs, high-dose IVIG (1 g/kg over 4 h) has been shown to reduce serum bilirubin levels and the need for blood exchange transfusion with ABO or Rh hemolytic diseases.

  5. Synthetic blood group trisaccharides. Their use is currently investigational, but early studies have shown a decrease in exchange transfusion rates in severe ABO hemolytic disease when A or B trisaccharides were administered.

VIII. Prognosis. For infants with ABO incompatibility, the overall prognosis is excellent. Timely recognition and appropriate management of the rare infant with aggressive ABO hemolytic disease may avoid any potential morbidity or severe hemolytic anemia and secondary hyperbilirubinemia and the inherent risks associated with exchange transfusion and with the use of blood products.

ANEMIA

I. **Definition.** Anemia developing during the neonatal period (0–28 days of life) in infants of >34 weeks' gestational age is indicated by a central venous hemoglobin <13 g/dL or a capillary hemoglobin <14.5 g/dL.

II. **Normal physiology.** At birth, normal values for the central venous hemoglobin in infants of >34 weeks' gestational age are 14–20 g/dL, with an average value of 17 g/dL. Reticulocyte count in the cord blood of infants ranges from 3–7%. The average mean corpuscular volume of RBCs is 107 fL. Premature infants have slightly lower hemoglobin and higher mean corpuscular volume and reticulocyte counts. In healthy term infants, hemoglobin values remain unchanged until the third week of life and then decline, reaching a nadir of 11 g/dL at 8–12 weeks. This is known as the "physiologic anemia of infancy." In preterm infants, this decline is more profound, reaching a nadir of 7–9 g/dL at 4–8 weeks. This exaggerated physiologic anemia of prematurity is related to a combination of decreased RBC mass at birth, increased iatrogenic losses from laboratory blood sampling, shorter RBC life span, inadequate erythropoietin production, and rapid body growth. In the absence of clinical complications associated with prematurity, infants will remain asymptomatic during this process.

III. **Pathophysiology.** Anemia in the newborn infant results from one of three processes: (1) loss of RBCs, or hemorrhagic anemia, the most common cause; (2) increased destruction of RBCs, or hemolytic anemia; or (3) underproduction of RBCs, or hypoplastic anemia.

A. **Hemorrhagic anemia**
1. **Antepartum period** (1 in 1000 live births)
    a. **Loss of placental integrity.** Abruptio placentae, placenta previa, or traumatic amniocentesis (acute or chronic) may result in loss of placental integrity.
    b. **Anomalies of the umbilical cord or placental vessels.** Velamentous insertion of the umbilical cord occurs in 10% of twin gestations and almost all gestations with three or more fetuses. Communicating vessels (vasa praevia), umbilical cord hematoma (1 in 5500 deliveries), or entanglement of the cord by the fetus may also cause hemorrhagic anemia.
    c. **Twin-twin transfusion.** This is observed only in monozygotic multiple births. In the presence of a monochorial placenta, 13–33% of twin pregnancies are associated with twin-twin transfusion. The difference in hemoglobin concentration between twins is >5 g/dL. The survival rate for twin-twin transfusion diagnosed before 28 weeks' gestation is 21%. The anemic donor twin may develop congestive heart disease, whereas the recipient plethoric twin may manifest signs of the hyperviscosity syndrome.
2. **Intrapartum period**
    a. **Fetomaternal hemorrhage.** Fetomaternal hemorrhage occurs in 30–50% of pregnancies. The risk is increased with preeclampsia-eclampsia, with the need for instrumentation, and with cesarean section. In ~8% of pregnancies, the volume of the hemorrhage is >10 mL.
    b. **Cesarean section.** In elective cesarean deliveries, there is a 3% incidence of anemia. The incidence is increased in emergency cesarean

deliveries. Delay in cord clamping beyond 30 s is associated with an increased risk of fetomaternal hemorrhage.

   c. **Traumatic rupture of the umbilical cord.** Rupture may occur if delivery is uncontrolled or unattended.

   d. **Failure of placental transfusion.** Failure is usually caused by umbilical cord occlusion (eg, a nuchal cord or an entangled or prolapsed cord) during vaginal delivery. Blood loss may be 25–30 mL in the newborn.

   e. **Obstetric trauma.** During a difficult vaginal delivery, occult visceral or intracranial hemorrhage may occur. It may not be apparent at birth. Difficult deliveries are more common with large for gestational age infants, breech presentation, or difficult extraction.

3. **Neonatal period**

   a. **Enclosed hemorrhage.** Hemorrhage severe enough to cause neonatal anemia suggests obstetric trauma, severe perinatal distress, or a defect in hemostasis.

      i. **Caput succedaneum** is relatively common and may result in benign hemorrhage.

      ii. **Cephalhematoma** is found in up to 2.5% of births. It is associated with vacuum extraction and primiparity (5% risk of associated linear nondepressed skull fracture).

      iii. **Intracranial hemorrhage** may occur in the subdural, subarachnoid, or subependymal space.

      iv. **Visceral parenchymal hemorrhage** is uncommon. It is usually the result of obstetric trauma to an internal organ, most commonly the liver but also the spleen, kidneys, or adrenal glands.

   b. **Defects in hemostasis.** Defects in hemostasis may be congenital, but more commonly hemorrhage occurs secondary to consumption coagulopathy, which may be caused by the following:

      i. **Congenital coagulation factor deficiency.**

      ii. **Consumption coagulopathy**

         (a) Disseminated congenital or viral infection.

         (b) Bacterial sepsis.

         (c) Intravascular embolism of thromboplastin (as a result of a dead twin, maternal toxemia, necrotizing enterocolitis, or others).

      iii. **Deficiency of vitamin K–dependent coagulation factors** (factors II, VII, IX, and X)

         (a) Failure to administer vitamin K at birth usually results in a bleeding diathesis at 3–4 days of age.

         (b) Use of antibiotics may interfere with the production of vitamin K by normal gastrointestinal flora.

      iv. **Thrombocytopenia**

         (a) Immune thrombocytopenia may be isoimmune or autoimmune.

         (b) **Congenital thrombocytopenia with absent radii** is a syndrome frequently associated with hemorrhagic anemia in the newborn.

   c. **Iatrogenic blood loss.** Anemia may occur if blood loss resulting from repeated venipuncture is not replaced routinely. Symptoms may develop if a loss of >20% occurs within a 48-h period.

B. **Hemolytic anemia**

   1. **Immune hemolysis**

      a. **Isoimmune hemolytic anemia** is caused mostly by Rh incompatibility.

      b. **Autoimmune hemolytic anemia.**

   2. **Nonimmune hemolysis**

      a. **Bacterial sepsis may cause primary microangiopathic hemolysis.**

      b. **Congenital TORCH** (*t*oxoplasmosis, *o*ther, *r*ubella, *c*ytomegalovirus, and *h*erpes simplex virus) infections (see Chapter 68).

3. **Congenital erythrocyte defect**
   a. **Metabolic enzyme deficiency**
      i. Glucose-6-phosphate dehydrogenase (G6PD) deficiency.
      ii. Pyruvate kinase deficiency.
   b. **Thalassemia.** Hemolytic anemia secondary to thalassemia has invariably been associated with homozygous α-thalassemia and presents at birth. The disorders in β-thalassemia become apparent only after 2–3 months of age.
   c. **Hemoglobinopathy** may be characterized as unstable hemoglobins or congenital Heinz body anemias.
   d. **Membrane defects** are usually autosomal dominant.
      i. **Hereditary spherocytosis** (1 in 5000 neonates) commonly presents with jaundice and less often with anemia.
      ii. **Hereditary elliptocytosis** (1 in 2500 neonates) rarely presents in the newborn infant.
4. **Systemic diseases**
   a. Galactosemia.
   b. Osteopetrosis.
5. **Nutritional deficiency.** Vitamin E deficiency occurs with chronic malabsorption but usually does not present until after the neonatal period.
C. **Hypoplastic anemia**
   1. **Congenital disease**
      a. Diamond-Blackfan syndrome (congenital hypoplastic anemia).
      b. Atransferrinemia.
      c. Congenital leukemia.
      d. Sideroblastic anemia.
   2. **Acquired disease**
      a. Infection. Rubella and syphilis are the most common causes.
      b. Aplastic crisis.
      c. Aplastic anemia.
IV. **Clinical presentation**
   A. **Symptoms and signs.** The four major forms of neonatal anemia may be demonstrated by determination of the following factors: (1) age at presentation of anemia, (2) associated clinical features at presentation, (3) hemodynamic status of the infant, and (4) presence or absence of compensatory reticulocytosis.
      1. **Hemorrhagic anemia.** Hemorrhagic anemia is often dramatic in clinical presentation when acute but may be more subtle when chronic. Both forms have significant rates of perinatal morbidity and mortality if they remain unrecognized. Neither form has significant elevation of bilirubin levels or hepatosplenomegaly.
         a. **Acute hemorrhagic anemia** presents at birth or with internal hemorrhage after 24 h. There is pallor not associated with jaundice and often without cyanosis (<5 g of deoxyhemoglobin) and unrelieved by supplemental oxygen. Tachypnea or gasping respirations are present. Vascular instability ranges from decreased peripheral perfusion (a 10% loss of blood volume) to hypovolemic shock (20–25% loss of blood volume). There is also decreased central venous pressure and poor capillary refill. Normocytic or normochromic RBC indices are present, with reticulocytosis developing within 2–3 days of the hemorrhagic event.
         b. **Chronic hemorrhagic anemia** presents at birth with unexplained pallor, often without cyanosis (<5 g of deoxyhemoglobin), and unrelieved by supplemental oxygen. Minimal signs of respiratory distress are present. The central venous pressure is normal or increased. Microcytic or hypochromic RBC indices are present, with compensatory reticulocytosis. The liver is often enlarged because of compensatory extramedullary erythropoiesis. Hydrops fetalis or stillbirth may occur

with failure of compensatory reticulocytosis or intravascular volume maintenance.

c. **Asphyxia pallida** (severe neonatal asphyxia) is not associated with hemorrhagic anemia at presentation. This disorder must be distinguished clinically from acute hemorrhage because specific immediate therapy is needed for each disorder. Asphyxia pallida presents at birth with pallor and cyanosis, which improves with supplemental oxygen delivery, respiratory failure, bradycardia, and normal central venous pressure.

2. **Hemolytic anemia.** Jaundice is often seen before diagnostic levels of hemoglobin are obtained, in part because of the compensatory reticulocytosis that is invariably present. The infant usually presents with pallor after 48 h of age. However, severe Rh isoimmune disease or homozygous α-thalassemia presents at birth with severe anemia and, in many cases, hydrops fetalis. Unconjugated hyperbilirubinemia of >10–12 mg/dL, tachypnea, and hepatosplenomegaly may be seen with hemolytic anemia.

3. **Hypoplastic anemia.** Hypoplastic anemia is uncommon. It is characterized by presentation after 48 h of age, absence of jaundice, and reticulocytopenia.

4. **Other forms of anemia**
   a. **Anemia associated with twin-twin transfusion.** If chronic hemorrhage is occurring, there is often a >20% difference in the birth weights of the two infants, the donor being the smaller twin.
   b. **Occult (internal) hemorrhage**
      i. **Intracranial hemorrhage.** Signs include a bulging anterior fontanelle and neurologic signs (eg, a change in consciousness, apnea, or seizures).
      ii. **Visceral hemorrhage.** Most commonly, the liver has been injured. An abdominal mass or distention is seen.
      iii. **Pulmonary hemorrhage.** Partial or total radiographic opacification of a hemithorax and bloody tracheal secretions are seen.

B. **History**
1. **Anemia at birth**
   a. **Hemorrhagic anemia.** There may be a history of third-trimester vaginal bleeding or amniocentesis. Hemorrhagic anemia may be associated with multiple gestation, maternal chills or fever postpartum, and nonelective cesarean section.
   b. **Hemolytic anemia** may be associated with intrauterine growth retardation (IUGR) and Rh-negative mothers.
2. **Anemia presenting after 24 h of age** is often associated with obstetric trauma, unattended delivery, precipitous delivery, perinatal fetal distress, or a low Apgar score.
3. **Anemia presenting with jaundice** suggests hemolytic anemia. There may be evidence of drug ingestion late in the third trimester; IUGR; a family member with splenectomy, anemia, jaundice, or cholelithiasis; maternal autoimmune disease; or Mediterranean or Asian ethnic background.

V. **Diagnosis**
A. **Obligatory initial studies**
1. Hemoglobin.
2. RBC indices
   a. **Microcytic or hypochromic RBC indices** suggest fetomaternal or twin-twin hemorrhage or α-thalassemia (mean corpuscular volume <90 fL).
   b. **Normocytic or normochromic RBC indices** are suggestive of acute hemorrhage, systemic disease, intrinsic RBC defect, or hypoplastic anemia.

3. **Reticulocyte count** (corrected). The following formula is used:

Corrected reticulocyte count =

$$\frac{\text{Observed reticulocyte count} \times \text{Observed hematocrit}}{\text{Normal hematocrit for age}}$$

An elevated reticulocyte count is associated with antecedent hemorrhage or hemolytic anemia. A low count is seen with hypoplastic anemia.
4. **Blood smear**
   a. **Spherocytes** are associated with ABO isoimmune hemolysis or hereditary spherocytosis.
   b. **Elliptocytes** are seen in hereditary elliptocytosis.
   c. **Pyknocytes** may be seen in G6PD deficiency.
   d. **Schistocytes or helmet cells** are most often seen with consumption coagulopathy.
5. **Direct antiglobulin test (direct Coombs' test).** This test is positive in isoimmune or autoimmune hemolysis.
B. **Other selected laboratory studies**
   1. **Isoimmune hemolysis.** The blood type and Rh type should be determined and an eluate of neonatal cells prepared.
   2. **Fetomaternal hemorrhage.** The **Kleihauer-Betke test** should be performed. Using an acid elution technique, a maternal blood smear is stained with eosin. Fetal RBCs stain darkly. Adult RBCs do not stain and appear as "ghost cells." ABO incompatibility between mother and infant will result in an increased clearance rate of fetal cells from the maternal circulation, giving a falsely low result. Because various conditions may lead to a false-negative result, new and more accurate flow cytometry techniques can be used when the index of suspicion for fetomaternal transfusions is elevated.
   3. **Pulmonary hemorrhage.**
   4. **Congenital hypoplastic or aplastic anemia.** Bone marrow aspiration is usually indicated.
   5. **TORCH infection**
      a. Skull and long-bone films.
      b. IgM levels.
      c. Acute or convalescent serologic.
      d. Urine culture for cytomegalovirus.
   6. **Consumption coagulopathy**
      a. Prothrombin time (PT) and partial thromboplastin time (PTT).
      b. Platelet count.
      c. Thrombin time (TT) or fibrinogen assay.
      d. Factor V and factor VIII levels.
      e. Fibrin split products.
   7. **Occult hemorrhage**
      a. Pathologic examination of the placenta.
      b. Cranial or abdominal ultrasonography will help identify the site of bleeding.
   8. **Intrinsic RBC defect**
      a. RBC enzyme studies.
      b. Analysis of the globin chain ratio.
      c. Studies of RBC membrane.
VI. **Management.** Treatment of neonatal anemia may involve, individually or in combination, simple replacement transfusion, exchange transfusion, nutritional supplementation, or treatment of the underlying primary disorder.
A. **Simple replacement transfusion**
   1. **Indications**
      a. Acute hemorrhagic anemia.

b. Ongoing deficit replacement.

c. Maintenance of effective oxygen-carrying capacity. There are no universally accepted guidelines; however, those presented next are fairly representative of most common practice.

  i. Hematocrit <35% with severe cardiopulmonary disease (eg, intermittent positive-pressure ventilation with mean airway pressure >6 cm H_2O).

  ii. Hematocrit <30%

    (a) With mild to moderate cardiopulmonary disease (FIO_2 >35%, continuous positive airway pressure).

    (b) Significant apnea (>9–12 h, or requiring bag-and-mask ventilation).

    (c) "Symptomatic anemia": weight gain <10 g/kg/day at full caloric intake and heart rate >180 beats/min persisting for 24 h.

    (d) If undergoing major surgery.

  iii. Hematocrit <21%: asymptomatic but with low reticulocyte count.

2. Emergency transfusion at birth only

  a. Use type O, Rh-negative packed RBCs.

    i. Adjust the hematocrit to 50%.

    ii. If a medical emergency exists, blood that has not been cross-matched may be given.

    iii. Blood drawn from the placental vein and heparinized (1 unit/mL) can be used if given through a blood filter. If time permits, blood may be cross-matched to the mother's blood.

  b. Alternative replacement fluids include fresh-frozen plasma, 5% albumin in saline, and dextran. Timely infusion of packed RBCs or partial exchange transfusion should follow.

  c. Perform umbilical vein catheterization to a depth of 2–3 cm or until free blood flow is established (see Chapter 27).

  d. Measure the central venous pressure, if time and technical capabilities allow, after advancing the catheter to the level of T6–T9.

  e. Draw initial blood samples for diagnostic studies. Obtain a hemogram and differential, blood type and Rh type, direct Coombs' test, and, if indicated, total bilirubin levels. In a medical emergency, transfusion may be started before the results of laboratory testing are known.

  f. Infuse 10–15 mL/kg of replacement fluid over 10–15 min if emergency measures are needed. Once the infant's status has stabilized, reassess the diagnostic studies, physical examination, and obstetric history.

  g. Calculate the RBC volume. Under controlled circumstances or if simple transfusion is indicated, calculate the volume of packed RBCs needed to achieve the desired increase in RBC mass (see p 275).

  h. The volume of a single transfusion should not exceed 10 mL/kg unless the central venous pressure is monitored.

B. Exchange transfusion

  1. Indications

    a. Chronic hemolytic anemia or hemorrhagic anemia with increased central venous pressure.

    b. Severe isoimmune hemolytic anemia with circulating sensitized RBCs and isoantibody.

    c. Consumption coagulopathy.

  2. Technique. See Chapter 21 for the technique of exchange transfusion in neonates.

C. Nutritional replacement

  1. Iron. Iron replacement is useful in the following situations:

    a. Fetomaternal hemorrhage of significant volume.

    b. Chronic twin-twin transfusion (in the donor twin).

    c. Incremental external blood loss (if unreplaced).
    d. Preterm infant (<36 weeks' gestational age).
  2. Folate (especially with serum levels <0.5 ng/mL)
    a. Premature infants weighing <1500 g or <34 weeks' gestational age.
    b. Chronic hemolytic anemias or conditions involving "stress erythropoiesis."
    c. Infants receiving phenytoin (Dilantin).
  3. Vitamin E. Preterm infants of <34 weeks' gestational age, unless they are being breast-fed.
D. Prophylactic
  1. Recombinant human erythropoietin (r-HuEPO). High doses of erythropoietin are capable of increasing neonatal erythropoiesis and have very little adverse side effect. It has been shown to decrease the requirement for "late" transfusions (those required past the age of 2–3 weeks); it will not compensate for the anemia secondary to phlebotomy losses. Its use in the very low birth weight infant continues to be *controversial* because the severity of anemia in this group can be more effectively minimized by a restrictive policy for blood sampling and the use of micromethods in the laboratory. The need for transfusions is also reduced when a consistent "protocolized" approach for transfusions is available in the neonatal intensive care unit. It has been also argued that what needs to be avoided, more than the transfusion itself, is the exposure to multiple donors. The allocation of a single donor for each high-risk infant, for a 42-day period, is the most effective way to reach that former goal. Early and late strategies have been used for erythropoietin treatment.
    a. Early. Starting on day 1 or 2, 1200–1400 units/kg/week. r-HuEPO is added to the total parenteral nutrition solution, and 1 mg/kg/day of iron is added.
    b. Late. 500–700 units/kg/week given 3–5 times/week subcutaneously. Supplemental oral iron needs to be provided at 3 mg/kg/day in 3 divided doses. The iron dose is increased to 6 mg/kg/day as soon as the infant is tolerating full enteral feeds.
  2. Nutritional supplementation
    a. Elemental iron, 1–2 mg/kg/day, beginning at 2 months of age and continuing through 1 year of age.
    b. Folic acid, 1–2 mg/week for preterm infants; 50 μg/day for term infants.
    c. Vitamin E, 25 IU/day, until a corrected age of 4 months is reached.
E. Treatment of selected disorders
  1. Consumption coagulopathy
    a. Treat the underlying cause (eg, sepsis).
    b. Give blood replacement therapy. Perform exchange transfusion or give fresh-frozen plasma, 10 mL/kg every 12–14 h. Platelet concentrate, 1 unit, may be used as a substitute for plasma transfusion.
    c. Perform coagulation studies. Monitor the PTT, PT, and fibrinogen levels and the platelet count.
  2. Immune thrombocytopenia
    a. Isoimmune thrombocytopenia
      i. Consider performing cesarean section if the diagnosis has been confirmed and there is an older sibling with immune thrombocytopenia (75% risk of recurrence).
      ii. Give maternal washed platelets when indicated for bleeding diathesis in an infant with a platelet count <20,000–30,000/μL. Exchange transfusion may be used as an alternative.
      iii. Corticosteroid therapy and IVIG are *controversial.*
    b. Autoimmune thrombocytopenia
      i. Consider performing cesarean section if the maternal platelet count is <100,000/μL or the fetal platelet count is <50,000/μL.

ii. Use of corticosteroids is *controversial*. Under the conditions just mentioned, consider giving corticosteroids to the mother several weeks before delivery. Transfusion of random donor platelets may be given when indicated.

POLYCYTHEMIA AND HYPERVISCOSITY

I. **Definitions.** Polycythemia is increased total RBC mass. Polycythemic hyperviscosity is increased viscosity of the blood resulting from, or associated with, increased numbers of RBCs.
   A. **Polycythemia.** Polycythemia of the newborn is defined as a central venous hematocrit >65%. The clinical significance of this value results from the curvilinear relationship between the circulating RBC volume (hematocrit) and whole blood viscosity. Above a hematocrit of 65%, blood viscosity, as measured in vitro, rises exponentially.
   B. **Hyperviscosity.** Hyperviscosity is the cause of clinical symptoms in infants presumed to be symptomatic from polycythemia. Many polycythemic infants are also hyperviscous, but this is not invariably the case. The terms *polycythemia* and *hyperviscosity* are not interchangeable.
II. **Incidence**
   A. **Polycythemia.** Polycythemia occurs in 2–4% of the general newborn population. Half of these patients are symptomatic, although it is not at all certain whether their symptoms are caused by polycythemia.
   B. **Hyperviscosity.** Hyperviscosity without polycythemia occurs in 1% of normal (nonpolycythemic) newborns. In infants with a hematocrit of 60–64%, one fourth have hyperviscosity.
III. **Pathophysiology.** Clinical signs attributed to hyperviscosity may result from the regional effects of hyperviscosity, including tissue hypoxia, acidosis, and hypoglycemia, and from the formation of microthrombi within the microcirculation. An important caveat, however, is that the same clinical signs may result from coexisting perinatal circumstances in the presence or absence of hyperviscosity. Potentially affected organs include the central nervous system, the kidneys and adrenal glands, the cardiopulmonary system, and the gastrointestinal tract. Blood viscosity is dependent on the interaction of frictional forces in whole blood. These forces are defined as **shear stress** and **shear rate,** a measure of blood flow velocity. The frictional forces identified within whole blood and their relative contributions to hyperviscosity in the newborn include the following:
   A. **Hematocrit.** Increase in the hematocrit is the most important single factor contributing to hyperviscosity in the neonate. An increased hematocrit results from either an absolute increase in circulating RBC volume or a decrease in plasma volume.
   B. **Plasma viscosity.** A direct linear relationship exists between plasma viscosity and the concentration of plasma proteins, particularly those of high molecular weight, such as fibrinogen. Term infants and, to a greater degree, preterm infants have low plasma fibrinogen levels compared with adults. Consequently, except for the rare case of primary hyperfibrinogenemia, plasma viscosity does not contribute to increased whole blood viscosity in the neonate. Under normal conditions, low plasma fibrinogen levels and, correspondingly, low plasma viscosity actually may protect the microcirculation of the neonate by facilitating perfusion and contributing to low whole blood viscosity.
   C. **RBC aggregation.** Aggregation of erythrocytes occurs only in areas of low blood flow and is usually limited to the venous microcirculation. Because fibrinogen levels are typically low in term and preterm infants, RBC aggregation does not contribute significantly to whole blood viscosity in newborn infants. There is some concern that the use of adult fresh-frozen plasma for partial exchange transfusion in neonates might critically alter the concentra-

tion of fibrinogen and paradoxically raise whole blood viscosity within the microcirculation.
  D. **Deformability of RBC membrane.** There are apparently no differences among term infants, preterm infants, and adults in terms of the membrane deformability of erythrocytes.
IV. **Risk factors**
  A. **Conditions that alter incidence**
    1. **Altitude.** There is an absolute increase in RBC mass as part of physiologic adaptation to high altitude.
    2. **Neonatal age.** The normal pattern of fluid shifts during the first 6 h of life is away from the intravascular compartment. The period of maximum physiologic increase in the hematocrit occurs at 2–4 h of age.
    3. **Obstetric factors.** A delay in cord clamping beyond 30 s or stripping of the umbilical cord, if that is the prevailing practice, will result in a higher incidence of polycythemia.
    4. **High-risk delivery.** High-risk delivery is associated with an increased incidence of polycythemia, particularly if precipitous or uncontrolled.
  B. **Perinatal processes**
    1. **Enhanced fetal erythropoiesis.** Elevated erythropoietin levels result from a direct stimulus, usually related to fetal hypoxia, or from altered regulation of erythropoietin production.
      a. **Placental insufficiency**
        i. Maternal hypertensive disease (preeclampsia-eclampsia) or primary renovascular disease.
        ii. Abruptio placentae (chronic recurrent).
        iii. Postmaturity.
        iv. Cyanotic congenital heart disease.
        v. IUGR.
        vi. Maternal cigarette smoking.
      b. **Endocrine disorders.** Increased oxygen consumption is the suggested mechanism by which hyperinsulinism or hyperthyroxinemia creates fetal hypoxemia and stimulates erythropoietin production.
        i. Infant of a diabetic mother (>40% incidence of polycythemia).
        ii. Infant of a mother with gestational diabetes (>30% incidence of polycythemia).
        iii. Congenital thyrotoxicosis.
        iv. Congenital adrenal hyperplasia.
        v. Beckwith-Wiedemann syndrome (secondary hyperinsulinism).
      c. **Genetic trisomies** (trisomies 13,18, and 21).
    2. **Hypertransfusion.** Conditions that enhance placental transfusion at birth may create hypervolemic normocythemia, which evolves into hypervolemic polycythemia as the normal pattern of fluid shift occurs. A larger transfusion may create hypervolemic polycythemia at birth, with signs present in the infant. Conditions associated with hypertransfusion include the following:
      a. **Delay in cord clamping.** Placental vessels contain up to one third of the fetal blood volume, half of which will be returned to the infant within 1 min after birth. Representative blood volumes for term infants with a variable delay in cord clamping are as follows:
        • 15-s delay, 75–78 mL/kg.
        • 60-s delay, 80–87 mL/kg.
        • 120-s delay, 83–93 mL/kg.
      b. **Gravity.** Positioning the infant below the placental bed (>10 cm below the placenta) enhances placental transfusion via the umbilical vein. Elevation of the infant >50 cm above the placenta will prevent placental transfusion.
      c. **Maternal use of medications.** Drugs that enhance uterine contractility—specifically oxytocin—do not significantly alter the gravitational

effects on placental transfusion during the first 15 s after birth. With further delay in clamping of the cord, however, blood flow toward the infant will accelerate to a maximum at 1 min of age.

d. **Cesarean section.** In cesarean delivery, there is usually a lower risk of placental transfusion if the cord is clamped early because of the absence of active uterine contractions in most cases and because of gravitational effects.

e. **Twin-twin transfusion.** Interfetal transfusion (**parabiosis syndrome**) is observed in monochorionic twin pregnancy with an incidence of 15%. The recipient twin, on the venous side of the anastomosis, becomes polycythemic, and the donor, on the arterial side, becomes anemic. Simultaneous venous hematocrits obtained after delivery differ by >12–15%, and both twins will have a high risk of intrauterine or neonatal death and increased neurologic morbidity.

f. **Maternal-fetal transfusion.** Approximately 10–80% of normal newborn infants receive a small volume of maternal blood at the time of delivery. The "reverse" Kleihauer-Betke acid elution technique (see p 338) will document maternal RBC "ghosts" on a neonatal blood smear. With large transfusions, the test will be positive for several days. Because various conditions may lead to a false-negative test result, new and more accurate flow cytometry techniques can be used when the index of suspicion for fetomaternal transfusions is elevated.

g. **Intrapartum asphyxia.** Prolonged fetal distress enhances the net umbilical blood flow toward the infant until cord clamping occurs, and acidosis may encourage capillary leak and reduced plasma volume.

V. **Clinical presentation.** Clinical signs observed in polycythemia are nonspecific and reflect the regional effects of hyperviscosity within a given microcirculation. The conditions listed next may occur independently of polycythemia or hyperviscosity and must be considered in the differential diagnosis.

A. **Central nervous system.** There may be an altered state of consciousness, including lethargy and decreased activity, hyperirritability, proximal muscle hypotonia, vasomotor instability, and vomiting. Seizures, thromboses, and cerebral infarction are extraordinarily rare.

B. **Cardiopulmonary system.** Respiratory distress and tachycardia may be present. Congestive heart failure with cardiomegaly may be seen but is rarely clinically prominent. Pulmonary hypertension may occur but is not usually severe unless other predisposing factors are present.

C. **Gastrointestinal tract.** Feeding intolerance occurs occasionally. Necrotizing enterocolitis has been reported but rarely without other factors (eg, IUGR), which casts doubt on the primary cause.

D. **Genitourinary tract.** Oliguria, acute renal failure, renal vein thrombosis, or priapism may occur.

E. **Metabolic disorders.** Hypoglycemia, hypocalcemia, or hypomagnesemia may be seen.

F. **Hematologic disorders.** There may be hyperbilirubinemia, thrombocytopenia, or reticulocytosis (with enhanced erythropoiesis only).

VI. **Diagnosis**

A. **Venous (not capillary) hematocrit.** Polycythemia is present when the central venous hematocrit is ≥65%.

B. **The following screening studies may be used:**
1. A cord blood hematocrit >56% suggests polycythemia.
2. A warmed capillary hematocrit ≥65% suggests polycythemia.

VII. **Management.** Clinical management of the polycythemic infant is more expectant now than a decade ago. Studies and reviews have created much doubt about any long-term benefits of partial exchange transfusion (PET). Consequently, PET should probably be performed only on infants in whom significant morbidity is in question.

A. **Asymptomatic infants.** Only expectant observation is required for virtually all asymptomatic infants. The possible exception is an infant with a central venous hematocrit of >75%, but even in this group the risks of central catheter insertion probably outweigh the benefits of PET.

B. Symptomatic infants. When the central venous hematocrit is ≥65%, PET may ameliorate acute signs of polycythemia or hyperviscosity. Whether treatment of a self-limited problem justifies the risks of central catheter insertion and an exchange procedure is debatable, however. For the procedure for partial exchange transfusion, see Chapter 21.

VIII. Prognosis. The long-term outcome of infants with polycythemia or hyperviscosity and response to PET is as follows:

   A. A causal relationship exists between PET and an increase in gastrointestinal tract disorders and necrotizing enterocolitis.

   B. Older randomized controlled prospective studies of polycythemic and hyperviscous infants indicate that PET may reduce but not eliminate the risk of neurologic sequelae. More recent data suggest that no benefits accrue from PET.

   C. Infants with "asymptomatic" polycythemia have an increased risk for neurologic sequelae, but normocythemic controls with the same perinatal histories have a similarly increased risk.

Rh INCOMPATIBILITY

I. Definition. Isoimmune hemolytic anemia of variable severity may result when Rh incompatibility develops between an Rh-negative mother previously sensitized to the Rh (D) antigen and her Rh-positive fetus. The onset of clinical disease begins in utero as the result of active placental transfer of maternal IgG-Rh antibody. It is manifested as a partially compensated, moderate to severe hemolytic anemia at birth, with unconjugated hyperbilirubinemia developing in the early neonatal period.

II. Incidence. Historically, Rh hemolytic disease of the newborn accounted for up to one third of symptomatic cases seen and was associated with detectable antibody in ~15% of Rh-incompatible mothers. The use of Rh immunoglobulin (RhoGAM) prophylaxis has reduced the incidence of Rh sensitization to <1% of Rh-incompatible pregnancies. Other alloimmune antibodies have become relatively more important as a cause of hemolysis. Anti-c, Kell, Duffy (Fy), and less commonly anti-C and anti-E may cause severe hemolytic disease of the newborn. This cannot be prevented by the use of D antigen–specific Rh immunoglobulin.

III. Pathophysiology. Initial exposure of the mother to the Rh antigen occurs most often during parturition, miscarriage, abortion, and ectopic pregnancy. Invasive investigative procedures such as amniocentesis, chorionic villus sampling, and fetal blood sampling also increase the risk of fetal transplacental hemorrhage and alloimmunization. Recognition of the antigen by the immune system ensues after initial exposure, and reexposure to the Rh antigen will induce a maternal anamnestic response and elevation of specific IgG-Rh antibody. Active placental transport of this antibody and immune attachment to the Rh antigenic sites on the fetal erythrocyte are followed by extravascular hemolysis of erythrocytes within the fetal liver and spleen. The rate of the hemolytic process is proportionate in part to the levels of the maternal antibody titer but is more accurately reflected in the antepartum period by elevation of the amniotic fluid bilirubin concentration and in the postpartum period by the rate of rise of unconjugated bilirubin. In contrast to ABO incompatibility, the greater antigenicity and density of the Rh antigen loci on the fetal erythrocyte will facilitate progressive, rapid clearance of fetal erythrocytes from the circulation. A demonstrable phase of spherocytosis will be absent. Compensatory reticulocytosis and shortening of the erythrocyte generation time, if unable to match the often high rate of hemolysis in utero, will result in anemia in the newborn infant and a risk of multiple systemic complications.

IV. Risk factors
  A. Birth order. The first-born infant is at minimum risk (<1%) unless sensitization has occurred previously. Once sensitization has occurred, subsequent pregnancies are at a progressive risk for fetal disease.
  B. Fetomaternal hemorrhage. The volume of fetal erythrocytes entering the maternal circulation correlates with the risk of sensitization. The risk is ~8% with each pregnancy but ranges from 3–65%, depending on the volume of fetal blood (0.1 to >5 mL) that passes into the maternal circulation.
  C. ABO incompatibility. Coexistent incompatibility for either the A or B blood group antigen will reduce the risk of maternal Rh sensitization to 1.5–3.0%. Rapid immune clearance of these fetal erythrocytes after their entry into the maternal circulation exerts a partial protective effect. It confers no protection once sensitization has occurred.
  D. Obstetric factors. Cesarean section or trauma to the placental bed during the third stage of labor increases the risk of significant fetomaternal transfusion and subsequent maternal sensitization.
  E. Gender. Male infants are reported to have an increased risk of more severe disease than females, although the basis for this observation is unclear.
  F. Ethnicity. Approximately 15% of whites are Rh-negative compared with 7% of blacks and almost 0% in Asiatic Chinese and Japanese. The risk to the fetus varies accordingly.
  G. Maternal immune response. A significant proportion of Rh-negative mothers (10–50%) fail to develop specific IgG-Rh antibody despite repeated exposure to Rh antigen.
V. Clinical presentation
  A. Symptoms and signs
    1. **Jaundice.** Unconjugated hyperbilirubinemia is the most common presenting neonatal sign of Rh disease, usually appearing within the first 24 h of life.
    2. **Anemia.** A low cord blood hemoglobin at birth reflects the relative severity of the hemolytic process in utero and is present in ~50% of cases.
    3. **Hepatosplenomegaly.** Enlargement of the liver and spleen is seen in severe hemolysis, sometimes occurring in association with ascites, with an increased risk for splenic rupture.
    4. **Hydrops fetalis.** Severe Rh disease has a historical association with hydrops fetalis and at one time was its most common cause. Clinical features in the fetus include progressive hypoproteinemia with ascites or pleural effusion, or both; severe chronic anemia with secondary hypoxemia; and cardiac failure. There is an increased risk of late fetal death, stillbirth, and intolerance of active labor. The neonate frequently has generalized edema, notably of the scalp, which can be detected by antepartum ultrasonography; cardiopulmonary distress often involving pulmonary edema and severe surfactant deficiency; congestive heart failure; hypotension and peripheral perfusion defects; cardiac rhythm disturbances; and severe anemia with secondary hypoxemia and metabolic acidosis. Currently, nonimmune conditions are more commonly associated with hydrops fetalis. Secondary involvement of other organ systems may result in hypoglycemia or thrombocytopenic purpura.
VI. Diagnosis. Obligatory screening in an infant with unconjugated hyperbilirubinemia includes the following studies:
  A. Blood type and Rh type (mother and infant). These studies establish the likelihood of Rh incompatibility and will exclude the diagnosis if the infant is Rh-negative, with one exception (see section VI,C, on the direct Coombs' test).
  B. Reticulocyte count. Elevated reticulocyte levels, adjusted for the degree of anemia and gestational age in preterm infants, reflect the degree of compensation and support a diagnosis of an ongoing hemolytic process. Normal values are 4–5% for term infants and 6–10% for preterm infants (30–36

weeks' gestational age). In symptomatic Rh disease, expected values are 10–40%.

C. **Direct antiglobulin (Coombs') test.** A strongly positive direct Coombs' test indicates that fetal RBCs are coated with antibodies and is diagnostic of Rh incompatibility in the presence of the appropriate setup and an elevated reticulocyte count. If Rh immunoglobulin was given at 28 weeks' gestation, subsequent passive transfer of antibody will result in a false-positive direct Coombs' test without associated reticulocytosis. Very rarely, a strongly positive direct Coombs' test will be associated with a falsely Rh-negative infant when all fetal RBC Rh antigenic sites are covered by a high titer of maternal antibodies.

D. **Blood smear.** Polychromasia and normoblastosis proportionate to the reticulocyte count are typically present. Spherocytes are not usually present. The nucleated RBC count will often be >10 per 100 white blood cells.

E. **Bilirubin levels.** Progressive elevation of unconjugated bilirubin on serial testing provides an index of the severity of the hemolytic process. An elevated direct fraction is most likely to be secondary to a laboratory artifact in the first 3 days of life and should not be subtracted from the total bilirubin when making management decisions. In the most severely affected infant, particularly those who are hydropic, the intense extramedullary erythropoiesis may cause hepatocellular dysfunction and biliary canalicular obstruction with significant elevated direct bilirubin by 5–6 days of age.

F. **Bilirubin-binding capacity tests.** Correlation between measurements of serum albumin, free bilirubin, bilirubin saturation index, and reserve binding capacity and outcome has been variable. The role of these values in directing the management of patients remains unclear.

G. **Glucose and blood gas levels** should be monitored closely.

H. **Supplementary laboratory studies.** Supportive diagnostic studies may be required when the basis of the hemolytic process remains unclear.

1. **Direct Coombs' test in the mother.** This study should be negative in Rh disease. This test can be positive in the presence of maternal autoimmune hemolytic disease, particularly collagen vascular disease.

2. **Indirect antiglobulin titer (indirect Coombs' test).** This test detects the presence of antibodies in the maternal serum. Rh-positive RBCs are incubated with the serum being tested for the presence of anti-D. If present, the RBCs now coated with anti-D are agglutinated by an antihuman globulin serum reflecting a positive indirect antiglobulin (Coombs') test result. The reciprocal of the highest dilution of maternal serum that produces agglutination is the indirect antiglobulin titer.

3. **Carbon monoxide (CO).** The severity of Rh disease may be determined by measurement of endogenous CO production. When heme is catabolized to bilirubin, CO is produced in equimolar amounts. Hemoglobin binds the CO to form carboxyhemoglobin (CO Hb) and then is finally excreted in the breath. CO Hb levels are increased in neonates with hemolysis. CO Hb levels >1.4% have correlated with an increased need for exchange transfusion.

VII. **Management**

A. **Antepartum treatment.** Verification of the Rh-negative status at the first prenatal visit may be obtained by the following measures:

1. **Maternal antibody titer.** Once an IgG-Rh antibody has been identified, it is important to determine the titer. Serial antibody titer determinations are required every 1–4 weeks (depending on the gestational age) during pregnancy. Invasive fetal testing becomes indicated when the titer is above a critical level, usually between 1:8 and 1:16. A negative antibody screen (indirect Coombs' test) signifies absence of sensitization. This test should be repeated at 28–34 weeks' gestation.

2. **RhoGAM.** Current obstetric guidelines suggest giving immunoprophylaxis at 28 weeks' gestation in the absence of sensitization.

3. **Amniocentesis.** If maternal antibody titers indicate a risk of fetal death (usual range, 1:16–1:32), amniocentesis should be performed. To reasonably predict the risk of moderate to severe fetal disease, serial determinations of amniotic fluid bilirubin levels present photometrically at 450 nm are plotted on standard graphs according to gestational age. Readings falling into very high zone II or zone III indicate that hydrops will develop within 7–10 days. Zone I indicates no fetal hemolytic disease or no anemia.

4. **Ultrasonography.** As a screening study in pregnancies at risk, serial fetal ultrasound examinations allow detection of scalp edema, ascites, or other signs of developing hydrops fetalis.

5. **Intrauterine transfusion.** Based on the studies just mentioned, intrauterine transfusion may be indicated because of possible fetal demise or the presence of fetal hydrops. This procedure must be performed by an experienced team. The goal is maintenance of effective erythrocyte mass within the fetal circulation and maintenance of the pregnancy until there is a reasonable chance for successful extrauterine survival of the infant.

6. **Glucocorticoids.** If premature delivery is anticipated, glucocorticoids should be given to accelerate fetal lung maturation.

7. **Reduction of maternal antibody level.** Intensive maternal plasma exchange and high-dose IVIGs have been reported as being of value in the severely alloimmunized pregnant woman to reduce circulating maternal antibodies levels by >50%.

B. **Postpartum treatment**

1. **Resuscitation.** Moderately to severely anemic infants with or without hydropic features are at risk for high-output cardiac failure, hypoxemia secondary to decreased oxygen-carrying capacity or surfactant deficiency, and hypoglycemia. These infants may require immediate single-volume exchange blood transfusion at delivery to improve oxygen-carrying capacity, mechanical support of ventilation, and an extended period of monitoring for hypoglycemia.

2. **Cord blood studies.** A cord blood bilirubin level >4 mg/dL or a cord hemoglobin <12 g/dL, or both, usually suggests moderate to severe disease. The cord blood is used for these and initial screening studies, including blood typing, Rh typing, and Coombs' test.

3. **Serial unconjugated bilirubin studies.** Determination of the rate of increase in unconjugated bilirubin levels will provide an index of the severity of the hemolytic process and the need for exchange transfusion. Commonly used guidelines include a rise of >0.5 mg/dL/h or >5 mg/dL over 24 h within the first 2 days of life or projection of a serum level that will exceed a predetermined "exchange level" for a given infant (usually 20 mg/dL in term infants).

4. **Phototherapy.** In severe Rh hemolytic disease, phototherapy is used only as an adjunct to exchange transfusion. Phototherapy decreases bilirubin levels and reduces the number of total exchange transfusions required. Phototherapy should be started if bilirubin rises 0.5 mg/dL/h or if total bilirubin exceeds 10, 12, or 14 mg/dL at 12, 18, or 24 h of life, respectively.

5. **Exchange transfusion.** (For the procedure, see Chapter 21.) Exchange transfusion is indicated if the unconjugated bilirubin level is likely to reach a predetermined "exchange level" for that patient. Optimally, exchange transfusion is done well before this exchange level is reached to minimize the risk of entry of unconjugated bilirubin into the central nervous system. Consideration should be given to irradiation of blood before the transfusion is given, particularly in preterm infants or infants expected to require multiple transfusions, to reduce the risk of graft-versus-host disease.

6. **Heme oxygenase inhibitors** (metalloporphyrins) are currently investigational. The enzyme heme oxygenase catalyzes the rate-limiting step in bilirubin production, the conversion of heme to biliverdin.
7. **IVIG.** Postnatal treatment may be effective by blocking neonatal reticuloendothelial Fc receptors and thus decrease hemolysis of the antibody-coated Rh-positive RBCs.
C. **RhoGAM prophylaxis.** Most cases of incompatibility involve the D antigen. RhoGAM given at 28 weeks' gestation or within 72 h of suspected Rh antigen exposure, or both, will reduce the risk of sensitization to <1%; the recommended dosage should be well in excess of the amount of Rh antigen transfused. In massive fetomaternal hemorrhage, however, conventional doses may be insufficient. The amount of fetal blood entering the maternal circulation may be estimated using the Kleihauer-Betke acid elution technique (p 338) during the immediate postpartum period.

No treatment equivalent to RhoGAM is available for maternal Rh sensitization to non-D antigens, notably C and E antigens. These antigens, however, are significantly less antigenic than the D antigen, clinical manifestations of incompatibility are frequently milder, and the risk of severe disease is considerably less.

D. **Hydrops fetalis.** Skilled resuscitation and anticipation of selective systemic complications may prevent early neonatal death.
1. **Isovolumetric partial exchange transfusion** with type O Rh-negative packed erythrocytes will raise the hematocrit and improve the oxygen-carrying capacity (see Chapter 21).
2. **Central arterial and venous catheterization** may be performed to provide the following measures:
   a. **Isovolumetric exchange transfusion.**
   b. **Monitoring of arterial blood gas levels and central venous and systemic blood pressures.**
   c. **Monitoring of fluid and electrolyte balance,** particularly renal and hepatic function, calcium/phosphorus ratio, and serum albumin levels as well as appropriate hematologic studies and serum bilirubin levels.
3. **Positive-pressure mechanical ventilation.** This measure may include increased levels of positive end-expiratory pressure, if pulmonary edema is present, as a means of stabilizing alveolar ventilation. Treatment with exogenous surfactant may be considered in particular when the infant is judged to be not fully mature.
4. **Therapeutic paracentesis or thoracentesis** may be performed to remove fluid that may further compromise respiratory effort. Excessive removal of ascitic fluid may lead to systemic hypotension.
5. **Volume expanders** may be necessary, in addition to erythrocytes, to improve peripheral perfusion defects. This should be done with caution because most hydropic infants are hypotensive or poorly perfused because of hypoxic heart failure rather than hypovolemia, or both.
6. **Drug treatment** may include diuretics such as furosemide for pulmonary edema and pressor agents such as dopamine (for dosages, see Chapter 80). In the case of cardiac rhythm disturbances, appropriate drugs may be used if indicated.
7. **Electrocardiography or echocardiography** may be needed to determine whether cardiac abnormalities are present.

VIII. **Prognosis.** Prenatal mortality for infants at risk of anti-D Rh isoimmunization is currently ~1.5% and has decreased significantly over the past two decades. Antenatal immune prophylaxis and improved management techniques, including amniotic fluid spectrophotometry, intrauterine transfusion, and advances in neonatal intensive care, have been largely responsible for this reduction. Isolated cases of severe isoimmunization still occur because of isoimmunization by other than anti-D antibody or failure to receive immune prophylaxis and may exhibit the full spectrum of disease, including an increased risk of stillbirths and early neonatal morbidity and mortality.

THROMBOCYTOPENIA AND PLATELET DYSFUNCTION

I. **Definition.** Thrombocytopenia is defined as a platelet count less than 150,000/ μL, although a few normal neonates may have counts as low as 100,000/μL in the absence of clinical disease. The best measure of platelet function is the standardized (Ivy) bleeding time (1.5–5.5 min). During the first week of life, bleeding times are shorter than those in adults.

II. **Normal platelet physiology.** The rate of platelet production and turnover in neonates is similar to that of older children and adults. The platelet life span is 7–10 days, and the mean platelet count is >200,000/μL. Platelet counts are slightly lower in low birth weight infants, in whom platelet counts <100,000/μL have occasionally been observed in the absence of a clinical disorder. Low platelet counts should nonetheless be investigated in low birth weight infants. Platelet counts vary according to the method of determination. Phase microscopy determinations are generally 25,000–50,000/μL lower than those obtained by direct microscopy.

III. **Etiology**
   A. **Thrombocytopenia**
      1. **Maternal disorders causing thrombocytopenia in infant**
         a. Drug use (eg, heparin, quinine, hydralazine, tolbutamide, and thiazide diuretics).
         b. Infections (eg, TORCH infections, bacterial or viral infections).
         c. Disseminated intravascular coagulation (DIC).
         d. Severe hypertension (HELLP syndrome [*h*emolysis, *e*levated *l*iver enzymes, *l*ow *p*latelet count]).
         e. Antiplatelet antibodies
            i. Antibodies against maternal and fetal platelets (autoimmune thrombocytopenia).
               (a) Idiopathic thrombocytopenic purpura (ITP).
               (b) Drug-induced thrombocytopenia.
               (c) Systemic lupus erythematosus.
               (d) Gestational or *incidental* thrombocytopenia
            ii. Antibodies against fetal platelets (isoimmune thrombocytopenia).
               (a) Neonatal alloimmune thrombocytopenia (mostly anti-HPA-1a alloantibodies).
               (b) Isoimmune thrombocytopenia associated with erythroblastosis fetalis.
      2. **Placental disorders causing thrombocytopenia in infant (rare)**
         a. Chorioangioma.
         b. Vascular thrombi.
         c. Placental abruption.
      3. **Neonatal disorders causing thrombocytopenia**
         a. Decreased platelet production or congenital absence of megakaryocytes.
            i. Isolated.
            ii. Thrombocytopenia–absent radius syndrome (TAR).
            iii. Fanconi's anemia.
            iv. Rubella syndrome.
            v. Congenital leukemia.
            vi. Trisomies 13, 18, or 21.
         b. Increased platelet destruction
            i. Increased platelet consumption occurs in many sick infants not associated with any specific pathologic state. This form of thrombocytopenia is the most common hemostatic abnormality in the

newborn admitted to neonatal intensive care. About 20% of new-borns admitted to the NICU experience thrombocytopenia; for 20% of those, counts are <50,000/μL. This form of thrombocytopenia, generally present by 2 days of life, reaches a nadir by 4 days and usually recovers to normal by 10 days of life.

    ii. Pathologic states associated with increased platelet destruction
       (a) Bacterial and *Candida* sepsis.
       (b) TORCH infections.
       (c) DIC.
       (d) Birth asphyxia.
       (e) Necrotizing enterocolitis.
       (f) Platelet destruction associated with giant hemangioma (Kasabach-Merritt syndrome).

B. Platelet dysfunction
  1. Drug-induced platelet dysfunction
    a. Maternal use of aspirin.
    b. Indomethacin.
  2. Metabolic disorders
    a. Phototherapy-induced metabolic abnormalities.
    b. Acidosis.
    c. Fatty acid deficiency.
    d. Maternal diabetes.
  3. Inherited thrombasthenia (Glanzmann's disease).

IV. Clinical presentation
  A. Symptoms and signs. It is important to carefully assess the general condition of the infant. A "sick"-appearing newborn implies a very different approach for the investigation and treatment of thrombocytopenia (such as sepsis) than the infant who otherwise appears healthy (such as with most case of alloimmune thrombocytopenia).
    1. Generalized superficial petechiae are often present, particularly in response to minor trauma or pressure or increased venous pressure. Platelet counts are usually <60,000/μL.
    2. Gastrointestinal bleeding, mucosal bleeding, or spontaneous hemorrhage in other sites may be occurring with platelet counts <20,000/μL.
    3. Intracranial hemorrhage may occur with severe thrombocytopenia.
    4. Large ecchymoses and muscle hemorrhages are more likely to be due to coagulation disturbances than to platelet disturbances.
    5. Petechiae in normal infants tend to be clustered on the head and upper chest, do not recur, and are associated with normal platelet counts. They are a result of a transient increase in venous pressure during birth.

  B. History
    1. There may be a family history of thrombocytopenia or history of intracranial hemorrhage in a sibling.
    2. Maternal drug ingestion may be a factor.
    3. A history of infection should be noted.
    4. Previous episodes of bleeding may have occurred.

  C. Placental examination. The placenta should be carefully examined for evidence of chorioangioma, thrombi, or abruptio placentae.

  D. Physical examination
    1. Petechiae and bleeding should be noted.
    2. Physical malformations may be present in TAR syndrome, rubella syndrome, giant hemangioma, or trisomy syndromes.
    3. Hepatosplenomegaly may be caused by viral or bacterial infection or congenital leukemia.

V. Diagnosis
  A. Laboratory studies
    1. Newborn studies
      a. Neonatal platelet count: Thrombocytopenia diagnosed from a capillary sample should be confirmed by a repeated count from a sample

obtained from a peripheral vein and by careful examination of a peripheral blood smear.
 b. Complete blood count.
 c. Blood typing.
 d. Coombs' test.
 e. Coagulation studies.
 f. Other studies (if indicated).
   i. TORCH titers.
   ii. Bacterial cultures.
   iii. Bone marrow studies if decreased platelet production is present.
2. **Maternal studies**
 a. Test for maternal thrombocytopenia. A low maternal count suggests autoimmune thrombocytopenia or inherited thrombocytopenia (X-linked recessive thrombocytopenia or autosomal dominant thrombocytopenia).
 b. Maternal serum and whole blood sample for rapid HPA-1a (PI^{A1}) phenotyping plus screen for anti-HPA-1a (PI^{A1}) alloantibodies.
B. Decreased platelet production versus increased platelet destruction
1. **Decreased platelet production**
 a. Platelet size is normal.
 b. Platelet survival time is normal.
 c. Megakaryocytes are decreased in a bone marrow sample.
 d. A sustained increase in the platelet count over a period of 4–7 days is seen after platelet transfusion.
2. **Increased platelet destruction**
 a. Platelet size is increased.
 b. Platelet survival time is decreased.
 c. Megakaryocytes in the bone marrow are normal or increased.
 d. There is little or no sustained increase in platelet count after platelet transfusion.
VI. Management
A. Obstetric management of maternal autoimmune thrombocytopenia
1. Treatment is aimed at prevention of intracranial hemorrhage during vaginal delivery.
2. There is an increased risk of severe neonatal thrombocytopenia and intracranial hemorrhage if antibody is present in the maternal plasma or if fetal scalp platelet counts are <50,000/μL.
3. Cesarean delivery may be indicated.
4. Administering corticosteroids to the mother has sometimes been described as beneficial.
B. Management of isoimmune thrombocytopenia
1. Transfuse platelets lacking the incompatible antigen. Although these platelets are usually obtained from the mother, transfusion of unmatched platelets from a random donor may be helpful if matched platelets cannot be obtained.
2. Intravenous gamma globulin may be useful (see Chapter 80 for dosage and other pharmacologic information).
3. The risk of recurrence in siblings is >75%. In subsequent pregnancies, the administration of corticosteroids and intravenous gamma globulin weekly during the third trimester may be effective (see Chapter 80 for dosage and other pharmacologic information). Some may receive in utero platelet transfusions. Most infants are delivered by cesarean section.
C. Treatment of infants with thrombocytopenia
1. Treat the underlying cause (eg, sepsis). If drugs are the cause, stop administration.
2. Platelet transfusions are indicated if active bleeding is occurring with any degree of thrombocytopenia or if there is no active bleeding but platelet counts are <20,000/μL. It may be desirable to transfuse "sick" premature

infants if the platelet count is <50,000/μL. Random donor platelets are given in a dosage of 10–20 mL/kg of standard platelet concentrates. The plasma in platelets should be ABO and Rh compatible with the infant's RBCs. The platelet count should increase to >100,000/μL. Platelet count should be repeated 1 h posttransfusion. Failure to achieve or sustain a rise in platelet count suggests a destructive process. Washed maternal platelets may need to be used for infants with alloimmune thrombocytopenia.

3. Exchange transfusion is given for immune thrombocytopenia. The platelet count may rise only transiently. There is considerable risk involved.

4. Prednisone, 2 mg/kg/day, may also be beneficial in immune thrombocytopenia.

5. Interleukin-11 (Neumega), a hematopoietic growth factor, and recombinant thrombopoietin have been used in adults for the prevention of severe thrombocytopenia. No data are presently available on its safety and efficacy in neonates.

REFERENCES

Alpay F et al: High-dose intravenous immunoglobulin therapy in neonatal immune haemolytic jaundice. *Acta Paediatr* 1999;88:216.

American Academy of Pediatrics: Commentary: neonatal jaundice and kernicterus. *Pediatrics* 2001;108:763.

Bifano EM, Curran TR: Minimizing donor blood exposure in the neonatal intensive care unit: current trends and future prospects. *Clin Perinatol* 1995;22:657.

Black VD, Lubchenco LO: Neonatal polycythemia and hyperviscosity. *Pediatr Clin North Am* 1982;29:1137.

Black VD et al: Neonatal hyperviscosity: randomized study of effect of partial plasma exchange transfusion on long-term outcome. *Pediatrics* 1985;75:1048.

Blanchette VS, Rand ML: Platelet disorders in newborn infants: diagnosis and management. *Semin Perinatol* 1997;21:53.

Bowman JM: Immune hemolytic disease. In Nathan DG, Orkin S (eds): *Hematology of Infancy and Childhood,* 5th ed. Saunders, 1998.

Bowman JM: Rh erythroblastosis fetalis. *Semin Hematol* 1975;12:189.

Bussel JB et al: Antenatal treatment of neonatal alloimmune thrombocytopenia. *N Engl J Med* 1988;319:1374.

Castle V et al: Frequency and mechanism of neonatal thrombocytopenia. *J Pediatr* 1986;108: 749.

Davis BH: Detection of fetal red cells in fetomaternal hemorrhage using a fetal hemoglobin monoclonal antibody by flow cytometry. *Transfusion* 1998;38:749.

Dickerman JF: Anemia in the newborn infant. *Pediatr Rev* 1984;6:131.

Glader BE: Erythrocyte disorders in infancy. In Avery ME, Taeusch HW (eds): *Schaffer's Diseases of the Newborn,* 5th ed. Saunders, 1984.

Gollin YG, Copel JA: Management of the Rh-sensitized mother. *Clin Perinatol* 1995;22:545.

Gross S et al: The blood and hematopoietic system. In Fanaroff AA, Martin RJ (eds): *Behrman's Neonatal Perinatal Medicine,* 3rd ed. Mosby, 1983.

Klemperer MR: Hemolytic anemias: immune defects. In Miller DR et al (eds): *Blood Diseases of Infancy and Childhood,* 5th ed. Mosby, 1984.

Lee DA et al: Reducing blood donor exposure in low birth weight infants by use of older, unwashed packed red blood cells. *J Pediatr* 1995;126:280.

Linderkamp O: Placental transfusion: determinants and effects. *Clin Perinatol* 1982;9:559.

Linderkamp O et al: Contributions of red cells and plasma to blood viscosity in preterm and full-term infants and adults. *Pediatrics* 1984;74:45.

Martin JN et al: Autoimmune thrombocytopenic purpura: current concepts and recommended practices. *Am J Obstet Gynecol* 1984;150:86.

Martinez JC: Control of severe hyperbilirubinemia in full-term newborns with the inhibitor of bilirubin production Sn-mesoporphyrin. *Pediatrics* 1999;103:1.

Mentzer WC: Polycythemia and hyperviscosity syndrome in newborn infants. *Clin Haematol* 1978;7:63.

Miller DR: Normal values and examination of the blood: perinatal period, infancy, childhood, and adolescence. In Miller DR et al (eds): *Blood Diseases of Infancy and Childhood,* 5th ed. Mosby, 1984.

Naiman JL: Disorders of the platelets. In Oski FA, Naiman JL (eds): *Hematologic Problems in the Newborn,* 3rd ed. Saunders, 1982a.

Naiman JL: Erythroblastosis fetalis. In Oski FA, Naiman JL (eds): *Hematologic Problems in the Newborn,* 3rd ed. Saunders, 1982b.

Oh W: Neonatal polycythemia and hyperviscosity. *Pediatr Clin North Am* 1986;33:523.

Ohls R et al: Effects of early erythropoietin therapy on the transfusion requirements of preterm infants below 1250 gm birth weight: a multicenter, randomized, controlled trial. *Pediatrics* 2001;108:934.

Oski FA: Hematologic problems. In Avery GD (ed): *Neonatology, Pathophysiology, and Management of the Newborn,* 2nd ed. Lippincott, 1981.

Oski FA: Hydrops fetalis. In Avery ME, Taeusch HW (eds): *Schaffer's Diseases of the Newborn,* 5th ed. Saunders, 1984.

Oski FA, Naiman JL (eds): *Hematologic Problems in the Newborn,* 3rd ed. Saunders, 1982a.

Oski FA, Naiman JL: Polycythemia and hyperviscosity in the neonatal period In Oski FA, Naiman JL (eds): *Hematologic Problems in the Newborn,* 3rd ed. Saunders, 1982b.

Pearson HA: Posthemorrhagic anemia in the newborn. *Pediatr Rev* 1982;4:40.

Pearson HA, McIntosh S: Neonatal thrombocytopenia. *Clin Haematol* 1978;7:111.

Peddle LJ: The antenatal management of the Rh sensitized woman. *Clin Perinatol* 1984;11:251.

Peterec SM. Management of neonatal Rh disease. *Clin Perinatol* 1995;22:561.

Polesky HF: Diagnosis, prevention and therapy in hemolytic diseases of the newborn. *Clin Lab Med* 1982;2:107.

Rothenberg T: Partial plasma exchange transfusion in polycythaemic neonates. *Arch Dis Child* 2002;86:60.

Ryan G, Morrow HJ: Fetal blood transfusion. *Clin Perinatol* 1994;21:573.

Shannon K: Recombinant human erythropoietin in neonatal anemia. *Clin Perinatol* 1995;22:627.

Shohat M et al: Neonatal polycythemia: I. Early diagnosis and incidence related to time of sampling. *Pediatrics* 1984;73:7.

Sola et al: Evaluation and treatment of thrombocytopenia in the neonatal intensive care unit. *Clin Perinatol* 2000;27:655.

Stockman JA III: Overview of the state of the art of Rh disease: history, current clinical management, and recent progress. *J Pediatr Hematol Oncol* 2001;23:554.

Stuart MJ: Platelet function in the neonate. *Am J Pediatr Hematol Oncol* 1979;1:227.

Vreman HJ, Wong RJ, Stevenson DK: Alternative metalloporphyrins for the treatment of neonatal jaundice. *J Perinatol* 2001;21(Suppl 1):5119.

62 Cardiac Abnormalities

CONGENITAL HEART DISEASE

The diagnostic dilemma of the newborn with congenital heart disease must be resolved quickly because therapy may prove lifesaving for some of these infants. Congenital heart disease occurs in ~1% of live-born infants. Nearly half of all cases of congenital heart disease are diagnosed during the first week of life. The most frequently occurring anomalies seen during this first week are patent ductus arteriosus (PDA), D-transposition of the great arteries, hypoplastic left heart syndrome (HLHS), tetralogy of Fallot, and pulmonary atresia.

I. **Classification.** Symptoms and signs in newborns with heart disease permit grouping according to levels of arterial oxygen saturation. Further classification (based on other physical findings and laboratory tests) facilitates delineation of the exact cardiac lesion present.

   A. **Cyanotic heart disease.** Infants with cyanotic heart disease are usually unable to achieve a Pao_2 of >100 mm Hg after breathing 100% inspired oxygen for 10–20 min.

   B. **Acyanotic heart disease.** Infants with acyanotic heart disease will achieve Pao_2 levels of >100 mm Hg under the same conditions as noted in Congenital Heart Disease, section I,A.

II. **Cyanotic heart disease** (Table 62–1)

   A. **100% oxygen test.** Because of intracardiac right-to-left shunting, the newborn with cyanotic congenital heart disease (in contrast to the infant with pulmonary disease) is unable to raise the arterial saturation, even in the presence of increased ambient oxygen.

      1. **Determine Pao_2 while the infant is on room air.**

      2. **Give 100% oxygen for 10–20 min by mask, hood, or endotracheal tube.**

      3. **Obtain an arterial blood gas level while the infant is breathing 100% oxygen.**

   B. **Cyanosis.** Care must be taken in evaluating cyanosis by skin color because polycythemia, jaundice, racial pigmentation, or anemia may make clinical recognition of cyanosis difficult.

   C. **Murmur.** The infant with cyanotic congenital heart disease often does not have a distinctive murmur. In fact, the most serious of these anomalies may not be associated with a murmur at all.

   D. **Other studies.** Cyanotic infants may be further classified on the basis of pulmonary circulation on chest x-ray and electrocardiographic findings.

   E. **Diagnosis and treatment.** Table 62–1 outlines the diagnosis and treatment of cyanotic heart disease.

   F. **Specific cyanotic heart disease abnormalities**

      1. **D-transposition of the great arteries** is the most common cardiac cause of cyanosis in the first year of life, with a male-female ratio of 2:1. The aorta comes from the right ventricle, and the pulmonary artery from the left ventricle, with resultant separate systemic and pulmonary circuits. With modern newborn care, the 1-year survival rate approaches 80%.

         a. **Physical examination.** Typical presentation is a large, vigorous infant with cyanosis but little or no respiratory distress. There may be no murmur or a soft, systolic ejection murmur.

         b. **Chest x-ray study.** This study may be normal, but typically it reveals a very narrow upper mediastinal shadow ("egg on a stick" appearance).

TABLE 62-1. CYANOTIC CONGENITAL HEART DISEASE (Pao₂ <100 mm Hg in 100% Fio₂)

	Decreased blood flow with small heart (or normal heart)		Decreased pulmonary blood flow with large heart		Increased pulmonary blood flow with small heart	Increased pulmonary blood flow with large heart		Normal pulmonary blood flow, with normal-sized heart. No thymus
Chest x-ray								
ECG	RVH	LVH, LAD	LVH, normal axis	RBBB	RVH	RVH or normal	LVH or normal	Normal
Differential diagnosis	Pulmonary atresia with VSD, TOF	Tricuspid atresia	Pulmonary atresia with intact septum	Ebstein's anomaly	TAPVR	HLHS	TGA with VSD, truncus arteriosus	TGA
Physical examination	Short, soft ejection murmur may only be heard in back	Faint PDA murmur or systolic murmur of small VSD	Systolic and diastolic murmurs at xiphoid TS/TI	Widely split S₂, scratchy diastolic murmur at xiphoid	No murmur. Quadruple rhythm often secondary to pulmonary ejection sound, split S₂, diastolic filling sound	Poor peripheral pulses	Systolic murmur	No murmur
Treatment	If Pao₂ is low, start PGE₁ infusion. Then perform further cardiac evaluation. Operation may or may not be needed.				Consider PGE₁ infusion. Then perform further cardiac evaluation. Operation may or may not be needed.			Immediate balloon septostomy

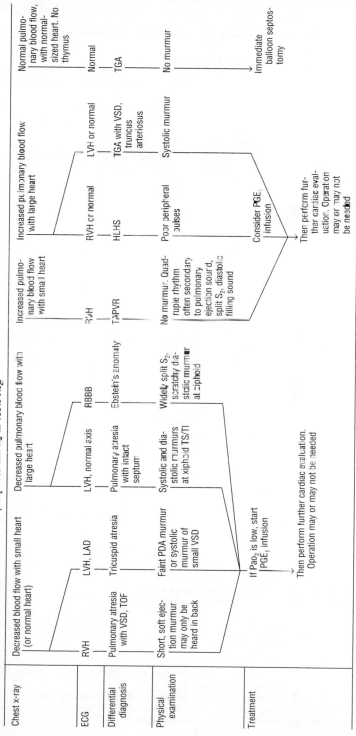

ECG, electrocardiography; HLHS, hypoplastic left heart syndrome; LAD, left axis deviation; LVH, left ventricular hypertrophy; PDA, patent ductus arteriosus; PGE₁, prostaglandin E₁; RBBB, right bundle branch block; RVH, right ventricular hypertrophy; TAPVR, total anomalous pulmonary venous return; TGA, transposition of the great arteries; TOF, tetralogy of Fallot; TS, tricuspid stenosis; VSD, ventricular septal defect.

c. **Electrocardiography (ECG).** There are no characteristic ECG findings.

d. **Echocardiography is diagnostic.** Typical findings include branching of the anterior great vessel into the innominate, subclavian, and carotid vessels and branching of the posterior great vessel into the right and left pulmonary arteries.

e. **Cardiac catheterization.** Like echocardiography, this study is diagnostic and often therapeutic as outlined next in Congenital Heart Disease, section II,F,1,f.

f. **Treatment.** If severe hypoxia or acidosis occurs, urgent balloon atrial septostomy can be done under echocardiogram guidance in the nursery. Cardiac catheterization with balloon septostomy and subsequent arterial switch operation are methods of treatment.

2. **Tetralogy of Fallot.** Tetralogy of Fallot is characterized by four anomalies: pulmonary stenosis, ventricular septal defect, overriding aorta, and right ventricular hypertrophy (RVH). There is a slight male predominance. Cyanosis usually signifies complete or partial atresia of the right ventricular overflow tract or extremely severe pulmonary stenosis with hypoplastic pulmonary arteries. The degree of right ventricular outflow obstruction is inversely proportional to pulmonary blood flow and directly proportional to the degree of cyanosis. Tetralogy of Fallot with absent pulmonary valve may present with respiratory distress or poor feeding (because of compression of the esophagus or bronchi by the large pulmonary arteries).

   a. **Physical examination.** The patient is cyanotic with a systolic ejection murmur along the left sternal border. Loud murmurs are associated with more flow across the right ventricular outflow tract and milder degrees of desaturation. Softer murmurs are associated with less flow and more hypoxia.

   b. **Chest x-ray study.** The chest x-ray film reveals a small, often "boot-shaped" heart, with decreased pulmonary vascular markings. A right aortic arch is seen in ~20% of these infants.

   c. **ECG.** The ECG may be normal or may demonstrate RVH. The only sign of RVH may be an upright T wave in V_4R or V_1 after 72 h of age.

   d. **Echocardiography** is usually diagnostic, with the demonstration of an overriding aorta, ventricular septal defect (VSD), and small right ventricular outflow tract.

   e. **Treatment.** Pulmonary blood flow may be ductal-dependent with severe cyanosis and may respond to ductal dilation using prostaglandin E_1 (see Chapter 80). This measure allows more flexibility for planning cardiac catheterization and surgical correction. Surgery (shunting or total correction) may be palliative.

III. **Acyanotic heart disease** (Table 62–2)

   A. **100% oxygen test.** See Congenital Heart Disease, section II,A.

   B. **Murmur.** The infant who is not cyanotic will have either a heart murmur or symptoms of congestive heart failure.

   C. **Diagnosis and treatment** (see Table 62–2)

   D. **Specific acyanotic heart disease abnormalities**

   1. **VSD** is the most common congenital heart abnormality, with equal sex distribution. Murmurs can be heard at birth but typically appear between 3 days and 3 weeks of age. Congestive heart failure is unusual before 4 weeks of age but may develop earlier in premature infants. Symptoms and physical findings vary with patient age and defect size. Spontaneous closure occurs in half of the patients. Surgical correction is reserved for large, symptomatic VSD only.

   2. **Atrial septal defect (ASD)** is not an important cause of morbidity or mortality in infancy. Occasionally, congestive heart failure can occur in infancy but not usually in the neonatal period.

TABLE 62–2. ACYANOTIC CONGENITAL HEART DISEASE ($Pao_2 > 100$ mm Hg in 100% Fio_2)

	Normal pulmonary blood flow with normal-sized heart		Normal pulmonary blood flow with large heart			Increased pulmonary blood flow with large heart	
Chest x-ray							
ECG	RHV or normal	LVH or normal	Normal arrhythmia or complete heart block	LVH	RVH or LVH	RVH	LAD
Differential diagnosis	Valvular PS	Noncritical valvular AS VDS PDA	Intrauterine arrhythmia	AV malformation Common sites are head, liver, placenta AS, critical	AV valve insufficiency Primary myocardial disease (including EFE)	HLHS, coarctation of aorta	AV canal
Physical examination	SEM	SEM-AS VSD, no murmur PDA, continuous murmur	May be hydropic or normal	AV malformation, usually continuous murmur over site Increased pulses Critical AS, decreased pulses Not much murmur	TI, MI Pansystolic murmur with rumble EFE gallop	HLHS; poor pulses, perfusion, and color; gallop Coarctation of aorta, decreased femoral pulses	SEM, diastolic rumble
Treatment	Observe	Observe	Treat arrhythmia with drugs or cardioversion May need furosemide Congenital complete heart block may need pacemaker	AV malformation, ultrasound, CT scanning, angiography AS: PGE₁ infusion Digoxin, furosemide	Digoxin, furosemide	Anticongestives if in heart failure HLHS: consider PGE₁ infusion	Observe Anticongestives if in heart failure

Further cardiac evaluation

AS, aortic stenosis; AV canal, atrioventricular canal; AV malformation, arteriovenous malformation; AV valve, atrioventricular valve; CT, computed tomography; ECG, electrocardiogram; EFE, endocardial fibroelastosis; HLHS, hypoplastic left heart syndrome; LAD, left axis deviation; LVH, left ventricular hypertrophy; MI, myocardial infarction; PDA, patent ductus arteriosus; PGE₁, prostaglandin E₁; PS, pulmonary stenosis; RVH, right ventricular hypertrophy; SEM, systolic ejection murmur; TI, tricuspid incompetence; VSD, ventricular septal defect.

3. **Endocardial cushion defects** include ostium primum–type ASD with or without a cleft mitral valve and an atrioventricular (AV) canal. These defects are commonly associated with multiple congenital anomalies, especially Down syndrome. If marked AV valve insufficiency is present, the patient may have congestive heart failure at birth or in the neonatal period.
   a. **Physical examination.** On physical examination, a systolic murmur resulting from atrioventricular (AV) valve insufficiency may be heard. Cyanosis may be present but is often not severe. Infants with severe pulmonary artery hypertension may have little or no murmur.
   b. **Chest x-ray study.** Variable findings may include a dilated pulmonary artery or a large heart secondary to atrial dilatation.
   c. **ECG.** Left axis deviation (left superior vector) is *always* found; the PR interval may be long, or there may be an RSR´ pattern in V_4R and V_1.
   d. **Echocardiography** is usually diagnostic; the echocardiogram usually demonstrates a common AV valve with inlet VSD or a defect in the septum primum with an abnormal mitral valve.
   e. **Treatment.** Congestive heart failure is treated with diuretics and digoxin (for dosages, see Chapter 80); early cardiac catheterization with corrective surgery may be needed to prevent pulmonary vascular obstructive disease.

IV. **Hypoplastic left heart syndrome (HLHS)** occurs in both cyanotic and acyanotic forms. In 15% of cases, the foramen ovale is intact and thus prevents mixing at the atrial level, causing cyanosis. Infants with mixing at the atria are acyanotic. HLHS accounts for 25% of all cardiac deaths during the first week of life.
   A. **Physical examination.** The infant is typically pale and tachypneic, with poor perfusion and poor to absent peripheral pulses. A loud single S_2 is present, usually with a gallop and no murmur. There is hepatomegaly, and metabolic acidosis is usually present by 48 h of age.
   B. **ECG** demonstrates small or absent left ventricular forces.
   C. **Chest x-ray study.** Moderate cardiomegaly is present, often with large main pulmonary artery shadow.
   D. **Echocardiography.** A diagnostic study demonstrates a small or slit-like left ventricle with a hypoplastic ascending aorta.
   E. **Treatment.** Systemic blood flow is ductal-dependent; therefore, prostaglandin E_1 is of value. Surgical correction is done in two or three stages. The first is palliation (the Norwood procedure), redirecting the blood flow so that the right ventricle serves as the "systemic ventricle," and a surgically constructed "shunt" provides pulmonary blood flow. Successful outcome is influenced by gestational age (term infants do much better than preterm infants) and the presence of other major anomalies. The second stage (the Fontan procedure) directs systemic venous return directly to the pulmonary circulation, and the ASD is closed. The Fontan procedure may be done in two stages. Neonatal cardiac transplantation is a second option, but shortage of organs is a significant deterrent. Compassionate care (keeping the infant comfortable until death) may be appropriate in some instances.

V. **Associated anomalies and syndromes** (Table 62–3). No discussion of heart disease in neonates would be complete without the inclusion of common multiple congenital anomaly (MCA) syndromes associated with heart defects. Many times, recognition of MCA syndromes will facilitate identification of the heart defect. Syndromes that tend to present after the newborn period have not been included.

VI. **Teratogens and heart disease.** Several teratogens associated with congenital heart disease have been identified (Table 62–4), although there is not a 100% relationship between exposure and heart defects. A history of teratogen exposure may help in the diagnosis.

VII. **Abnormal situs syndromes.** Syndromes of abnormal situs relationships are associated with congenital heart disease. For example, an infant with situs inversus

TABLE 62–3. CONGENITAL ANOMALIES ASSOCIATED WITH DEFECTS

Congenital anomaly	Heart defect
Chromosomal Anomaly	
Trisomy 21 (Down syndrome)	Atrioventricular canal, ventricular septal defect
Triomies 13, 15, and 18	Ventricular septal defect, patent ductus arteriosus
Syndrome associated with 4p−	Atrial septal defect, ventricular septal defect
Syndrome associated wtih 5p− (cri du chat syndrome)	Variable
XO (Turner's syndrome)	Coarctation of aorta, aortic stenosis
Syndromes with predominantly skeletal defects[a]	
Ellis–van Creveld syndrome	Atrial septal defect, single atrium
Laurence-Moon-Biedl syndrome	Tetralogy of Fallot, ventricular septal defect
Carpenter's syndrome	Patent ductus arteriosus, ventricular septal defect
Holt-Oram syndrome	Atrial septal defect, ventricular septal defect
Fanconi's syndrome	Patent ductus arteriosus, ventricular septal defect
Thrombocytopenia–absent radius syndrome	Atrial septal defect, tetralogy of Fallot
SYNDROMES WITH CHARACTERISTIC FACIES[a]	
Noonan's syndrome (long arm of chromosome 12)	Pulmonary stenosis
DiGeorge syndrome (chromosome 22 deletion)	Tetralogy of Fallot, aortic arch anomalies
Smith-Lemli-Opitz syndrome	Ventricular septal defect, patent ductus arteriosus
de Lange's syndrome	Tetralogy of Fallot, ventricular septal defect
Goldenhar's syndrome	Tetralogy of Fallot, variable
Williams syndrome	Supravalvular aortic stenosis, peripheral pulmonary artery stenosis
Asymmetric crying facies	Variable

[a]Not all infants with these syndromes have heart defects.

totalis and dextrocardia has the same incidence of congenital heart disease as the general population. If, however, there is disparity between thoracic and abdominal situs, the incidence of congenital heart disease is >90%. (Check the chest x-ray film to see whether the cardiac apex and the stomach bubble are on the same side.) Some of these syndromes involve bilateral left-sidedness (two bilobed lungs or multiple spleens) and complex cyanotic congenital heart disease, whereas others have bilateral right-sidedness (two trilobed lungs or an absent spleen) and complex cyanotic congenital heart disease.

TABLE 62–4. TERATOGENS ASSOCIATED WITH HEART DEFECTS

Teratogen	Heart defect
Drugs	
Alcohol	Ventricular septal defect, tetralogy of Fallot, atrial septal defect
Anticonvulsants	Variable, ventricular septal defect, tetralogy of Fallot
Retinoic acid	Aortic arch anomalies
Lithium	Ebstein's anomaly of the tricuspid valve
Environmental agents	
Irradiation	Variable
High altitude	PDA, other variable
Maternal factors	
Diabetes	Variable
Maternal lupus	Complete (3rd degree) AV block
Maternal PKU	Ventricular septal defect, coarctation
Infections	
Rubella syndrome	PDA, peripheral pulmonary stenosis
Other viruses	Variable

AV, artrioventricular; PDA, patent ductus arteriosus; PKU, phenylketonuria.

VIII. General principles of management

A. Fetal echocardiography

1. **General considerations.** Fetal echocardiography is now possible in many centers. The optimal gestational age to perform echocardiography is between 18 and 24 weeks, when structural abnormalities and arrhythmias can be detected. With early detection of cardiac abnormalities, arrangements can be made for delivery at a center with pediatric cardiac and surgical facilities. If the anomaly is not consistent with life, some families may elect termination of pregnancy.

2. **Indications**
   a. **Maternal factors.** Oligohydramnios or polyhydramnios, diabetes, collagen vascular disease, teratogen exposure, or a previous child with congenital heart disease (Table 62–5).
   b. **Fetal factors.** Suspected cardiac abnormality on obstetric ultrasound examination, pleural fluid, pericardial fluid, heart rate abnormalities, intrauterine growth retardation (IUGR), or other abnormality on obstetric ultrasound examination.
   c. **Genetic factors.** Familial history of chromosomal disorders or congenital heart disease.

B. Emergency therapy.
Once the specific lesion has been identified as emergent, a decision about therapy must be made. If, for example, one is confronted with a very cyanotic infant with no murmur, a normal chest x-ray film, and a normal ECG and believes that the diagnosis of D-transposition of the great arteries is likely, it is necessary to prepare for a **balloon septostomy.**

C. Prostaglandins.
As a general principle, if an infant is cyanotic and has decreased pulmonary blood flow, the Pao_2 will be improved by promoting flow through the ductus arteriosus via a drip of **prostaglandin E₁** (alprostadil, or Prostin VR Pediatric). Maintaining patency of the ductus will enable stabilization of the infant and subsequent catheterization or surgery to be planned on an urgent rather than emergent basis. Similarly, if poor peripheral pulses and acidosis from poor perfusion are present, infusion of prostaglandin, using the same dose, will open the ductus arteriosus and allow right ventricular blood flow to augment the systemic circulation. This measure is beneficial in critical aortic stenosis, coarctation of the aorta, and HLHS. (For dosage and other pharmacologic information, see Chapter 80.)

D. Antiarrhythmic drugs.
Rapid arrhythmias may occur during intrauterine life or after delivery. Arrhythmias are a cause of fetal hydrops and intrauterine death; most often, the rhythm disturbance is a rapid supraventricular tachycardia with a 1:1 ventricular response. Occasionally, atrial flutter with 2:1 block presents before or just after birth. **Digitalis** has been a successful an-

---

TABLE 62–5. INDICATIONS FOR FETAL ECHOCARDIOGRAM

Maternal conditions
  Diabetes
  Collagen vascular disease
  Maternal drug/teratogen exposure
Family conditions
  History of congenital heart disease
  History of chromosomal or genetic abnormalities
Fetal conditions
  Abnormal fetal heart rate
  Suspected cardiac malformation on screening ultrasonogram
  Presence of other malformations on ultrasonogram
  Oligo- or polyhydramnios
  Evidence of hydrops fetalis
  Intrauterine growth retardation

tiarrhythmic agent in this situation, but treatment with adenosine or electrical cardioversion is also sometimes necessary.
  E. **Pacemaker.** Fetal hydrops can result from congenital complete heart block. If cardiovascular demise is imminent, **temporary transvenous ventricular pacing may be lifesaving.** It should be followed by urgent surgical placement of a permanent pacemaker. Mothers may have anti-Rho or anti-LA antibodies.

PATENT DUCTUS ARTERIOSUS

I. **Definition.** The ductus arteriosus is a large vessel that connects the main pulmonary trunk (or proximal left pulmonary artery) with the descending aorta, some 5–10 mm distal to the origin of the left subclavian artery. In the fetus, it serves to shunt blood away from the lungs and is essential (closure in utero may lead to fetal demise or pulmonary hypertension). In full-term healthy newborns, functional closure of the ductus occurs rapidly after birth. Final functional closure occurs in almost half of full-term infants by 24 h of age, in 90% by 48 h, and in all by 96 h after birth. PDA refers to failure of the closure process and continued patency of this fetal channel.

II. **Incidence.** Incidence varies according to means of diagnosis (eg, clinical signs vs echocardiography).
  A. **Factors associated with increased incidence of PDA**
    1. **Prematurity.** Incidence is inversely related to gestational age. PDA is found in ~45% of infants <1750 g; in infants weighing <1000 g, the incidence is closer to 80%.
    2. **Respiratory distress syndrome (RDS) (and surfactant treatment).** The presence of RDS is associated with an increased incidence of PDA, and this is correlated with the severity of RDS. After surfactant treatment, there is an increased risk of a clinically symptomatic PDA; moreover, surfactant may lead to an earlier clinical presentation of a PDA.
    3. **Fluid administration.** Increased intravenous fluid load in the first few days of life is associated with an increased incidence of PDA.
    4. **Asphyxia.**
    5. **Congenital syndromes.** PDA is present in 60–70% of infants with congenital rubella syndrome. Trisomy 13, trisomy 18, Rubinstein-Taybi syndrome, and XXXXX (Penta X) syndrome are associated with an increased incidence of PDA.
    6. **High altitude.** Infants born at high altitude have an increased incidence of PDA.
    7. **Congenital heart disease.** PDA may occur as part of a congenital heart disease (eg, coarctation, pulmonary atresia with intact septum, transposition of the great vessels, or total anomalous pulmonary venous return).
  B. **Factors associated with a decreased incidence of PDA**
    1. **Antenatal steroid administration.**
    2. **IUGR.**
    3. **Prolonged rupture of membranes.**
III. **Pathophysiology.** In the fetus, the ductus is essential to divert blood flow from the high-resistance pulmonary circulation to the descending aorta. After birth, functional closure of the ductus occurs within hours (but up to 3–4 days). Complete anatomic closure with fibrosis and permanent sealing of the lumen takes up to 2–3 weeks. An increase in Pao_2, as occurs with ventilation after birth, constricts the ductus in mature animals. Other factors, such as the release of vasoactive substances (eg, acetylcholine), may contribute to the postnatal closure of the ductus under physiologic conditions. Of paramount importance, however, is the dilatory effects of prostaglandins (E_1 and E_2) and prostacyclin on the ductus. Inhibitors of prostaglandin synthesis produce constriction of the ductus. Thus, the patency or closure of the ductus depends on the balance between the

various constricting effects (eg, of oxygen) and the relaxing effects of various prostaglandins. The effects of oxygen and prostaglandins vary at different gestational ages. Oxygen has less of a constricting effect with decreasing gestational age.

On the other hand, the sensitivity of the ductus to the relaxing effects of prostaglandin E_2 is greatest in immature animals (and decreases with advancing gestational age). In term infants, responsiveness is lost shortly after birth, but this does not occur in the immature ductus. Indomethacin constricts the immature ductus more than it does the close-to-term ductus. The magnitude and direction of the ductus shunt are related to the vessel size (diameter and length), the pressure difference between the aorta and the pulmonary artery, and the ratio between the systemic and pulmonary vascular resistances. The clinical features associated with a left-to-right ductal shunt depend on the magnitude of the shunt and the ability of the infant to handle the extra volume load. Left ventricular output is increased by the extra volume return. The increase in pulmonary venous return causes an increase in ventricular diastolic volume (preload). Left ventricular dilation will result, with an increase in left ventricular end-diastolic pressure and a secondary increase in left atrial pressure. This may eventually result in left heart failure with pulmonary edema. Eventually, these changes may lead to right ventricular failure. With a PDA, there is also a redistribution of systemic blood flow secondary to retrograde aortic flow (ductal steal, or "runoff"). Renal and mesenteric blood flows are thus reduced, as is cerebral blood flow.

IV. **Clinical signs and presentation.** The initial presentation may be at birth but is usually on days 1–4 of life. The cardiopulmonary signs and symptoms are as follows:

  A. **Heart murmur.** The murmur is usually systolic and is heard best in the second or third intercostal space at the left sternal border. The murmur may be continuous also and sometimes may be heard only intermittently. Frequently, it may be necessary to disconnect the infant from mechanical ventilation to appreciate the murmur.

  B. **Hyperactive precordium.** The increased left ventricular stroke volume may result in a hyperactive precordium.

  C. **Bounding peripheral pulses and increased pulse pressure.** The increased stroke volume with diastolic runoff through the PDA may lead to these signs.

  D. **Hypotension.** PDA is associated with decreased mean arterial blood pressure. In some infants (particularly those of extremely low birth weight), hypotension may be the earliest clinical manifestation of a PDA, sometimes without a murmur (ie, the "silent" PDA).

  E. **Respiratory deterioration.** Respiratory deterioration after an initial improvement in a small premature infant with RDS should arouse suspicion of a PDA. The deterioration may be gradual (days) or brisk (hours) but is usually not sudden (as in pneumothorax). PDA may similarly complicate the respiratory course of chronic lung disease.

  F. **Other signs.** These may include tachypnea, crackles, or apneic spells. If the PDA is untreated, the left-to-right shunt may lead to heart failure with frank pulmonary edema and hepatomegaly.

V. **Diagnosis**

  A. **Echocardiography.** Two-dimensional echocardiography combined with Doppler ultrasonography is by far the most sensitive means of diagnosing a PDA. The ductus can be directly visualized, and the direction of flow may be demonstrated. In addition, echocardiography can assess the secondary effects of the PDA (eg, left atrial and ventricular size) and contractility. The echocardiogram will also rule out alternative or additional cardiac diagnoses.

  B. **Radiologic studies.** On initial presentation, the chest film may be unremarkable, especially if the PDA has occurred against a background of preexisting RDS. Later, pulmonary plethora and increased interstitial fluid may be noted with subsequent florid pulmonary edema. True cardiomegaly is usually a later sign, but a gradual increase in heart size may often be appreciated if serial films are available. An increase in pulmonary fluid in an infant with previously improving or stable respiratory status should raise the possibility of PDA.

VI. **Management**

A. **Ventilatory support.** Respiratory distress secondary to a PDA may require intubation and mechanical ventilation. If the infant is already ventilated, the PDA may lead to increased ventilatory requirements. These should be determined by blood gases. Increasing positive end-expiratory pressure is helpful in controlling pulmonary edema.

B. **Fluid restriction.** Decreasing fluid intake as far as possible will decrease the PDA shunt as well as the accumulation of fluid in the lungs. Increased fluid intake in the first few weeks of life is associated with increased risk of patency of the ductus in premature infants with RDS.

C. **Increasing hematocrit (Hct).** Increasing Hct above 40–45% will decrease the left-to-right shunt. Frequently, an increase in Hct will abate some of the signs of the PDA (eg, the murmur may disappear).

D. **Indomethacin.** This is a prostaglandin synthetase inhibitor that has proved to be effective in promoting ductal closure. Its effectiveness is limited to premature infants and also decreases with increasing postnatal age; thus, it will have limited efficacy beyond 3–4 weeks of age, even in premature infants. There are essentially three approaches to administering indomethacin for ductal closure in premature infants: (1) prophylactic, (2) early symptomatic, and (3) late symptomatic. (**Note:** There are minor variations in dosage regimens, and what follows are guidelines.)

1. **Prophylactic indomethacin.** Indomethacin, 0.1 mg/kg/dose, is given intravenously (infused over 20 min) every 24 h from the first day of life for 6 days. In this regimen, indomethacin is given prophylactically to all infants <1250 g birth weight who have received surfactant for RDS (before any clinical signs suggestive of PDA). It would also be appropriate to limit this regimen to infants with RDS who are <1000 g birth weight. Clinical trials have shown that this treatment is safe and effective in reducing the incidence of symptomatic PDA in these infants. The major drawback is that up to 40% of these infants probably would never have had a symptomatic PDA and hence did not require treatment. A 2000 study by Narayanan et al found that indomethacin given prophylactically for the first 3 days of life had a greater rate of permanent ductus closure.

2. **Early symptomatic indomethacin.** Infants are given indomethacin, 0.2 mg/kg intravenously (infused over 20 min). Second and third doses are given 12 and 36 h after the first dose. The second and third doses are 0.1 mg/kg/dose if the infant is <1250 g birth weight and <7 days old. If the infant is either >7 days old or >1250 g, then the second and third doses are also 0.2 mg/kg/dose. Indomethacin is given if there is any clinical sign of a PDA (eg, a murmur) and before there are signs of overt failure. This is usually on days 2–4 of life.

3. **Late symptomatic indomethacin.** Infants are given indomethacin when signs of congestive failure appear (usually at 7–10 days). Dosage is as described in Patent Ductus Arteriosus, section VI,D,2. The problem with this approach is that if indomethacin fails to constrict the ductus significantly, there is less opportunity for a second trial of indomethacin and the infant is likely to require surgery.

4. **Ductus reopening and indomethacin failure.** In 20–30% of infants, the ductus will reopen after the first course of indomethacin. In such cases, a second course of indomethacin may be worthwhile because a significant proportion of these infants will have their PDA closed with this course. The ductus is more likely to reopen in infants of very low gestational age

and in those who had received a greater amount of fluids previously. Infection and necrotizing enterocolitis (NEC) are also risk factors for ductus reopening (and may be contraindications for indomethacin).

5. **Complications of indomethacin**
   a. **Renal effects.** Indomethacin causes a transient decrease in the glomerular filtration rate and urine output. In such cases, fluid intake should be reduced to correct for the decreased urine output, which should improve with time (usually within 24 h).
   b. **Gastrointestinal bleeding.** Stools may be heme-positive after indomethacin. This is transient and usually of no clinical significance. Indomethacin is a mesenteric vasoconstrictor, but the PDA itself also decreases mesenteric blood flow. In the trials of indomethacin, there has been no increased incidence of NEC in the infants treated with this drug.
   c. **Platelet function.** Indomethacin impairs platelet function for 7–9 days regardless of platelet number. In the various trials of indomethacin, there has been no increased incidence of intraventricular hemorrhage (IVH) associated with the drug, and there is no evidence that it extends the degree of preexisting IVH. Nevertheless, it may be unwise to impose additional platelet dysfunction in infants who are also significantly thrombocytopenic.

6. **Contraindications for indomethacin**
   a. **Serum creatinine >1.7 mg/dL.**
   b. **Frank renal or gastrointestinal bleeding** or generalized coagulopathy.
   c. **NEC.**
   d. **Sepsis.** All anti-inflammatory drugs should be withheld if there is sepsis. Indomethacin may be given once this is under control.

E. **Ibuprofen.** This is another nonselective cyclooxygenase inhibitor that has been shown to close the ductus in animals. Clinical studies have suggested that ibuprofen is as effective as indomethacin for the treatment of PDA in preterm infants. It has an advantage in that it does not reduce mesenteric and renal blood flow as much as indomethacin and is associated with fewer renal side effects. The dose used is an initial dose of 10 mg/kg followed by 2 doses of 5 mg/kg each after 24 and 48 h. There is less experience with the use of ibuprofen, and it has not been sufficiently studied in preterm infants <27 weeks' gestation.

F. **Surgery.** Surgery should be performed in patients with a hemodynamically significant PDA in whom medical treatment has failed or in whom there is a contraindication to the use of indomethacin. Surgical mortality is low (<1%).

VII. **PDA in the full-term infant.** PDA accounts for ~10% of all congenital heart disease in full-term infants. The PDA in a full-term infant is structurally different, and this may explain why it does not respond appropriately to the various stimuli for closure. Indomethacin is usually ineffective. The infant should be monitored carefully, and surgical ligation should be considered at the earliest signs of significant congestion. Even without signs of failure, the PDA should be ligated before 1 year of age to prevent endocarditis and pulmonary hypertension.

PERSISTENT PULMONARY HYPERTENSION OF THE NEWBORN

I. **Definition.** Persistent pulmonary hypertension of the newborn (PPHN) is a condition characterized by marked pulmonary hypertension resulting from elevated pulmonary vascular resistance (PVR) and altered pulmonary vasoreactivity, leading to right-to-left extrapulmonary shunting of blood across the foramen ovale and the PDA. It is associated with a wide array of cardiopulmonary disorders that may also cause intrapulmonary shunting. When this disorder is of un-

known cause and is the primary cause of cardiopulmonary distress, it is often called "idiopathic PPHN" or persistent fetal circulation.
II. **Pathophysiology.** PPHN may be the result of (1) underdevelopment of the lung together with its vascular bed (eg, congenital diaphragmatic hernia and hypoplastic lungs); (2) maladaptation of the pulmonary vascular bed to the transition occurring around the time of birth (eg, various conditions of perinatal stress, hemorrhage, aspiration, hypoxia, and hypoglycemia); and (3) maldevelopment of the pulmonary vascular bed in utero from a known or unknown cause. It is convenient to think in terms of this basic pathologic classification. However, the clinical manifestations of PPHN are often not attributable to a single physiologic or structural entity, and many disorders exhibit more than one underlying pathology. Often, even when there is evidence of perinatal or postnatal stress (eg, meconium aspiration), the underlying cause of PPHN had been secondary to an In utero process of some duration.

Preacinar arteries are already present in the lungs by 18 weeks' gestation; thereafter, respiratory units are added with further growth of the appropriate arteries. Muscularization of the peripheral pulmonary arteries is related to differentiation of pericytes and to recruitment of fibroblasts and is influenced by numerous trophic factors (eg, neuropeptides, fibroblast growth factors, and insulin-like growth factors). In addition, the growth, differentiation, and adaptation of the pulmonary vascular bed are also influenced by changes that occur in the connective tissue matrix (eg, elastin and collagen). The lungs of infants with PPHN contain many undilated precapillary arteries, and pulmonary arterial medial thickness is increased. There may be extension of muscle in small and peripheral arteries that are normally nonmuscular. After a few days, there is already evidence of structural remodeling with connective tissue deposition.

In the fetus, PVR is high, and only 5–10% of the combined cardiac output flows into the lungs. After birth, with expansion of the lungs, there is a sharp drop in PVR and pulmonary blood flow increases about 10-fold. The factors that are responsible for maintaining high PVR in the fetus and for effecting the acute reduction in PVR that occurs after birth are incompletely understood. Fetal and neonatal pulmonary vascular tone is modulated through a balance between vasconstrictive (eg, leukotrienes and thromboxanes) and vasodilatory (eg, adenosine and prostaglandin I_2) stimuli. The endothelins are vasoactive peptides that play an important role in regulating pulmonary vascular tone through their action on at least two receptor types. It has become clear that the endothelium (and its interaction with vascular smooth muscle cells) plays a crucial role in regulating pulmonary vascular tone. In particular, endothelial cells secrete endothelium-derived relaxing factors that mediate pulmonary vasodilation. Nitric oxide (NO) has been identified as the most important of these relaxing factors. There is a reciprocal relationship between many of the humoral mediators of pulmonary vasoregulation and the structural remodeling that occurs with PPHN. For example, NO and prostacyclin have antiproliferative effects on smooth muscle cells, and NO also inhibits smooth muscle cell migration (in vitro).
III. **Associated factors.** The following factors or conditions may be associated with PPHN:
   A. **Lung disease.** Meconium aspiration; RDS; pneumonia; pulmonary hypoplasia; cystic lung disease, including congenital cystic adenomatoid malformation and congenital lobar emphysema; diaphragmatic hernia; and congenital alveolar capillary dysplasia.
   B. **Systemic disorders.** Polycythemia, hypoglycemia, hypoxia, acidosis, hypocalcemia, hypothermia, and sepsis.
   C. **Congenital heart disease.** Particularly, total anomalous venous return, HLHS, transient tricuspid insufficiency (transient myocardial ischemia), coarctation of the aorta, critical aortic stenosis, endocardial cushion defects, Ebstein's anomaly, transposition of the great arteries, endocardial fibroelastosis, and cerebrovenous malformations.

D. Perinatal factors. Asphyxia, perinatal hypoxia, and maternal ingestion of aspirin or indomethacin.

E. Miscellaneous. Central nervous system disorders, neuromuscular disease, and upper airway obstruction.

IV. Clinical features. The primary finding is respiratory distress with cyanosis (confirmed by demonstrating hypoxemia). This may occur despite adequate ventilation. Other clinical findings are highly variable and depend on the severity, stage, and other associated disorders (particularly pulmonary and cardiac diseases).

A. Respiratory. Initial respiratory symptoms may be limited to tachypnea, and onset may be at birth or within 4–8 h of age. In addition, in an infant with pulmonary disease, PPHN should be suspected as a complicating factor when there is marked lability in oxygenation. These infants will have significant decreases in pulse oximetry readings with routine nursing care or minor stress (eg, movement or noise). Furthermore, a minor decrease in inspired oxygen concentration may lead to a surprisingly large decrease in arterial oxygenation (eg, the $AaDo_2$ gradient changes more rapidly and is more labile than that seen in the normal course of progression of uncomplicated RDS or other pulmonary disease).

B. Cardiac signs. Physical findings may include a prominent right ventricular impulse, a single second heart sound, and a murmur of tricuspid insufficiency. In extreme cases, there may be hepatomegaly and signs of heart failure.

C. Radiography. The chest film may show either cardiomegaly or a normal-sized heart. If there is no associated pulmonary disease, the film may show normal or diminished pulmonary vascularity. If there is also a parenchymal lung disorder, the degree of hypoxemia may be out of proportion to the radiographic measure of severity of the pulmonary disease.

D. Other. Thrombocytopenia has been reported to be present in as many as 60% of infants with PPHN. The specificity of this finding is unknown. Once the diagnosis is suspected, certain tests are either strongly suggestive or supportive of PPHN.

V. Diagnosis. PPHN is essentially a diagnosis of exclusion.

A. Differential oximeter readings. In the presence of right-to-left shunting of blood via the PDA, the Pao_2 in preductal blood (eg, from the right radial artery) is higher than that in the postductal blood (obtained from left radial, umbilical, or tibial arteries). Hence, simultaneous preductal and postductal monitoring of oxygen saturation is a useful indicator of right-to-left shunting at the ductal level. However, it is important to note that PPHN cannot be excluded if no difference is found, because the right-to-left shunting may be predominantly at the atrial level (or the ductus may not be patent at all). A difference >5% between preductal and postductal oxygen saturations is considered indicative of a right-to-left ductal shunt. A difference >10–15 mm Hg between preductal and postductal Pao_2 is also considered suggestive of a right-to-left ductal shunt. Preductal and postductal oxygenation should be assessed simultaneously.

B. Hyperventilation test. PPHN should be considered if marked improvement in oxygenation (>30 mm Hg increase in Pao_2) is noted on hyperventilating the infant (lowering $Paco_2$ and increasing pH). When a "critical" pH value is reached (often ~7.55 or greater), PVR decreases, there is less right-to-left shunting, and Pao_2 increases. This test may differentiate PPHN from cyanotic congenital heart disease. Little or no response is expected in infants with the latter diagnoses. It has been suggested that infants subjected to this test should be hyperventilated for 10 min. Prolonged hyperventilation is not recommended, however, particularly in premature infants (see later discussion).

C. Radiography. Clear lung fields or only minor disease in the face of severe hypoxemia is strongly suggestive of PPHN, if cyanotic congenital heart disease has been ruled out. In an infant with significant pulmonary parenchymal disease, a chest film is of little help in diagnosing PPHN (although it is indicated for other reasons). In an infant with rapidly worsening oxygenation, the major value of a chest film is in the exclusion of alternative diagnosis (eg, pneumothorax or pneumopericardium).

D. **Echocardiography.** This is often essential in distinguishing cyanotic congenital heart disease from PPHN because the latter is frequently a diagnosis of exclusion. Furthermore, whereas all the other previously mentioned signs and tests are suggestive, echocardiography (together with Doppler studies) can provide confirmatory evidence that is often diagnostic. The first question that needs to be answered is whether the heart is structurally normal. Then the pulmonary artery pressure can be assessed indirectly by measuring the acceleration time of the systolic flow in the main pulmonary artery, by measuring the velocity of the tricuspid regurgitant jet, and by measuring ductal shunt velocities. Echocardiography (with Doppler) will also provide information about shunting at the atrial and ductal levels. Echocardiography can also be used to assess ventricular output and contractility (both of which may be depressed in infants with PPHN).

VI. Management

A. **Prevention.** Adequate resuscitation and support from birth may presumably prevent or ameliorate, to some degree, PPHN when it may occur superimposed on a preexisting condition. An example is adequate and timely ventilation of an asphyxiated infant with appropriate attention to temperature control.

B. **General management.** Infants with PPHN clearly require careful and intensive monitoring. Fluid management is important because hypovolemia will aggravate the right-to-left shunt. However, once normovolemia can be assumed, there is no known benefit to be gained from repeated administration of either colloids or crystalloids. Normal serum glucose and calcium should be maintained because hypoglycemia and hypocalcemia will aggravate PPHN. Temperature control is also crucial. Significant acidosis should be avoided. It is useful to use two pulse oximeters: one preductal and one postductal.

C. **Minimal handling.** Because infants with PPHN are extremely labile with significant deterioration after seemingly "minor" stimuli, this aspect of care deserves special mention. Endotracheal tube suctioning, in particular, should be performed only if indicated and not as a matter of routine. Noise level and physical manipulation should be kept to a minimum.

D. **Mechanical ventilation.** This is often needed to ensure adequate oxygenation and should first be attempted using "conventional" ventilation. The goal is to maintain adequate and stable oxygenation using the lowest possible mean airway pressures. The lowest possible positive end-expiratory pressure should also be sought. Hyperventilation should, if possible, be avoided and, as a guide, arterial P_{CO_2} values should be kept >30 mm Hg if possible; even levels of 40–50 mm Hg are acceptable if this does not compromise oxygenation (see Persistent Pulmonary Hypertension of the Newborn, section VI,I, on alkalinization). Initially, it would be wise to ventilate with 100% inspired oxygen concentration. Weaning should be gradual and in small steps. In those infants who cannot be adequately oxygenated with conventional ventilation, high-frequency oscillation (HFO) should be considered early. There are a few reports (albeit uncontrolled) suggesting that the use of HFO is of benefit and may even prevent some neonates from requiring extracorporeal membrane oxygenation (ECMO).

E. **Surfactant.** In infants with RDS, administration of surfactant is associated with a fall in PVR. Surfactant may also be of benefit in various other pulmonary disorders (eg, meconium aspiration), although it is unknown whether its actions in these is related to a reduction in PVR.

F. **Pressor agents.** Some infants with PPHN have reduced cardiac output. In addition, increasing systemic blood pressure will reduce the right-to-left shunt. Hence, at least normal blood pressure should be maintained, and some recommend maintaining blood pressure of ≥40 mm Hg. Dopamine is the most commonly used drug for this purpose. Dobutamine has the disadvantage, in this context, that, although it may improve cardiac output, it has less of a pressor effect than dopamine. A simple nonpharmacologic measure to increase systemic vascular resistance is to inflate blood pressure cuffs on all four extremities. In a small study using this technique, inflating the blood pressure cuffs was associated with a 10- to 25- mm Hg increase in arterial oxygen tension. Moreover, administration of tolazoline to these infants resulted in a further 10- to 20-mm Hg increase and did not precipitate hypotension (see Rhodes et al, 1995).

G. **Sedation.** The lability of these infants has been mentioned previously, and hence sedation is commonly used. Nembutal (1–5 mg/kg) or Versed (0.1 mg/kg) is frequently used, and analgesia with morphine (0.05–0.2 mg/kg) is also used.

H. **Paralyzing agents.** The use of these agents is *controversial*. It is reasonable to use a paralyzing agent in infants who have not responded to sedation and are still labile or who appear to "fight" the ventilator. Pancuronium is the drug most commonly used, although it may increase PVR to some extent and worsen ventilation-perfusion mismatch. Vecuronium (0.1 mg/kg) has also been used.

I. **Alkalinization.** In the past, it had been noted that hyperventilation, with the resulting hypocapnia, improved oxygenation secondary to pulmonary vasodilation. Subsequently, it was shown that the beneficial effect of hypocapnia was actually a result of the increased pH rather than of the low $Paco_2$ values achieved. Furthermore, follow-up of infants with PPHN had suggested that hypocapnia was related to poor neurodevelopmental outcome (especially sensorineural hearing loss). Hypocapnia is known to reduce cerebral blood flow. Hence, it may be advisable to increase pH using an infusion of sodium bicarbonate (0.5–1 mEq/kg/h) if possible. Serum sodium should be monitored so as to avoid hypernatremia. Improvement in oxygenation is often seen with arterial pH 7.50–7.55 (sometimes levels as high as 7.65 are required).

J. **Intravenous pulmonary vasodilators.** Various intravenous pulmonary vasodilators have been tried in the past (tolazoline, prostaglandin E_1, prostacyclin, nitroglycerin, nitroprusside, and others). All of these are also systemic vasodilators and often cause systemic hypotension with little, if any, net benefit. Tolazoline is probably the most commonly used drug of this class. It is an α-adrenergic antagonist with histaminergic action. It is given as a loading dose of 1–2 mg/kg followed by continuous infusion of 1–2 mg/kg/h. It should be given with both volume support and pressor drugs close at hand in case systemic hypotension occurs. Some advocate its use only in conjunction with simultaneous infusion of pressors as a prophylactic measure. Side effects of tolazoline are hypotension, oliguria, seizures, thrombocytopenia, and gastrointestinal hemorrhage, but some of these effects may have resulted from the severity of the infant's underlying condition. It is possible that a lower dosage of tolazoline may be effective as a pulmonary vasodilator while reducing the incidence of side effects (which are dose-related). A loading dose of 0.5 mg/kg has been recommended, followed by infusion of 0.5 mg/kg/h. Tolazoline is effective in 10–50% of newborns with PPHN, but the rate of complications is close to 70%. Two intravenous drugs that have been reported as successful pulmonary vasodilators with minimal systemic effects are **magnesium sulfate** and **adenosine.** The experience with **magnesium sulfate** has been uncontrolled, and some animal studies have shown other findings. Nevertheless, magnesium appears to be worthy of further study. Adenosine has been tried in full-term infants with PPHN in a controlled randomized study. It was found to improve oxygenation in some of the infants in whom it was tried and was without detrimental systemic hemodynamic effects. It thus appears promising.

K. Inhalational Nitric Oxide (iNO)

1. **Background.** A number of studies have shown that NO, when given by inhalation, reduces PVR and improves oxygenation in a significant proportion of infants with PPHN, both term and preterm. The administration of iNO to infants with PPHN reduces the number requiring ECMO. Oxygenation can also improve during iNO therapy via mechanisms additional to its effect of reducing extrapulmonary right-to-left shunting. Inhaled NO can also improve oxygenation by redirecting blood from poorly aerated or diseased lung regions to better aerated distal air spaces (which are better exposed to the inhaled drug), thereby improving ventilation-perfusion mismatching. Although the benefits of iNO have been demonstrated in full-term neonates with pulmonary hypertension, iNO treatment of preterm infants with pulmonary hypertension is more controversial. In some studies, iNO treatment in premature infants with severe hypoxemic respiratory failure was found to improve oxygenation and reduce the number of ventilator days. On the other hand, no effect on survival or bronchopulmonary dysplasia were demonstrated in trials of preterm infants given iNO. Further trials in premature infants will be required to determine the benefits of iNO, and some are in progress.

2. **Physiology.** NO is a colorless gas with a half-life of seconds. Exogenous inhaled NO diffuses from alveoli to pulmonary vascular smooth muscle and produces vasodilation by the same mechanism as endothelium-derived NO. Excess NO diffuses into the bloodstream, where it is rapidly inactivated by binding to hemoglobin and subsequent metabolism to nitrates and nitrites. This rapid inactivation thereby limits its action to the pulmonary vasculature.

3. **Toxicity.** NO reacts with oxygen to form other oxides of nitrogen and, in particular, NO_2 (nitrogen dioxide). The latter may produce toxic effects and hence must be removed from the respiratory circuit (this can be done by using an adsorbent). When NO combines with hemoglobin, it forms methemoglobin, and this is also of potential concern. In the several large trials that have been completed, methemoglobinemia has not been a significant complication at NO doses <20 ppm. The rate of accumulation of methemoglobin depends on both the dose and duration of NO administration. Even when using doses >20 ppm, clinically significant methemoglobinemia does not appear to be a frequent complication. NO inhibits platelet adhesion to endothelium. Hence, another potential complication is the prolongation of bleeding time described at NO doses of 30–300 ppm. In a small study of premature infants treated with inhaled NO, no change in bleeding time occurred. NO may also have an adverse effect on surfactant function, but this appears to require much higher doses than those relevant in clinical applications. On the contrary, low-dose NO also has antioxidant effects, and these may be potentially beneficial. Because of these potential complications, when administering NO, NO_2 levels should be monitored. Also, blood methemoglobin concentration should be measured. Follow-up studies have shown no increase in adverse clinical outcome, at 1 year of age, associated with iNO compared with controls.

4. **Dosage and administration.** Available evidence supports the use of doses of iNO beginning at 20 ppm. There is little to be gained by administering higher doses because only a few patients will respond to these higher doses after not having responded to a dose of 20 ppm. Higher doses may significantly increase the rate of methemoglobinemia. There is no agreement as to the duration of treatment and criteria of discontinuation of iNO. The basic criterion for weaning of iNO is the achievement of adequate oxygenation and stability of the patient without evidence of rebound pulmonary hypertension. To that end, iNO is usually weaned gradually, and the patient's need for oxygen and hemodynamic status

are assessed after each stepwise reduction in iNO dose. An example of a practical protocol is to wean iNO if the patient can maintain a PaO_2 of >60 mm Hg when fractional inspired O_2 is <0.6. If a reduction in iNO dose is followed by a need to increase FiO_2 by more than, for example, 10–15%, then the weaning process is halted. Doppler echocardiographic assessment may be used to assist in the process of weaning, and other protocols have been used.

5. **Other inhalational drugs.** The idea of effecting selectivity by route of administration has seen some "old" drugs revisited, with systemic effects avoided by administering these drugs by inhalation. Thus, clinical success with inhaled prostacyclin has been reported, and animal studies with inhaled tolazoline have been carried out.

L. **ECMO** (see Chapter 11). ECMO may be indicated for term or near-term infants with PPHN who fail to respond to conventional therapy and who meet ECMO entry criteria. The survival rate with ECMO is reportedly >80%, although only the most severely afflicted infants are referred for this treatment.

VII. **Prognosis.** The overall survival rate appears to be >70–75%. There is, however, a marked difference in survival and long-term outcome according to the cause of the PPHN. More than 80% of term or near-term neonates with PPHN are expected to have an essentially normal neurodevelopmental outcome. Abnormal long-term outcome in PPHN survivors (and a high incidence of sensorineural hearing loss) has been reported to correlate with duration of hyperventilation. However, the relationship may not be causal because prolonged hyperventilation may simply be a marker for the severity of PPHN and hypoxic insult. Survivors of idiopathic PPHN usually have no residual lung or heart disease. Very low birth weight infants with PPHN accompanying severe RDS have a much higher rate of mortality, and there are few data on the long-term outcome of the survivors.

REFERENCES

Abu-Osba YK: Treatment of persistent pulmonary hypertension of the newborn: update. *Arch Dis Child* 1991;66:74.

Allan LD et al: Prospective diagnosis of 1,006 consecutive cases of congenital heart disease in the fetus. *J Am Coll Cardiol* 1994;23:1452.

Barrington KJ, Finer NN: Inhaled nitric oxide for respiratory failure in preterm infants. *Cochrane Database Syst Rev* 2001;4:CD000509.

Bifano EM, Pfannensteil A: Duration of hyperventilation and outcome in infants with persistent pulmonary hypertension. *Pediatrics* 1988;81:657.

Clarke WR: The transitional circulation: physiology and anesthetic implications. *J Clin Anesth* 1990;2:192.

Clyman RI: Ductus arteriosus: current theories of prenatal and postnatal regulation. *Semin Perinatol* 1987;11:64.

Clyman RI: Recommendations for the postnatal use of indomethacin: an analysis of four separate treatment strategies. *J Pediatr* 1996;128:601.

Clyman RI, Campbell D: Indomethacin therapy for patent ductus arteriosus: when is prophylaxis not prophylactic? *J Pediatr* 1987;111:718.

Clyman RI: Ibuprofen and patent ductus arteriosus. *N Engl J Med* 2000;343:728.

Cotton RB et al: Symptomatic patent ductus arteriosus following prophylactic indomethacin: a clinical and biochemical appraisal. *Biol Neonate* 1991;60:273.

Couser RJ et al: Prophylactic indomethacin therapy in the first twenty-four hours of life for the prevention of patent ductus arteriosus in preterm infants treated prophylactically with surfactant in the delivery room. *J Pediatr* 1996;128:631.

Cvetnic WG, Sills JH: Neonatal lung disease. *Clin Anesth* 1992;6:395.

Cvetnic WG et al: Intermittent mandatory ventilation with continuous negative pressure compared with positive end-expiratory pressure for neonatal hypoxemia. *J Perinatol* 1992;12:316.

Dallopiccol B et al: A mendelian basis of congenital heart defects. *Cardiol Young* 1996;6:264.

Edwards AD et al: Effects of indomethacin on cerebral hemodynamics in very preterm infants. *Lancet* 1990;335:1491.

Evans N: Diagnosis of patent ductus arteriosus in the preterm newborn. *Arch Dis Child* 1993; 68:58.

Evans N, Moorcraft J: Effect of patency of the ductus arteriosus on blood pressure in very preterm infants. *Arch Dis Child* 1992;67:1169.

Finer NN, Barrington KJ: Nitric oxide in respiratory failure in the newborn infant. *Semin Perinatol* 1997;21:426.

Fowlie PW: Prophylactic indomethacin: systemic review and meta-analysis. *Arch Dis Child* 1996; 74:F81.

Geggel RL: Inhalational nitric oxide: a selective pulmonary vasodilatory for treatment of persistent pulmonary hypertension of the newborn. *J Pediatr* 1993;123:76.

Gonzalez A et al: Influence of infection on patent ductus arteriosus and chronic lung disease in premature infants weighing 1000 grams or less. *J Pediatr* 1996;128:470.

Hallmann M, Kankaanpaa K: Evidence of surfactant deficiency in persistence of the fetal circulation. *Eur J Pediatr* 1980;134:129.

Hammerman C: Patent ductus arteriosus. *Clin Perinatol* 1995;22:457.

Hammerman C et al: Prostanoids in neonates with persistent pulmonary hypertension. *J Pediatr* 1987;110:470.

Hoffman GM et al: Inhaled nitric oxide reduces the utilization of extracorporeal membrane oxygenation in persistent pulmonary hypertension of the newborn. *Crit Care Med* 1997; 25:352.

Jenkins PC et al: A comparison of treatment strategies for hypoplastic left heart syndrome using decision analysis. *J Am Coll Cardiol* 2001;38:1181.

Keszler M et al: Severe respiratory failure after elective repeat cesarean delivery: a potentially preventable condition leading to extracorporeal membrane oxygenation. *Pediatrics* 1992; 89:670.

Kinsella JP, Abman SH: Inhalational nitric oxide therapy for persistent pulmonary hypertension of the newborn. *Pediatrics* 1993;91:997.

Kinsella JP, Abman SH: Inhaled nitric oxide in the premature infant: animal models and clinical experience. *Semin Perinatol* 1997;21:418.

Kinsella JP, Abman SH: Clinical approach to inhaled nitric oxide therapy in the newborn with hypoxemia. *J Pediatr* 2000;136:717.

Knight DB: The treatment of patent ductus arteriosus in preterm infants: a review and overview of randomized trials. *Semin Neonatol* 2001;6:63.

Kohelet D et al: High-frequency oscillation in the rescue of infants with persistent pulmonary hypertension. *Crit Care Med* 1988;16:510.

Konduri GG et al: Adenosine infusion improves oxygenation in term infants with respiratory failure. *Pediatrics* 1996;97:295.

Lipkin PH et al: Neurodevelopmental and medical outcomes of persistent pulmonary hypertension in term newborns treated with nitric oxide. *J Pediatr* 2002;140:306.

Mahony L et al: Prophylactic indomethacin therapy for patent ductus arteriosus in very-low-birthweight infants. *N Engl J Med* 1982;306:506.

Marino MS, Wernovsky G: Preoperative and postoperative care of the infant with critical congenital heart disease. In Avery GB et al (eds): *Neonatology,* 5th ed. Lippincott Williams & Wilkins, 1999.

Marron MJ et al: Hearing and neurodevelopmental outcome in survivors of persistent pulmonary hypertension of the newborn. *Pediatrics* 1992;90:392.

Meinert CL: Extracorporeal membrane oxygenation trials. *Pediatrics* 1990;85:365.

Morin FC III, Stenmark KR: Persistent pulmonary hypertension of the newborn. *Am J Respir Crit Care Med* 1995;151:2010.

Murphy JD et al: The structural basis of persistent pulmonary hypertension of the newborn infant. *J Pediatr* 1981;98:962.

Nagashima M et al: Cardiac arrhythmias in healthy children revealed by 24-hour ambulatory ECG monitoring. *Pediatric Cardiol* 1987;8:102.

Narayanan M et al: Prophylactic indomethacin: factors determining permanent ductus arteriosus closure. *J Pediatr* 2000;136:330.

Patole SK, Finer NN: Experimental and clinical effects of magnesium infusion in the treatment of neonatal pulmonary hypertension. *Magnesium Res* 1995;8:373.

Perry LW et al: Infants with congenital heart disease: the cases. In Ferencz C et al (eds): *Epidemiology of Congenital Heart Disease: The Baltimore-Washington Infant Heart Study 1981–1989.* Futura, 1993.

Pezzati M et al: Effects of indomethacin and ibuprofen on mesenteric and renal blood flow in preterm infants with patent ductus arteriosus. *J Pediatr* 1999;135:733.

Reller MD et al: The timing of spontaneous closure of the ductus arteriosus in infants with respiratory distress syndrome. *Am J Cardiol* 1990;66:75.

Renfro WH et al: Criteria for use of indomethacin injection in neonates. *Clin Pharm* 1993;12:232.

Rhodes J et al: Effect of blood pressure cuffs on neonatal circulation: their potential application to newborns with persistent pulmonary hypertension. *Pediatr Cardiol* 1995;16:20.

Roberson DA, Silverman NH: Color Doppler flow mapping of the patent ductus arteriosus in very low birthweight neonates: echocardiographic and clinical findings. *Pediatr Cardiol* 1994; 15:219.

Rosenberg AA: Outcome in term infants treated with inhaled nitric oxide. *J Pediatr* 2002;140:284.

Rosenthal A: Hypoplastic left heart syndrome. In JH Moller, JIE Hoffman (eds): *Pediatric Cardiovascular Medicine*, 1st ed. Churchill Livingston, 2000.

Satur CR et al: Day case ligation of patent ductus arteriosus in preterm infants: a 10-year review. *Arch Dis Child* 1991;66:477.

Schreiber MD et al: Increased arterial pH, not decreased $Paco_2$, attenuates hypoxia-induced pulmonary vasoconstriction in newborn lambs. *Pediatr Res* 1986;20:113.

Stefano JL et al: Closure of the ductus arteriosus with indomethacin in ventilated neonates with respiratory distress syndrome. Effects of pulmonary compliance and ventilation. *Am Rev Respir Dis* 1991;143:236.

UK Collaborative ECMO Trial Group: Extra-corporeal membrane oxygenation (ECMO): the UK collaborative neonatal ECMO trial. *Lancet* 1996;348:75.

Van Bel F et al: Contribution of color Doppler flow imaging to the evaluation of the effect of indomethacin on neonatal cerebral hemodynamics. *J Ultrasound Med* 1990;9:107.

Van Overmeire et al: A comparison of ibuprofen and indomethacin for closure of patent ductus arteriosus. *N Engl J Med* 2000;343:674.

Varnholt V et al: High frequency oscillatory ventilation and extracorporeal membrane oxygenation in severe persistent pulmonary hypertension of the newborn. *Eur J Pediatr* 1992;151:769.

Varvarigou A et al: Early ibuprofen administration to prevent patent ductus arteriosus in premature newborn infants. *JAMA* 1996;275:539.

Walsh-Sukys MC: Persistent pulmonary hypertension of the newborn. The black box revisited. *Clin Perinatol* 1993;20:127.

Walther FJ et al: Persistent pulmonary hypertension in premature neonates with severe respiratory distress syndrome. *Pediatrics* 1992;90:899.

Weigel TJ, Hageman JR: National survey of diagnosis and management of persistent pulmonary hypertension of the newborn. *J Perinatol* 1990;10:369.

Weiss H et al: Factors determining reopening of the ductus arteriosus after successful clinical closure with indomethacin. *J Pediatr* 1995;127:466.

Zanardo V et al: Early screening and treatment of "silent" patent ductus arteriosus in prematures with RDS. *J Perinatal Med* 1991;19:291.

63 Common Multiple Congenital Anomaly Syndromes

The neonatal intensive care unit (NICU) is a busy place where quick decisions must often be made. For many disorders, treatment is the same regardless of the underlying problem. However, in the management of multiple congenital anomaly (MCA) syndromes, the neonatologist must deal with complex clinical issues calling for a wide range of diagnostic skills. Without a correct diagnosis of MCA syndrome, many available forms of therapy go underused and others may be tried, although they will be relatively ineffective. Furthermore, unrealistic counseling may be given about prognosis and recurrence risk.

Only a few MCA syndromes are life-threatening in the neonatal period. It is important to note, however, that malformations are the most common cause of death at this critical point in the life span.

An MCA syndrome can be defined as multiple primary defects (eg, malformation, anomaly) in different geographic but not necessarily different embryologic body areas. Multiple anomalies can sometimes occur within a geographic/embryologic field such as the midline as in holoprosencephaly, in which hypotelorism and cleft lip/palate often occur in association with the midline brain defect. Subtle anomalies are no less important diagnostically and often require close scrutiny of the parents' and siblings' features.

I. **Clinical presentation.** Table 63–1 lists symptoms and signs that should alert the clinician to the possibility of cryptogenic malformations or disorders. Obviously, if overt malformations are present, an MCA syndrome will be immediately recognized and diagnostic efforts will shortly follow. However, if external features of the disorder are subtle or nonspecific and the usual procedures associated with intensive newborn support have been started, findings may go unrecognized early. Each manifestation listed in Table 63–1 is more common in infants with MCA syndromes. Tables 63–2 through 63–5 list the more common neonatal MCA syndromes, many of which share some of the features set forth in Table 63–1.

II. **General approach to diagnosis.** The diagnostic approach to malformations in neonates is no different from that in older children, except that the effects of delivery and excess baby fat must be considered. Because so many of these children are intubated and have protective eye patches, the face may be obscured. Early and accurate documentation of physical characteristics, including photographs, is essential. If the infant is critically ill, confirmatory tests (chromosome studies, renal or brain ultrasonography, brain computed tomography/magnetic resonance imaging [CT/MRI] scan, or echocardiography) become a priority equal in importance to ongoing therapy.

The basis of diagnosis of MCA syndromes in the neonate is knowing which disorders are most common plus documenting the physical manifestations and appropriate exclusion tests such as chromosomal analysis. This somewhat "overkill" approach is necessary because a significant percentage of infants with MCA syndromes die in the neonatal period, often before a diagnosis is made, and because the parents in such cases often refuse to permit autopsy. Diagnostic problems also occur because immediate efforts tend to emphasize therapy. Nevertheless, diagnosis will often facilitate or guide therapy in a more efficient manner. If clinical geneticists or dysmorphologists are locally available, they should be asked to examine the infant as soon as possible after delivery. If specialists in these fields are not available, a telephone call to a university medical center for expert advice is often useful.

TABLE 63-1. SYMPTOMS AND SIGNS IN NEONATES THAT MIGHT INDICATE CRYPTOGENIC MULTIPLE CONGENITAL ANOMALY SYNDROME

Prenatal
Oligohydramnios
Polyhydramnios
Decreased or unusual fetal activity
Abnormal fetal problem/position

Postnatal
Abnormalities of size: SGA or LGA, microcephaly or macrocephaly, large or irregular abdomen, small chest, limb-trunk disproportion, asymmetry
Abnormalities of tone: hypotonia, hypertonia
Abnormalities of position: joint contractures, fixation of joints in extension, hyperextension of joints
Midline aberrations: hemangiomas, hair tufts, dimples or pits
Problems of secretion, excretion, or edema: no urination, no passage of meconium, chronic nasal or oral secretions, edema (nuchal, pedal, generalized, ascites)
Symptoms: unexplained seizures, resistant or unexplained respiratory distress
Metabolic disorders: resistant hypoglycemia, unexplained hypo- or hypercalcemia, polycythemia, hyponatremia, thrombocytopenia

SGA, small for gestational age; LGA, large for gestational age.

III. **Chromosomal syndromes.** Chromosomal syndromes are by far the most common MCA syndromes diagnosed in the neonatal period (see Table 63–2).
   A. **Trisomy 21 (Down syndrome)**
      1. **Incidence.** Trisomy 21 is by far the most common MCA syndrome, occurring in about 1 in 600 live births. Only ~80% of cases are diagnosed accurately in the newborn nursery, which means that there is a 20% rate of diagnostic error for this most common cause of MCA and mental retardation. The reason for missing the diagnosis is probably that most of the features of trisomy 21 may occur as isolated features in otherwise normal infants.
      2. **Physical findings.** Findings include hypotonia, upward eye slant, epicanthus, hypotelorism, a tendency to protrude the tongue, Brushfield's spots, a single transverse palmar crease, redundant nape of neck skin, and short, incurved fifth fingers. Although each of these features may occur in normal individuals, it is the combination of features forming a recognizable pattern that usually permits early diagnosis.
      3. **Associated anomalies** include congenital heart defects, particularly of the atrioventricular canal, and increased frequency of duodenal atresia, esophageal atresia, and imperforate anus. Patients may have many immediate medical problems because of these anomalies.
      4. **Hypotonia** may be associated with breathing difficulties, poor swallowing, and aspiration.
   B. **Trisomy 18 (Edwards' syndrome)**
      1. **Incidence.** About 1 in 5000 live births.
      2. **Morbidity.** Highly lethal within the first 3 months of life. Ten percent survive the first year.

TABLE 63-2. THE MOST COMMON CHROMOSOME DISORDERS DIAGNOSED IN THE NEONATAL PERIOD

Trisomy 21 (Down syndrome)
Trisomy 18 (Edwards' syndrome)
Trisomy 13 (Patau's syndrome)
45,X (Turner's syndrome)

3. **Physical findings.** Manifested by prenatal and postnatal growth deficiency, micrognathia, overlapping digits, congenital heart disease (95% incidence, usually complex), abnormal ears, short sternum, ptosis, rocker-bottom clubfeet, and generalized hypertonicity.
4. **Other anomalies** of <10% frequency include tracheoesophageal fistula or esophageal atresia, hemivertebra, radial hypoplasia or aplasia, omphalocele, and spina bifida.
C. **Trisomy 13 (Patau's syndrome)**
1. **Incidence.** About 1 in 7000 live births.
2. **Morbidity.** Highly lethal within the first 3 months of life. Survival beyond the first year is rare.
3. **Physical findings.** Manifested by cleft lip and palate, polydactyly, scalp cutis aplasia, a bulbous nose, microphthalmos, and congenital heart disease (95% frequency, usually complex).
4. **Other anomalies** include cystic kidneys, hooked penis (in males), midline cleft lip with holoprosencephaly, and rocker-bottom clubfeet.
D. **45,X (Turner's) syndrome**
1. **Incidence.** About 1 in 2000 live-born females.
2. **Morbidity.** The 45,X syndrome is usually compatible with survival if the child reaches term. Ninety-five percent of conceptions are miscarried or stillborn.
3. **Physical findings.** Neck webbing, pedal and nuchal edema, shield chest, coarctation of the aorta, and short stature are the hallmarks of this disorder.
IV. **Nonchromosomal syndromes** (see Table 63–3)
A. **Oligohydramnios sequence (Potter's oligohydramnios sequence)**
1. **Incidence.** This syndrome is the second most common MCA (1 in 4000 live births). Most cases are nonsyndromic and have a 2–7% recurrence risk, depending on the specific urinary tract defect. Some may be associated with the prune-belly syndrome (absent abdominal musculature, urinary tract abnormalities, and cryptorchidism) if the kidneys were hydronephrotic early in gestation and later decompress, leaving a wrinkled abdomen and the effects of oligohydramnios (pulmonary hypoplasia and Potter's sequence). About 5% of cases are part of an MCA syndrome with primary defects outside the urinary system.
2. **Morbidity.** Almost all of these infants die.
3. **Pathophysiology.** Renal agenesis leads to decreased production of amniotic fluid (oligohydramnios). Deficient amniotic fluid is believed to be responsible for associated pulmonary hypoplasia.
4. **Clinical presentation**
   a. **History.** The history of oligohydramnios must be solicited from the obstetrician. Anuria is typically present in the newborn.
   b. **Placental examination.** The placenta must be examined for yellowish plaques (amnion nodosum).
   c. **Physical findings.** Unexplained and highly refractory respiratory distress coupled with pneumothoraces, clubfeet, hyperextensible fingers, large cartilage-deficient ears, lower inner eye folds, and a beak nose are classic manifestations associated with prolonged and severe oligohydramnios.

TABLE 63–3. THE MOST COMMON NONCHROMOSOMAL DEFORMATION OR DISRUPTION SEQUENCES DIAGNOSED IN THE NEONATAL PERIOD

Potter's oligohydramnios sequence
Amniotic band syndrome
Arthrogryposis
Pierre Robin sequence

5. **Diagnosis** is usually confirmed by renal ultrasonography and autopsy disclosure of the urinary tract abnormality. It is advisable to perform chromosome studies on the propositus to exclude a chromosomal basis for the disorder. The recurrence risk depends on the specific syndrome diagnosis. Parents should have renal ultrasonograms. Future pregnancies should be monitored by ultrasonography unless the risk of recurrence is definitely ruled out.

B. **Amniotic band syndrome**
   1. **Incidence.** About 1 in 2000 to 1 in 4000 live births. Because in some newborns many body areas are involved and because the bands dissipate before delivery in 90% of cases, the diagnosis is often missed or a misdiagnosis is made.
   2. **Pathophysiology.** This syndrome is poorly understood, but the effects of early amnion rupture with entanglement of body parts in bands or strands of amnion are well appreciated. The resulting biomechanical forces can cause deformities of the limbs, digits, and craniofacies. Viscera that are normally outside the fetus in early embryonic development may be hindered in their return, giving rise to omphalocele and other anomalies.
   3. **Physical findings**
      a. **Extremities.** Limb and digit amputations, constrictions, and distal swellings.
      b. **Craniofacies.** Facial clefts and encephaloceles.
      c. **Viscera.** Omphalocele, gastroschisis, and ectopia cordis.
   4. **Placental examination.** It is always important to examine the placenta, but especially so in these cases. The amnion is often small, absent, or rolled into strands. Not all amniotic bands cause intrauterine problems. Ultrasound studies of routine pregnancies have identified amniotic bands that were not attached to the fetus. Follow-up of these pregnancies has revealed normal newborns.
   5. **Management.** Surgical removal of the constricting band and plastic surgical reconstruction should be done if possible.

C. **Arthrogryposis (multiple joint fixations)**
   1. **Incidence.** About 1 in 3000 live births.
   2. **Pathophysiology.** Ninety percent of children with arthrogryposis have a neurologic (brain or spinal cord) basis for the disorder. Many syndromes associated with fetal inactivity (akinesia) may be characterized by arthrogryposis also, because normal fetal joint development depends on adequate fetal movement.
   3. **Clinical presentation.** The newborn infant is afflicted by a combination of joint contractures, joint extensions, and joint dislocations. Those with arthrogryposis of central nervous system (CNS) origin are at increased risk for aspiration and inadequate respiratory movement.
   4. **Management.** Early treatment and rehabilitation can result in remarkable improvement.

D. **Pierre Robin sequence**
   1. **Incidence.** About 1 in 8000 live births.
   2. **Pathophysiology.** The basis of this sequence is severe hypoplasia of the mandible, which does not support the tongue. The accompanying glossoptosis results in severe upper airway obstruction and early intrauterine cleft palate.
   3. **Clinical presentation.** These infants have a short jaw (micrognathia) or receding chin associated with cleft palate. Respiratory distress secondary to upper airway obstruction may occur. Low-set ears are also present.
   4. **Differential diagnosis.** Many syndromes (eg, Stickler or Catel-Manzke) have the craniofacial features of Pierre Robin sequence. If noncraniofacial primary defects (malformations) are seen, an MCA syndrome other than Pierre Robin sequence is present. Some syndromes (eg, Stickler syndrome) may be manifested only by craniofacial features in infancy. Exami-

nations for myopia and malar flattening should be done to support a diagnosis of Stickler syndrome rather than Pierre Robin sequence.

5. **Management.** Positioning the infant in the prone position with the head lower than the rest of the body works in mild cases. Obturators made from a cast of the palate work in mild to severe cases when the infant accepts the apparatus. Intubation, tracheostomy, and suturing of the tongue tip to the lower gingiva are effective temporary measures for glossoptosis when nothing else works. As the mandible grows out, the glossoptosis eventually will resolve. Oral feedings may result in choking or respiratory distress, and gavage feedings or gastrostomy tube feedings may be needed. Most cases of Pierre Robin sequence are nonsyndromic and have little or no recurrence risk.

V. **Miscellaneous syndromes** (see Table 63–4)

A. **VATER association**

1. **Incidence.** About 1 in 5000 live births.
2. **Clinical presentation.** Major features include vertebral anomalies, anal atresia, tracheoesophageal fistula, esophageal atresia, and radial defects. The *V* in *VATER* can also represent vascular (cardiac) defects and the *R*, renal defects, because these two areas are also commonly involved. The presence of additional features, such as atresia of the small intestine and occasional hydrocephalus, rules out a diagnosis of VATER association. This nonrandom association is usually not of genetic origin and requires exclusion of other similar disorders, including chromosomal syndromes.

B. **CHARGE association**

1. **Incidence.** Although it does not occur as frequently as the VATER association, the CHARGE (coloboma, heart disease, choanal atresia, retarded growth and development with or without CNS anomalies, genital anomalies with or without hypogonadism, ear abnormalities or deafness) association is common, occurring in 1 in 10,000 to 1 in 15,000 live-born infants. CHARGE often presents as a medical emergency because about half of the patients have choanal atresia, serious heart defects, and swallowing difficulties.
2. **Clinical presentation**

a. **Choanal atresia.** The infant may present with unexplained respiratory distress. The posterior nares can be blocked unilaterally or bilaterally as well as being stenotic.

b. **Associated anomalies.** Patients with CHARGE association also have heart defects, small ears, retinal colobomas, and cleft lip and palate; males have micropenis. A smaller percentage have unilateral facial palsies and swallowing difficulties, the latter potentially as lethal as choanal atresia. Postnatal growth deficiency and psychomotor delay round out the major features of this nonrandom and nongenetic association.

3. **Diagnosis.** Any newborn with unexplained breathing difficulties should have nasogastric tubes passed through its nasal passages, particularly if there are multiple congenital anomalies. Exclusion of other similar entities

TABLE 63–4. OTHER MCA SYNDROMES OF SPECIAL INTEREST IN THE NEONATE

VATER association
CHARGE association
Lethal short-limb, short-rib dwarfism
DiGeorge association
Beckwith's syndrome

MCA, multiple congenital anomaly.

and chromosomal disorders is essential before the diagnosis of CHARGE association can be accepted.

C. **Lethal short-limb, short-rib dwarfism (skeletal dysplasia)**
   1. **Incidence.** About 1 in 5000 live births.
   2. **Pathophysiology.** The three most common lethal dwarfing conditions are achondrogenesis, thanatophoric dysplasia, and type II osteogenesis imperfecta. However, at least seven other disorders can be lethal in neonates. All of these disorders are of genetic origin.
   3. **Clinical presentation.** These conditions commonly present clinical and diagnostic difficulties in neonates. Recognition of disproportionate parameters in a newborn with respiratory distress should immediately suggest the possibility of a lethal dwarfing condition. Because many newborns have a substantial amount of fat, chest size may be difficult to assess.
   4. **Diagnosis.** If the "babygram" (chest and abdominal x-ray film) shows a small chest and long-bone metaphyseal or epiphyseal abnormalities, a potentially lethal dwarfing condition is present and accurate diagnosis is essential for prognosis and recurrence risk. A full skeletal x-ray study is mandatory in all cases. The presence of specific anomalies (eg, polydactyly, nail dysplasia, camptodactyly, cleft lip and palate, ear cysts, encephalocele, fractures, ambiguous genitalia, craniosynostosis, macrocephaly, hypoplastic midface, and intestinal atresia) helps to quickly narrow the diagnostic possibilities. The x-ray films and the pattern of bone abnormalities are usually pathognomonic for a specific disorder.

D. **DiGeorge association/syndrome**
   1. **Clinical presentation**
      a. **Physical findings** include heart defects (usually conotruncal in nature); small, abnormally shaped ears; and mild nonspecific facial dysmorphology.
      b. **Laboratory findings** usually consist of hypocalcemia secondary to absence or hypoplasia of the parathyroid glands. Hypocalcemia is often diagnosed before other features are recognized, and this finding should immediately stimulate a search for abnormalities of the heart and craniofacial area. A decreased lymphocyte count may also be seen.
   2. **Associated anomalies.** Total or partial thymic absence is a cryptic feature of DiGeorge syndrome that should be investigated because it may be the most serious of all the abnormalities.
   3. **Etiology.** A chromosomal deletion at the 22q11 region is responsible for DiGeorge syndrome in >80% of cases. A sometimes indistinguishable disorder, velocardiofacial syndrome has a deletion in the same region. The velocardiofacial syndrome has a higher frequency of cleft palate and a more distinctive facies.

E. **Beckwith's syndrome**
   1. **Clinical presentation**
      a. **Physical findings** typically include macroglossia and omphalocele, but ~20% of patients have only one or neither of these two features. Unilateral limb hypertrophy may also be seen.
      b. **Laboratory findings.** Refractory hypoglycemia is frequently present regardless of the presence of external features and should immediately raise the possibility of Beckwith's syndrome.
   2. **Management.** Making the diagnosis early in the postnatal period and immediate institution of aggressive hypoglycemic therapy may prevent mental retardation.

VI. **Teratogenic malformations** (see Table 63–5)
   A. **Fetal alcohol syndrome (FAS)** may be suspected on the basis of the phenotype alone (short palpebral fissures; epicanthal folds; a flat nasal bridge; a long, simple philtrum; a thin upper lip; and small, hypoplastic nails) or may present only as a small for gestational age infant. It may also present with mi-

TABLE 63-5. TERATOGENIC SYNDROMES COMMONLY SEEN IN NEONATES

Fetal alcohol syndrome
Fetal hydantoin syndrome
Fetal valproate syndrome
Fetal cocaine syndrome
Fetal Accutane syndrome
Infant of a diabetic mother
Infant of a myotonic dystrophy mother
Infectious diseases

crocephaly. FAS also has an increased association with congenital heart defects. A thorough history of maternal drug intake is important to rule out a teratogenic cause of multiple anomalies and mental retardation.

B. **Fetal hydantoin syndrome** is characterized by a typical facies (a broad, low nasal bridge; hypertelorism; epicanthal folds; ptosis; and prominent, malformed ears), and these infants also have a high incidence of absence or hypoplasia of the fifth fingernail and toenail.

C. **Fetal valproate syndrome** was recognized in 1982, after establishing an association of neural tube defects (ie, spina bifida) in offspring of mothers taking valproic acid. Other anomalies comprising the fetal valproate syndrome include prominent or fused metopic suture, trigonocephaly, epicanthal folds, midface hypoplasia, anteverted nostrils, oral cleft, heart defect, hypospadias, clubfeet, and psychomotor retardation.

D. **Fetal cocaine syndrome** is characteristically seen in small for gestational age infants, who may show hyperirritability or withdrawal symptomatology. There is an increased incidence of genitourinary tract anomalies such as hydronephrosis, hypospadias, and prune-belly sequence and CNS abnormalities such as microcephaly, porencephaly, and infarction. There have been reports of gastrointestinal and cardiac anomalies. No well-established facial phenotype is proven at this time.

E. **Fetal Accutane (isotretinoin) syndrome** is caused by maternal exposure to isotretinoin, which is a synthetic retinoid (13-*cis*-retinoic acid) used for severe cystic acne. Fetal malformations that result include microtia, hydrocephalus, nonspecific facial aberrations, and an increased incidence of cardiac defects. About 25% of exposed fetuses will be adversely affected. Megadoses of vitamin A may give the same adverse fetal effects.

F. **Infants of diabetic mothers (IDMs)**
1. **Incidence.** These infants are at 3 times the risk for malformations compared with the offspring of nondiabetic mothers. IDMs present with anomalies in ~1 in 2000 consecutive deliveries.
2. **Clinical presentation.** The well-known malformations are sacral agenesis, femoral hypoplasia, heart defects, and cleft palate. Others include preaxial radial defects, microtia, cleft lip, microphthalmos, holoprosencephaly, microcephaly, anencephaly, spina bifida, hemivertebra, urinary tract defects, and hallucal polydactyly. Some IDMs have many anomalies, which may not be recognized as related to maternal diabetes. Improved diabetic control during gestation dramatically reduces the incidence of IDM-related malformations but does not reduce it back to baseline.

G. **Infants of mothers with myotonic dystrophy** are often born with clubfeet, multiple joint contractures, hypotonia, and myopathic facial gestalt. This occurs only when the mother has myotonic dystrophy and the infant also received the gene (usually at the q13.3 locus of chromosome 19). Such children can appear very dysmorphic and die from poor respiratory effort. Any child with these features, particularly severe unexplained hypotonia, should have gene studies for myotonic dystrophy. The mother should also be carefully examined for subtle myotonia, cataracts, and myopathic face.

H. **Infectious (prenatal) diseases** such as rubella, cytomegalovirus, and toxoplasmosis can cause anomalies such as microcephaly, hydro-/macrocephaly, cataracts, microphthalmia, and heart defects. These defects can be confused by single gene or chromosome abnormalities. Any neonate who has these features with no obvious cause should have TORCH studies and a brain scan.

VII. **Genetic counseling** for MCA syndromes is complex and requires a great deal of bona fide sensitivity. First, it is important to have a secure diagnosis, if one is possible. The next step is to establish the parents' understanding of the entire situation and what they have been told by other professionals. Be sure you know what questions the parents want answers to before the factual counseling begins. Do not give excessive details relative to the facts and try to avoid specific predictions, particularly regarding timing and the presence or absence of certain problems relative to the future. Leave some degree of hope, but be honestly realistic, particularly if the parents clearly demand it. Assume frequent follow-up counseling sessions, and outline a long-term program for the child's care and evaluations. Recurrence risk figures and the availability of prenatal diagnosis for subsequent pregnancies are mandatory areas to cover. Remember: You may well view the child's problems much differently than the parents do. Consequently, work with the family from their perspective.

REFERENCES

Aase JM: *Diagnostic Dysmorphology.* Plenum, 1990.
Cadle RG et al: The prevalence of genetic disorders, birth defects and syndromes in central and eastern Kentucky. *Kentucky Med Assoc J* 1996;94:237.
Cunniff C et al: Contribution of heritable disorders to mortality in the pediatric intensive care unit. *Pediatrics* 1995;95:678.
Hall BD: The twenty-five most common multiple congenital anomaly syndromes. In Kaback MM (ed): *Genetic Issues in Pediatric, Obstetric, and Gynecologic Practice.* Year Book, 1981.
Hall BD: The state of the art of dysmorphology. *Am J Dis Child* 1993;147:1184.
Hall BD: Chromosomal abnormalities. In Berg BO (ed): *Principles of Child Neurology.* McGraw-Hill, 1996.
Jones KL: *Smith's Recognizable Patterns of Human Malformation,* 5th ed. Saunders, 1997.
Lynfield R, Eaton RB: Teratogen update: Congenital toxoplasmosis. *Teratology* 1995;52:176.
Marchini C et al: Correlations between individual clinical manifestations and CTG repeat amplification in myotonic dystrophy. *Clin Pediatr* 2002;57:74.

64 Hyperbilirubinemia

Hyperbilirubinemia is a common transitional finding occurring in 60–70% of term newborns and almost all premature infants. An elevation of serum bilirubin concentration >2 mg/dL is found in virtually all newborns in the first several days of life. Jaundice becomes clinically apparent at serum bilirubin concentration of >5 mg/dL.

Bilirubin is the end product of the catabolism of heme and is produced primarily by the breakdown of red blood cell hemoglobin. Other sources of heme include heme-containing proteins such as myoglobin, cytochromes, and nitric oxide synthase. Bilirubin exists in several forms in the blood but is predominantly bound to serum albumin. Free unconjugated bilirubin, and possibly other forms, can enter the central nervous system (CNS) and become toxic to cells if concentration is great enough. The precise mechanism is unknown.

Inside liver cells, unconjugated bilirubin is bound to ligandin, Z protein, and other binding proteins; it is conjugated by uridine diphosphoglucuronyl transferase (UDPGT). Conjugated bilirubin is water-soluble and can be excreted in the urine, but most of it is rapidly excreted as bile into the intestine. Conjugated bilirubin is further metabolized by bacteria in the intestine and excreted in the feces.

Hyperbilirubinemia presents in the neonate as either unconjugated hyperbilirubinemia or conjugated hyperbilirubinemia. The two forms involve different pathophysiologic causes with distinct potential complications.

UNCONJUGATED (INDIRECT) HYPERBILIRUBINEMIA

I. **Definition.** When the rate of bilirubin production exceeds the rate of bilirubin elimination, the end result is an increase in the total serum bilirubin (TSB) concentration, resulting in the clinical condition of hyperbilirubinemia, often called jaundice.

II. **Classification and pathophysiology.** The causes of unconjugated hyperbilirubinomia are listed in Table 64–1.

A. **Physiologic jaundice.** In almost every newborn infant, particularly premature infants, a physiologic elevation of serum unconjugated bilirubin develops during the first week of life, usually in the second or third day, and resolves spontaneously. Jaundice that develops in the first 24 h of life is to be considered pathologic until proven otherwise.

1. **Exclusion criteria**
   a. **Unconjugated bilirubin level** >12.9 mg/dL in the term infant.
   b. **Unconjugated bilirubin level** >15 mg/dL in the preterm infant. (Threshold level may vary depending on the gestational age and birth weight of infant)
   c. **Bilirubin level** increasing at a rate >5 mg/dL/day.
   d. **Jaundice** in the first 24 h of life.
   e. **Conjugated bilirubin level** >2 mg/dL.
   f. **Clinical jaundice** persisting >1 week in full-term infants or >2 weeks in preterm infants.

2. **Physiology**
   a. **Full-term infant.** Serum unconjugated bilirubin progressively rises to a mean peak of 5–6 mg/dL by the third day of life in both white and black infants and a peak of 10 mg/dL at 3–4 days in Asian babies. Figure 64–1 shows hour-specific nomogram with predictive value for subsequent hyperbilirubinemia.

TABLE 64–1. CAUSES OF UNCONJUGATED HYPERBILIRUBINEMIA

Physiologic jaundice
Hemolytic anemia
  Congenital: red blood cell defects (hereditary spherocytosis, infantile pyknocytosis, pyruvate kinase defi-
  ciency, G6PD deficiency, and thalassemia)
  Acquired: blood group incompatibilities (ABO or Rh incompatibility), infection, and drug-induced hemolysis
Polycythemia
Blood extravasation
Defects of conjugation
  Congenital: Crigler-Najjar syndrome (types I and II), Gilbert syndrome
  Acquired: Lucey-Driscoll syndrome
Breast-feeding and breast milk jaundice
Metabolic disorders: galactosemia, hypothyroidism
Increased enterohepatic circulaton of bilirubin
Substances/disorders affecting binding of bilirubin to albumin: drugs, fatty acids in nutritional products,
asphyxia, acidosis, sepsis, hypothermia, hyperosmolality, hypoglycemia

G6PD, glucose-6-phosphate dehydrogenase.

    b. Preterm neonates. Liver function is less mature, and jaundice is more
    frequent and pronounced. A peak concentration of 10–12 mg/dL is
    reached by the fifth day of life.
  3. Mechanisms. A number of mechanisms have been suggested.
    a. Increased bilirubin load because of the larger red blood cell volume,
    the shorter life span of red blood cells, and increased enterohepatic re-
    circulation of bilirubin in newborn infants.
    b. Defective uptake by the liver as a result of decreased concentration of
    bilirubin binding proteins, such as ligandin.
    c. Defective conjugation because of reduced glucuronyl transferase ac-
    tivity in the term newborn; even more pronounced in premature infants.

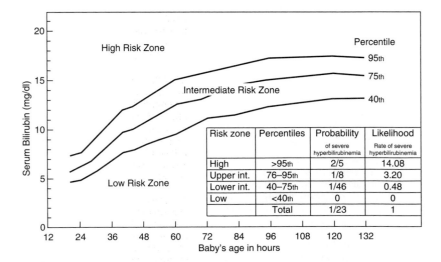

Risk zone	Percentiles	Probability	Likelihood
		of severe hyperbilirubinemia	Rate of severe hyperbilirubinemia
High	>95th	2/5	14.08
Upper int.	76–95th	1/8	3.20
Lower int.	40–75th	1/46	0.48
Low	<40th	0	0
	Total	1/23	1

FIGURE 64–1. Hour-specific bilirubin nomogram with the predictive ability of the predischarge bilirubin
value for subsequent severe hyperbilirubinemia, >95th percentile tract. Reproduced with permission from
Bhutani VK,, Johnson LH. Jaundice technologies; prediction of hyperbilirubinemia in term and near term
newborns. J Perinatol 2001;21:576

d. **Impaired excretion into bile.**
e. **Overall impairment/immaturity of liver function.**
B. **Hemolytic anemia**
  1. **Red blood cell defects.** Hemolytic anemia may result from a congenital red blood cell defect such as hereditary spherocytosis, infantile pyknocytosis, pyruvate kinase deficiency, glucose-6-phosphate dehydrogenase (G6PD) deficiency, thalassemia, or vitamin K-induced hemolysis.
  2. **Acquired hemolytic anemia** may be seen in blood group incompatibilities, such as ABO or Rh incompatibility between infant and mother. It may also be associated with the use of certain drugs (eg, sulfonamides) or with infection.
C. **Polycythemia.** The liver may not have the capacity to metabolize the increased bilirubin load presented by the increased blood volume.
D. **Blood extravasation.** Sequestration of blood within body cavities can result in increased bilirubin and thus overload the bilirubin degradation pathway. It may be seen with cephalhematoma, intracranial and pulmonary hemorrhage, subcapsular hematoma of the liver, excessive ecchymoses or petechiae, occult gastrointestinal hemorrhage, and large hemangiomas (ie, Kasabach-Merritt syndrome).
E. **Defects of conjugation**
  1. **Congenital deficiency of glucuronyl transferase**
    a. **Crigler-Najjar syndrome type I.** A severe form of uridine diphosphate (UPD) glucuronyl transferase deficiency that is inherited as an autosomal recessive disorder. It is unresponsive to phenobarbital therapy and has a poor prognosis.
    b. **Crigler-Najjar syndrome type II.** Moderate deficiency of UDP-glucuronyl transferase. It is responsive to phenobarbital therapy.
    c. **Gilbert syndrome** is a mild form of UDP-glucuronyl transferase deficiency and is inherited as an autosomal dominant condition, is benign, and is relatively common. It is responsive to phenobarbital, although no specific therapy is necessary.
  2. **Glucuronyl transferase inhibition**
    a. **Drugs** such as novobiocin.
    b. **Lucey-Driscoll syndrome.** An unspecified maternal gestational hormone, found in the infant's serum interferes with the conjugation of bilirubin. This problem appears to resolve spontaneously; however, in extreme cases, exchange transfusions may be required to avoid kernicterus.
F. **Breast milk jaundice (late onset)** is a result of the prolongation of increased enterohepatic recirculation of bilirubin because of a factor in human milk that promotes intestinal absorption. It is characterized by a higher peak (10–30 mg/dL, peaking by days 10–15 of life) and a slower decline in the serum bilirubin concentration that can last for several weeks. It rarely appears before the end of the first week of life for term or preterm infants. Interruption of breast-feeding for 24–48 h at unacceptable bilirubin levels results in a rapid decline. Resumption of breast-feeding increases bilirubin levels slightly but usually below previous levels. Breast milk jaundice may recur in 70% of future pregnancies.
G. **Metabolic disorders.** Galactosemia, hypothyroidism, and maternal diabetes may be associated with unconjugated hyperbilirubinemia.
H. **Increased enterohepatic recirculation** of unconjugated bilirubin as a result of pathologic conditions such as cystic fibrosis, gastrointestinal obstruction (ie, pyloric stenosis, duodenal atresia, annular pancreas), and ileus may result in exaggerated jaundice. Blood swallowed during delivery and decreased caloric intake may also be contributing factors.
I. **Substances and disorders affecting binding of bilirubin to albumin.** Certain drugs occupy bilirubin-binding sites on albumin and increase the amount of free unconjugated bilirubin that can cross the blood-brain barrier. Drugs in

which this effect may be significant include aspirin and sulfonamides. Chloral hydrate is shown to compete for hepatic glucuronidation with bilirubin and thus increase serum unconjugated bilirubin. Common drugs used in the neonates such as penicillin and gentamicin have also been shown to compete with bilirubin for albumin binding sites. Fatty acids in nutritional products (eg, Intralipid) may also influence bilirubin binding to albumin, as may asphyxia, acidosis, sepsis, hypothermia, hyperosmolality, and hypoglycemia.

III. Morbidity

A. **General.** Unconjugated bilirubin in high concentration can cross the blood-brain barrier, penetrating the brain cells. This has been associated with neuronal dysfunction and death. Bilirubin is toxic to the brain in several ways. It has been shown to depress O_2 consumption and at high concentration uncouples oxidative phosphorylation. Severe hyperbilirubinemia can cause long-term neurologic sequelae; however, the safety of moderate degree of hyperbilirubinemia has been debated. One study has shown that moderate hyperbilirubinemia (13.6–26.0 mg/dL) may be associated with an increase in minor neurologic dysfunction.

B. **Encephalopathy**

1. **Transient.** Early bilirubin-induced neurologic dysfunction is transient and reversible. **Auditory brainstem evoked responses (ABRs)** show significant prolongation of latency of specific wavelengths. These changes may be reversed with either exchange transfusions or with spontaneous decrease in bilirubin levels. More recent data suggest that with marked hyperbilirubinemia, complete recovery of the ABR may be delayed. The auditory system serves as an objective window in looking at the CNS in cases of severe hyperbilirubinemia, which can be used as an early predictor of bilirubin encephalopathy.

2. **Bilirubin encephalopathy.** This is a preventable lifelong neurologic sequelae of untreated hyperbilirubinemia. It is a clinically worsening encephalopathy (over 24 h) caused by bilirubin toxicity to the basal ganglia and various brainstem nuclei.

   a. **Acute phase.** A severely jaundiced infant develops lethargy, hypotonia, and poor sucking response. If left untreated, the infant becomes hypertonic and may develop fever and a high-pitched cry. Decerebrate posturing can occur at the end stage of the disease.

   b. **Chronic phase.** Survivors usually develop choreoathetoid cerebral palsy, hearing loss, dental dysplasia and paralysis of upward gaze, and, less often, mental retardation.

C. **Kernicterus.** A postmortem diagnosis of pathologic findings of bilirubin toxicity in the brain.

1. **Staining and necroses of neurons** in the basal ganglia, hippocampal cortex, subthalamic nuclei, and cerebellum. Cerebral cortex is usually spared.

2. **Bilirubin toxicity to the brain** may be reversible if bilirubin levels fall before saturation of the CNS nuclei occurs.

3. **Controversy exists over bilirubin levels** considered at risk for kernicterus. In nonhemolytic states, and otherwise healthy term infants, levels of >25 mg/dL are considered to place the patient at risk.

4. **Kernicterus registry.** Kernicterus is not a reportable condition in the United States; therefore, its prevalence is not known. A pilot registry at a Pennsylvania hospital documented 90 cases from January 1984–June 2001.

IV. Clinical presentation

A. **History**

1. **Family history.** Family history of jaundice, anemia, splenectomy, or metabolic disorders is significant. A history of a sibling with jaundice may suggest blood group incompatibility, breast milk jaundice, or G6PD deficiency. A familial tendency of neonatal hyperbilirubinemia is present regardless of breast-feeding and other risk factors.

2. **Maternal history.** Neonatal jaundice is increased with a history of maternal diabetes or infection. Use of oxytocin, sulfonamides, antimalarials, and nitrofurantoins by the mother may initiate hemolysis in G6PD-deficient infants. Delivery trauma, asphyxia, delayed cord clamping, and prematurity are associated with an increased risk of hyperbilirubinemia in the infant.

3. **Infant's history.**
   a. **Breast-feeding.** Poor breast-feeding may result in poor caloric intake, leading to "starvation jaundice." (See prior discussion of breast milk jaundice).
   b. **Factors affecting the gastrointestinal tract,** such as obstruction, deoreaced motility (ileus), and delayed passage of meconium
   c. **Check for clinical symptoms** such as vomiting and lethargy. Metabolic disorders, infection, and bowel obstruction can present in this manner.

B. **Signs and symptoms.** Clinical jaundice is visible when the serum bilirubin level approaches 5–7 mg/dL. Jaundice is often apparent first in the face, especially the nose, and then descending to the torso and lower extremities as the degree of jaundice increases. Jaundice can be demonstrated in some infants by pressing lightly on the skin with a finger. The yellow color is seen more easily in the "fingerprint" area than in the surrounding skin. These signs should not appear within the first 24 h after birth in otherwise healthy infants.

Besides confirming the presence of jaundice, physical examination may also be helpful in determining the cause of hyperbilirubinemia. Areas of bleeding such as cephalhematoma, petechiae, or ecchymoses indicate blood extravasation. Hepatosplenomegaly may signify hemolytic disease, liver disease, or infection. Physical signs of prematurity, intrauterine growth retardation, and postmaturity may be helpful in elucidating a cause for hyperbilirubinemia. Plethora is seen with polycythemia, pallor with hemolytic disease, and large infants with maternal diabetes, all of which are associated with hyperbilirubinemia. Omphalitis, chorioretinitis, microcephaly, and petechial and purpuric lesions suggest infectious causes of increased serum bilirubin.

C. **Neurologic examination.** The appearance of abnormal neurologic signs heralds the onset of early bilirubin encephalopathy. Initial signs include lethargy, poor feeding, vomiting, and hypotonia. The persistently hyperbilirubinemic infant may go on to experience seizures (see section III,B above). The progression of neurologic changes parallels the stages of bilirubin encephalopathy from acute to chronic and irreversible changes.

V. **Diagnosis**

A. **Laboratory studies.** Hyperbilirubinemia should be investigated whenever pathologic causes are suspected. The presence of a serum bilirubin level of ≥13 mg/dL in any infant requires initial evaluation.

1. **Total and direct bilirubin**
   a. **Direct bilirubin** = conjugated fraction.
   b. **Indirect bilirubin** = unconjugated fraction. Derived by subtracting direct fraction from TSB.

2. **Complete blood cell count and reticulocyte count.** A low hemoglobin or hematocrit associated with a high reticulocyte count and the presence of nucleated red blood cells is highly suggestive of hemolytic anemia. Polycythemia is defined as a venous blood hematocrit >65%. (*Use of capillary blood samples may cause underestimation of venous bilirubin values when the bilirubin value is >10 mg/dL).* Total white blood cell count with differential and platelet count may help detect sepsis. The peripheral blood smear aids in the diagnosis of hereditary spherocytosis and other red blood cell defects.

3. **Blood type and Rh status in mother and infant.** ABO and Rh incompatibility can be easily diagnosed by comparing infant and maternal blood types.

4. **Direct Coombs' test.** The test is usually positive in infant's with isoimmunization disorders. This test does not correlate with the severity of jaundice.

5. **Measurement of serum albumin** may help to assess total bilirubin binding sites available and whether there is a need for an albumin infusion.
6. **Other laboratory tests.** The urine should be tested for reducing substances (to rule out galactosemia if the infant is receiving a galactose-containing formula) and for infectious agents. If hemolysis is present, in the absence of ABO or Rh incompatibility, further testing by hemoglobin electrophoresis, G6PD screening, or osmotic fragility testing may be required to diagnose red blood cell defects. Persistent jaundice (>2 weeks of life) may require these types of investigation as well as additional tests for thyroid and liver function, blood and urine cultures, and metabolic screening workup, such as plasma amino acid and urine organic acid measurements.
B. **Radiologic studies** for suspected intestinal obstruction or blood extravasation into internal organs and ultrasonography of the head to document intracranial or subdural hemorrhage might be indicated.
C. **Transcutaneous bilirubinometry (TcB).** Measures the degree of yellow color in the skin and subcutaneous tissues by selective wavelength reflection. Data suggest that this methodology is an effective adjunct to nursing assessment in the term infant. A TcB value of >13 mg/dL should be correlated with TSB.
D. **Expired carbon monoxide breath analyzer.** End-tidal carbon monoxide (CO) corrected for ambient CO (ETCO$_2$). An equimolar amount of CO is produced for every molecule of bilirubin formed from the degradation of heme; therefore, measurement of CO in end-tidal breath is an index of total bilirubin production. The method can alert the attending physician to the presence of hemolysis irrespective of the timing of jaundice.
VI. **Management.** Three methods of treatment are commonly used to decrease the level of unconjugated bilirubin: exchange transfusion, phototherapy, and pharmacologic therapy. As noted, however, *controversy* persists as to what levels of serum bilirubin warrant therapy, especially in otherwise healthy full-term infants.
A. **Phototherapy** (see also Chapter 39)
  1. **Indication.** Most infants with pathologic jaundice are treated with phototherapy when it is believed that bilirubin levels could enter the toxic range.
    a. **Practice parameters.** The American Academy of Pediatrics (AAP) is currently revising the guidelines for management of hyperbilirubinemia. The concern for kernicterus is being reemphasized by the Subcommittee on Hyperbilirubinemia pending the full assessment and analysis of the new approaches to the jaundiced infant. It is important to remember that the current AAP guidelines are meant for healthy term newborn infants with no evidence of hemolysis. Although there is continuing uncertainty about which TSB level warrants exchange transfusions, the authors suggest that in an otherwise healthy term newborn a TSB level of 20 mg/dL at 48 h of life may be treated initially with phototherapy. If the TSB decreases by 1–2 mg/dL within 4–6 h of starting phototherapy, exchange transfusion may not be necessary.
    b. **In preterm** and sick term infants, a more conservative approach is usually adopted.
  2. **Using phototherapy effectively.**
    a. **Light source.** The most effective light source currently available for phototherapy is that provided by blue fluorescent tubes. Bilirubin absorbs light maximally in the blue range (420–500 nm). Blue lamps with narrow spectral range (420–480 nm) are most effective. The blue light reflection does interfere with skin color assessment and has been reported to cause dizziness and nausea in those caring for these patients. Addition of a daylight fluorescent tube tempers these side effects. Energy output or irradiance is a second variable that influences the efficacy of phototherapy. Radiometer measurements should be

minimally 5 $\mu W/cm^2/nm$, with saturation for bilirubin degradation at ~11 $\mu W/cm^2/nm$.

b. Distance from the light to the infant. Light intensity is a function of the distance from the light source; therefore, light source should be as close to the infant as possible (12–16 inches).

c. Surface area. The larger the skin surface area exposed, the more effective is the phototherapy. The availability of fiberoptic pads (biliblankets) make it easy to increase exposed skin area to the bili-lights. In preterm infants, this type of "double-phototherapy" (overhead light plus bili-blanket) is almost twice as effective as single phototherapy. Fiberoptic phototherapy blankets (bili-blankets) can be wrapped around or placed just beneath the infant.

3. Supportive management. The infant's eyes should be covered with opaque patches for overhead lamp phototherapy. However, this is not necessary when using only fiberoptic light source. Animal experiments have shown retinal damage occurring as a result of phototherapy. To maximize exposure, infants should be naked in servocontrolled incubators. Phototherapy does increase insensible fluid losses. For infants weighing <1500 g, increase fluids by 0.5 mL/kg/h; for those weighing >1500 g, increase by 1 mL/kg/h. Overhydration does not increase bilirubin elimination.

4. Termination of phototherapy. Phototherapy is stopped when the following criteria are met:

a. The bilirubin level is low enough to eliminate the risk of kernicterus.

b. The infant is old enough to handle the bilirubin load.

5. Complications. Phototherapy is simple, safe, and inexpensive. Complications are very rare but should not be overlooked.

a. The retinal effects of phototherapy on the exposed infant's eyes are unknown. However, animal studies suggest that retinal degeneration may occur. Thus, eye shields must be used.

b. Increased insensible fluid loss increases fluid requirements by 25%. In addition, stools may be looser and more frequent. Use of fiberoptic phototherapy results in lower insensible loss.

c. Bronze baby syndrome. With conjugated hyperbilirubinemia, phototherapy causes photodestruction of copper porphyrins, causing urine and skin to become bronze.

d. Congenital erythropoietic porphyria is a rare syndrome in which phototherapy is contraindicated. Exposure to visible light of moderate to high intensity will produce severe bullous lesions on exposed skin and may lead to death.

B. Exchange transfusion (see also Chapter 21). Exchange transfusion is used when the risk of kernicterus for a particular infant is significant. A double-volume exchange replaces 85% of the circulating red blood cells and decreases the bilirubin level to about half of the preexchange value. Besides removing bilirubin, an exchange transfusion can be used to correct severe anemia.

1. General guidelines. It appears that no specific level of bilirubin can be considered safe or dangerous for all infants because patient-to-patient variations exist for the permeability of the blood-brain barrier. The practice parameters published by the AAP in October 1994 recommend exchange transfusions in healthy term newborns at TSB 25–30 mg/dL. The debate for upper limits of serum bilirubin is directed to full-term infants with no evidence for associated disease.

Low birth weight infants are excluded from these considerations. The authors suggest that each institution and its practicing physicians must establish their criteria for phototherapy and exchange transfusion by gestational age, weight groups, postnatal age, and infant's condition consistent with current standard of pediatric practice.

2. Factors that may affect the decision to perform exchange transfusion include the infant's maturity, birth weight, age, rate of rise in bilirubin levels

(>0.5 mg/dL/h), and presence of hypoxia, acidosis, sepsis, or hypoproteinemia.

3. **Albumin transfusions** may be useful if bilirubin levels are >20 mg/dL and serum albumin levels are <3 g/dL. Infusion of 1 g of albumin 1 h before exchange transfusion may improve the yield of bilirubin removal. Fluid volume and cardiovascular status must be carefully considered before giving albumin.

C. **Pharmacology**
   1. **Phenobarbital therapy**
      a. **Action.** Phenobarbital affects the metabolism of bilirubin by increasing the concentration of ligandin in liver cells, inducing production of glucuronyl transferase, and enhancing bilirubin excretion. Because it takes 3–7 days to become effective, phenobarbital is usually not helpful in treating unconjugated hyperbilirubinemia in the newborn infant. The administration of phenobarbital to newborns at the time that jaundice is first noted or even at birth is less effective than administration to mothers during pregnancy for ≥2 weeks before delivery.
      b. **Indications.** It may be useful to give phenobarbital 1–2 weeks before delivery to a pregnant mother whose fetus has **documented hemolytic disease** to aid in reducing bilirubin levels in the affected neonate. Phenobarbital is also used to treat type II glucuronyl transferase deficiency and Gilbert syndrome in the infant.
   2. **Metalloporphyrins.** A synthetic heme analog, metalloporphyrins have been shown to inhibit heme oxygenase (HO), the rate-limiting enzyme in the catabolism of heme. By acting as a competitive inhibitor, the metalloporphyrins decrease the production of bilirubin. Tin-mesoporphyrin (SnMP) is a potent HO inhibitor that has been extensively studied. It has been reported to be effective as a single intramuscular injection (6 mmol/ kg) in two patients with hemolytic disease, resulting in a significant drop in TSB concentration, thereby avoiding the need for exchange transfusion. Another report has shown that a single dose of SnMP can prevent the development of severe hyperbilirubinemia in newborn infants with G6PD deficiency. The only untoward effect noted was a non-dose-dependent, mild, transient erythema when used in conjunction with phototherapy in a preterm infant.
   3. **Supportive management.** Most breast-fed infants do not develop bilirubin levels of ≥20 mg/dL in the first 8 days of life. For infants 6–8 days old, breast-fed and otherwise well, **consider interrupting breast-feeding** for 48 h and use phototherapy if the bilirubin is >18 mg/dL.

CONJUGATED (DIRECT) HYPERBILIRUBINEMIA

I. **Definition.** Conjugated hyperbilirubinemia is a sign of hepatobiliary dysfunction. It usually appears in the newborn infant after the first week of life, when the indirect hyperbilirubinemia of physiologic jaundice has receded. When the direct bilirubin level is >2.0 mg/dL or is >20% of the TSB, it is clinically significant.

II. **Classification.** Conjugated hyperbilirubinemia is caused by a defect or insufficiency in bile secretion, biliary flow, or both, resulting in an inability to remove conjugated bilirubin from the body. It is always pathologic. The term **cholestasis** is used to describe the group of disorders associated with bilirubin excretion and is associated with a rise in serum conjugated bilirubin levels and usually bile salts and phospholipids. Causes of conjugated hyperbilirubinemia are listed in Table 64–2.

A. **Extrahepatic biliary disease**
   1. **Biliary atresia** is the single most common cause of neonatal cholestasis, with an estimated incidence of 1:10,000 live births. It is the reason for 50–60% of liver transplantations in children worldwide. Its cause is poorly

TABLE 64-2. CAUSES OF CONJUGATED HYPERBILIRUBINEMIA

Extrahepatic biliary disease
  Biliary atresia
  Choledochal cyst
  Bile duct stenosis
  Spontaneous perforation of the bile duct
  Cholelithiasis
  Neoplasms
Intrahepatic biliary disease
  Intrahepatic bile duct paucity (syndromic or nonsyndromic)
  Progressive intrahepatic cholestasis
  Inspissated bile
Hepatocellular disease
  Metabolic and genetic defects
    α_1-antitrypsin deficiency, cystic fibrosis, Zellweger's syndrome, Dubin-Johnson and Rotor's syndromes, galactosemia
  Infections
  Total parenteral nutrition
  Idiopathic neonatal hepatitis
  Neonatal hemochromatosis
Miscellaneous
  Shock Hypoperfusion State, ECMO
INTRAHEPATIC CHOLESTASIS WITH NORMAL BILE DUCTS
Infection
  Viral: hepatitis B virus; non-A, non-B hepatitis virus; cytomegalovirus; herpes simplex virus; coxsackievirus, Epstein-Barr virus; adenovirus
  Bacterial: *Treponema pallidum*, *Escherichia coli*, group B streptococcus, *Staphylococcus aureus*, *Listeria*; urinary tract infection caused by *F. coli* or *Proteus* spp, pneumococcus
  Other: *Toxoplasma gondii*
Genetic disorders and inborn errors of metabolism: Dubin-Johnson syndrome, Rotor's syndrome, galactosemia, hereditary fructose intolerance, tyrosinemia, α_1-antitrypsin deficiency, Byler disease, recurrent cholestasis with lymphedema, cerebrohepatorenal syndrome, congenital erythropoietic porphyria, Niemann-Pick disease, Menkes' kinky hair syndrome
Idiopathic neonatal hepatitis (giant cell hepatitis)
Total parenteral nutrition-induced cholestasis

understood. It can be associated with polysplenia, cardiovascular defects, and situs inversus.

2. **Choledochal cysts** are dilatations of extrahepatic biliary tree. Diagnosis is by ultrasonography or nuclear medicine scanning.

3. **Other extrahepatic biliary diseases** are bile duct stenosis, spontaneous perforation of bile duct, cholelithiasis, and neoplasm. These are uncommon conditions in neonates. Cholelithiasis in infancy is usually related to other underlying conditions such as hemolysis, anatomic malformation, use of medications (furosemide), or prolonged use of parenteral nutrition. Cholecystectomy is rarely indicated.

B. **Intrahepatic biliary disease**

1. **Intrahepatic bile duct paucity.** This condition may be *syndromic* or *nonsyndromic*. The syndromic form is called Alagille's syndrome (arteriohepatic dysplasia). This is characterized by a constellation of features such as cholestasis, cardiovascular findings (pulmonary artery stenosis), butterfly vertebrae, ocular findings (posterior embryotoxon), and characteristic facies. Liver biopsy shows a paucity of interlobular bile ducts. Transmitted as autosomal dominant, this disorder has been assigned to chromosome 20p12, a region of the chromosome containing the *JAGGED1* gene.

2. **Progressive intrahepatic cholestasis.** These patients have chronic intrahepatic cholestasis but with different pathogenesis and prognosis. Clinical features include chronic persistent hepatocellular cholestasis, exclusion of

other identifiable disorders, occurrence consistent with autosomal recessive inheritance, and a combination of clinical, biochemical, and histologic features. (See Haber & Lake, 1990, for detailed classification and description.)

3. **Inspissated bile.** Infants with moderate to severe hemolytic disease can develop bilirubin overload and resulting cholestasis. Clinically, hepatosplenomegaly is often prominent and liver enzymes are normal or slightly elevated. Cholestasis may persist up to 4 weeks; however, if it persists beyond 4 weeks, it should not be attributed to bilirubin overload alone.

C. **Hepatocellular disease**

1. **Metabolic and genetic defects.** A significant number of identifiable metabolic and genetic abnormalities can present with hepatocellular dysfunction.

    a. **α_1-Antitrypsin deficiency.** This is an autosomal recessive condition characterized by accumulation of α_1-antitrypsin in the hepatocyte, resulting in subsequent hepatocellular necrosis. There are several phenotypes; however, only the homozygous Pi (protease inhibitor) ZZ and, rarely, MZ types have been associated with liver disease in infancy. Most patients experience jaundice in the first 8 weeks of life. Fifty to 70% of patients will go into remission by 6 months. Otherwise, the clinical course is highly variable; some patients develop progressive liver failure.

    b. **Cystic fibrosis.** Cholestasis can be an initial presentation of cystic fibrosis in infancy. Most of these infants will also have meconium ileus. Liver biopsy of these patients will show excessive biliary mucus, inspissated bile, mild inflammatory changes, and fibrosis. Patients who had resolved neonatal jaundice are not at greater risk for liver disease later in life over other cystic fibrosis patients.

    c. **Zellweger's or cerebrohepatorenal syndrome.** This is a peroxisomal disorder and is characterized by the absence of peroxisomes and deranged mitochondria. It is inherited as an autosomal recessive trait and presents in the neonatal period with cholestasis, hepatomegaly, profound hypotonia, and dysmorphic features. Diagnosis is confirmed by the presence of abnormal levels of very-long-chain fatty acid in the serum. Prognosis is very poor. Most infants die within 1 year. Survivors beyond 1 year of age have severe mental retardation and seizures.

    d. **Dubin-Johnson and Rotor's syndromes.** These syndromes are rarely diagnosed in the neonatal period, although they can initially present with cholestasis during that period. Dubin-Johnson syndrome is a nonhemolytic conjugated hyperbilirubinemia caused by deficiency in the canalicular secretion of conjugated bilirubin. Liver biopsy is normal except for the presence of pigmented granules. Rotor's syndrome is believed to be the result of a disturbance in the hepatic storage of anions, characterized by lifelong presence of mild conjugated hyperbilirubinemia. Liver biopsy is normal, but unlike Dubin-Johnson no pigment accumulation is noted. Both conditions are inherited as autosomal recessive and have an excellent prognosis.

    e. **Galactosemia.** This is an autosomal recessive disorder resulting from a deficiency of galactose-1-phosphate uridyltransferase activity. Incidence is about 1:100,000. It is characterized by presence of cholestasis, hepatomegaly, hypoglycemia, cataracts, vomiting, and failure to thrive. *Escherichia coli* sepsis is the most devastating complication in the newborn period. The two other enzymes, namely galactokinase and UDP galactose-4-epimerase, that are involved in the galactose metabolic pathway are less common causes of galactosemia. The pathologic consequences are thought to be secondary to accumulation of toxic metabolite, galactose-1-phosphate. Galactosemia must be rapidly excluded in infants with early-onset cholestasis, with associated eme-

sis, acidosis, and gram-negative sepsis (particularly *E. coli*). These infants, while on lactose-containing formula, will have galactose in the
urine, resulting in a positive reducing substance in the urine (Clinitest)
but negative urine test for glucose (glucose oxidase).

f. **Other metabolic and genetic disorders.** Tyrosinemia, fructosemia,
Niemann-Pick disease, Gaucher's disease, Wolman's disease, and
glycogenosis type IV are other metabolic and genetic disorders that
may present with cholestasis as an additional finding in the neonatal
period.

2. **Infection.**
   a. **Congenital infcotion.** Congenitally acquired infections have a spectrum of manifestations but are usually asymptomatic. Congenital infection usually presents with other stigmata of the disease. Vertical transmission of hepatitis viruses (B and C) is generally asymptomatic, but
   clinical hepatitis, including hepatic failure, may develop at about 2
   months of age. Coxsackievirus, Epstein-Barr virus, and adenovirus are
   known causes of neonatal hepatitis with elevated conjugated fractions.
   b. **Sepsis.** Direct bacterial infection of the liver may occur with overwhelm-
   ing sepsis. Toxic cholestasis with no direct invasion of the liver by microorganisms may be seen with urinary tract infection, particularly with
   E. coli urosepsis.

3. **Total parenteral nutrition (TPN) cholestasis.** The frequency, not necessarily the severity, of cholestasis is partly a function of the degree of prematurity. Cholestasis develops in >50% of infants with birth weight of
   <1000 g and <10% of term infants after prolonged hyperalimentation. No
   precise cause has been found; however, the most significant contributing
   factor was thought to be the lack of enteral feeding. The resumption of normal enteral feeds has been associated with improvement of cholestasis in
   1–3 months, with no or little residual fibrosis and normal hepatic function.

4. **Idiopathic neonatal hepatitis (Table 64–3).** This diagnosis applies when
   known infectious, metabolic, and genetic causes have been ruled out.
   Jaundice and hepatosplenomegaly are major physical findings. Liver
   biopsy demonstrates giant cell transformation, increased extramedullary
   hematopoiesis, and inflammation. Prognosis is fair.

5. **Miscellaneous.**
   a. **Neonatal hemochromatosis (NH).** Also known as neonatal iron storage disease, this condition results from liver disease of intrauterine
   onset. It is associated with extrahepatic deposits of stainable iron. Patients present with hepatocellular synthetic insufficiency (hypoalbuminemia, coagulopathy, and low fibrinogen) with end-stage liver disease.
   Prognosis is very poor and is almost always fatal.
   b. **Shock or hypoperfusion.** Multiorgan involvement is not uncommon in
   cases of perinatal asphyxia or shock/hypoperfusion state.

TABLE 64–3. CLINICAL FINDINGS ASSOCIATED WITH EXTRAHEPATIC BILIARY ATRESIA (EHBA)
AND IDIOPATHIC NEONATAL HEPATITIS (INH)

Variable	EHBA	INH
Jaundice at birth	Never	Rarely
Jaundice presentation	2–4 weeks	2–4 weeks
Dark yellow urine	Yes	Yes
Hepatomegaly	Yes	Yes
Splenomegaly	Sometimes (signifies cirrhosis)	More commonly than with EHBA
Acholic stool	Yes	Transient/incomplete
Alpha-fetoprotein (serum, infant)	May be absent	Frequently (+)

     c. **Extracorporeal membrane oxygenation (ECMO).** Infants on ECMO may show an increase in the prevalence and severity of cholestasis.

III. **Clinical presentation.** The classic clinical manifestations of neonatal cholestasis include jaundice, acholic stools, and dark urine. Other findings may include hepatomegaly, splenomegaly, pruritus, failure to thrive, decreased feeding/ appetite, ascites, and portal hypertension. Unfortunately, individual signs and symptoms cannot differentiate between intra- versus extrahepatic disease. The combination of clinical and historical findings can lead to possible causes. The presence of nonhepatic findings will provide helpful clues to specific diagnosis, such as the following:

    A. **Alagille's syndrome.** Cardiovascular findings (peripheral pulmonic stenosis), vertebral anomalies, ocular findings (posterior embryotoxon), and peculiar facies.

    B. **Zellweger's syndrome or cerebrohepatorenal syndrome.** Profound hypotonia, seizures, and dysmorphic features.

    C. **Congenital infections.** Microcephaly, intracranial calcifications, intrauterine growth retardation.

    D. **Galactosemia.** Failure to thrive, vomiting, cataracts, and Gram-negative bacterial sepsis (*E. coli*).

    E. **TPN-induced cholestasis.** History of prematurity and prolonged use of hyperalimentation.

IV. **Diagnosis**

    A. **Laboratory studies**

      1. **Bilirubin levels (total and direct).**

      2. **Liver function tests.** Serum glutamic oxaloacetic transaminase (SGOT [aspartate transaminase, or AST]), serum glutamic pyruvic transaminase (SGPT [alanine transaminase, or ALT]), and alkaline phosphatase may be helpful in monitoring the course of the disease.

      3. **Prothrombin time and partial thromboplastin time** may be reliable indicators of liver function.

      4. **γ-Glutamyl transpeptidase, 5′-nucleotidase, and serum bile acids** are also usually elevated in cholestasis. Once the diagnosis of cholestasis is made, measurement of these markers of cholestasis may not add any further information.

      5. **A complete blood cell count and reticulocyte count** may be helpful if hepatitis is a possibility because hemolysis may be found.

      6. **Serum cholesterol, triglycerides, and albumin levels.** Triglyceride and cholesterol levels may aid in nutritional management and assessment of liver failure. Albumin is a long-term indicator of hepatic function.

      7. **Ammonia levels** should be checked if liver failure is suspected.

      8. **Serum glucose levels** should be checked if the infant appears ill.

      9. **Urine testing for reducing substances** is a simple screening test that should always be performed to detect for metabolic disease.

     10. **TORCH (*t*oxoplasmosis, *r*ubella, *c*ytomegalovirus [CMV], and *h*erpes simplex virus) titers and urine cultures for CMV.** The use of TORCH titers should be guided by the clinical presentation, keeping in mind that CMV infection may be asymptomatic and congenital syphilis is treatable. CMV immunoglobulins M and G (IgM and IgG), Venereal Disease Research Laboratory (VDRL), and IgM-specific titers for herpes simplex, rubella, and toxoplasmosis may be useful in some cases.

     11. **Alpha-fetoprotein (AFP).**

     12. **Other tests.** More specific tests are indicated in the investigation of the specific causes of conjugated hyperbilirubinemia.

       a. **Hepatitis.** The maternal hepatitis B surface antigen (HBsAg) status should be known, and the infant should also be tested.

       b. **Sepsis.** If bacterial sepsis or urinary tract infection is suspected, appropriate cultures should be obtained.

       c. **Metabolic disorders**

i. **Galactosemia and hereditary fructose intolerance.** The urine should be tested for non-glucose-reducing substances. Enzymes involved in these disorders can also be assayed in the blood.

ii. **Tyrosinemia.** High concentrations of tyrosine and methionine, and their metabolic derivatives, will be seen in the urine.

iii. **α_1-Antitrypsin deficiency.** Decreased serum α_1-antitrypsin concentration and liver biopsy showing periodic acid–Schiff (PAS)-positive cytoplasmic granules with variable degrees of hepatic necrosis and fibrosis.

iv. **Cystic fibrosis.** A sweat test may diagnose cystic fibrosis.

B. **Radiologic studies.** Diagnosis of biliary atresia and other forms of extrahepatic biliary obstruction by 8 weeks of age is required to prevent progression of the disease.

1. **Ultrasonography.** This is used to view the liver parenchyma and to diagnose dilatation of the biliary tree; in extrahepatic obstruction, half of the infants will have dilated proximal ducts within the liver. Choledochal cysts are seen. An inability to identify the gallbladder on ultrasonography may result from obliteration of its lumen in biliary atresia. However, the presence of a gallbladder does not rule out biliary atresia. Because this test is simple and noninvasive and because of the reported coexistence of certain cholestatic diseases, we highly recommend that all infants with cholestasis have this diagnostic test done.

2. **Hepatobiliary imaging.** Contrast agents are taken up by the liver and excreted into the bile. HIDA (hepatobiliary iminodiacetic acid), EHIDA (ethyl hepatobiliary iminodiacetic acid), and PIPIDA (*p*-isopropylacetanilideiminodiacetic acid) are technetium labeled and provide a clear image of the biliary tree after intravenous injection. **Neonatal hepatitis, hyperalimentation**, and **septo-optic dysplasia** are reported causes of absent gastrointestinal contrast excretion and must be considered in the diagnosis of biliary atresia. Administration of phenobarbital, 5 mg/kg/day for 5 days, in conjunction with hepatobiliary scanning may be helpful in distinguishing infants who do not have biliary atresia. Excretion of the contrast medium may improve after phenobarbital treatment.

C. **Other studies**

1. **Percutaneous liver biopsy.** This is a safe procedure in experienced hands. Biopsy findings must be correlated with clinical and laboratory data.

2. **Exploratory laparotomy** with operative cholangiogram is sometimes indicated to correct biliary atresia, especially if the just-mentioned tests are not diagnostic.

V. **Management** (see also Chapter 38)

A. **Medical management**

1. **General plan.** In cholestatic jaundice, promotion of bile flow and prevention of malnutrition, vitamin deficiencies, and bleeding are goals of treatment.

2. **Pharmacologic management.** Phenobarbital and cholestyramine will promote bile flow and decrease serum bilirubin and bile salt levels. Cholestyramine is a nonabsorbable anion exchange resin that irreversibly binds salts in the intestine. This leads to increased fecal excretion of bile salts and increased hepatic synthesis of bile salts from cholesterol, which may lower serum cholesterol levels. **Actigall** (ursodeoxycholic acid) has also been successfully used in conjunction with phenobarbital and cholestyramine.

B. **Dietary management**

1. **Medium-chain triglycerides (MCT).** Long-chain triglycerides are poorly absorbed in the absence of sufficient bile salts. Therefore, infants with cholestasis often require a diet that includes MCTs, which can be absorbed without the action of bile salts. Formulas containing MCTs include Portagen and Pregestimil. Breast-fed cholestatic infants should be given supplemental MCT.

2. **Vitamin supplementation.** Fat malabsorption will also interfere with maintenance of adequate levels of fat-soluble vitamins in these infants. Supplementation of vitamins A, D, E, and K is suggested. Extra vitamin K supplementation may be necessary if a bleeding tendency develops.

3. **Dietary restrictions.** Removal of galactose plus lactose and fructose plus sucrose may prevent the development of cirrhosis and other manifestations of galactosemia and hereditary fructose intolerance, respectively. Dietary restrictions may also be used to treat tyrosinemia but usually are less successful. Most other metabolic causes of cholestatic jaundice have no specific therapy.

C. **Surgical management**

1. **Laparotomy with biopsy.** If extrahepatic biliary obstruction is strongly suspected after completion of an appropriate evaluation, exploratory laparotomy should be performed with operative cholangiography and liver biopsy. Operative examination should be performed by surgeons prepared to proceed with corrective procedures if necessary. Other causes of extrahepatic biliary obstruction that may be diagnosed and treated during exploratory laparotomy include choledochal cyst, spontaneous rupture of the bile duct, lymph node enlargement, tumors, annular pancreas, pancreatic and hepatic cysts, and hemangioendothelioma of the pancreas or liver. Inspissated bile syndrome caused by cystic fibrosis also requires surgical removal of tenacious bile from the bile ducts.

2. **Kasai procedure.** Surgical procedure such as Kasai portoenterostomy should be done to establish biliary drainage in patients diagnosed with biliary atresia. Optimal results are obtained if the procedure is done before 8 weeks of age. If the Kasai procedure is successful, most infants will have deterioration of liver function over time and eventually need a liver transplant. The procedure is used as a bridge to transplantation.

3. **Liver transplantation.** When end-stage liver disease is inevitable, liver transplantation is considered. Biliary atresia is the most common indication for liver transplantation in the United States. Overall, the success of liver transplantation has improved significantly, with reports of 5-year survival rate of >80%. Some centers report a 1-year survival rate close to 90%.

D. **Other treatments**

1. **Infectious diseases.** Some of the infectious causes of hepatitis, such as hepatitis B virus, herpes simplex virus, congenital syphilis, and bacterial infections, have specific therapeutic regimens. Most other forms of infectious hepatitis resolve with no specific therapy.

2. **TPN-induced conjugated hyperbilirubinemia** will usually resolve once TPN is stopped. The decision to continue TPN (with or without trace elements) in an infant with cholestasis must be carefully considered. Resumption of normal enteral feeds is associated with clearing of cholestasis in 4–12 weeks.

REFERENCES

Abramson O, Rosenthal P: Current status of liver transplantation. *Clin Liv Dis* 2000;4:533.

American Academy of Pediatrics: Practice parameter: management of hyperbilirubinemia in the healthy term newborn. *Pediatrics* 1994;94:558.

Bhutani VK, Johnson LH: Jaundice technologies: prediction of hyperbilirubinemia in term and near-term newborns. *J Perinatol* 2001;21:S76.

Cashore WJ: The neurotoxicity of bilirubin. *Clin Perinatol* 1990;17:437.

Connolly AM, Volpe JJ: Clinical features of bilirubin encephalopathy. *Clin Perinatol* 1990;17:371.

Ebbesen A: Transcutaneous bilirubinometry in neonatal intensive care units. *Arch Dis Child* 1996;75:F53.

Funato M et al: Follow-up study of auditory brainstem responses in hyperbilirubinemic newborns treated with exchange transfusions. *Acta Paediatr Japon* 1996;38:17.

Gartner LM, Herschel M: The management of breastfeeding: jaundice and breastfeeding. *Pediatr Clin North Am* 2001;48:389.

Haber BA, Lake AM: Cholestatic jaundice in the newborn. *Clin Perinatol* 1990;17:483.

Halamek L, Stevenson D: Neonatal jaundice and liver disease. In Fanaroff AA, Martin RJ (eds): *Neonatal-Perinatal Medicine—Diseases of the Fetus and Infant,* 6th ed. Mosby, 1997.

Kappas A et al: A single dose of Sn-mesoporphyrin prevents development of severe hyperbilirubinemia in glucose-6-phosphate dehydrogenase-deficient newborns. *Pediatrics* 2001; 108:25.

Kappas A et al: Sn-mesoporphyrin interdiction of severe hyperbilirubinemia in Jehovah's Witness newborns as an alternative to exchange transfusion. *Pediatrics* 2001;108:1374.

Kernicterus in full-term infants—United States 1994–1998. *MMWR Morb Mortal Wkly Rep* 2001;50:491.

Martinez JC et al: Hyperbilirubinemia in the breast-fed newborn: a controlled trial of four interventions. *Pediatrics* 1993;91:470.

Ruchala P et al: Validating assessment of neonatal jaundice with transcutaneous bilirubin measurements. *Neonal Network* 1996;15:33.

Schuman AJ, Karush G: Fiber optic vs. conventional home phototherapy for neonatal hyperbilirubinemia. *Clin Pediatr* 1992;31:345.

Shapiro SM, Nakamura H: Bilirubin and the auditory system. *J Perinatol* 2001;21:S52.

Soorani-Lunsing I et al: Are moderate degrees of hyperbilirubinemia in healthy term neonates really safe for the brain? *Pediatr Res* 2001;50:701.

Stevenson DK et al: Prediction of hyperbilirubinemia in near term and term infants. *Pediatrics* 2001;108:31.

Watchko JF, Oski FA: Kernicterus in preterm newborns: past, present, and future. *Pediatrics* 1992;90:707.

65 Inborn Errors of Metabolism With Acute Neonatal Onset

Inborn errors of metabolism (IEMs) are a group of disorders that are of great importance to physicians treating newborns. The immediate diagnosis and appropriate treatment of these conditions are directly linked to the patient's outcome to the extremes of avoiding death or irreversible brain damage. Nonetheless, many pediatricians feel overwhelmed by the number and complexity of these disorders (Table 65–1) and the interpretation of laboratory tests needed to diagnose these conditions. This may result in a lack of confidence when evaluating infants for IEMs, commonly combined with fears that among the numerous disorders the correct diagnosis may be missed. This chapter, therefore, concentrates on the symptom patterns, laboratory tests and their interpretation, and initial stabilization of the patient rather than details of the specific biochemical and genetic defects and special treatment measures of IEMs. Usually, the patient's ongoing treatment is supervised by a geneticist specially trained in biochemical genetics.

I. **Classification**
   A. **Classification by time of onset.** Because of the nature of this manual, we concentrate here on metabolic disorders with onset in the neonatal period and early infancy. Be aware, however, that onset of a disease in later infancy or even in adolescence and adulthood does not exclude the diagnosis of an IEM. It is also important to realize that, even with comprehensive and well-organized neonatal screening programs, a number of IEMs will clinically present before they are detected by screening tests or before the test result is available to the treating physicians.

   One development has been the use of **tandem mass spectrometry** in newborn screening. Through this technique, multiple metabolic defects, many of which previously required specific targeted testing, can be detected through the analysis of a routine blood spot sample. The feasibility and cost-effectiveness of this technique for routine screening are currently being evaluated by a number of U.S. state and international screening programs, while a few programs have implemented tandem mass spectrometry at this time.

   B. **Classification by clinical presentation.** Subdividing IEMs by clinical presentation may be the most useful approach to aid in establishing the correct diagnosis, and this classification system serves as the basis for the more detailed sections of this chapter. IEMs may present with the following:

   - **Encephalopathy with or without metabolic acidosis.**
   - **Impairment of liver function.**
   - **Impairment of cardiac function.**
   - **Dysmorphic syndromes.**
   - **Less commonly, nonimmune hydrops fetalis.**

   Note that some syndromes with dysmorphic features are now known to be IEMs (eg, Smith-Lemli-Opitz syndrome or Zellweger syndrome [see sections VIII,A and B]). Other classic examples of IEMs are discussed only briefly because they are clinically asymptomatic in the neonatal period (eg, phenylketonuria [PKU]). Note that some **skeletal dysplasias** and disorders affecting bone and cartilage formation (not discussed here) are, strictly speaking, also IEMs (eg, rhizomelic chondrodysplasia punctata and hypophosphatasia).

TABLE 65–1. INBORN ERRORS OF METABOLISM PRESENTING IN THE NEONATAL PERIOD AND INFANCY

Disorders of carbohydrate metabolism
Galactosemia
Fructose-1,6-bisphosphatase deficiency
Glycogen storage disease (types IA, IB, II, III, and IV)
Hereditary fructose intolerance

Disorders of amino acid metabolism
Maple syrup urine disease
Nonketotic hyperglycinemia
Hereditary tyrosinemia
Pyroglutamic acidemia (5-oxoprolinuria)
Hyperornithinemia-hyperammonemia-homocitrullinemia syndrome
Lysinuric protein intolerance
Methylene tetrahydrofolate reductase deficiency
Sulfite oxidase deficiency

Disorders of organic acid metabolism
Methylmalonic acidemia
Propionic acidemia
Isovaleric acidemia
Multiple carboxylase deficiency
Glutaric acidemia type II (multiple acyl-CoA dehydrogenase deficiencies)
HMG-CoA lyase deficiency
3-Methylcrotonoyl-CoA carboxylase deficiency
3-Hydroxyisobutyric aciduria

Disorders of pyruvate metabolism and the electron transport chain
Pyruvate carboxylase deficiency
Pyruvate dehydrogenase deficiency
Electron transport chain defects

Disorders of the urea cycle
Ornithine-transcarbamylase deficiency
Carbamyl phosphate synthetase deficiency
Transient hyperammonemia of the neonate (unclear cause)
Argininosuccinate synthetase deficiency (citrullinemia)
Argininosuccinate lyase deficiency
Arginase deficiency
N-Acetylglutamate synthetase deficiency

Lysosomal storage disorders
GM_1 gangliosidosis type I (β-galactosidase deficiency)
Gaucher's disease (glucocerebrosidase deficiency)
Niemann-Pick disease types A and B (sphingomyelinase deficiency)
Wolman's disease (acid lipase deficiency)
Mucopolysaccharidosis type VII (β-glucuronidase deficiency)
I-cell disease (mucolipidosis type II)
Sialidosis type II (neuraminidase deficiency)
Fucosidosis

Peroxisomal disorders
Zellweger syndrome
Neonatal adrenoleukodystrophy
Single enzyme defects of the peroxisomal β-oxidation
Rhizomelic chondrodysplasia punctata
Infantile Refsum's disease

Miscellaneous disorders
Adrenogenital syndrome (21-hydroxylase and other deficiencies)
Disorders of bilirubin metabolism (Crigler-Najjar syndrome and others)
Pyridoxine-dependent seizures
α_1-Antitrypsin deficiency
Fatty acid oxidation disorders (short, medium, and long chain)
Cholesterol biosynthesis defects (Smith-Lemli-Opitz syndrome)
Disorders of protein glycosylation (carbohydrate-deficient glycoprotein syndromes)
Neonatal hemochromatosis

HMG, 3-hydroxy-3-methylglutaryl; CoA, coenzyme A.

C. **Classification according to the biochemical basis of the disease.** A concept that divides IEMs according to their biochemical characteristics helps in understanding the pathogenesis of symptoms and different approaches to treatment.

II. **Incidence.** By some estimates, IEMs may account for as much as 20% of disease among full-term infants not known to have been born at risk. Cumulatively, an IEM may be present in >1 in 500 live births.

III. **Pathophysiology.** Metabolic processes are catalyzed by genetically encoded enzyme proteins. When these enzymes are lacking or deficient in function, **substrates accumulate** and may be converted to products not usually present. In addition, end products of the normal pathway will be deficient. Symptoms may result from an increased level of the normal substrate (eg, in urea cycle disorders, the substrate ammonia is toxic and leads to cerebral edema, central nervous system [CNS] dysfunction, and eventually death). Additionally, a **lack of normal end products** of metabolism can lead to symptoms (eg, lack of cortisol in 21-hydroxylase deficiency [see Chapter 60]). The **alternative products may interfere with normal metabolic processes** (eg, accumulated propionyl-CoA may participate in reactions normally using acetyl-CoA in propionic acidemia). Finally, an **inability to degrade end products** of a metabolic pathway may lead to symptoms (eg, myocardial dysfunction in **glycogen storage disease** type II or hepatomegaly in glycogen storage disease type I). The time of clinical presentation often relates to the question of whether the symptoms are caused by metabolites that are able to diffuse prenatally across the placenta. These are usually of low molecular weight and, therefore, prenatally removed from the fetus and cleared by the maternal metabolism.

IV. **General clinical presentation, signs, and symptoms.** Although there are several specific situations, listed next, in which an IEM must be considered, the safest guideline for clinical practice is that **an IEM should be considered in any sick newborn.** The newborn has a "limited repertoire" of symptoms that are often nonspecific. The differential diagnosis of symptoms such as **poor feeding, lethargy, hypotonia, vomiting, hypothermia, seizures, and disturbances of breathing** is extensive. Although the diagnosis of sepsis is often at the top of the differential diagnosis list, it is important for a timely diagnosis and in the best interest of the patient to evaluate for other causes, including IEMs, at the same time that laboratory investigations are initiated to rule out sepsis. This can be accomplished with a relatively small number of laboratory tests readily available in most hospitals, as discussed in the following sections.

A high index of suspicion for an IEM must be maintained under the following circumstances:

A. A history of **unexplained neonatal deaths in the family** (prior siblings or male infants on the mother's side of the family).

B. Infants who are the **offspring of consanguineous matings** (because of the higher incidence of autosomal recessive conditions; autosomal recessive inheritance is common among IEMs).

C. **Onset of signs and symptoms after a period of good health** that may be as short as hours.

D. It is not uncommon for infants with an IEM to have experienced an **uneventful perinatal and newborn course** before the manifestation of symptoms.

E. Symptoms may also be related to the introduction and progression of **enteral feedings.**

F. **Failure of usual therapies** to alleviate the symptoms or **inability to prove a suggested diagnosis** such as sepsis, CNS hemorrhage, or other congenital or acquired conditions.

G. **Progression of symptoms.**

H. Although patients with an IEM might, for reasons unrelated to the IEM, be born prematurely, they are **typically full-term** infants. An exception is the diagnosis of transient hyperammonemia of the neonate, which is typically made in preterm infants. Although this condition is discussed in this chapter, it should be pointed out that the exact cause of the hyperammonemia in these patients remains unclear and may well be related to prematurity rather than being a typical IEM.

Signs and symptoms seen in different IEMs are summarized in Table 65–2. Table 65–3 lists some of the conditions with which infants with IEM have been misdiagnosed. Keep in mind that **symptoms may overlap** with frequent neonatal conditions; for example, a child with an IEM may have transient tachypnea of the neonate or be at high risk for sepsis for unrelated reasons! In rare exceptions, two conditions may be present with a causative relationship. A typical example is the frequently quoted but still unexplained increased incidence of *Escherichia coli* sepsis in infants with galactosemia.

To guide the clinician in the diagnostic workup, signs and symptoms are discussed further for four different clinical presentations. Flow diagrams in Figures 65–1 and 65–2 are also designed to assist in the diagnostic workup. Details regarding the different laboratory tests are outlined in section XI.

V. **Inborn errors presenting with encephalopathy.** Encephalopathies associated with IEMs are clinically often indistinguishable from those caused by a hypoxic-ischemic insult or other CNS insult (hemorrhage or infectious disease). **Abnormal tone** (hypotonia as well as hypertonia may be of central origin) and **abnormal movements and seizures** clearly indicate CNS involvement. Clinically, seizures may present as lip smacking, tongue thrusting, bicycling movements of the lower extremities, opisthotonos, tremors, or generalized tonic-clonic movements. The **electroencephalographic changes** may be as specific as the clinical presentation with diffuse burst suppression pattern. Once the encephalopathy is diagnosed, careful **evaluation of the acid-base status** is mandatory.

- A group of IEMs present with usually severe metabolic acidosis.
- When interpreting the venous or arterial blood gas of a newborn, the **alterations in respiratory status** that are so frequent in this patient group must be taken into careful consideration. An isolated respiratory acidosis is likely pulmonary, and a mixed acidosis, especially shortly after delivery, may be related to perinatal events.
- The findings of a **severe and prolonged metabolic acidosis** or **respiratory alkalosis,** on the other hand, must be interpreted while asking the following question: Is there any diagnosis other than an IEM that would be accompanied by a severe acidosis that is specific or proven (eg, sepsis with bacteremia or hypovolemic shock)? If not, it is mandatory to evaluate whether **acidic metabolites** (eg, the excessive production of lactic acid) could be the cause of the imbalance. When considering compensatory mechanisms (eg, respiratory correction of a metabolic acidosis), remember that the resulting blood gas should reflect a mixed acid-base status.
- An **isolated respiratory alkalosis** is usually not explained by a pulmonary disease. A more likely mechanism is a central disturbance of the respiratory pattern, and **hyperammonemia** should be ruled out in this situation. Ammonia directly stimulates the respiratory center, resulting in primary hyperventilation, which in turn leads to respiratory alkalosis.

In addition to an arterial or venous blood gas, the following tests (for details, see section XI) should be done as part of the **acute evaluation** of patients with encephalopathy: (1) serum electrolytes with calculation of the anion gap, (2) ammonia level, and (3) initiate urine collection and store urine refrigerated or, ideally, frozen.

Other causes of encephalopathy should be assessed by appropriate studies (eg, imaging studies, sepsis workup, or lumbar puncture) as indicated and outlined in other sections of this manual. If cerebrospinal fluid (CSF) is obtained, it is wise to freeze a sample for possible future testing (eg, ~1–2 mL for CSF amino acids to rule out nonketotic hyperglycinemia [NKH]). If an IEM remains a diagnostic possibility after the acute evaluation, the analysis of plasma amino acids and urine organic acids should be arranged.

TABLE 65-2. SIGNS AND SYMPTOM COMPLEXES SUGGESTING CLASSES OF METABOLIC DISORDERS

Neurologic (hypotonia, lethargy, poor sucking, seizures, coma)
Glycogen storage disease, galactosemia, organic acidemias, hereditary fructose intolerance, maple syrup urine disease, urea cycle disorders, hyperglycinemia, pyridoxine dependency, peroxisomal disorders, carbohydrate-deficient glycoprotein syndromes

Hepatomegaly
Lysosomal storage diseases, galactosemia, hereditary fructose intolerance, glycogen storage disease, tyrosinemia, α_1-antitrypsin deficiency, Gaucher's disease, Niemann-Pick disease, Wolman's disease, fatty acid oxidation defects

Hyperbilirubinemia
Galactosemia, hereditary fructose intolerance, tyrosinemia, α_1-antitrypsin deficiency, Crigler-Najjar syndrome, and other disorders of bilirubin metabolism

Nonimmune hydrops
Gaucher's disease, Niemann-Pick disease, GM_1 gangliosidosis, carbohydrate-deficient glycoprotein syndromes

Cardiomegaly
Glycogen storage disease type II, fatty acid oxidation defects

Macroglossia
GM_1 gangliosidosis, glycogen storage disease type II

Abnormal odor
Maple syrup urine disease (odor of maple syrup or burnt sugar)
Isovaleric acidemia, glutaric acidemia (odor of sweaty feet)
HMG-CoA lyase deficiency (odor of cat urine)

Abnormal hair
Argininosuccinic acidemia, lysinuric protein intolerance, Menkes' kinky hair syndrome

Hypoglycemia
Galactosemia, hereditary fructose intolerance, tyrosinemia, maple syrup urine disease, glycogen storage disease, methylmalonic acidemia, propionic acidemia, fatty acid oxidation defects

Ketosis
Organic acidemias, tyrosinemia, methylmalonic acidemia, maple syrup urine disease

Metabolic acidosis
Galactosemia, hereditary fructose intolerance, maple syrup urine disease, glycogen storage disease, organic acidemias

Hyperammonemia
Urea cycle defects, transient hyperammonemia of the neonate, organic acidurias, HMG-CoA lyase deficiency, fatty acid oxidation disorders

Neutropenia
Organic acidemias, especially methylmalonic acidemia and propionic acidemia; nonketotic hyperglycinemia, carbamyl phosphate synthetase deficiency

Thrombocytopenia
Organic acidemias, lysinuric protein intolerance

Dysmorphic features
Glutaric aciduria type II, 3-hydroxyisobutyric aciduria, Smith-Lemli-Opitz syndrome, peroxisomal disorders, carbohydrate-deficient glycoprotein syndromes

Renal cysts
Glutaric aciduria type II, peroxisomal disorders

Abnormalities of the eye (eg; glaucoma, retinopathy)
Galactosemia, lysosomal storage disorders, peroxisomal disorders

HMG, 3-hydroxy-3-methylglutaryl; CoA, coenzyme A.

TABLE 65-3. MISDIAGNOSES OF METABOLIC DISEASE IN THE NEWBORN INFANT

Sepsis (bacterial or viral)
Asphyxia
Gastrointestinal tract obstruction
Hepatic failure, hepatitis
Central nervous system catastrophe
Persistent pulmonary hypertension
Myocardiopathy
Neuromuscular disorder

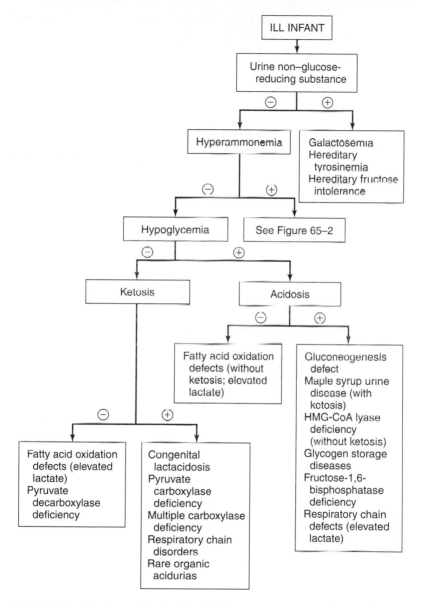

FIGURE 65–1. Algorithm for the diagnosis of metabolic disorders of acute onset (guideline only; for details, see text and references).

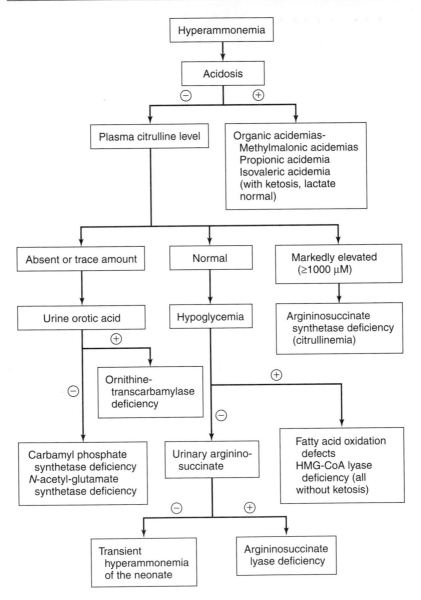

FIGURE 65–2. Algorithm for the differential diagnosis of hyperammonemia (guideline only; for details, see text and references).

Although the **differential diagnosis** of IEMs associated with encephalopathy is extensive, the following conditions are discussed in more detail because of either their frequency or clinical significance. (Items A–D, below, are typically without severe metabolic acidosis at presentation; items E and F are typically associated with a severe metabolic acidosis.)

A. **Urea cycle defects** (and transient hyperammonemia of the neonate). **Hyperammonemia** (not caused by liver failure) in a neonate leaves **three major diagnostic possibilities.**

- A primary defect of one of the enzymes of the urea cycle (that degrades ammonia produced in the metabolism of amino acids).
- An organic acidemia as an underlying cause with secondary impairment of the urea cycle (see section V,E).
- **Transient hyperammonemia of the neonate (THAN),** a condition usually seen in premature infants.

Information regarding the diagnostic workup of patients with hyperammonemia is outlined in Figure 65–2. Quantitative measurement of plasma amino acids and orotic acid is necessary to establish the exact diagnosis. Urine organic acids should also be examined. Initial treatment is similar, independent of the final diagnosis (see section XII,A). Immediate transfer to a facility able to perform hemodialysis is strongly advised once hyperammonemia is detected. The use of medication such as sodium phenylacetate and butyrate should be supervised by a biochemical geneticist. The most common urea cycle defect is **ornithine-transcarbamylase deficiency (OTC),** which is transmitted in an X-linked recessive fashion. Newborn patients are, therefore, usually male. **Female heterozygotes** can be symptomatic, depending on the X-chromosome inactivation pattern in the liver, but females usually present later in life. It is important to note that a mother heterozygous for OTC deficiency may develop symptoms (hyperammonemia) at the time of delivery because of the metabolic stresses of labor and delivery. The other urea cycle defects are inherited in an autosomal recessive fashion, **carbamyl phosphate synthetase deficiency** being the second most common. In some defects (eg, argininosuccinate lyase deficiency), substitution of **arginine** (intravenous arginine hydrochloride) may alleviate symptoms; arginine becomes secondarily deficient as a metabolite of the cycle located after the deficient reaction. Long-term **protein restriction** is necessary (see section XII,B,1). Acute treatment of **THAN** is similar to that of inborn errors of the urea cycle, but deficiency of the metabolic pathway is temporary and normal protein intake is tolerated later in life. The **outcome** (especially in regard to CNS damage) is much more favorable for THAN compared with the inherited defects, even if the diagnosis is made early and treatment is initiated in a timely fashion.

B. **Maple syrup urine disease (MSUD)**
1. Accumulation of **branched-chain amino acids (leucine, isoleucine, and valine)** is secondary to a defect in the decarboxylase involved in the catabolism of these amino acids. 2-Keto metabolites of the three amino acids also accumulate. Leucine is the amino acid that has been implied to be neurotoxic.
2. Presentation is commonly after the second week of life but may be as early as at 24 h of age and, therefore, may precede **neonatal screening** test results. Typical symptoms are feeding intolerance, lethargy, signs of encephalopathy such as hypotonia or posturing, abnormal movements, or frank seizures (late in the course). **Typical odor** (maple syrup or "burnt sugar") may not be prominent, and metabolic acidosis is a late presentation of untreated MSUD.
3. Diagnosis is by quantitative amino acid analysis (elevated leucine, isoleucine, valine, and glycine) and detection of 2-keto metabolites in urine organic acid analysis. The 2,4-dinitrophenylhydrazine (DNPH) test may be available (see Table 65–5).
4. **Concept of treatment.** Restrict all protein acutely while providing high amounts of glucose and fluid (see section XII,A). Later, provide formula low in leucine, valine, and isoleucine with restriction of natural protein. Use dialysis as acute therapy if severe encephalopathy has

developed. Some patients may show response to thiamine (see section XII,B,3).
C. **Nonketotic hyperglycinemia**
1. A typical presentation for NKH is a patient suffering from a severe encephalopathy that is rapidly progressing and eventually results in respiratory arrest, but standard evaluation for IEMs and other causes of this presentation does not reveal any abnormalities (no acidosis, hypoglycemia, or hyperammonemia and no other organ system affected).
2. Hyperglycinemia in plasma is typical but may not be pronounced in young infants because of decreased renal reabsorption of this amino acid. In addition, other IEMs also result in increased blood glycine levels, such as MSUD (which is sometimes referred to as ketotic hyperglycinemia). This diagnostic situation is one of the few indications for urine amino acids to detect the high renal glycine excretion.
3. A more specific diagnostic test is to determine the CSF–plasma glycine ratio, because an elevation of glycine in the CSF is specific for NKH. A CSF–blood glycine ratio of >0.08 is considered abnormal.
4. Treatment options remain limited at this point. Restoration of normal glycine levels in blood can be achieved (through hydration or the use of sodium benzoate [see section XII,A,5]), but the glycine accumulation in CSF remains unaffected. Several medications (dextromethorphan, diazepam, and even strychnine) have been used to try to affect the CNS symptomatology but have achieved only limited success.
5. Patients may survive, because the respiratory depression has the potential to improve, but severe brain damage is the rule. A few patients with a transient form of NKH have been reported.
D. **Peroxisomal disorders**
1. Multiple peroxisomal disorders (typically the defects of peroxisome biogenesis [eg, Zellweger syndrome and neonatal adrenoleukodystrophy] and some of the peroxisomal single enzyme defects [eg, multifunctional enzyme deficiency]) present with encephalopathy in the neonatal period. Patients are extremely floppy as a result of severe central hypotonia and develop seizures (usually within the first week of life). Hepatomegaly, renal and hepatic cysts, or retinal abnormalities may also be found.
2. Most peroxisomal defects can be detected by analysis of very long-chain fatty acids (VLCFAs) (with carbon chains of 24 and more) in plasma. To fully exclude a peroxisomal defect, additional studies such as plasmalogen levels in red blood cells, phytanic acid, and others (see section XI,C,7) are necessary.
E. **Organic aciduria/acidemias (OAs).** This group of IEMs is complex, and many clinicians feel overwhelmed by the biochemical details regarding these conditions. Relevant clinical information is as follows:
1. Many OAs present later in infancy. Three conditions commonly present in the neonatal period and are clinically nearly indistinguishable: **methylmalonic acidemia, propionic acidemia,** and **isovaleric acidemia.** Diagnostic landmarks are encephalopathy with severe acidosis, hyperammonemia, and seizures; an unusual odor (most noticeable in urine [see Table 65–2]) may be noted, and neutropenia may occur. More OAs are listed in Table 65–1.
2. Analysis of plasma amino acids and urine organic acids is the appropriate diagnostic evaluation for OAs. Interpretation of these tests by an experienced biochemical geneticist familiar with the clinical presentation of the patient is strongly recommended.
3. If this diagnosis is suspected, the following treatment should be initiated: hydration and glucose infusion (both at least 1½ times the maintenance level), treatment of hyperammonemia (see section XII,A), and careful correction of metabolic acidosis with bicarbonate while ensuring appropriate ventilation. Involvement of a geneticist in the diagnostic workup and treatment is strongly recommended.

  4. Some OAs may partially respond to vitamins (see section XII,B,3).
F. Congenital lactic acidosis (LA)
  1. LA may be difficult to differentiate clinically from hypoxic-ischemic encephalopathy, sepsis, and other conditions that result in metabolic acidosis, poor perfusion, and shock. Clinical hints that the acidosis may be due to LA are severity of the acidosis, **growth retardation** resulting in birth of a small for gestational age infant, some mild **dysmorphic features,** and anatomic abnormalities of the brain. **Multiorgan disease** not explained by other causes (eg, hypertrophic cardiomyopathy or cataracts) may occur.
  2. Once an increase of lactic acid is found, determination of the **lactate–pyruvate ratio** will further guide the diagnostic process (see section XI,C,1). The common biochemical concept of metabolic disorders leading to LA is a deficiency to provide energy through aerobic metabolism, which depends on conversion of pyruvate to metabolites of the citrate cycle and an intact mitochondrial respiratory chain.
  3. Some possible causes of LA in a neonate are **pyruvate dehydrogenase (PDH) defect, pyruvate carboxylase defect,** and **mitochondrial electron transport chain defects** (most common are defects of complex I or IV).
  4. Be aware that PDH deficiency is one of the rare exceptions to the treatment approach to provide high levels of glucose to the patient; the LA may worsen.
  5. Hypoglycemia with LA may be a presentation of a glycogen storage disease (see section VI,F).
G. Other rare but significant IEMs with encephalopathy include the following:
  I. **Fatty acid oxidation disorders with dicarboxylic aciduria.** Although the most common fatty acid oxidation defect (medium-chain acyl-CoA dehydrogenase deficiency [MCAD]) does rarely cause illness in a neonate, SCAD or LCAD (short- and long-chain acyl-CoA dehydrogenase deficiencies, respectively) may present in the neonatal period (see section VII,A).
  2. Multiple carboxylase deficiency.
  3. Holocarboxylase synthetase deficiency.
  4. Glutaric acidemia type II (a defect of the electron transport flavoprotein or its dehydrogenase).
  5. Pyroglutamic acidemia (5-oxoprolinuria, a defect in glutathione synthetase).
  6. Molybdenum cofactor deficiency (xanthine deficiency or sulfite oxidase deficiency). One diagnostic clue to xanthine oxidase deficiency may be a significantly low plasma uric acid level. A commercial test is available to determine urine sulfite excretion in urine.
  7. HMG-CoA lyase deficiency.
  8. Pyridoxine-dependent seizures are a rare condition for which treatment is available. Patients present with seizures in the neonatal period or in early infancy that are refractory to treatment with anticonvulsants but show dramatic improvement with administration of vitamin B_6 (100 mg of pyridoxine intravenously).
  9. Carbohydrate-deficient glycoprotein syndromes may also present with acute encephalopathy, seizures, and stroke-like episodes. Patients are usually hypotonic. **Cerebellar atrophy** appears to be common. Psychomotor development is delayed later in life and ataxia, dyskinesia, and muscle weakness become prominent. **Severe feeding problems and failure to thrive** are typical; intractable diarrhea in a neonate has been reported. **Unusual fat pads in the buttock area and inverted nipples** are believed to be quite characteristic findings.
    These autosomal recessive conditions are characterized by **defects in the glycosylation of proteins** (see section XI,C,9 for diagnostic test-

ing). They are multisystem disorders. Other than neurologic involvement, hepatic dysfunction with abnormal liver enzymes, pericardial effusions, nephrotic syndrome, nonimmune hydrops, and facial dysmorphic features (broad nasal bridge, prominent jaw and forehead, large ears, strabismus) have been described in infants.

VI. **Inborn errors presenting with liver disease.** Several IEMs result in liver disease that may present in the neonatal period with the following:

- Liver enlargement.
- Jaundice.
- Hepatocellular dysfunction.
- Hypoglycemia.

The initial evaluation in these patients consists of routine tests (eg, bilirubin levels, glucose measurement, liver function tests, and imaging studies). Considering that the liver is the main organ of amino acid metabolism, it becomes evident that analysis of plasma amino acid patterns may give additional information regarding liver function; this is a more elaborate and expensive test, however. Many synthetic functions of the liver can be partially evaluated by routine tests such as glucose, cholesterol, total protein, and albumin levels. The following conditions are discussed in more detail because of either their frequency or clinical significance.

A. **Galactosemia** will not present in an affected newborn until the patient is receiving galactose. Breast milk and most formulas contain **lactose** (a disaccharide of glucose and galactose); most soy formulas do not. Typical symptoms are **hyperbilirubinemia** (which may be unconjugated initially but later becomes mainly conjugated). Then signs of **liver dysfunction** (which may include **coagulopathy, hypoglycemia, hypoalbuminemia, and ascites**) and **hepatomegaly** develop. **Cataracts** may be diagnosed as early as the disease manifests in the neonatal period. If undetected, symptoms may proceed to include encephalopathy with cerebral edema, metabolic acidosis (hyperchloremia and hypophosphatemia), and renal dysfunction. Patients with galactosemia have an increased risk for *E. coli* **sepsis** (reasons remain unclear). **Testing urine** for reducing substances is an initial screening test (see section XI,B,7). If galactose has been discontinued, reducing substance testing is insufficient and blood tests must be used to make the diagnosis. Galactosemia is due to a defect in either **galactose-1-phosphate uridyltransferase (GALT)** (classic galactosemia) or UDP galactose 4-epimerase (rare variant); red blood cells are used to measure GALT activity, or accumulation of galactose-1-phosphate is measured. Treatment consists of galactose restriction in the diet; the diet is relatively strict and difficult to follow. Even if compliance with the diet is good, many patients show **developmental delays** and females suffer **ovarian failure** later in life.

B. **Hepatorenal tyrosinemia.** Tyrosinemia type I, or hepatorenal tyrosinemia, usually presents in infancy but has been described in neonates who developed **severe liver dysfunction,** including hyperbilirubinemia, hypoglycemia, hyperammonemia, coagulopathy, hypoalbuminemia with ascites, and anasarca. This IEM also causes renal disease with mainly tubular dysfunction (amino aciduria or glucosuria) and results in hypophosphatemia and hyperchloremic metabolic acidosis. **Cardiomyopathy** can also develop, so that the clinical presentation may overlap with disorders of fatty acid metabolism. Although altered tyrosine levels are also found with liver dysfunction as a result of other causes, the presence of **succinylacetone** in urine is a finding specific for tyrosinemia (see section XI,C,4). Plasma cysteine might be low; plasma alpha-fetoprotein may be markedly increased. The only long-term treatment option is liver transplantation.

C. **α_1-Antitrypsin deficiency (AATD).** This IEM presents as **hyperbilirubinemia,** which is usually prolonged and conjugated (with signs of cholestasis) but may resolve spontaneously within the first 6 months of life. These children may then not present again clinically until **liver cirrhosis** with portal hypertension has developed. An adult manifestation of AATD is the development of **emphysema** as early as in the third or fourth decade of life, a disease process much accelerated by smoking. The cause of AATD is a mutation in the *AATD* gene (designated as **Z mutation**), which, in homozygous carriers, results in deficiency of AATD, which is an inhibitor of an elastase, a degrading enzyme of neutrophils. The defect in this enzyme inhibition results in destruction of pulmonary or hepatic tissue. Diagnosis is confirmed by **genotyping** and is routinely available in most hospitals because of the frequency with which the test is performed in the workup of adults with emphysema. Although the symptoms during early life may resolve spontaneously and not all patients develop liver and lung manifestations, the neonatologist or pediatrician has the opportunity to ensure a diagnosis early in life, possibly enabling the patient to prevent serious disease later through behavior modification.

D. **Inborn errors of bilirubin metabolism.** Inherited defects in the metabolism of bilirubin include defects in conjugation (**Crigler-Najjar syndrome**) and uptake and excretion of bilirubin (**Dubin-Johnson and Rotor's syndromes**). These conditions result in either indirect or direct hyperbilirubinemia and are discussed in more detail in Chapter 64.

E. **Fatty acid oxidation (FAO) disorders** may present with a combination of encephalopathy and cardiac and liver dysfunction. These conditions are discussed in more detail in section VII,A. The liver dysfunction may be mild with less severe hypoalbuminemia and coagulopathy than in other IEMs. The clinical presentation is dominated by severe and generalized hypotonia and cardiomyopathy. Succinylacetone will be negative, whereas tyrosine metabolites may be present in urine organic acids. Analysis of an **acetyl carnitine profile** is helpful in making the diagnosis (see section XI,C,5).

F. **Glycogen storage disease type I (von Gierke's disease).** The clinical presentation of glycogen storage disorders in the newborn period may be limited to **hypoglycemia,** which is usually severe and may be accompanied by LA. In von Gierke's disease, the hypoglycemia is unresponsive to glucagon injection. Liver enlargement and dysfunction usually develop shortly thereafter (as soon as within 1–2 weeks). Glycogen storage disorders are diagnosed by liver biopsy with enzyme analysis.

G. **Peroxisomal disorders.** Patients with disorders of peroxisomal biogenesis such as Zellweger syndrome and neonatal adrenoleukodystrophy develop hepatomegaly early in life that usually progresses to fibrosis and cirrhosis. The clinical presentation is usually dominated by central hypotonia and seizures (see section V,D).

H. **Others.** Other inherited conditions that may present with hepatocellular dysfunction, sometimes as early as in the neonatal period, are as follows:
1. **Neonatal hemochromatosis.**
2. **Hereditary fructose intolerance.**
3. **Defects in carnitine metabolism.**
4. **Other glycogen storage diseases.**
5. **Lysosomal storage disorders** (Niemann-Pick disease may present with neonatal hepatitis).
6. **Carbohydrate-deficient glycoprotein syndromes** (see section V,G,9).

VII. **Inborn errors presenting with impairment of cardiac function**
A. **FAO disorders** are subdivided according to the length of the carbon chain of the fatty acids that accumulate: SCAD, MCAD, and LCAD acyl-CoA deficiency. All of these except MCAD are associated with severe **cardiomyopathy** usually resulting in cardiac failure. In addition to cardiomyopathy, patients may also suffer from **encephalopathy** and **myopathy; hepatomegaly** also occurs, and with low glucose intake or intercurrent illnesses patients characteristically develop **hypoketotic hypoglycemia.** Acetyl carnitine profile analysis by mass spectrometry helps to establish the diagnosis, which is

then confirmed by enzyme assays in cultured fibroblasts. Treatment of FAO disorders consists of avoidance of prolonged periods without carbohydrate intake. Secondary **carnitine deficiency** may develop, and oral carnitine may be indicated. Although medium-chain triglycerides are contraindicated in MCAD, they may be a good source of energy in the other conditions.
  B. **Pompe's disease.** The cardiomyopathy of Pompe's disease may (although not typically) present as early as in the neonatal period. Of diagnostic help are **electrocardiographic changes,** some of which are fairly characteristic: shortening of the PR interval, marked left-axis deviation, T-wave inversion, and enlarged QRS complexes. The diagnosis is confirmed by measurement of the deficient enzyme (α-glucosidase or acid maltase) in leukocytes or cultured fibroblasts.
  C. **Hepatorenal tyrosinemia.** Type I tyrosinemia may present with cardiomyopathy in addition to liver and renal tubular dysfunction (see section VI,B).
  D. **Carbohydrate-deficient glycoprotein syndromes** (see section V,G,9). Pericardial effusions have been observed in affected patients.
VIII. **Inborn errors presenting as dysmorphic syndromes.** Several dysmorphic syndromes are now known to be due to an underlying metabolic defect. With the ongoing progress in developmental biology, cell biology, and human genetics, it is likely that more and more conditions initially described as syndromes will eventually be found to be IEMs or genetic conditions secondary to other molecular mechanisms. Examples of disorders in this category include the following:
  A. **Smith-Lemli-Opitz syndrome.** The main clinical signs of this relatively common syndrome, with an estimated frequency of 1 in 20,000, are as follows:

  • **Growth deficiency** (usually postnatal) and microcephaly.
  • **Dysmorphic features,** including a high forehead, ptosis, epicanthal folds, strabismus, rotated and low-set ears, a nose with a wide tip, and micrognathia.
  • **Hypospadias** in males.
  • **Syndactyly** of the second and third toes.

  Other signs are cataracts and hypotonia. Patients show significant psychomotor retardation. The metabolic basis of Smith-Lemli-Opitz syndrome is a defect in 7-dehydrocholesterol dehydrogenase, resulting in an accumulation of 7-dehydrocholesterol and typically low cholesterol levels in plasma. Treatment trials with cholesterol substitution are currently being performed.
  B. **Zellweger syndrome and other peroxisomal disorders.** Although Zellweger syndrome and **neonatal adrenoleukodystrophy** were initially described based on clinical characteristics, they are now known to be disorders of peroxisome biogenesis, as is **infantile Refsum's disease.** These three conditions are believed to be clinically different phenotypes of the same underlying defect, all due to defects in peroxisomal biogenesis and function (hence the use of the term *Zellweger spectrum*); typical findings are as follows:

  • **Dysmorphic features,** including a high forehead, a wide and flat nasal bridge, epicanthal folds, and dysplastic ears; the fontanelles are wide open.
  • Severe **hypotonia, seizures,** and lack of psychomotor development.
  • **Hepatomegaly** with fibrosis.
  • **Ocular abnormalities** (corneal clouding, cataract, and retinal changes).
  • **Punctate calcifications** of the skeleton.
  • Small **renal cortical cysts.**

  The diagnosis is established by measurement of VLCFAs and other biochemical parameters affected by peroxisomal dysfunction (see section XI,C,8).
  Patients with some classic IEMs may also have (usually mild) dysmorphic features, as discussed next.

C. **Pyruvate dehydrogenase (PDH) deficiency.** Patients with congenital LA (see section V,F) resulting from PDH deficiency often display dysmorphic features, including a high and prominent forehead, a widened nasal bridge, a small anteverted nose, and dysmorphic and enlarged ears.

D. **Carbohydrate-deficient glycoprotein syndromes** (see section V,G,9). Dysmorphic features include broad nasal bridge, prominent jaw and forehead, large ears, and strabismus. **Unusual fat pads in the buttock area and inverted** nipples are believed to be quite characteristic findings.

IX. **Nonimmune hydrops in IEMs.** Although the differential diagnosis of nonimmune hydrops is extensive and this condition is discussed in other sections of this manual, two groups of inherited disorders that can present with hydrops are briefly mentioned here.

A. **In the inherited hematologic conditions** (eg, glucose-6-phosphate dehydrogenase deficiency and pyruvate kinase deficiency), the hydrops is related to anemia and heart failure.

B. The mechanism by which **lysosomal storage disorders** result in hydrops is unclear. Cases of hydrops have been reported in **GM₁ gangliosidosis, Gaucher's disease, Niemann-Pick disease,** and other genetic conditions with disturbed lysosomal function. If any of these conditions are considered, the presence of **hepatomegaly, dysostosis multiplex,** and abnormal **vacuolated mononuclear cells** in the peripheral blood smear warrant the involvement of a geneticist and consequent specific enzymatic assays using white blood cells or fibroblasts.

C. **Carbohydrate-deficient glycoprotein syndromes** (see section V,G,9).

X. **Phenylketonuria.** Although PKU is an IEM of foremost interest because of its frequency and well-established treatment that prevents the extreme mental retardation characteristic of untreated PKU, it is not discussed in detail here because **untreated PKU does not cause symptoms in the neonate.** Even though the patient is clinically well, **irreversible brain damage** occurs as a result of accumulating phenylalanine and its metabolites. Patients, therefore, benefit enormously from detection by neonatal screening for PKU.

A. If an **abnormal neonatal screening** for PKU is reported, formula or breast milk must be discontinued and hydration provided (short-term enteral feedings with electrolyte solutions are feasible; intravenous therapy is usually not mandated). The patient should immediately (within hours) be referred to a geneticist for further evaluation (including differentiation between classic PKU and hyperphenylalaninemia), initiation of diet, and family education, training, and counseling.

B. Occasionally, the clinician will take care of a **child of a mother with PKU;** considering that this child is an obligate heterozygote for PKU combined with the high frequency of the PKU allele in the general population (1 in 20), this child has a 1 in 80 risk of being affected, and measurement of phenylalanine after enteral feedings are established is mandatory. Although institutional practices vary, many geneticists recommend early quantitative amino acid analysis rather than routine newborn screening in this scenario. Newborns of affected mothers with insufficient treatment manifest with **microcephaly, congenital heart disease,** and **mental deficiencies** (even if the infant is not homozygous for PKU).

XI. **Diagnostic tests**

A. **Prenatal.** The ability to diagnose IEMs prenatally has increased in recent years. Biochemical methods (eg, detection of metabolites in amniotic fluid and enzyme assays using cultured cells) as well as DNA analysis (mutation detection) are used. Diagnostic procedures routinely available are **chorionic villus sampling** and **amniocentesis.** In some centers, analysis of **fetal cells in maternal circulation** or **testing of preimplantation embryos** may also be offered. In some cases, in utero treatment can be achieved (eg, dietary control in maternal PKU or experimental therapies such as fetal stem cell treatment). Otherwise, appropriate therapies can begin quickly subsequent to delivery of the infant. Prenatal counseling is essential so that parents are well informed and able to make an educated decision regarding continuation of the pregnancy.

B. Postnatal tests routinely available. Although some of these laboratory tests and their significance in aiding the diagnostic process have already been discussed, details regarding the specifics of these tests and their interpretations are briefly outlined here. Please refer also to Tables 65–4 through 65–6.

1. **Blood cell count with differential, hemoglobin, and platelets.** Be aware that neutropenia (especially when accompanied by metabolic acidosis) not only is typically found in sepsis and poor perfusion but may be indicative of an organic acidopathy (most common are propionic acidemia, methylmalonic acidemia, and isovaleric acidemia). These IEMs are accompanied by hyperammonemia; measurement of an ammonia level is mandatory in a newborn with acidosis with no established diagnosis.

2. **Blood gas.** Interpretation of the acid-base status is important in the differential diagnosis and has already been discussed (see section V). IEMs must be especially considered in the scenario of a severe metabolic acidosis or a mainly respiratory alkalosis. Ammonia measurement is indicated in this situation to rule out an organic aciduria with secondary hyperammonemia or a urea cycle defect causing a respiratory alkalosis as a result of the direct stimulation of the respiratory center by ammonia with hyperventilation. Be aware that excess heparin in a blood gas specimen may mimic a metabolic acidosis. Those specimens that are not instantly processed should be stored in ice water.

3. **Electrolyte determination.** In addition to the interpretation of the different electrolyte components, an **anion gap** should be calculated. The concentration of negatively and positively charged electrolytes is compared: Add the sodium and potassium levels (in mEq/L) and subtract the sum of the chloride and bicarbonate concentrations. An excess of negatively charged ions (eg, metabolites found in an organic acidopathy) is suggested if the anion gap is >17 mEq/L. Be aware that in a hemolyzed specimen potassium is released from cells that will distort the anion gap calculation (artificially increased).

   Disturbance of electrolytes is also found in other inherited conditions (eg, adrenogenital syndrome [see Chapter 60]).

4. **Ammonia level.** Although the measurement of ammonia levels can be of foremost importance in making the diagnosis of an IEM, this test is unfortunately very susceptible to artifacts, resulting in a false elevation of ammonia levels. Several precautions must be strictly followed to avoid incorrect test results.

   a. The specimen must be placed on ice at the bedside.
   b. Timely processing of the sample is mandatory; this demands immediate transfer to the laboratory with instant preparation of the sample for analysis. If samples have to be stored, the blood must be centrifuged and the plasma maintained at −20 °C. Without strict adherence to these precautionary measures, false elevation by as much as 60–100 mcg/dL may occur. Levels in the neonate may normally be as high as up to 80 mcg/dL. IEMs typically result in levels in the hundreds and thousands. If a result is equivocal, a repeat measurement must be done while considering that the hyperammonemia in IEM most likely will be progressive.

5. **Liver function tests.** Transaminases (aspartate aminotransferase [SGOT] and alanine aminotransferase [SGPT]) are released from hepatocytes with cell damage. Conjugated bilirubin and alkaline phosphatase are elevated with cholestasis. Cholesterol, albumin, and coagulation factor levels reflect the synthetic function of the liver. The plasma amino

TABLE 65–4. LABORATORY FINDINGS SUGGESTIVE OF METABOLIC DISEASE

Variable	Galactosemia	Glycogen storage disease	Maple syrup urine disease	Nonketotic hyperglycinemia	Glutaric acidemia type II	Organic acidemia	Disorders of pyruvate metabolism	Disorders of the urea cycle	Transient hyperammonemia of the newborn
Hypoglycemia	+	+	±	−	±	±	±	−	−
Metabolic acidosis with or without elevated anion gap	+	±	+	−	±	+	+	±	±
Respiratory alkalosis	−	−	−	−	−	−	−	+	+
Hyperammonemia	−	−	−	−	−	±	−	−	±
Jaundice	+	±	−	−	−	±	−	−	−
Urine ketones	−	±	+	−	−	+	±	−	−
Urine abnormal odor or color	−	−	+	−	−	+	−	−	−
Neutropenia or thrombocytopenia	−	−	−	−	−	+	−	−	−

Guidelines only; for details, see text and references.

TABLE 65–5. PROCEDURES FOR URINE TESTS HELPFUL IN THE DIAGNOSIS OF METABOLIC DISEASE

Clinitest (Ames)
1. Mix 5 drops of urine and 10 drops of water in a clean test tube. Add 1 tablet. Fifteen seconds after the end of the reaction, gently shake the test tube.
2. Compare the color after the reaction with the chart supplied. A negative test gives a blue color. Tests that produce green, brown, yellow, or red solutions may indicate the presence of carbohydrate-reducing substances (eg, glucose or galactose), amino acids, or a variety of exogenous drugs.

Acetest (Ames)
1. Place 1 tablet on a clean white filter paper. Apply 1 drop of urine; wait 30 s.
2. The test is positive only if the tablet turns purple. The result is coded as a small, moderate, or large amount of ketones by comparison to a color chart.

Ketostix (Ames)
1. Dip the reagent strip into urine.
2. Compare the color to the chart on the bottle.

Dinitrophenylhydrazine (DNPH)
1. Mix 10 drops of reagent (refrigerated solution of 100 mg of 2,4-dinitrophenylhydrazine in 100 mL of 2 N HCl) with 1 mL of urine.
2. Yellow-white precipitates indicate the presence of keto acids. This test is usually highly positive with maple syrup urine disease, although it may be positive with glycogen storage disease, fructose-1,6-bisphosphatase deficiency, organic acidemias, phenylketonuria, or tyrosinemia.

---

acid pattern is affected by liver dysfunction. Ammonia levels are increased in liver failure.

6. **Urine testing for ketones.** The presence of ketones in the urine of a neonate should always be considered abnormal. One of the IEMs that typically results in strongly positive testing is MSUD.

7. **Urine testing for reducing substances.** Most laboratories perform testing for reducing substances. In some institutions, the test may be performed by the physician or nurses themselves. Use the Clinitest (non-enzyme) assay. The main indication in the neonate is suspected galactosemia. A negative test does not rule out the diagnosis (is the child receiving galactose?). Even a few hours of galactose restriction (eg, a sick patient taking nothing by mouth and on parenteral glucose solution) may result in a negative test. Consider which enteral nutrition the patient is receiving; for example, soy formulas are often galactose free, whereas breast milk is not. Chemistry reminder: Lactose ("milk sugar") is a disaccharide of glucose and galactose.

C. **Laboratory testing more specific for IEMs.** Although some of the following tests might still be available through laboratories at larger hospitals, we consider them to be a second line of more specific tests. One reason is that, dealing with newborn patients, a concern is always to limit the amount of blood that is obtained from the patient. The following tests are, therefore, usually performed to further evaluate a specific diagnosis or abnormalities found on previous testing or to confirm a diagnosis that is clinically suspected.

A helpful resource to localize a laboratory for a specific genetic test, biochemical or molecular, is the **GeneTests data base,** which is maintained through the University of Washington (http://www.genetests.org).

1. **Lactic acid level and lactate–pyruvate ratio.** Determination of lactate and pyruvate levels may be indicated in the evaluation of patients with severe metabolic acidosis. When excess lactate is present, the anion gap (see section XI,B,3) is elevated. Of practical importance is that a specimen for measurement of lactic acid is best obtained from a central line or arterial specimen because even short stasis of blood (venous sampling using a tourniquet) may result in a significant increase in lac-

tate. The lactate–pyruvate ratio is normal (15/20) in PDH deficiency and defects of gluconeogenesis (glycogen storage diseases) and elevated to >25 in pyruvate decarboxylase deficiency and mitochondrial defects of the electron transport chain.

2. **Amino acid analysis.** Amino acid analysis must be quantitative to aid in the diagnosis of IEMs. Note that amino acid analysis of urine is not a test usually indicated in the evaluation of newborns. There are only a few indications for this test, such as to rule out cystinuria in pediatric patients with renal calculi or to demonstrate a high renal glycine excretion in a patient suspected of having NKH (see section V,C). **Plasma amino acid results** are best evaluated (in a sample obtained after a 4-h fast) by concentrating on certain patterns of abnormalities (see Table 65–6) rather than on single abnormal values that may be nutritional or artifacts (eg, taurine is often increased with delayed analysis of the sample). As suggested for urine organic acid analysis, evaluation by an experienced biochemical geneticist who is aware of the clinical presentation and nutritional status of the patient is strongly recommended.

    Plasma amino acid analysis not only is indicated in classic IEMs of amino acid metabolism (eg, MSUD or PKU) but also helps evaluate urea cycle defects because several metabolites of the urea cycle are chemically amino acids (eg, citrulline, arginine, and ornithine) (see Table 65–6 and Figure 65–2). Conditions resulting in hyperammonemia often show elevated glutamine levels (glutamine synthesis incorporates ammonia).

    At least 1–2 mL of blood should be obtained. Laboratories usually request heparinized blood or samples without additives. If processed immediately, samples should be sent on ice. If analysis is to be deferred to a later time, serum or plasma should be separated and frozen.

3. **Urine organic acid analysis.** This analytic test, in which urine organic acids are extracted and analyzed by gas chromatography and mass spectrometry, requires extensive knowledge of biochemical genetics for interpretation and is, therefore, usually performed by laboratories specializing in biochemical genetics. In expert hands, this test can provide an enormous amount of information. Details are far beyond the scope of this manual, but some information is nonetheless helpful for the clinician: Urine organic acid analysis helps to establish the diagnosis of **OAs.** The most common of this large group of disorders are methylmalonic acidemia, propionic acidemia, and isovaleric acidemia (see section V,E). Specific metabolites found are listed in Table 65–6. Most laboratories request at least 5–10 mL of "fresh" urine. As soon as the specimen is collected, it should either be transported to the laboratory on ice or frozen at –20 °C.

4. **Succinylacetone in urine.** This test is specific for hepatorenal tyrosinemia. A sample is collected and used to wet a filter paper (as used for the routine neonatal screening tests). After air drying, the sample can be forwarded to the testing laboratory by mail or carrier services.

5. **Acetyl carnitine profile.** Fatty acids that are metabolized in the mitochondrion (all but VLCFAs with carbon chains of 24 or longer that are metabolized in the peroxisome) are conjugated with carnitine to facilitate their transport into the mitochondrion. The acetyl carnitine profile is assessed by specialized biochemical genetics laboratories using mass spectrometry. Dried whole blood spot samples placed on filter paper cards provided by neonatal screening programs are used. Total and free carnitine plasma levels can be measured, usually using plasma from heparinized blood.

6. **Tandem mass spectrometry (TMS).** TMS detects a large number of disorders of amino and organic acid metabolism as well as fatty acid oxidation defects. This makes it a valuable tool for newborn screening; in

TABLE 65–6. ANALYSIS OF AMINO AND ORGANIC ACIDS IN PLASMA AND URINE

Variable	Organic acids	Amino acids
Isovaleric acidemia	Isovalerylglycine	Normal
	3-Hydroxyisovalerate	
Propionic acidemia	3-Hydroxypropionate	Elevated glycine
	Methylcitrate	
Methylmalonic acidemia	Methylmalonate	Elevated glycine
Multiple carboxylase deficiency	3-Methylcrotonyl	Normal
	3-Hydroxyisovalerate	
	3-Hydroxypropionate	
Glutaric acidemia, type II	Glutaric acid	Elevated lysine
	2-Hydroxyglutarate	
	Ethylmalonate	
	2-Hydroxyisovalerate	
5-Oxoprolinuria (pyroglutamic acidemia)	Pyroglutamate	Normal or elevated oxoproline
Nonketotic hyperglycinemia	Normal	Elevated glycine

addition, however, TMS may also be used in the individual diagnostic evaluation of infants presenting with symptoms suggestive of an inborn error of metabolism. Testing is usually easily done (blood spot samples mailed to laboratories) and usually quite cost-effective.

7. **Galactosemia testing.** To measure galactose-1-phosphate levels and GALT activity, whole blood is usually requested by the laboratory because the metabolites and enzyme are localized in the erythrocytes. Blood must be obtained before blood transfusions. An alternative in already transfused patients is to evaluate the heterozygous parents of the patient, because heterozygote detection is possible with the enzymatic assay.

8. **Peroxisomal function tests.** Measurement of VLCFAs is done by gas chromatography. Normally, only trace amounts of fatty acids with carbon chains of 24 carbons or more are detectable. Measurement of VLCFAs, therefore, detects all peroxisomal disorders that affect the degradation of these compounds. Note that VLCFAs will be normal in a small subgroup of patients with peroxisomal defects (eg, rhizomelic chondrodysplasia punctata). Tests assessing other aspects of peroxisomal function (eg, plasmalogens, phytanic acid, or pipecolic acid measurements) may be necessary. Most of these analyses are done on plasma obtained from EDTA blood. The red blood cell pellet of the sample should also be sent to the laboratory (separated) because plasmalogen levels are evaluated in red blood cells. Samples do not need to be frozen.

9. **Transferrin electrofocusing analysis.** A suspected diagnosis of carbohydrate-deficient glycoprotein syndromes (see section V,G,9) is confirmed by electrofocusing analysis of a glycoprotein, usually transferrin. The measurement of transferrin levels is inappropriate as a diagnostic test for these conditions (levels usually normal).

D. **Postmortem evaluation when an IEM is suspected.** If an IEM is suspected as a possible cause of death in a newborn or young infant, we recommend obtaining the following samples postmortem:

1. **Blood.** Blood should be collected. If no central access was established, a postmortem cardiac puncture may be necessary to obtain a sufficient sample. Serum as well as plasma should be frozen. Also, keep the red blood cell pellets (not frozen). EDTA blood and blood spots on filter paper may allow isolation of DNA or RNA later for mutation analysis.

2. **Urine.** Collect urine, if possible, and freeze it at –20 °C. If no urine could be obtained but urine organic acid analysis is indicated, swabs of the

bladder surface can be obtained on autopsy to attempt urine organic acid analysis.

3. **Skin.** Three to 4 mm should be taken as a full-thickness sterile biopsy (cleansed with alcohol, not iodine). Store in a sterile culture medium. If this is not available, serum from the patient may be used). Do not freeze the specimen, and transport it immediately to the tissue culture laboratory for fibroblast culture and storage.

4. **CSF.** If not performed before death, a lumbar puncture can be obtained postmortem. This procedure may be indicated to rule out infection or an IEM. In addition to obtaining cultures, we recommend freezing a 1- to 2-mL specimen at −20 °C.

5. **A percutaneous liver biopsy** may be performed to obtain a specimen early (freeze for enzyme analysis) or if the family did not consent to a full autopsy.

6. **A full autopsy and consultation with a geneticist** (even postmortem) may be helpful if an IEM is suspected. The geneticist may give special recommendations for postmortem specimens to be obtained on autopsy (eg, frozen or specially prepared samples rather than standard formalin processing).

XII. **Management.** For most IEMs, therapy is currently restricted to dietary measures and in some cases special medications and vitamin substitutions. In some metabolic disorders, **liver or bone marrow transplantation** may be an option.

A. **Acute care while awaiting results of diagnostic studies**

1. **Supportive care** following the standards of neonatal and intensive care includes securing an airway, respiration, and circulation and establishing intravenous access. General measures may also include correction of the acid-base balance, electrolyte abnormalities, and hydration status. Assisted ventilation may be required in severely affected neonates, and aggressive antibiotic therapy is frequently indicated because of the overlap in symptomatology with infectious disorders.

2. **Nutritional measures.** An acutely ill newborn will receive nothing by mouth. For almost all IEMs, a supply of sufficient glucose to avoid a catabolic state is indicated. Try to achieve a caloric intake of 80–100 kcal/kg/day. Eliminate protein acutely (24–48 h) but not over prolonged periods, because breakdown of endogenous protein may otherwise occur and may worsen the patient's clinical status. Intravenous lipids may be contraindicated in certain FAO defects.

3. **Hemodialysis or peritoneal dialysis** may be needed to remove toxic metabolites and in cases in which acidosis is intractable. Exchange transfusions are not effective, and early transfer to a facility where hemodialysis is possible is mandatory in these situations (eg, hyperammonemia).

4. **Vitamin treatment.** Several IEMs have vitamin-responsive forms. Often, a combination of vitamin cofactors (vitamin B_{12}, biotin, riboflavin, thiamine, pyridoxine, and folate) is considered while specific test results are still outstanding. Give vitamins only after appropriate specimens have been obtained for full metabolic investigation and after consultation with a geneticist. **Carnitine substitution** may be indicated in some patients (eg, FAO defects or OAs).

5. **Medications to treat hyperammonemia.** In patients with hyperammonemia, several medications can be used to provide an alternative pathway for ammonia excretion. These include **sodium phenylacetate, sodium phenylbutyrate,** and **sodium benzoate.** Because of the intrinsic side effects, different indications, coordination with nutritional interventions, and frequent dosage adjustments necessary, the use of these medications should be initiated and supervised by an experienced biochemical geneticist.

B. Long-term therapy

1. **Diet.** One of the classic principles for the treatment of IEMs is the restriction of the substance leading to the accumulation of a toxic metabolite (eg, phenylalanine in PKU). In some disorders (eg, urea cycle defects), the overall protein intake is restricted. Careful monitoring is necessary to avoid essential amino acid deficiencies.

2. **Provision of a deficient substance.** This is effective when the deficient product is readily available and can reach the appropriate tissue (eg, cortisol and mineralocorticoid in 21-hydroxylase deficiency). Carnitine replacement may be needed in organic acidurias because carnitine is lost through renal excretion of metabolites bound to carnitine.

3. **Vitamin therapy.** Large doses of specific cofactors may increase the activity of partially deficient enzymes: vitamin B_6 (homocystinuria), vitamin B_{12} (methylmalonic acidemia), biotin (multiple carboxylase deficiency), thiamine (MSUD), and riboflavin (glutaric acidemia II).

4. **Supportive therapy** may help to reduce the morbidity associated with specific IEMs. Splinting may reduce deformities in mucopolysaccharidoses. Splenectomy may be indicated for thrombocytopenia associated with Gaucher's disease.

5. **Long-term therapy.** Genetic disorders require lifelong nutritional, medical, and laboratory monitoring by a team of specialists in these disorders. Many times, intercurrent illnesses and stress may precipitate the recurrence of symptoms.

6. **Early intervention and special education programs** may be beneficial in those disorders characterized by intellectual impairment. Families may find a forum for their concerns and stresses in **family support groups.**

7. As mentioned, **liver and bone marrow transplantation** may be a treatment option in some IEMs.

REFERENCES

Antoun H et al: Cerebellar atrophy: an important feature of carbohydrate deficient glycoprotein syndrome type 1. *Pediatr Radiol* 1999;29:194.

Brusilow SW, Maestri NE: Urea cycle disorders: diagnosis, pathophysiology, and therapy. *Adv Pediatr* 1996;43:127.

Burton BK: Inborn errors of metabolism: the clinical diagnosis in early infancy. *Pediatrics* 1987; 79:359.

Carpenter KH, Wiley V: Application of tandem mass spectrometry to biochemical genetics and newborn screening. *Clin Chim Acta* 2002;322:1.

Clarke JTR: *A Clinical Guide to Inherited Metabolic Diseases.* Cambridge University Press, 1996.

Clayton PT, Thompson E: Dysmorphic syndromes with demonstrable biochemical abnormalities. *J Med Genet* 1988;25:463.

Clayton PT et al: Hypertrophic obstructive cardiomyopathy in a neonate with the carbohydrate-deficient glycoprotein syndrome. *J Inherit Met Dis* 1992;15:857.

de Koning TJ et al: Recurrent nonimmune hydrops fetalis associated with carbohydrate-deficient glycoprotein syndrome. *J Inherit Metab Dis* 1998;21:681.

GeneTests-GeneClinics: *Medical Genetics Information Resource 1993–2002.* University of Washington and Children's Health System, Seattle. Retrieved from http://www.geneclinics.org and http://www.genetests.org.

Goodman SL: Inherited metabolic disease in the newborn: approach to diagnosis and treatment. *Adv Pediatr* 1986;33:197.

Goodman SL, Greene CL: Inborn errors as causes of acute disease in infancy. *Semin Perinatol* 1991;15:31.

Hicks JM, Young DS: *DORA 1997–99. The Directory of Rare Tests.* American Association for Clinical Chemists, 1997.

Hudak ML et al: Differentiation of transient hyperammonemia of the newborn and urea cycle enzyme defects by clinical presentation. *J Pediatr* 1985;107:712.

Iafolla AK, McConkie-Rosell A: Prenatal diagnosis of metabolic disease. *Clin Perinatol* 1990;17: 761.

Imtiaz F et al: Genotypes and phenotypes of patients in the UK with carbohydrate-deficient glycoprotein syndrome type 1. *J Inherit Metab Dis* 2000;23:162.

Kuretz R et al: Neonatal jaundice and coagulopathy. *J Pediatr* 1985;107:982.

Morris AA, Turnbull DM: Metabolic disorders in children. *Curr Opin Neurol* 1994;7:535.

National Organization for Rare Disorders (NORD): *NORD Resource Guide*, 3rd ed. NORD, 1997.

Poggi-Travert F et al: Clinical approach to inherited peroxisomal disorders. *J Inherit Metab Dis* 1995;18(suppl 1):1.

Rinaldo P, Matern D: Disorders of fatty acid transport and mitochondrial oxidation: challenges and dilemmas of metabolic evaluation. *Genet Med* 2000;2:338.

Roe CR: Inherited disorders of mitochondrial fatty acid oxidation: a new responsibility for the neonatologist. *Semin Neonatol* 2002;7:37.

Saudubray JM, Charpentier C: Clinical phenotypes: diagnosis/algorithms. In Scriver CR et al (eds): *The Metabolic and Molecular Basis of Inherited Disease*, 7th ed. McGraw-Hill, 1995;327.

Saudubray JM et al: Clinical approach to the inherited metabolic disorders in neonates. *Biol Neonate* 1990;58(suppl 1):44.

Scriver CR et al (eds): *The Metabolic and Molecular Basis of Inherited Disease*, 7th ed. McGraw-Hill, 1995.

Seashore MR, Rinaldo P: Metabolic disease of the neonate and young infant. *Semin Perinatol* 1993;17:318.

Servidei S et al: Hereditary metabolic cardiomyopathies. *Adv Pediatr* 1994;41:1.

van der Knaap WS et al: Congenital nephrotic syndrome: a novel phenotype of type I carbohydrate-deficient glycoprotein syndrome. *J Inherit Met Dis* 1996;19:787.

Waber L: Inborn errors of metabolism. *Pediatr Ann* 1990;19:105.

Ward JC: Inborn errors of metabolism of acute onset in infancy. *Pediatr Rev* 1990;11:205.

Wraith JE: Diagnosis and management of inborn errors of metabolism. *Arch Dis Child* 1989;64:1410.

Zytkovicz TH et al: Tandem mass spectrometric analysis for amino, organic, and fatty acid disorders in newborn dried blood spots: a two-year summary from the New England newborn screening program. *Clin Chem* 2001;47:1945.

66 Infant of a Diabetic Mother

Good control of maternal diabetes is the key factor in determining fetal outcome. Data indicate that perinatal morbidity and mortality rates in the offspring of women with diabetes mellitus have improved with dietary management and insulin therapy. However, when adequate control of diabetes has not been accomplished, the physician must be aware of possible complications in the infant, including hypoglycemia, hypocalcemia, hypomagnesemia, perinatal asphyxia, respiratory distress syndrome (RDS), other respiratory illnesses, hyperbilirubinemia, polycythemia, renal vein thrombosis, macrosomia, birth injuries, and congenital malformations. Because of better current understanding of the pathophysiology of diabetic pregnancies, these complications can be recognized and treated.

I. **Classification**
   A. **White's classification.** In earlier descriptions of diabetic pregnancies, physicians relied on White's classification (Table 66–1). This nomenclature is based on the age at onset, duration of the disorder, and complications. It is currently used chiefly to compare groups of infants delivered.
   B. **The Expert Committee on the Diagnosis and Classification of Diabetes Mellitus.** Table 66–2 presents the nomenclature of the Expert Committee. It replaces the National Diabetes Data Group classification.

II. **Incidence.** Insulin-dependent diabetes occurs in 0.5% of all pregnancies. In addition, 1–3% of women exhibit biochemical abnormalities during pregnancy consistent with gestational diabetes.

III. **Pathophysiology**
   A. **Macrosomia.** Macrosomia is the classic presentation of the infant of a diabetic mother (IDM). It is the result of biochemical events along the maternal hyperglycemia-fetal hyperinsulinemia pathway, as described by Pedersen (1971). Infants born to mothers described by White's classification as having class A (insulin-dependent), B, C, or D diabetes are often macrosomic. Complications are minimal in gestational diabetes and in class A diabetes controlled by diet.
   B. **Small for gestational age.** Mothers with renal, retinal, or cardiac diseases are more likely to have small for gestational age or premature infants, poor fetal outcome, fetal distress, or fetal death.
   C. **Specific disorders frequently encountered in IDMs**
      1. **Metabolic disorders**
         a. **Hypoglycemia** is defined as a blood glucose level <35 mg/dL in a preterm or term infant. It is present in up to 40% of IDMs, most commonly in macrosomic infants. It usually presents within 1–2 h after delivery. According to Pedersen (1971), at birth the transplacental glucose supply is terminated, and, because of high concentrations of plasma insulin, blood glucose levels fall. Mothers with well-controlled blood glucose levels have fewer infants with hypoglycemia. Hypoglycemia in SGA infants born to mothers with diabetic vascular disease is caused by decreased glycogen stores; it appears 6–12 h after delivery.
         b. **Hypocalcemia.** Serum calcium levels <2 mg/dL associated with symptoms or <6 mg/dL without symptoms—or an ionized calcium level <3 mg/dL—are considered hypocalcemic. The incidence is up to 50% of IDMs (Rosenn & Tsang, 1991). The severity of hypocalcemia is related to the severity of maternal diabetes and involves decreased function of the parathyroid glands (Tsang et al, 1979). Serum calcium levels are lowest at 24–72 h of age.

TABLE 66-1. WHITE'S CLASSIFICATION OF DIABETES

Class	Description
A	Chemical diabetes with a positive glucose tolerance test before or during pregnancy
B	Onset after age 20; <10 years' duration
C	Onset at age 10–19 years
D1	Onset before age 10 years
D2	Duration >20 years
D3	Calcification of vessels of the leg
D4	Benign retinopathy
D5	Hypertension
E	Calcification of pelvic vessels (not used)
F	Nephropathy
G	Pregnancy failures
H	Vascular lesions developing in childbearing years; includes patients with cardiopathy
R	Malignant retinopathy

Based on data from White P: Diabetes mellitus in pregnancy. *Clin Perinatol* 1974;1:331. Appears with permission from Elsevier Science.

c. **Hypomagnesemia.** A serum magnesium level <1.52 mg/dL in any in fant indicates hypomagnesemia. It is related to maternal hypomagnesemia and the severity of maternal diabetes.

2. **Cardiorespiratory disorders**
   a. **Perinatal asphyxia.** Perinatal asphyxia occurs in up to 25% of IDMs It may result from prematurity, cesarean delivery, intrauterine hypoxia caused by maternal vascular disease, or macrosomia.
   b. **Hyaline membrane disease or RDS**
      i. **Incidence.** The incidence has decreased to only 3% of IDMs because of better management of diabetes during pregnancy (Frantz & Epstein, 1979). Most cases are the result of premature delivery, delayed maturation of pulmonary surfactant production, or delivery by elective cesarean section.
      ii. **Fetal lung maturity.** Pulmonary surfactant production in the IDM is deficient or delayed principally in class A, B, and C diabetics. Fetal

TABLE 66-2. NOMENCLATURE OF THE EXPERT COMMITTEE ON THE DIAGNOSIS AND CLASSIFICATION OF DIABETES MELLITUS

Class	Description
Type I diabetes:	Beta cell destruction leading to absolute insulin deficiency.
Type II diabetes:	May range from predominantly insulin resistance with relative insulin deficiency to a predominantly secretory defect with insulin resistance.
Other specific types:	Genetic defects, diseases of exocrine pancreas, endocrinopathies, drug or chemical induced, infections, genetic syndromes.
Gestational diabetes mellitus:	Any degree or glucose intolerance with onset or first recognition during pregnancy. Diagnosis requires at least 2 abnormal plasma glucose values on a 3-h oral glucose tolerance test (100 g of glucose). Fasting: 95 mg/dL 1 h: 180 mg/dL 2 h: 155 mg/dL 3 h: 140 mg/dL

Based on data from: Expert Committee on the Diagnosis and Classification of Diabetes Mellitus: Report. *Diabetes Care* 2002;25:55.

hyperinsulinism may adversely affect the lung maturation process in the IDM by antagonizing the action of cortisol (Smith et al, 1975).

iii. Cesarean section. Infants delivered by elective cesarean section are at risk for RDS because of decreased prostaglandin production and increased pulmonary vascular resistance (Csaba et al, 1978).

c. **Other causes of respiratory distress**

i. **Transient tachypnea of the newborn** occurs especially after elective cesarean section. This disorder may or may not require oxygen therapy and usually responds by 72 h of age.

ii. **Hypertrophic cardiomyopathy** occurs in up to 50% of IDMs (Way et al, 1979). It occurs secondary to increased fat and glycogen deposition in the myocardium and may lead to congestive heart failure.

3. **Hematologic disorders**

a. **Hyperbilirubinemia.** Bilirubin production is apparently increased in the IDM secondary to prematurity, macrosomia, hypoglycemia, and polycythemia.

b. **Polycythemia and hyperviscosity.** The cause of polycythemia is unclear but may be related to increased levels of erythropoietin in the IDM, increased red blood cell production secondary to chronic intrauterine hypoxia in mothers with vascular disease, and intrauterine placental transfusion resulting from acute hypoxia during labor and delivery.

c. **Renal venous thrombosis** is a rare complication most likely caused by hyperviscosity, hypotension, or disseminated intravascular coagulation. It is usually diagnosed by ultrasonography and may present with hematuria and an abdominal mass.

4. **Morphologic and functional problems**

a. **Macrosomia and birth injury**

i. **Macrosomia** is caused by fetal hyperglycemia, resulting in increased glucose uptake in insulin-sensitive tissues. It is seen in the offspring of gestational and class A, B, and C diabetics. Macrosomia is rarely seen in the other classes because of maternal vascular disease.

ii. **Birth injury.** Macrosomia may lead to shoulder dystocia, which may cause birth asphyxia. Birth injuries include fractures of the clavicle or humerus, Erb's palsy, phrenic nerve palsy, and, rarely, central nervous system injury.

b. **Congenital malformations.** Congenital malformations occur in 6.4% of IDMs (Molsted-Pedersen, 1980), a much higher incidence than in the general population. It is suspected that poor diabetic control in the first trimester is associated with a higher percentage of congenital malformations. Congenital malformations now account for up to 50% of perinatal deaths and include cardiac defects (eg, transposition of the great vessels, ventricular septal defect, or atrial septal defect), renal defects (eg, agenesis), gastrointestinal tract defects (eg, small left colon syndrome or situs inversus), neurologic defects (eg, anencephaly or meningocele syndrome), skeletal defects (eg, hemivertebrae or caudal regression syndrome), unusual facies, and microphthalmos.

IV. **Risk factors.** The following factors or conditions may be associated with an increased risk for problems in IDMs:

A. **Maternal class of diabetes**

1. **In gestational diabetes and class A diabetes controlled by diet alone,** infants have few complications.

2. **Women with class A diabetes controlled with insulin and class B, C, and D diabetes** are prone to deliver macrosomic infants if diabetes is inadequately controlled.

3. **Diabetic women with renal, retinal, cardiac, and vascular disease** have the most severe fetal problems.

B. **Hemoglobin A$_{1C}$.** To decrease perinatal morbidity and mortality rates, the diabetic woman should attempt to achieve good metabolic control before conception. Elevated hemoglobin A$_{1C}$ levels during the first trimester appear to be associated with a higher incidence of congenital malformations (Yinnen et al, 1984).

C. **Diabetic ketoacidosis.** Pregnant women with insulin-dependent diabetes are apt to develop diabetic ketoacidosis. The onset of this complication may be life-threatening for the mother and fetus or may lead to preterm delivery.

D. **Preterm labor.** Premature onset of labor in a diabetic woman is a serious problem because of the increased likelihood of RDS in the fetus. Furthermore, β-sympathomimetic agents used to prevent preterm delivery may be associated with maternal hyperglycemia, hyperinsulinemia, and acidosis.

E. **Immature fetal lung profile.** Diabetic women who present at 36 weeks' gestation or later should undergo amniocentesis to evaluate fetal lung maturity. A mature lecithin–sphingomyelin ratio may not ensure normal respiratory function in the IDM. However, the presence of phosphatidylglycerol in the amniotic fluid is more apt to be associated with normal neonatal respiratory function (see also Chapter 1).

V. **Clinical presentation**
A. **At birth,** the infant may be large for gestational age or, if the mother has vascular disease, small for gestational age. The size of most infants is appropriate for gestational age; however, if macrosomia is present, birth trauma may occur.

B. **After birth,** hypoglycemia can present as lethargy, poor feeding, apnea, or jitteriness in the first 6–12 h after birth. Jitteriness that occurs after 24 h of age may be the result of hypocalcemia or hypomagnesemia. Signs of respiratory distress secondary to immature lungs can be noted on examination. Cardiac disease may be present as an enlarged cardiothymic shadow on a chest x-ray film or by physical evidence of heart failure. Gross congenital anomalies may be noted on physical examination.

VI. **Diagnosis**
A. **Laboratory studies.** The following tests must be closely monitored in the IDM:
1. **Serum glucose levels** should be checked at delivery and at ½, 1, 1½, 2, 4, 8, 12, 24, 36, and 48 h of age. Glucose levels should be checked with Chemstrip-bG or Dextrostix. Readings <40 mg/dL on Chemstrip-bG or <45 mg/dL on Dextrostix should be verified by serum glucose measurements.
2. **Serum calcium levels** should be obtained at 6, 24, and 48 h of age. If serum calcium levels are low, serum magnesium levels should be obtained because they may also be low.
3. **The hematocrit** should be checked at birth and at 4 and 24 h of age.
4. **Serum bilirubin levels** should be checked as indicated by physical examination.
5. **Other tests.** Arterial blood gas levels, complete blood cell counts, cultures, and Gram stains should be obtained as clinically indicated.
B. **Radiologic studies** are not necessary unless there is evidence of cardiac, respiratory, or skeletal problems.
C. **Electrocardiography and echocardiography** should be performed if hypertrophic cardiomyopathy or a cardiac malformation is suspected.

VII. **Management**
A. **Initial evaluation.** Upon delivery, the infant should be evaluated in the usual manner. In the transitional nursery, blood glucose levels and the hematocrit should be obtained. The infant should be observed for jitteriness, tremors, convulsions, apnea, weak cry, and poor sucking. A physical examination

should be performed, paying particular attention to the heart, kidneys, lungs, and extremities.

B. Continuing evaluation. Over the first several hours after delivery, the infant should be assessed for signs of respiratory distress. During the first 48 h, observe for signs of jaundice and for renal, cardiac, neurologic, and gastrointestinal tract abnormalities.

C. Metabolic management
  1. **Hypoglycemia.** See Chapter 43.
  2. **Hypocalcemia**
     a. **Calcium therapy.** Symptomatic infants should receive 10% calcium gluconate intravenously. The infusion should be given slowly to prevent cardiac arrhythmias, and the infant should be monitored for signs of extravasation. After the initial dose, a maintenance dose is given by continuous intravenous infusion. The hypocalcemia should respond in 3–4 days; until then, serum calcium levels should be monitored every 12 h.
     b. **Magnesium maintenance therapy.** Magnesium is usually added to intravenous fluids or given orally as magnesium sulfate 50%, 0.2 mL/kg/day (4 mEq/mL).

D. Management of cardiorespiratory problems
  1. **Perinatal asphyxia.** Close observation for fetal distress should continue (see Chapter 73).
  2. **Hyaline membrane disease.** Obtaining amniotic fluid for a fetal lung maturity profile can decrease the incidence of hyaline membrane disease. However, some infants must be delivered even if the lung profile is immature.
  3. **Cardiomyopathy.** The treatment of choice is with propranolol (for dosage information, see Chapter 80). Digoxin is contraindicated because of possible ventricular outflow obstruction.

E. Hematologic therapy
  1. **Hyperbilirubinemia.** Frequent monitoring of serum bilirubin levels may be necessary. Phototherapy and exchange transfusion for infants with hyperbilirubinemia are discussed in Chapter 64.
  2. **Polycythemia.** See Chapter 61.
  3. **Renal venous thrombosis.** Treatment consists of fluid restriction and close monitoring of electrolytes and renal status. Supportive therapy is indicated to ensure adequate blood circulation. Nephrectomy is usually only a last resort in unilateral disease.

F. Management of morphologic and functional problems
  1. **Macrosomia and birth injury**
     a. **Fractures of the extremities** should be treated with immobilization.
     b. **Erb's palsy** can be treated with range-of-motion exercises.
  2. **Congenital malformations.** If a gross malformation is discovered, a specialist should be consulted.

VIII. Prognosis. Less morbidity and mortality occur with adequate control during the diabetic pregnancy. Preconceptual counseling is used as an adjunct to preventive health care of the diabetic patient. The known pregnant diabetic is currently receiving better health care than before, but the challenge is early identification of women with biochemical abnormalities of gestational diabetes. The risk of subsequent diabetes in the infants of these women is at least 10 times greater than in the normal population.

REFERENCES

Csaba et al: Relationship of maternal treatment with indomethacin to persistence of fetal circulation syndrome. *J Pediatr* 1978;92:484.
Cummins M, Norrish M: Follow-up of children of diabetic mothers. *Arch Dis Child* 1980;55:259.

Expert Committee on the Diagnosis and Classification of Diabetes Mellitus: Report. *Diabetes Care* 2002;25:S5.

Frantz IO III, Epstein MF: Fetal lung development in pregnancies complicated by diabetes. In Merkatz IR, Adam PAJ (eds): *The Diabetic Pregnancy: A Perinatal Perspective*. Grune & Stratton, 1979.

Hollingsworth DR: Diabetes. In Hollingsworth DR, Resnik R (eds): *Medical Counseling Before Pregnancy*. Churchill, 1988.

Kitzmiller JL et al: Management of diabetes and pregnancy. In Kozak GP (ed): *Clinical Diabetes Mellitus*. Saunders, 1982.

Kulovich MV, Gluck L: The lung profile: 2. Complicated pregnancy. *Am J Obstet Gynecol* 1979; 135:64.

Molsted-Pedersen L: Pregnancy and diabetes: a survey. *Acta Endocrinol Suppl* 1980;238:13.

Pedersen J: *The Pregnant Diabetic and Her Newborn*, 2nd ed. Williams & Wilkins, 1971.

Rosenn B, Tsang RC: The effects of maternal diabetes on the fetus and neonate. *Ann Clin Lab Sci* 1991;21(suppl 3):153.

Smith BT et al: Insulin antagonism of cortisol action on lecithin synthesis by cultured fetal lung cells. *J Pediatr* 1975;87:953.

Tsang RC et al: Diabetes and calcium: calcium disturbances in infants of diabetic mothers. In Merkatz IR, Adam PAJ (eds): *The Diabetic Pregnancy: A Perinatal Perspective*. Grune & Stratton, 1979.

Way GL et al: The natural history of hypertrophic cardiomyopathy in infants of diabetic mothers. *J Pediatr* 1979;95:1020.

White P: Diabetes mellitus in pregnancy. *Clin Perinatol* 1974;1:331.

Yinnen K et al: Risk of minor and major fetal malformations in diabetics with high haemoglobin A_{1c} values in early pregnancy. *BMJ* 1984;289:345.

67 Infant of a Drug-Abusing Mother

I. **Definition.** An infant of a drug-abusing mother (IDAM) is one whose mother has taken drugs that may potentially cause neonatal withdrawal symptoms. The constellation of signs and symptoms associated with withdrawal is called the neonatal withdrawal syndrome. Table 67–1 lists drugs that have been associated with this syndrome.

II. **Incidence.** Maternal drug abuse has increased over the past decade. It is estimated that ~5–10% of deliveries nationwide are to women who have abused drugs (excluding alcohol) during pregnancy. The incidence is considerably higher in inner-city hospitals.

III. **Pathophysiology.** Drugs of abuse are of low molecular weight and are usually water-soluble and lipophilic. These features facilitate their transfer across the placenta and accumulation in the fetus and amniotic fluid. The half-life of drugs is usually prolonged in the fetus compared with an adult. Most drugs of abuse either bind to various central nervous system (CNS) receptors or affect the release and reuptake of various neurotransmitters. This may have a long-lasting trophic effect on developing dendritic structures. In addition, some drugs are directly toxic to fetal cells. The developing fetus may also be affected by the direct physiologic effects of a drug. Many of the fetal effects of cocaine, including its putative teratogenic effects, are thought to be due to its potent vasoconstrictive property.

Some drugs appear to have a partially beneficial effect. The incidence of respiratory distress syndrome (RDS) is decreased after maternal use of heroin and possibly also cocaine. These effects are probably a reflection of fetal stress rather than a direct maturational effect of these drugs. Particularly in the case of cocaine, the decreased incidence of RDS is more than offset by the considerable increase in preterm deliveries after its use. The major concern in IDAMs is the long-term outcome. The importance of direct and indirect effects of drugs on the developing CNS predominates, and the risks of drug abuse far outweigh the benefits.

IV. **Limitations of studies on drug abuse.** Existing studies on the neonatal effects of drug exposure in utero are subject to many confounding factors. Many studies have relied on the history obtained from the mother, which is notoriously inaccurate. In addition to recall bias, there is a considerable incentive to withhold information. Testing of urine for drugs of abuse does not reflect drug exposure throughout pregnancy and does not provide quantitative information. Many women who abuse drugs are multiple drug abusers and also drink alcohol and smoke cigarettes. It is thus difficult to isolate the effects of any one drug. Social and economic deprivation is common among drug abusers, and this factor not only confounds perinatal data but has a major effect on long-term studies of infant outcome.

V. **Risk factors.** Associated with an increased incidence of drug abuse are the following.
   A. **Poor social and economic circumstances.**
   B. **Poor antenatal care.**
   C. **Teenage or unwed mothers.**
   D. **Poor education.**

VI. **Associated conditions**
   A. **Infectious diseases** (hepatitis B, syphilis, and other sexually transmitted diseases).
   B. **HIV-positive serology.**
   C. **Multiple drug abuse.**

TABLE 67-1. DRUGS CAUSING NEONATAL WITHDRAWAL SYNDROME

Opiates	Barbiturates	Miscellaneous
Codeine	Butalbital	Alcohol
Heroin	Phenobarbital	Amphetamine
Meperidine	Secobarbital	Chlordiazepoxide
Methadone		Clomipramine
Morphine		Cocaine
Pentazocine		Desmethylimipramine
Propoxyphene		Diazepam
		Diphenhydramine
		Ethchlorvynol
		Fluphenazine
		Glutethimide
		Hydroxyzine
		Imipramine
		Meprobamate
		Phencyclidine

    D. Poor nutritional status.
    E. Anemia.
VII. Obstetric complications
    A. Premature delivery.
    B. Premature rupture of membranes.
    C. Chorioamnionitis.
    D. Fetal distress.
    E. Intrauterine growth retardation (IUGR).
    F. With cocaine use, the following may be present (in addition to the conditions just mentioned):
        1. Hypertension.
        2. Abruptio placentae.
        3. Cardiac: Arrhythmias, myocardial ischemia, and infarction.
        4. Cerebrovascular accident.
        5. Respiratory arrest.
        6. Fetal demise.
VIII. Diagnosis
    A. History. Many, if not most, drug abusers withhold this information. Details of the extent, quantity, and duration of abuse are unreliable. However, the history is the simplest and most convenient means of diagnosis.
    B. Laboratory tests. The most commonly used tests to detect drugs of abuse are immunoassays (enzymatic assays or radioimmunoassays). They are, however, subject to a low rate of false-negative and, because of cross-reactivity, false-positive testing. They are thus viewed as screening tests. When it is either medically or legally important, these tests should be supplemented by the more sensitive and specific chromatographic or mass spectrometric tests.
        1. Urine is easily obtained and is the most common substance used for drug testing. It reflects intake only in the last few days before delivery. Urine may be obtained from both the mother and the infant (in whom it may persist for a longer time).
            a. False-negative immunoassays may be due to dilution (low specific gravity) or high sodium chloride content (detected by high specific gravity). Various adulterants may also affect detection; this is unlikely in the neonate but may occur in maternal urine.
            b. False-positive immunoassays. Although these depend on the specific assay used, the following have been reported:
                i. Detected as morphine: Codeine (found in many cold and cough medications and in analgesics). About 10% of codeine is metabo-

lized to morphine in the liver. The consumption of baked goods containing poppy seeds (eg, bagels) can result in detectable amounts of morphine in the urine. These are "physiologic" false-positive results, but chromatography or mass spectrometry may determine the source by quantitative assays of other metabolites.

ii. **Detected as amphetamines:** Ranitidine, chlorpromazine, ritodrine, phenylpropanolamine, ephedrine, pseudoephedrine, phenylephrine, phentermine, and phenmetrazine. Some of these (eg, phenylpropanolamine, pseudoephedrine, and phenylephrine) are found in many over-the-counter preparations.

iii. **Very high concentrations of nicotine** (probably higher than those obtained in smokers) have shown false-positive in vitro testing for morphine and benzoylecgonine.

2. **Meconium** is easily obtained, and drugs may be found up to 3 days after delivery. It is a more sensitive test than urine for detecting drug abuse and reflects usage over a longer period than is detectable by urine testing. Its main disadvantage is that the specimen requires processing before testing and hence places an additional burden on the laboratory.

3. **Hair.** This is by far the most sensitive test available for detection of drug abuse. Hair grows at 1–2 cm/month; hence, maternal hair can be segmented and each segment analyzed for drugs. Thus, details of drug abuse throughout pregnancy may be obtained. There is a quantitative relationship between amounts of drug used and amounts incorporated in growing hair. Hair may be obtained from the mother or the infant (in whom it will reflect usage only during the last trimester). Hair may also be obtained from the infant a long time after delivery should symptoms occur that suggest in utero drug exposure that was previously unsuspected. The test requires processing before assay, is more expensive, and is currently not as widely available as other test methods.

IX. **Signs and symptoms of drug withdrawal** are listed in Table 67–2. These signs essentially reflect CNS "irritability," altered neurobehavioral organization, and abnormal sympathetic activation. Although each drug may have its own effects, these signs and symptoms must be noted for every IDAM (because of multiple drug abuse); conversely, drug abuse should be suspected in infants exhibiting these signs and symptoms.

TABLE 67–2. SIGNS AND SYMPTOMS OF NEONATAL ABSTINENCE

Hyperirritability
    Increased deep-tendon and primitive reflexes
    Hypertonus, hyperacusis
    Tremors
    High-pitched cry
Seizures
Wakefulness
Increased rooting reflex
Uncoordinated or ineffectual sucking and swallowing
Regurgitation and vomiting
Loose stools and diarrhea
Tachypnea, apnea
Yawning, hiccups
Sneezing, stuffy nose
Mottling
Fever
Failure to gain weight
Lacrimation

A scoring system has been devised for assessment of withdrawal signs. Commonly called the Finnegan score, after its originator, the score was devised for neonates exposed to opiates in utero. Its utility for assessing signs after exposure to other drugs or for guiding management in these cases has not been established, but it can be used as a guide. The scoring system is shown in Table 67–3.

No laboratory tests are routinely required in IDAMs (other than tests to confirm the diagnosis). Laboratory tests are required to rule out other causes of particular signs and symptoms (eg, calcium and glucose for cases of jerky movements) or to follow up and manage some particular complication of drug abuse appropriately.

X. **Specific drugs**

A. **Opiates.** Opiates bind to opiate receptors in the CNS, while part of the clinical manifestations of narcotic withdrawal result from α_2-adrenergic supersensitivity (particularly in the locus ceruleus). Infants born to opiate-addicted mothers show an increased incidence of IUGR and perinatal distress. Even when these infants are not small for gestational age, they have lower weight and a smaller head circumference compared with drug-free infants.

1. **Signs and symptoms of withdrawal occur in 60–90% of exposed infants.** The onset of symptoms may be minutes after delivery up to 1–2 weeks of age, but most infants will exhibit signs by 2–3 days of life. The onset of withdrawal may be delayed beyond 2 weeks in infants exposed to methadone (and parents should be appropriately informed).

2. **The clinical course is variable, ranging from mild symptoms of brief duration to severe symptoms.** The clinical course may be protracted, with exacerbations or recurrence of symptoms after discharge. Restlessness, agitation, tremors, wakefulness, and feeding problems may persist for 3–6 months. A blunted ventilatory response to carbon dioxide has been shown. There is a reduced incidence of both RDS and hyperbilirubinemia.

3. **Prognosis.** There are increased risks of sudden infant death syndrome (SIDS) and strabismus. A substantial proportion of children will demonstrate good catch-up growth by 1–2 years of age, although they may still be below the mean. There are limited data on long-term follow-up, but at 5–6 years of age these children appear to function within the normal range of mental and motor development. Some differences have been found in various behavioral, adaptive, and perceptual skills. Some children will require special education classes. A positive and reinforcing environment can improve infant outcome significantly.

B. **Cocaine.** Cocaine prevents the reuptake of neurotransmitters (epinephrine, norepinephrine, dopamine, and serotonin) at nerve endings and causes a supersensitivity or exaggerated response to neurotransmitters at the effector organs. It also affects the permeability of nerves to sodium ions. Cocaine is a CNS stimulant and a sympathetic activator with potent vasoconstrictive properties. It causes a decrease in uterine and placental blood flow with consequent fetal hypoxemia. It causes hypertension in the mother and the fetus with a reduction in fetal cerebral blood flow.

1. **Symptoms seen in neonates exposed to cocaine in utero** are irritability, tremors, hypertonia, a high-pitched cry, hyperreflexia, frantic fist sucking, feeding problems, sneezing, tachypnea, and abnormal sleep patterns. A specific cocaine withdrawal syndrome has not been described. The symptoms just mentioned may be a reflection of cocaine intoxication rather than withdrawal, and after an initial period of irritability and overactivity, a period of lethargy and decreased tone has been described.

2. *Controversial* **cocaine associations**

a. **In the neonate, the following have been described:** Necrotizing enterocolitis, transient hypertension, and reduced cardiac output (on the

TABLE 67–3. MODIFIED FINNEGAN'S SCORING SYSTEM FOR NEONATAL WITHDRAWAL

Signs and symptoms[a]	Score																
Cry																	
High-pitched	2																
Continuous	3																
Sleep hours after feed																	
1 h	3																
2 h	2																
3 h	1																
Moro reflex																	
Hyperactive	2																
Marked	3																
Tremors when disturbed																	
Mild	2																
Marked	3																
Tremors when undisturbed																	
Mild	3																
Marked	4																
Muscle tone increased																	
Mild	3																
Marked	6																
Convulsions	8																
Feedings																	
Frantic sucking of fists	1																
Poor feeding ability	1																
Regurgitation	1																
Projectile vomiting	1																
Stools																	
Loose	2																
Watery	3																
Fever																	
100–101 °F	2																
Over 101 °F	2																
Respiratory rate																	
>60/min	1																
Retractions	2																
Excoriations																	
Nose	1																
Knees	1																
Toes	1																
Frequent yawning	1																
Sneezing	1																
Nasal stuffiness	1																
Sweating	1																
Total scores per day	( )																

[a]Sign and symptoms are scored between feedings.
Once an objective score has been attained, a dose for treatment can be decided on.
From *Finnegan LP et al: A scoring system for evaluation and treatment of neonatal abstinence syndrome: a new clinical and research tool. In Morselli PL et al (editors):* Basic and Therapeutic Aspects of Perinatal Pharmacology. *Raven, 1975.*

first day of life); intracranial hemorrhages and infarcts; seizures; apneic spells; periodic breathing; abnormal electroencephalogram; abnormal brainstem auditory evoked potentials; abnormal response to hypoxia and carbon dioxide; and ileal perforation. These reports were mostly case reports or insufficiently controlled case series with numerous confounding factors (notably, various other perinatal and gestational risk factors, including multiple drug and alcohol usage). There are large case-control studies that have found no association between cocaine exposure and intraventricular hemorrhage. Despite earlier concerns, there does not appear to be an increased risk of SIDS.

    b. **Cocaine has been suggested as a teratogen.** Its teratogenic potential is presumed to be due to its vascular effects, although direct toxicity on various cell lines may also play a role. Numerous CNS anomalies as well as cardiovascular abnormalities, limb reduction defects, intestinal atresias, and other malformations have been attributed to cocaine. However, most of these associations were derived from case reports or series or poorly controlled studies, and a detailed examination of the data does not substantiate most of these teratogenic associations. An exception appears to be an increased risk of genitourinary tract defects associated with cocaine exposure during gestation. Moreover, there does not appear to be a dysmorphism recognizable as a "cocaine syndrome." Cocaine is associated with an increased incidence of spontaneous abortion, stillbirth, abruptio placentae, premature labor, and IUGR.

3. **Prognosis.** By 1 year of age, most infants will have achieved catch-up growth. At 3–4 years, there are problems with expressive and receptive speech, and children are reported to be hyperactive, distractable, and irritable and to have problems socializing. There are, however, very limited data, and many of these problems appear to be related to a deprived environment. A number of studies have found no major differences in intellectual abilities or academic achievement between children exposed to cocaine in utero and controls. Studies have suggested that cognitive deficits may be related to heavy cocaine exposure during gestation and that more sensitive and selective tests are required to detect such differences. These deficits were primarily those of poorer recognition memory and information processing. An intriguing study from Toronto assessed the neurodevelopment of adopted children who had been exposed in utero to cocaine. In a follow-up (14 months to 6½ years), the cocaine-exposed children caught up with the control subjects in weight and stature but not in head circumference. There were no significant differences between the two groups in global IQ, but the cocaine-exposed children had a lower score in verbal comprehension and expressive language. This is the first study to document measurable adverse outcome from in utero cocaine exposure, independent of postnatal home and environmental confounders; however, the effect of prenatal confounding factors such as alcohol could not be eliminated. More recent studies have sustained the debate as to whether cocaine is a behavioral teratogen. One longitudinal study (Singer et al, 2002) found that cocaine-exposed children had significant cognitive deficits and a doubling of the rate of developmental delay during the first 2 years of life, although there were no effects on motor outcomes. On the other hand, a systematic review (Frank et al, 1996) found that, among children ≤6 years, there is no convincing evidence that prenatal cocaine exposure is associated with specific developmental toxic effects that are different in severity, scope of kind from sequelae of multiple other confounding risk factors (such as tobacco, marijuana, alcohol, and environmental quality).

C. **Alcohol** is probably the foremost drug of abuse today. Ethanol is an anxiolytic-analgesic with a depressant effect on the CNS. Both ethanol and its metabolite, acetaldehyde, are toxic. Alcohol crosses the placenta and also impairs its function. The risk of affecting the fetus is related to alcohol dose, but there is a continuum of effects and no known safe limit. The risk that an alcoholic woman will have a child with fetal alcohol syndrome (FAS) is ~35–40%. However, even in the absence of FAS, and also with lower alcohol intakes, there is an increased risk of congenital anomalies and impaired intellect. It is estimated that alcohol is the major cause of congenital mental retardation today.

FAS consists of

- **Prenatal or postnatal growth retardation, CNS involvement** such as irritability in infancy or hyperactivity in childhood, developmental delay, hypotonia, or intellectual impairment
- **Facial dysmorphology:** microcephaly, microphthalmos, or short palpebral fissures, a poorly developed philtrum, a thin upper lip (vermilion border), and hypoplastic maxilla.

Numerous congenital anomalies have been described after exposure to alcohol in utero both with and without a full-blown FAS. CNS symptoms may appear within 24 h after delivery and include tremors, irritability, hypertonicity, twitching, hyperventilation, hyperacusis, opisthotonos, and seizures. Symptoms may be severe but are usually of short duration. Abdominal distention and vomiting are less frequent than with most other drugs of abuse. In premature infants of women who were heavy alcohol users (>7 drinks/week), there is an increased risk of both intracranial hemorrhage and white matter CNS damage.

D. Barbiturates. Symptoms and signs of withdrawal are similar to those observed in narcotic-exposed infants, but symptoms usually appear later. Most infants become symptomatic toward the end of the first week of life, although onset may be delayed up to 2 weeks. The duration of symptoms is usually 2–6 weeks.

E. Benzodiazepines. Symptoms are indistinguishable from those of narcotic withdrawal, including seizures. The onset of symptoms may be shortly after birth.

F. Phencyclidine (PCP). Symptoms usually begin within 24 h of birth, and the infant may show signs of CNS "hyperirritability" as in narcotic withdrawal. Gastrointestinal symptoms of withdrawal are less common. Very few studies have been done, but at 2 years of age these infants appear to have lower scores in fine motor, adaptive, and language areas of development. Although weight, length, and head circumference are somewhat reduced at birth, most children demonstrate adequate catch-up growth.

G. Marijuana. Studies have suggested a slightly shorter duration of gestation and somewhat reduced birth weight, but the extent of these differences was of no clinical importance. Although the drug may have some mild effect on a variety of newborn neurobehavioral traits, there is no evidence of long-term dysfunction.

XI. Treatment. Manifestations of drug withdrawal in many infants will resolve within a few days, and drug therapy is not required. Supportive care will suffice in many, if not most, infants. It is not appropriate to treat prophylactically infants of drug-dependent mothers. The infant's withdrawal score should be assessed to monitor the progression of symptoms and the adequacy of treatment.

A. Supportive care
   1. **Minimal stimulation.** Attempt to keep the infant in a darkened, quiet environment. Reduce other noxious stimuli.
   2. **Swaddling and positioning.** Use gentle swaddling with positioning that encourages flexion rather than extension.
   3. **Prevent excessive crying with a pacifier, cuddling, and so on.** Feedings should be on demand if possible, and treatment should be individualized based on the infant's level of tolerance.

B. Drug treatment. The general aim of treatment is to allow sleep and feeding patterns to be as close to normal as possible. When supportive care is insufficient to do this, or if symptoms are particularly severe, drugs are used. Indications for drug treatment are progressive irritability, continued feeding difficulty, and significant weight loss. A score >7 on the Finnegan score for three consecutive scorings (done every 2–4 h during the first 2 days) may also be regarded as an indication for treatment. However, the Finnegan score should not be followed slavishly and treated as a definitive laboratory value (eg, this is not like treating diabetes by monitoring blood and urine sugar levels). Many centers use the Finnegan score only every 12 h and increase the frequency of its application if the infant's scores rapidly escalate. Drugs used for withdrawal are discussed next. Additional treatment may be required for some symptoms (eg, dehydration or convulsions). With the exception of a few small trials comparing paregoric to phenobarbital for narcotic withdrawal, drug therapy is based largely on anecdotal evidence and hence is variable.

1. **Paregoric (camphorated opium tincture).** This has 0.4 mg/mL morphine equivalent and is thought to be more "physiologic" than nonnarcotic agents. Treated infants have a more physiologic sucking pattern, a higher calorie intake, and better weight gain than those treated with phenobarbital. Paregoric controls seizures related to narcotic withdrawal better than phenobarbital. It will control symptoms in >90% of infants with withdrawal after narcotic exposure. Potential disadvantages are due to other constituents present in the preparation: Camphor is a CNS stimulant, and paregoric also contains alcohol, anise oil, and benzoic acid, a metabolite of benzyl alcohol. In full-term infants, start with 0.2 mL every 3–4 h; if no improvement is seen within 4 h, increase the dose by 0.05-mL steps up to a maximum of 0.5 mL every 3–4 h. In premature infants, start 0.05 mL/kg every 4 h and increase with increments of 0.02 mL/kg every 4 h until symptoms are controlled, up to a maximum of 0.15 mL/kg every 4 h. Once the withdrawal score is stable for 48 h, the dosage may be tapered by 10% each day.

2. **Tincture of opium** is similar to paregoric and has the advantage of fewer additives than paregoric. It has 10 mg/mL morphine equivalent and should be diluted to provide the same (morphine) dosage as paregoric.

3. **Phenobarbital** is an adequate drug for controlling withdrawal from narcotics, especially those of irritability, fussiness, and hyperexcitability. It is not as effective as paregoric for control of gastrointestinal symptoms or seizures after narcotic exposure. It is not suitable for dose titration because of its long half-life. It is mainly useful for treatment of withdrawal from nonnarcotic agents. The dosage is a 20-mg/kg loading dose, followed by 4 mg/kg/day maintenance. Once symptoms have been controlled for 1 week, decrease the daily dose by 25% every week.

4. **Chlorpromazine** is quite effective in controlling symptoms of withdrawal from both narcotics and nonnarcotics. It has multiple untoward side effects (it reduces seizure threshold, cerebellar dysfunction, and hematologic problems) that make it potentially undesirable for use in neonates when alternatives can be used. The dosage is 3 mg/kg/day, divided into 3–6 doses/day.

5. **Clonidine** has been used for withdrawal from both narcotic and nonnarcotic agents. The dosage is 3–4 mcg/kg/day, divided into 4 doses/day.

6. **Diazepam** has been used to treat withdrawal from narcotics. One study showed a greater incidence of seizures after methadone withdrawal when infants were treated with diazepam rather than paregoric. When used to treat methadone withdrawal, it also impairs nutritive sucking more than does methadone alone. It may produce apnea when used with phenobarbital. It may be used for treatment of withdrawal from benzodiazepines and possibly also for the hyperexcitable phase after cocaine exposure. The dosage is 0.5–2 mg every 6–8 h.

7. **Combination therapy.** Coyle et al (2002) found that the combination of diluted tincture of opium (DTO) in combination with phenobarbital was superior to treatment with DTO alone. Patients given this combination spent less time with severe withdrawal and required less DTO, and duration of hospitalization was reduced by 48%.

C. **Long-term management.** If the infant is discharged after 4 days, an early appointment with the pediatrician should be arranged and the parents should be informed as to possible signs of delayed-onset withdrawal. During the first few years of life, infants exposed to drugs in utero may have various neurobehavioral problems. Minor signs and symptoms of drug withdrawal may continue for a few months after discharge. This places a difficult infant in a difficult home situation. There are a few reports of an increased incidence of child abuse in these circumstances. Thus, frequent follow-up visits and close involvement of social services may be required.

XII. **Breast-feeding.** The various drugs of abuse may be presumed to enter breast milk, and there have been reports of intoxication in breast-fed infants whose mothers had continued to abuse drugs. Mothers on low-dose methadone have been allowed to breast-feed, but this required close supervision and there was a constant concern that unsupervised weaning would precipitate withdrawal. The cautious course would be to dissuade these mothers from breast-feeding unless there is reasonable certainty that they will discontinue their habits.

XIII. **Warning.** Naloxone (Narcan) may precipitate acute drug withdrawal in infants exposed to narcotics. It should **not** be used in infants born to mothers suspected of abusing opiates.

REFERENCES

Azuma SD, Chasnoff IJ: Outcome of children prenatally exposed to cocaine and other drugs: a path analysis of three-year data. *Pediatrics* 1993;92:396.

Buehler BA et al: Teratogenic potential of cocaine. *Semin Perinatol* 1996;20:93.

Callahan CM et al: Measurement of gestational cocaine exposure: sensitivity of infants' hair, meconium, and urine. *J Pediatr* 1992;120:763.

Coyle MG et al: Diluted tincture of opium (DTO) and phenobarbital versus DTO alone for neonatal opiate withdrawal in term infants. *J Pediatr* 2002;140:561.

Day NL: Research on the effects of prenatal alcohol exposure—a new direction. *Am J Public Health* 1995;85:1614.

Dusick AM et al: Risk of intracranial hemorrhage and other adverse outcomes after cocaine exposure in a cohort of 323 very low birth weight infants. *J Pediatr* 1993;122:438.

Frank DA et al: Growth, development, and behavior in early childhood following prenatal cocaine exposure. A systematic review. *JAMA* 2001;285:1613.

Frank DA et al: Maternal cocaine use: impact on child health and development. *Curr Probl Pediatr* 1996;26:52.

Fried PA: Prenatal exposure to tobacco and marijuana: effects during pregnancy, infancy, and early childhood. *Clin Obstet Gynecol* 1993;36:319.

Hawley TL: The development of cocaine-exposed children. *Curr Probl Pediatr* 1994;24:259.

Holzman C et al: Perinatal brain injury in premature infants born to mothers using alcohol in pregnancy. *Pediatrics* 1995;95:66.

Howard BJ, O'Donnell KJ: What is important about a study of within-group differences of 'cocaine babies'? *Arch Pediatr Adolesc Med* 1995;149:663.

Jacobson SW et al: New evidence for neurobehavioral effects of in utero cocaine exposure. *J Pediatr* 1996;129:581.

Kain ZN et al: Cocaine exposure in utero: perinatal development and neonatal manifestations—review. *Clin Toxicol* 1992;30:607.

King TA et al: Neurologic manifestations of in utero cocaine exposure in near-term and term infants. *Pediatrics* 1995;96:259.

Little BB et al: Is there a cocaine syndrome? Dysmorphic and anthropometric assessment of infants exposed to cocaine. *Teratology* 1996;54:145.

Loebstein R, Koren G: Pregnancy outcome and neurodevelopment of children exposed in utero to psychoactive drugs: the Motherisk experience. *J Psychiatry Neurosci* 1997;22:192.

Lutiger B et al: Relationship between gestational cocaine use and pregnancy outcome: a meta-analysis. Teratology 1991;44:405.

Nulman I et al: Neurodevelopment of adopted children exposed in utero to cocaine. Can Med Assoc J 1994;151:1591.

Ostrea EM et al: Estimates of illicit drug use during pregnancy by maternal interview, hair analysis, and meconium analysis. J Pediatr 2001;138:344.

Ostrea EM ot al; Mortality within the first 2 years in infants exposed to cocaine, opiate, or cannabinoid during gestation. Pediatrics 1997;100:79.

Pierog S et al: Withdrawal symptoms in infants with the fetal alcohol syndrome. J Pediatr 1977; 90:630.

Pietrantoni M, Knuppel RA: Alcohol use in pregnancy. Clin Perinatol 1991;18:93.

Richardson GA et al: Pronatal cocaine exposure: effects on the development of school-age children. Neurotoxicol Teratol 1996;18:627.

Singer LT ot al: Cognitive and motor outcomes of cocaine-exposed infants. JAMA 2002;287: 1952.

Slutsker L: Risks associated with cocaine use during pregnancy. Obstet Gynecol 1992;79:778.

Stromland K, Hellstrom A· Fetal alcohol syndrome—an ophthalmological and socioeducational prospective study. Pediatrics 1996;97:845.

Theis JGW et al: Current management of the neonatal abstinence syndrome: a critical analysis of the evidence. Biol Neonate 1997;71:345.

Vega WA el al: Prevalence and magnitude of perinatal substance exposure in California. N Engl J Med 1993;329:850.

Volpe JJ: Effect of cocaine use on the fetus. N Engl J Med 1992;327:399.

68 Infectious Diseases

Isolation precautions for all infectious diseases, including maternal and neonatal precautions, breast-feeding, and visiting issues, can be found in Appendix G.

NEONATAL SEPSIS

I. **Definition.** Neonatal sepsis is a clinical syndrome of systemic illness accompanied by bacteremia occurring in the first month of life.

II. **Incidence.** The incidence of primary sepsis is 1–8 per 1000 live births and as high as 13–27 per 1000 for infants weighing <1500 g. The mortality rate is high (13–25%); higher rates are seen in premature infants and in those with early fulminant disease.

III. **Pathophysiology.** In considering the pathogenesis of neonatal sepsis, three clinical situations may be defined: early-onset, late-onset, and nosocomial disease.

A. **Early-onset disease** presents in the first 5–7 days of life and is usually a multisystem fulminant illness with prominent respiratory symptoms. Typically, the infant has acquired the organism during the intrapartum period from the maternal genital tract. In this situation, the infant is colonized with the pathogen in the perinatal period. Several infectious agents, notably treponemes, viruses, *Listeria,* and probably *Candida,* can be acquired transplacentally via hematogenous routes. Acquisition of other organisms is associated with the birth process. With rupture of membranes, vaginal flora or various bacterial pathogens may ascend to reach the amniotic fluid and the fetus. Chorioamnionitis develops, leading to fetal colonization and infection. Aspiration of infected amniotic fluid by the fetus or neonate may play a role in resultant respiratory symptoms. The presence of vernix or meconium impairs the natural bacteriostatic properties of amniotic fluid. Finally, the infant may be exposed to vaginal flora as it passes through the birth canal. The primary sites of colonization tend to be the skin, nasopharynx, oropharynx, conjunctiva, and umbilical cord. Trauma to these mucosal surfaces may lead to infection. Early-onset disease is characterized by a sudden onset and fulminant course that can progress rapidly to septic shock with a high mortality rate.

B. **Late-onset disease** may occur as early as 5 days of age; however, it is more common after the first week of life. Although these infants may have a history of obstetric complications, these are associated less frequently than with early-onset disease. These infants usually have an identifiable focus, most often meningitis in addition to sepsis. Bacteria responsible for late-onset sepsis and meningitis include those acquired after birth from the maternal genital tract as well as organisms acquired after birth from human contact or from contaminated equipment. Therefore, horizontal transmission appears to play a significant role in late-onset disease. The reasons for delay in development in clinical illness, the predilection for central nervous system (CNS) disease, and the less severe systemic and cardiorespiratory symptoms are unclear. Transfer of maternal antibodies to the mother's own vaginal flora may play a role in determining which exposed infants become infected, especially in the case of group B streptococcal infections.

C. **Nosocomial sepsis.** This form of sepsis occurs in high-risk newborn infants. Its pathogenesis is related to the underlying illness and debilitation of the infant, the flora in the neonatal intensive care (NICU) environment, and invasive monitoring and other techniques used in neonatal intensive care. Breaks in the natural barrier function of the skin and intestine allow this opportunistic organism to overwhelm the neonate. Infants, especially premature infants, have an increased susceptibility to infection because of underlying illnesses and immature immune defenses that are less efficient at localizing and clearing bacterial invasion.

D. Causative organisms. The principal pathogens involved in neonatal sepsis have tended to change with time. Primary sepsis must be contrasted with nosocomial sepsis. The agents associated with primary sepsis are usually the vaginal flora. Most centers report **group B streptococci (GBS)** as the most common, followed by **Gram-negative enteric organisms**, especially *Escherichia coli*. Other pathogens include *Listeria monocytogenes, Staphylococcus*, other **streptococci** (including the **enterococci**), **anaerobes**, and *Haemophilus influenzae*. In addition, many unusual organisms are documented in primary neonatal sepsis, especially in premature infants. The flora causing nosocomial sepsis vary in each nursery. **Staphylococci** (especially *Staphylococcus epidermidis*), gram-negative rods (including *Pseudomonas, Klebsiella, Serratia,* and *Proteus*) and fungal organisms predominate.

IV. Risk factors
  A. Prematurity and low birth weight. Prematurity is the single most significant factor correlated with sepsis. The risk increases in proportion to the decrease in birth weight.
  B. Rupture of membranes. Premature or prolonged (>18 h) rupture of membranes.
  C. Maternal peripartum fever (≥38 °C/100.4 °F) or infection. Chorioamnionitis, urinary tract infection (UTI), vaginal colonization with GBS, previous delivery of a neonate with GBS disease, perineal colonization with *E. coli*, and other obstetric complications.
  D. Amniotic fluid problems. Meconium-stained or foul-smelling, cloudy amniotic fluid.
  E. Resuscitation at birth. Infants who had fetal distress, were born by traumatic delivery, or were severely depressed at birth and required intubation and resuscitation.
  F. Multiple gestation.
  G. Invasive procedures. Invasive monitoring and respiratory or metabolic support.
  H. Infants with galactosemia (predisposition to *E. coli* sepsis), immune defects, or asplenia.
  I. Iron therapy (iron added to serum in vitro enhances the growth of many organisms).
  J. Other factors. Males are 4 times more affected than females, and the possibility of a sex-linked genetic basis for host susceptibility is postulated. Variations in immune function may play a role. Sepsis is more common in black than in white infants, but this may be explained by a higher incidence of premature rupture of membranes, maternal fever, and low birth weight. Low socioeconomic status is often reported as an additional risk factor, but again this may be explained by low birth weight. NICU staff and family members are often vectors for the spread of microorganisms, primarily as a result of improper hand washing.

V. Clinical presentation. The initial diagnosis of sepsis is, by necessity, a clinical one because it is imperative to begin treatment before the results of culture are available. Clinical signs and symptoms of sepsis are nonspecific, and the differential diagnosis is broad, including respiratory distress syndrome (RDS), metabolic diseases, hematologic disease, CNS disease, cardiac disease, and other infectious processes (ie, TORCH infections [see pp 441–442]). Clinical signs and symptoms most often mentioned include the following:
  A. Temperature irregularity. Hypo- or hyperthermia (greater heat output required by the incubator or radiant warmer to maintain a neutral thermal environment or frequent adjustments of the infant servocontrol probe).
  B. Change in behavior. Lethargy, irritability, or change in tone.

C. **Skin.** Poor peripheral perfusion, cyanosis, mottling, pallor, petechiae, rashes, sclerema, or jaundice.
D. **Feeding problems.** Feeding intolerance, vomiting, diarrhea (watery loose stool), or abdominal distention with or without visible bowel loops.
E. **Cardiopulmonary.** Tachypnea, respiratory distress (grunting, flaring, and retractions), apnea within the first 24 h of birth or of new onset (especially after 1 week of age), tachycardia, or hypotension, which tends to be a late sign.
F. **Metabolic.** Hypo- or hyperglycemia or metabolic acidosis.

VI. **Diagnosis**
A. **Laboratory studies**
  1. **Cultures.** Blood and other normally sterile body fluids should be obtained for culture. (In neonates <24 h of age, a sterile urine specimen is not necessary, given that the occurrence of UTIs is exceedingly rare in this age group.) Positive bacterial cultures will confirm the diagnosis of sepsis. Computer-assisted, automated blood culture systems have been shown to identify up to 94% of all microorganisms by 48 h of incubation. Results may vary because of a number of factors, including maternal antibiotics administered before birth, organisms that are difficult to grow and isolate (ie, anaerobes), and sampling error with small sample volumes (the optimal amount is 1–2 mL/sample). Therefore, in many clinical situations, infants are treated for "presumed" sepsis despite negative cultures, with apparent clinical benefit. Some *controversy* currently exists as to whether a spinal tap is needed in asymptomatic newborns being worked up for early-onset presumptive sepsis. Many institutions perform lumbar punctures only on infants who are clinically ill or who have documented positive blood cultures.
  2. **Gram's stain of various fluids.** Gram's staining is especially helpful for the study of CSF. Gram-stained smears and cultures of amniotic fluid or of material obtained by gastric aspiration are often performed. White blood cells in the samples can be maternal in origin, and their presence along with bacteria indicates exposure and possible colonization but not necessarily actual infection.
  3. **Adjunctive laboratory tests**
    a. **White blood cell count with differential.** These values alone are very nonspecific. There are references for total white blood cell count and absolute neutrophil count (probably a better measure) as a function of postnatal age in hours (see Chapter 54, particularly Tables 54–1 and 54–2). Neutropenia may be a significant finding with an ominous prognosis when associated with sepsis. The presence of immature forms is more specific but still rather insensitive. Ratios of bands to segmented forms >0.3 and of bands to total polymorphonuclear cells >0.1 have good predictive value, if present. A variety of conditions other than sepsis can alter neutrophil counts and ratios, including maternal hypertension and fever, neonatal asphyxia, meconium aspiration syndrome, and pneumothorax. Serial white blood cell counts several hours apart may be helpful in establishing a trend.
    b. **Platelet count.** A decreased platelet count is usually a late sign and is very nonspecific.
    c. **Acute-phase reactants** are a complex multifunctional group comprising complement components, coagulation proteins, protease inhibitors, C-reactive protein (CRP), and others that rise in concentration in the serum in response to tissue injury.
      i. **CRP** is an acute-phase reactant that increases the most in the presence of inflammation caused by infection or tissue injury. The highest concentrations of CRP have been reported in patients with bacterial infections, whereas moderate elevations typify chronic inflammatory conditions. Synthesis of acute-phase proteins by hepa-

tocytes is modulated by cytokines. Interleukin-1β (IL-1β), IL-6, IL-8, and tumor necrosis factor (TNF) are the most important regulators of CRP synthesis. After onset of inflammation, CRP synthesis increases within 4–6 h, doubling every 8 h, and peaks at about 36–50 h. Levels remain elevated with ongoing inflammation, but with resolution they decline rapidly due to a short half-life of 4–7 h. CRP is, therefore, superior to other acute-phase reactants that rise much slower. CRP demonstrates high sensitivity and negative predictive value. A single normal value cannot rule out infection because the sampling may have preceded the rise in CRP. Serial determinations are, therefore, indicated. CRP elevations in noninfected neonates have been seen with fetal hypoxia, RDS, and meconium aspiration. As well, a false-positive rate of 8% has been found in healthy neonates. Nonetheless, CRP is a valuable adjunct in the diagnosis of sepsis, monitoring the response to treatment, as well as guiding duration of treatment.

    ii. **The standard erythrocyte sedimentation rate** may be elevated but usually not until well into the illness and, therefore, is used rather infrequently in the initial workup.

    iii. **Cytokines IL-1β, IL-6, IL-8, and TNF** are produced primarily by activated monocytes and macrophages and are major mediators of the systemic response to infection. Studies have shown that combined use of IL-8 and CRP as part of the workup for bacterial infection reduces unnecessary antibiotic treatment.

    iv. **Surface neutrophil CD11** has been shown to be an excellent marker of early infection that correlates well with CRP but peaks earlier.

  d. **Miscellaneous tests.** Abnormal values for bilirubin, glucose, and sodium may, in the proper clinical situation, provide supportive evidence for sepsis.

B. Radiologic studies

  1. **A chest x-ray film** should be obtained in cases with respiratory symptoms, although it is often impossible to distinguish GBS or *Listeria* pneumonia from uncomplicated RDS. (GBS pneumonia may have associated pleural effusions.)

  2. **Urinary tract imaging. Imaging with renal ultrasound examination, renal scan, or voiding cystourethrography** should be part of the evaluation when UTI accompanies sepsis. Sterile urine for culture must be obtained by either a suprapubic (Chapter 17) or catheterized specimen (Chapter 18). Bag urine samples should not be used to diagnose UTI.

C. Other studies. Examination of the placenta and fetal membranes may disclose evidence of chorioamnionitis and thus an increased potential for neonatal infection.

VII. Management

A. GBS prophylaxis. GBS emerged as a major pathogen in the late 1960s and currently remains the most common cause of early-onset sepsis. Ten to 30% of pregnant women are colonized with GBS in the vaginal or rectal area. The incidence of infection has been estimated at 0.8–5.5/1000 live births (unchanged for the past three decades). Case fatality rate ranges from 5–15%. Consensus guidelines regarding management of GBS were published by Centers for Disease Control (CDC) in 1996 and were supported by American Association of Pediatrics and American College of Obstetricians and Gynecologists. The guidelines recommended one of two approaches: the prenatal screening approach (screening all pregnant women for GBS infection at 35–37 weeks' gestation and treatment of those women with positive cultures) and identifying women who present with risk factors and treating them during labor. To ensure appropriate treatment for neonates born to mothers who receive antibiotics for fever and presumed chorioamnionitis, as well as for those born to mothers who receive intrapartum antibiotic prophylaxis (IAP) because of GBS colonization, we are clinically using an algorithm in our hospital based on AAP guidelines, with some alterations based on our clinical experiences (Figure 68–1).

B. **Standard precautions** have been mandated by the U.S. Occupational Safety and Health Administration (OSHA) and apply to blood, semen, vaginal secretions, wound exudate, and cerebrospinal and amniotic fluids. Precautions include caution to prevent injuries when using or disposing of needles or other sharp instruments. Protective barriers appropriate for procedures should be used, including gloves, goggles, gowns, face shields, and other types of protection. Hands and exposed skin surfaces should be immediately and thoroughly washed after contamination with blood or other body fluids.

C. **Initial therapy.** Treatment is most often begun before a definite causative agent is identified. It consists of a **penicillin,** usually **ampicillin,** plus an **aminoglycoside** such as gentamicin. In nosocomial sepsis, the flora of the NICU must be considered; however, generally, staphylococcal coverage with **vancomycin plus either an aminoglycoside or a third-generation cephalosporin** is usually begun. Dosages are presented in Chapter 80.

D. **Continuing therapy** is based on culture and sensitivity results, clinical course, and other serial lab studies (eg, CRP). Monitoring for antibiotic toxicity is important as well as monitoring levels of aminoglycosides and vancomycin. When GBS is documented as the causative agent, a penicillin is the drug of choice; however, an aminoglycoside is often given as well because of documented synergism in vitro.

E. **Complications and supportive therapy**
  1. **Respiratory.** Ensure adequate oxygenation with blood gas monitoring, and initiate O_2 therapy or ventilator support if needed.
  2. **Cardiovascular.** Support blood pressure and perfusion to prevent shock. Use volume expanders, 10–20 mL/kg (normal saline, albumin, and blood), and monitor the intake of fluids and output of urine. Pressor agents such as dopamine or dobutamine may be needed (see Chapter 80).
  3. **Hematologic**
     a. **Disseminated intravascular coagulation (DIC).** With DIC, one may observe generalized bleeding at puncture sites, the gastrointestinal tract, or CNS sites. In the skin, large vessel thrombosis may cause gangrene. Laboratory parameters consistent with DIC include thrombocytopenia, increased prothrombin time, and increased partial thromboplastin time. There is an increase in fibrin split products or D-dimers. Measures include treating the underlying disease; fresh-frozen plasma, 10 mL/kg; vitamin K (Chapter 80); platelet infusion; and possible exchange transfusion (Chapter 21).
     b. **Neutropenia.** Multiple factors contribute to the increased susceptibility of neonates to infection, including developmental quantitative and qualitative neutrophil defects. Studies of infected neonates suggest that the use of recombinant human granulocyte colony–stimulating factor (rhG-CSF) or recombinant human granulocyte-macrophage colony–stimulating factor (rhGM-CSF) can partially counterbalance these defects and reduce morbidity and mortality. Further controlled studies with G-CSF and GM-CSF are required. Intravenous immunoglobulin (IVIG) does not appear useful as an adjunct to antibiotic therapy in serious neonatal infection.
  4. **CNS.** Implement seizure control measures (use phenobarbital, 20 mg/kg loading dose), and monitor for the syndrome of inappropriate antidiuretic hormone (SIADH) (decreased urine output, hyponatremia, decreased serum osmolarity, and increased urine specific gravity and osmolarity).

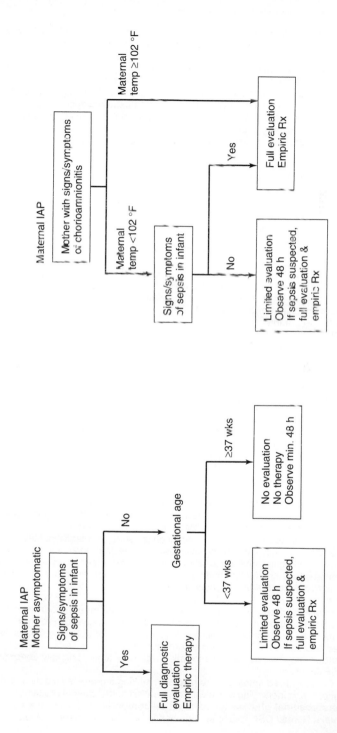

FIGURE 68–1. Management of the neonate after intrapartum antibiotic prophylaxis (IAP). Flow chart based on American Academy of Pediatrics guidelines with some alterations based on clinical experiences.

5. **Metabolic.** Monitor for and treat hypo- or hyperglycemia. Metabolic acidosis may accompany sepsis and is treated with bicarbonate and fluid replacement.
F. **Future developments.** Immunotherapy progress continues in the development of various hyperimmune globulins, monoclonal antibodies to the specific pathogens causing neonatal sepsis. They may prove to be significant adjuvants to the routine use of antibiotics for the treatment of sepsis. Research is also ongoing into blocking some of the body's own inflammatory mediators that result in significant tissue injury, including endotoxin inhibitors, cytokine inhibitors, nitric oxide synthetase inhibitors, and neutrophil adhesion inhibitors.

MENINGITIS

I. **Definition.** Neonatal meningitis is infection of the meninges and CNS in the first month of life. This is the most common time of life for meningitis to occur.
II. **Incidence.** The incidence is ~1 in 2500 live births. The **mortality rate** is 20–50%, and there is a high incidence ($\geq$ 50%) of neurodevelopmental sequelae in survivors.
III. **Pathophysiology.** In most cases, infection occurs because of hematogenous seeding of the meninges and CNS. In cases of CNS or skeletal anomalies (eg, myelomeningocele), there may be direct inoculation by flora on the skin or in the environment. Neonatal meningitis is often accompanied by **ventriculitis,** which makes resolution of infection more difficult. There is also a predilection for vasculitis, which may lead to hemorrhage, thrombosis, and infarction. Subdural effusions and brain abscess may also complicate the course.
   Most organisms implicated in neonatal sepsis also cause neonatal meningitis. Some have a definite predilection for CNS infection. **GBS** (especially type III) and the Gram-negative rods (especially *E. coli* with K1 antigen) are the **most common causative agents.** Other causative organisms include *L. monocytogenes,* other streptococci (enterococci), and other Gram-negative enteric bacilli (*Klebsiella, Enterobacter,* and *Serratia* spp).
   With CNS anomalies involving open defects or indwelling devices (eg, ventriculoperitoneal shunts), staphylococcal disease (*S. aureus* and *S. epidermidis*) is more common, as is disease caused by other skin flora, including streptococci and diphtheroids. Many unusual organisms, including fungi and anaerobes, have been described in case reports of neonatal meningitis in debilitated and normal neonates.
IV. **Risk factors.** Premature infants with sepsis have a much higher incidence (up to 3-fold) than term infants of CNS infection. Infants with CNS defects necessitating ventriculoperitoneal shunt procedures also are at increased risk.
V. **Clinical presentation.** The clinical presentation is usually nonspecific. Meningitis must be excluded in any infant being evaluated for sepsis or infection. Signs and symptoms of meningitis generally are similar to those reported for sepsis. A full or bulging fontanelle is often a late finding in meningitis. Syndrome of Inappropriate Antidiuretic Hormone (SIADH) may accompany meningitis.
VI. **Diagnosis**
   A. **Laboratory studies.** CSF examination is critical in the investigation of possible meningitis. Approximately 50% of all infants with positive CSF cultures for bacteria have negative blood cultures. The technique for obtaining fluid is discussed in Chapter 24. Normal values are found in Appendix D.
      1. **Culture** may be positive in association with normal or minimally abnormal CSF on inspection.
      2. **A Gram-stained** smear can be helpful in making a more rapid definitive diagnosis and identifying the initial classification of the causative agent.
      3. **Cerebrospinal glucose levels must be compared with serum glucose levels.** Normal CSF values are one half to two thirds of serum values.

4. **CSF protein** is usually elevated, although normal values for infants, especially preemies, may be much higher (up to 170 mg/dL) than in later life, and the test may be confounded by the presence of blood in the specimen.
5. **CSF pleocytosis** is variable. There are usually more cells with gram-negative rods than with GBS disease. Normal values range from 8–32 white blood cells in various studies, some of which may be polymorphonuclear cells. Pleocytosis (with neutrophils early) may also be an irritant reaction to CNS hemorrhage.
6. **Rapid antigen tests** are available for several organisms and should be done on spinal fluid.
7. **Ventricular tap,** with culture and examination fluid, is indicated in patients not responding to treatment.
B. **Radiologic studies**
1. **Cranial ultrasound examination** has been useful in the diagnosis of ventriculitis. (Echogenic strands can be seen in the ventricles.)
2. **Computed tomography (CT) scan** of the head may be indicated to rule out abscess, subdural effusion, or an area of thrombosis, hemorrhage, or infarction.
VII. **Management**
A. **Drug therapy.** For drug dosages and other pharmacologic information, see Chapter 80 *(Note:* Dosages for ampicillin, nafcillin, and penicillin G are doubled when treating meningitis.)
1. **Empiric therapy.** Optimal antibiotic selection depends on culture and sensitivity testing of causative organisms. **Ampicillin and gentamicin** are usually started as empiric therapy for suspected sepsis or meningitis. (For dosages, see Chapter 80.)
2. **Gram-positive meningitis (GBS and *Listeria*). Penicillin or ampicillin** is the drug of choice. These infections usually respond well to treatment. Administration for 14–21 days is indicated. (For dosages, see Chapter 80.)
3. **Staphylococcal disease. Nafcillin, methicillin, or vancomycin** should be substituted for penicillin or ampicillin as initial coverage. (For dosages, see Chapter 80.)
4. **Gram-negative meningitis.** The optimal treatment is still under investigation. Many organisms may be ampicillin-resistant, and penetration of CSF (even in the inflamed neonatal meninges) may be inadequate with aminoglycosides. Studies have shown no advantage to using intrathecal or intraventricular aminoglycosides. A better choice may be third-generation cephalosporins (eg, cefotaxime or cefuroxime). Currently, most clinicians would use **ampicillin plus cefotaxime** as initial therapy. In general, approximately 3 days are required to sterilize the CSF in infants with gram-negative meningitis, whereas in gram-positive meningitis sterilization usually occurs within 36–48 h. Follow-up CSF examination is recommended until sterility is documented. External ventricular drainage may be indicated in certain cases complicated by ventriculitis. Treatment should continue until 14 days after cultures are negative or for 21 days, whichever is longer.
B. **Supportive measures and monitoring for complications.** Head circumference should be measured daily, and transillumination of the head and neurologic examination should be performed frequently.

TORCH INFECTIONS

TORCH is an acronym (*t*oxoplasmosis; *o*thers such as syphilis, hepatitis B, coxsackievirus, Epstein-Barr, varicella-zoster virus (VZV), and human parvovirus; *r*ubella virus; *c*ytomegalovirus [CMV]; and *h*erpes simplex virus [HSV]) that denotes chronic nonbacterial perinatal infection. Herpetic disease in the neonate does not fit the pattern of chronic intrauterine infection but is traditionally grouped with the others. This group of infections may present in the neonate with similar clinical and laboratory findings (ie, small for gestational age, hepatosplenomegaly, rash, CNS manifestations, early jaundice, and low platelets), hence the usefulness of the TORCH concept.

TOXOPLASMOSIS

I. **Definition.** *Toxoplasma gondii* is an intracellular parasitic protozoan capable of causing intrauterine infection.
II. **Incidence.** The incidence of congenital infection is 1 in 1000 to 1 in 10,000 live births.
III. **Pathophysiology.** *T. gondii* is a coccidian parasite ubiquitous in nature. The primary natural host is the cat family. The organism exists in three forms: oocyst, tachyzoite, and tissue cyst (bradyzoites). The **oocysts** are excreted in cat feces. Ingestion of oocysts is followed by penetration of gastrointestinal mucosa by sporozoites and circulation of tachyzoites, the ovoid unicellular organism characteristic of acute infections. Most maternal organs, including the placenta, are "seeded" by the protozoan. Actual transmission to the fetus is by the transplacental-fetal hematogenous route. In the chronic form of the disease, organisms invade certain body tissues, especially those of the brain, eye, and striated muscle, forming bradyzoites.

Acute infection in the adult is often subclinical. If symptoms are present, they are generally nonspecific: mononucleosis-like illness with fever, lymphadenopathy, fatigue, malaise, myalgia, fever, skin rash, and splenomegaly. The vast majority of congenital toxoplasmosis cases are a result of acquired maternal primary infection during pregnancy; however, toxoplasmic reactivations can occur in immunosuppressed pregnant women and result in fetal infection. Placental infection occurs and persists throughout gestation. The infection may or may not be transmitted to the fetus. The later in pregnancy that infection is acquired, the more likely is transmission to the fetus (first trimester, 17%; second trimester, 25%; and third trimester, 65% transmission). Infections transmitted earlier in gestation are likely to cause more severe fetal effects (abortion, stillbirth, or severe disease with teratogenesis). Those transmitted later are more apt to be subclinical. Rarely, a parasite may be transmitted via an infected placenta during parturition. Infection in the fetus or neonate usually involves disease in one of two forms: infection of the CNS or the eyes, or infection of the CNS and eyes with disseminated infection. Seventy to 90% of infants with congenital infection are asymptomatic at birth. However, visual impairment, learning disabilities, or mental impairment becomes apparent in a large percentage of children months to several years later.
IV. **Risk factors.** *T. gondii* may be ingested during contact with soil or litter boxes contaminated with cat feces. It may also be transmitted in unpasteurized milk, in raw or undercooked meats (especially pork), and via blood product transfusion (white blood cells). Premature infants have a higher incidence of congenital toxoplasmosis than term infants (25–50% of cases in some series).
V. **Clinical presentation.** Congenital toxoplasmosis may be manifested as clinical neonatal disease, disease in the first few months of life, late sequelae or relapsed infection, or subclinical disease.
   A. **Clinical disease.** Those with evident clinical disease may have disseminated illness or isolated CNS or ocular disease. Late sequelae are primarily related to ocular or CNS disease. **Obstructive hydrocephalus, chorioretinitis, and intracranial calcifications** form the **classic triad** of toxoplasmosis.
   B. **Prominent signs and symptoms** in infants with congenital toxoplasmosis include chorioretinitis, abnormalities of CSF (high protein value), anemia, seizures, intracranial calcifications, direct hyperbilirubinemia, fever, hepatosplenomegaly, lymphadenopathy, vomiting, microcephaly or hydrocephalus,

diarrhea, cataracts, eosinophilia, bleeding diathesis, hypothermia, glaucoma, optic atrophy, microphthalmos, rash, and pneumonitis.
  C. **Associated findings.** Toxoplasmosis has been associated with congenital nephrosis, various endocrinopathies (secondary to hypothalamic or pituitary effects), myocarditis, erythroblastosis with hydrops fetalis, and isolated mental retardation.
  D. **Subclinical disease.** Subclinical infection is believed to be the most common. Studies of these infants (in whom infection is identified by serologic testing or documented maternal infection) indicate that a large percentage may have minor CSF abnormalities at birth and later develop visual or neurologic sequelae or learning disabilities.
VI. **Diagnosis**
  A. **Laboratory studies.** The diagnosis of congenital toxoplasmosis is most often based on clinical suspicion plus serologic tests; however, many hospital-based and commercial laboratories frequently are misinterpreted or inaccurate. This is particularly true of indirect fluorescence test for immunoglobulin (Ig)G and IgM antibodies and of enzyme-linked immunosorbent assay (ELISA) systems for quantitation of IgM specific antibodies. An FDA warning has been issued about misinterpretation of IgM serologies. The recommendation is that all suspected infections be confirmed in a reference laboratory setting such as the Palo Alto Medical Foundation (telephone: 650-853-4828).
    1. **Direct isolation of the organism from body fluids or tissues** requires inoculating blood, body fluids, or placental tissue into mice or tissue culture and is not readily available. Isolation of the organism from placental tissue correlates strongly with fetal infection.
    2. **Serologic tests.** *Toxoplasma*-specific IgM antibodies can be measured by indirect fluorescent antibody (IFA) test, ELISA, or IgM immunosorbent agglutination assay (IgM-ISAGA); usually become positive within 1–2 weeks of infection; and persist for months or years, especially when very sensitive assays such as double-sandwich IgM enzyme immunoassay (DS-IgM EIA) or IgM-ISAGA are used. If IgM titers are high and accompanied by high specific IgG titers of >1:512, as measured by IFA or Sabin-Feldman dye test, this suggests acute infection. IgA antibodies are found in >95% of patients with acute infections. *Toxoplasma*-specific IgE antibodies are found in almost all women who seroconvert during pregnancy.
    3. **Perinatal diagnosis** can be made by using polymerase chain reaction (PCR) amplification of the B_1 gene of *T. gondii* in a sample of amniotic fluid. DS-IgM EIA and ISAGA detect *Toxoplasma* IgM in >75–80% of infants with congenital infection.
    4. **CSF examination** should be performed in suspected cases. The most characteristic abnormalities are xanthochromia, mononuclear pleocytosis, and a very high protein level. Tests for CSF IgM to toxoplasmosis may also be performed.
  B. **Radiologic studies**
    1. **A cranial ultrasonogram or CT scan of the head** may demonstrate characteristic intracranial calcifications (speckled throughout the CNS, including the meninges).
    2. **Long-bone films** may show abnormalities, specifically, metaphyseal lucency and irregularity of the line of calcification at the epiphyseal plates without periosteal reaction.
  C. **Other studies. Ophthalmologic examination** characteristically shows chorioretinitis. Other ocular features are often present at some stages.
VII. **Management. Congenital toxoplasmosis** is a treatable infection, although at present it is not curable. Therapeutic agents are effective in killing the tachyzoite phase of the parasite but are not capable of eradicating encysted bradyzoites. Treatment of acute maternal toxoplasmosis appears to reduce the risk of fetal wastage and decreases the likelihood of congenital infection. In most cases, maternal infection is not suspected.

A. Treatment of symptomatic infants during the first 6 months of life consists of a combination of **pyrimethamine, sulfadiazine,** and **leucovorin calcium** supplements. Pyrimethamine (1 mg/kg orally) is administered in 1 or 2 divided doses daily or every other day after an initial loading dose of 2 mg/kg/day for 2 days. A 100-mg/kg/day dose of sulfadiazine is given orally in 2 divided daily doses. Leucovorin calcium (5 mg) is given intramuscularly (IM) every 3 days (some suggest 10 mg 3 times/week). After a 6-month regimen, treatment can be continued or modified to include 1-month courses of **spiramycin** alternating with 1-month courses of pyrimethamine, sulfadiazine, and leucovorin calcium for an additional 6 months. **Spiramycin** is a macrolide antibiotic related to erythromycin; it is given daily at a dose of 100 mg/kg/day in 2 divided oral doses. Corticosteroids are somewhat *controversial;* often prednisone or methylprednisolone (1.5 mg/kg/day orally in 2 divided doses) is given in infants with chorioretinitis or elevations in spinal fluid protein to decrease the inflammatory response. Infants with a symptomatic congenital toxoplasmosis are also treated for 1 year. They receive an initial 6-week course of pyrimethamine, sulfadiazine, and leucovorin calcium, followed by alternating courses of spiramycin for 6 weeks, and the other three drugs repeated for 4 weeks. Healthy infants born to mothers with gestational toxoplasmosis can be treated with a 4-week course of pyrimethamine, sulfadiazine, and leucovorin calcium. If a diagnosis of congenital toxoplasmosis is established later, chemotherapy is continued as delineated for infants with subclinical *T. gondii* infections. Infants treated with pyrimethamine and sulfadiazine require weekly blood counts, platelet counts, and urine microscopy to detect any adverse drug effects.

B. Prevention. Pregnant women should avoid eating raw meat or raw eggs and avoid exposure to cat litter boxes or cat feces.

RUBELLA

I. Definition. Rubella is a viral infection capable of causing chronic intrauterine infection and damage to the developing fetus.

II. Incidence. Rubella vaccine has virtually eliminated cases of congenital rubella syndrome (CRS) in the developed world. However, rubella can still be prevalent in nonvaccinated immigrant populations.

III. Pathophysiology. Rubella virus is an RNA virus that typically has an epidemic seasonal pattern of increased frequency in the spring. Epidemics have occurred at 6- to 9-year intervals, and major pandemics, every 10–30 years. Humans are the only known hosts, with an incubation period of ~18 days after contact. Virus is spread by respiratory secretions and is also spread from stool, urine, and cervical secretions. A live virus vaccine has been available since 1969. Five to 20% of women of childbearing age are susceptible to rubella. There is a high incidence of subclinical infections. Maternal viremia is a prerequisite for placental infection, which may or may not spread to the fetus. Most cases occur after primary disease, although a few cases have been described after reinfection.

The fetal infection rate varies according to the timing of maternal infection during pregnancy. If infection occurs at 1–12 weeks, there is an 81% risk of fetal infection; at 13–16 weeks, 54%; at 17–22 weeks, 36%; at 23–30 weeks, 30%; there is a rise to 60% at 31–36 weeks; and 100% in the last month of pregnancy. No correlation exists between the severity of maternal rubella and teratogenicity. However, the incidence of fetal effects is greater the earlier in gestation that infection occurs, especially at 1–11 weeks, when 90% of infected fetuses will be damaged, 50% during weeks 11–20 and 37% from 20–35 weeks, while at later gestational ages they occur only occasionally. The virus sets up chronic infection in the placenta and fetus. Placental or fetal infection may lead to resorption of the fetus, spontaneous abortion, stillbirth, fetal infection from multisystem disease, congenital anomalies, or inapparent infection.

The disease involves angiopathy as well as cytolytic changes. Other viral effects include chromosome breakage, decreased cell multiplication time, and mitotic arrest in certain cell types. There is little inflammatory reaction.

IV. Risk factors. Women of childbearing age who are rubella nonimmune.

V. Clinical presentation. Congenital rubella has a wide spectrum of presentations, ranging from acute disseminated infection to deficits and defects not evident at birth.

    A. Teratogenic effects. These include intrauterine growth retardation, congenital heart disease (patent ductus arteriosus or pulmonary artery stenosis), sensorineural hearing loss, cataracts or glaucoma, neonatal purpura, and dermatoglyphic abnormalities.

    B. Systemic involvement can be manifested by adonitis, hepatitis, hepatosplenomegaly, jaundice, anemia, decreased platelets with or without petechiae, bony lesions, encephalitis, meningitis, myocarditis, eye lesions (iridocyclitis or retinopathy), or pneumonia.

    C. Later-presenting defects. More than one half of all newborns with congenital rubella are normal at birth; however, the majority later develop one or more signs and symptoms of disease, including immunologic dyscrasias, hearing deficit, psychomotor retardation, autism, brain syndromes such as subacute sclerosing panencephalitis, diabetes mellitus, and thyroid disease.

VI. Diagnosis

    A. Laboratory studies

        1. Open cultures. The virus can be cultured for up to 1 year despite measurable antibody titer. The best specimens for viral recovery are from nasal pharyngeal swabs, conjunctival scrapings, urine, and CSF (in decreasing order of usefulness).

        2. CSF examination may reveal encephalitis with an increased protein-cellular ratio in some cases.

        3. Serologic studies are the mainstay of rubella diagnosis, but the disease itself may cause immunologic aberrations and delay the infant's ability to mount IgM or IgG responses. ELISA for IgM and IgG antibodies are the most commonly performed tests.

    B. Radiologic studies. Long-bone films may show metaphyseal radiolucencies that correlate with metaphyseal osteoporosis. This is caused by virus-induced inhibition of mitosis of bone-forming cells.

VII. Management. There is no specific treatment for rubella. Long-term follow-up is needed secondary to late-onset symptoms. Prevention consists of vaccination of the susceptible population (especially young children). Vaccine should not be given to pregnant women. Passive immunization does not prevent fetal infection when maternal infection occurs. Children with congenital rubella should be considered contagious until they are at least 1 year old, unless nasopharyngeal and urine cultures are repeatedly negative for rubella virus. Rubella vaccine virus can be isolated from breast milk in lactating women who have received vaccine. However, breast-feeding is not a contraindication to vaccination because there is no evidence that the vaccine virus is in any way harmful to the infant.

CYTOMEGALOVIRUS

I. Definition. CMV is a DNA virus and a member of the herpesvirus group.

II. Incidence. CMV is the most common cause of congenital infection in the United States and occurs in approximately 0.5–1.5% of all live births. This results in ~40,000 new cases in this country per year.

III. Pathophysiology. CMV is a ubiquitous virus that may be transmitted in secretions, including saliva, tears, semen, urine, cervical secretions, blood (white blood cells), and breast milk. Seroconversion and initial infection often occur around the time of puberty, and shedding of the virus may continue for a long time. CMV can also become latent and reactivate periodically. Ten to 30% of pregnant women have cervical colonization with CMV. CMV is capable of penetrating the placental barrier as well as the blood-brain barrier. Both primary and recurrent maternal CMV can lead to transmission of virus to the fetus. When primary maternal infection occurs during pregnancy, virus is transmitted to the fetus in about 35% of cases. The risk does not appear to vary significantly with gestational age at time of maternal infection. During recurrent infection, transmission rate is only 0.2–1.8%. More than 90% of infants born with CMV have subclinical infection. Symptomatic infants are usually born to women with primary infection. **Symptomatic infants have a mortality rate of 20–30%.** Maternal virus-infected leukocytes are the proposed vehicle of transplacental transmission to the fetus. Fetal viremia is spread by the hematogenous route. The primary target organs are the CNS, eyes, liver, lungs, and kidneys. Characteristic histopathologic features of CMV include focal necrosis, inflammatory response, formation of enlarged cells with intranuclear inclusions (cytomegalic cells), and the production of multinucleated giant cells. CMV may also be transmitted to the infant at delivery (with cervical colonization), via breast milk, and via transfusion of seropositive blood to an infant whose mother is seronegative. There is no definite evidence of CMV transmission among hospital personnel.

IV. **Risk factors.** CMV infection in neonates has been associated with lower socioeconomic status, drug abuse, and sexual promiscuity in the mother. Premature infants are more often affected than full-term infants. Transfusion with unscreened blood is an additional risk factor for neonatal disease.

V. **Clinical presentation**

   A. **Subclinical infection** is 10 times more common than clinical illness.

   B. **Low birth weight.** Maternal CMV infection is associated with low birth weight and small for gestational age infants even when the infant is not infected.

   C. **Classic CMV inclusion disease** consists of intrauterine growth retardation, hepatosplenomegaly with jaundice, abnormal liver function tests (LFTs), thrombocytopenia with or without purpura, and severe CNS disease (CNS and sensory impairments are seen in 50–90% of symptomatic newborns), including microcephaly, intracerebral calcifications (most characteristically in the subependymal area), chorioretinitis, and progressive sensorineural hearing loss (10–20% of cases). Other symptoms include hemolytic anemia and pneumonitis. By 2 years of age, 5–15% of infants who are asymptomatic at birth may experience serious sequelae, such as hearing loss or ocular abnormalities.

   D. **Late sequelae.** With subclinical infection, late sequelae such as mental retardation, learning disability, and sensorineural hearing loss have been attributed to CMV. Studies have now shown for children with asymptomatic congenital CMV infection a prevalence of sensorineural hearing loss of 7–15%. Approximately one half had bilateral loss, and 50% of affected children had progressive deterioration. Repeated auditory evaluation during the first 3 years is strongly recommended.

VI. **Diagnosis**

   A. **Laboratory studies**

      1. **Culture for demonstration of the virus.** The "gold standard" for CMV diagnosis is urine or saliva culture. Most urine specimens from infants with congenital CMV are positive within 48–72 h. Many laboratories now use a shell vial tissue culture technique with detection of CMV-induced antigens by monoclonal antibodies, allowing for identification of the virus within 18 h. Studies evaluating a rapid assay for detection of CMV in saliva as a screening method for congenital infection have shown it to be at least as sensitive a method for detecting congenital infection as for detection of viruria. Given that saliva can be collected with less difficulty and expense, it may eventually replace the current use of urine screening.

      2. **PCR** is used by some labs; however, it does not appear to offer any advantage over culture-based methods.

3. **Serologic tests** based on detection of IgM should not be used to diagnose congenital CMV because they are less sensitive and more subject to false-positive results than culture or PCR.
   B. **Radiologic studies.** Skull films or CT scans of the head may demonstrate characteristic intracranial calcifications.
VII. **Management**
   A. **Postdiagnosis evaluation.** CT scan of the brain, ophthalmologic examination, brainstem evoked responses (BER) hearing evaluation, complete blood cell count, platelet count, liver enzyme levels, bilirubin level, CSF for cell count, protein and glucose, CSF CMV culture, or test for CMV DNA.
   B. **Antiviral agents.** No antiviral agent is yet approved for treatment of congenital CMV. Ganciclovir has been shown in preliminary studies to be partially effective in the treatment of retinochoroiditis and pneumonitis in immunosuppressed patients; however, controlled studies of the treatment of congenital CMV infection are currently being performed, and subsequent 5-year follow-up will be required. Ganciclovir is mutagenic, teratogenic, and carcinogenic. Under life-threatening circumstances, a dose of 5–6 mg/kg intravenously (IV) every 8 h can be considered. A study to evaluate a CMV-specific monoclonal antibody is ongoing.
   C. **Prevention.** Efforts are focused primarily on the development of a safe vaccine. A phase II clinical trial of a recombinant subunit vaccine in young women is underway, and a new genetically engineered live virus vaccine entered phase I clinical trials. Affected infants may excrete the virus for months to years and are often a concern to personnel caring for them. Standard precautions, especially good hand washing after diaper changes, is particularly important for pregnant personnel.

HERPES SIMPLEX VIRUS

I. **Definition.** HSV is a DNA virus related to CMV, Epstein-Barr virus, and varicella virus and is among the most prevalent of all viral infections encountered by humans.
II. **Incidence.** The estimated rate of occurrence of neonatal HSV is 1 in 3000 to 1 in 10,000 deliveries per year.
III. **Pathophysiology.** Two serologic subtypes can be distinguished by antigenic and serologic tests: HSV-1 (orolabial) and HSV-2 (genital). Three quarters of neonatal herpes infections are secondary to HSV-2; the remainder are caused by HSV-1. HSV-1, however, is the cause of 7–50% of primary genital herpes infections. HSV infection of the neonate can be acquired at one of three times: intrauterine, intrapartum, or postnatal. Most infections (80%) are acquired in the intrapartum period as ascending infections with ruptured membranes (4–6 h is considered a critical period for this to occur) or by delivery through an infected cervix or vagina. The usual portals of entry for the virus are the skin, eyes, mouth, and respiratory tract. Once colonization occurs, the virus may spread by contiguity or via a hematogenous route. The incubation period is from 2–20 days. Three general patterns of neonatal HSV are disease localized to the skin, eyes, and mouth (SEM); CNS involvement (with or without SEM involvement); and disseminated disease (which also may include signs of the first 2 groups). Thirty-three percent of infants born vaginally to mothers with a primary infection will themselves have HSV compared with only 3–5% of those born to mothers with recurrent infection. Maternal antibody is not necessarily protective in the fetus.
IV. **Risk factors.** The risk of genital herpes infection may vary with maternal age, socioeconomic status, and number of sexual partners. Only ~25–33% of cases have signs or symptoms of genital herpes at the time of labor and delivery despite having active infection. The primary infection may be "active" for as long as 2 months. Many neonatal infections occur because of asymptomatic cervical shedding of virus, usually after a primary episode of HSV infection.

V. Clinical presentation. The disease may be localized or disseminated. Humoral and cellular immune mechanisms appear important in preventing initial HSV infections or limiting their spread. Infants with disseminated and SEM disease usually are brought in for medical attention within the first 2 weeks of life, whereas those with disease localized to the CNS usually are seen between the 2nd and 3rd weeks of life. More than 20% of infants with disseminated disease and 30–40% of infants with encephalitis will never have skin vesicles.

A. Localized infections involving the skin, eyes, or oral cavity usually manifest at 10–11 days of age and account for ~40% of neonatal herpes. **Skin lesions** vary from discrete vesicles to large bullous lesions and occasionally denude the skin. There is skin involvement in 90% of SEM cases. Assertive **mouth lesions** (~10% of SEM cases) with or without cutaneous involvement can be seen. **Ocular findings** include keratoconjunctivitis and chorioretinitis. Before the availability of effective antiviral agents, up to 30% of children with SEM disease experienced neurologic impairment. Even with treatment, there is still a risk of neurologic sequelae, usually manifested between 6 and 12 months of age. With SEM, there is increased morbidity with three or more recurrences in the first 6 months of life.

B. Disseminated disease carries the worst prognosis with respect to mortality and long-term sequelae. It involves the **liver and adrenal glands** as well as virtually any other organ. Approximately one half of these cases also have localized disease as described previously. Infants with disseminated HSV infection account for 25% of all neonatal herpes patients. Usually, they present at 9–11 days of age. Presentation may include the signs and symptoms of localized disease as well as anorexia, vomiting, lethargy, fever, jaundice (with abnormal LFTs), rash or purpura, apnea, respiratory distress, bleeding, and shock. Presentation with bleeding and cardiovascular collapse may be sudden and rapidly fatal. CNS involvement is present in two thirds of these patients. Without antiviral therapy, 80% or more die, and most go on to have serious neurologic sequelae. The mortality rate remains as high as 55%, even with appropriate treatment; however, 40–55% of survivors suffer long-term neurologic impairment.

C. Encephalitis. CNS involvement can present with or without SEM lesions. Clinical manifestations of encephalitis include seizures (focal and generalized), lethargy, irritability, tremors, poor feeding, temperature instability, a bulging fontanelle, and pyramidal tract signs. These infants usually present at 15–17 days of age (30–40% will have no herpetic skin lesions), and the mortality rate is ~17%; however, it may be as high as 50% in untreated patients. Of survivors, 40% have long-term neurologic sequelae, such as psychomotor retardation. CSF findings are variable: typically mild pleocytosis, increased protein, and slightly low glucose.

VI. Diagnosis

A. Laboratory studies

1. **Viral cultures.** The virus grows readily, with preliminary results available in 24–72 h. Cultures are usually obtained from conjunctiva, throat, feces, urine, nasal pharynx, and CSF. Surface cultures obtained before 24–48 h of life may indicate exposure without infection. Recovery of virus from spinal fluid and characteristic lesions indicates infection regardless of the age of the infant.

2. **Immunologic assays** to detect HSV antigen in lesion scrapings, usually using monoclonal anti-HSV antibodies in either an ELISA or fluorescent microscopy assay, are very specific and 80–90% sensitive.

3. **Tzanck smear.** Cytologic examination of the base of skin vesicles is with a Giemsa or Wright stain, looking for characteristic but nonspecific giant cells and eosinophilic intranuclear inclusions. This is only about 50% sensitive and is plagued with false-positive results as well.

4. **Serologic tests** are not helpful in the diagnosis of neonatal infection, until a test for HSV IgM is readily available.

5. **PCR** to detect HSV DNA is a very sensitive method, as high as 100% in diagnosing HSV within CSF. Contamination, however, can frequently occur with this technique.
6. **Lumbar puncture** should be performed in all suspected cases. Evidence of hemorrhagic CNS infection with increased white and red blood cells and protein is found. PCR should also be performed on CSF.
B. **Radiologic studies.** CT scan of the head may be useful in the diagnosis of CNS disease, but magnetic resonance imaging (MRI) and an electroencephalogram (multiple independent foci of periodic slow and sharp wave discharge) are probably better for detecting earlier disease. In the neonate, CNS disease is more diffuse than in older patients.
C. **Other tests.** Brain biopsy may be needed in certain cases to confirm the diagnosis; however, PCR testing of CSF may make this obsolete.

VII. **Management**
A. **Antepartum.** The American College of Obstetrics and Gynecology (ACOG) has revoked previous guidelines of weekly antenatal surveillance cultures of the lower genital tract, because this has little correlation with virus spreading at the time of delivery. Most infants with neonatal herpes are delivered to women with no history of infection and no lesions at the time of delivery. The current ACOG guidelines for management of genital herpes infection in pregnancy include, most importantly, that a history of genital herpes in a pregnant woman or in her partner(s) should be solicited and recorded in the prenatal record. If a positive history is obtained, take the following steps:
1. **Studies are ongoing to determine** whether acyclovir therapy should be given to pregnant women who have a primary episode of genital HSV as well as to women with active infection (primary or secondary) near or at time of delivery.
2. **If there are no visible lesions** at the onset of labor or prodromal symptoms, vaginal delivery is acceptable.
3. **Deliver by cesarean section (C-section)** in women who have clinically apparent HSV infection (definitely for primary infection and most experts also recommend in secondary infection as well). Debate exists if membranes have already been ruptured for >6 h. Most experts still recommend C-section. These studies, especially including evaluation of the efficacy, safety, and cost of acyclovir prophylaxis administration to mothers in late pregnancy, may change the current recommended delivery route.
B. **Neonatal treatment**
1. **Isolation.** The Committee on Infectious Diseases of the American Academy of Pediatrics currently recommends that infants with known infection or exposure to HSV be placed in contact isolation. (Herpesvirus is coated with a lipid layer and is easily killed with detergent soaps and water.) For possibly exposed infants or those at low risk of infection, isolation goals may be met by allowing infants to room-in with mothers, if careful hand washing is observed.
2. **Infants born to mothers with a genital lesion.** If it is a known recurrent lesion and the infant is asymptomatic, the infection rate is 1–3%. Educate the parents regarding the signs and symptoms of early herpes infection. Consider surface screen cultures of the infant at 24–48 h of age. Treat if symptoms develop or if the culture is positive. If maternal infection is primary, the risk to the infant is 33–50%; therefore, most clinicians recommend empiric acyclovir at birth after cultures have been obtained. Some support no treatment initially if the infant is asymptomatic, and obtain cultures at 24–48 h.
3. **Pharmacologic therapy.** The first-line drug of choice is acyclovir with current recommendations for high-dose therapy of 60 mg/kg/day for 21 days for CNS and disseminated disease. The second choice being vidarabine (which requires 12-h infusion with a large volume of fluid). For doses, see Chapter 80. Trifluridine is the treatment of choice for ocular HSV infection in the neonate.

4. **Feedings.** The infant may breast-feed as long as no breast lesions are present on the mother, and the mother should be instructed in good hand-washing technique.
5. **Parents** with orolabial herpes should wear a mask when handling the newborn and should not kiss or nuzzle the infant.

VIRAL HEPATITIS

Hepatitis may be produced by many infectious and noninfectious agents. Typically, viral hepatitis refers to several clinically similar diseases that differ in cause and epidemiology. These include hepatitis A, B, C, D (delta), and E. To date, perinatal transmission of hepatitis D and E has not been well documented. It is unlikely that hepatitis A or E will prove to be a problem because they are not characterized by a chronic carrier state.

The differential diagnosis of a newborn liver disease includes neonatal hepatitis (giant cell), biliary atresia, metabolic disorders, antitrypsin deficiency, iron storage disease, and other infectious agents that cause hepatocellular injury (eg, CMV, rubella, varicella, toxoplasmosis, *Listeria,* syphilis, and tuberculosis, as well as bacterial sepsis, which can cause nonspecific hepatic dysfunction). Table 68–1 outlines various hepatitis panel tests useful in the management of this disease.

HEPATITIS A

I. **Definition.** Hepatitis A (**infectious hepatitis**) is caused by RNA virus transmitted by the fecal-oral route. A high concentration of virus is found in stools of infected persons, especially during the late incubation and early symptomatic phases (and

TABLE 68–1. HEPATITIS TESTING

Specific test	Description
HAV	Etiologic agent of "infectious" hepatitis
Anti-HAV	Detectable at onset of symptoms; lifetime persistence
Anti-HAV-IgM	Indicates recent infection with HAV; positive up to 4–6 months postinfection
Anti-HAV-IgG	Signifies previous HAV infection; confers immunity
HBV	Etiologic agent of "serum" hepatitis
HBsAg	Detectable in serum; earliest indicator of acute infection or indicative of chronic infection if present >6 months
Anti-HBs	Indicates past infection with and immunity to HBV, passive antibody from HBIG, or immune response from HBV vaccine
HBeAg	Correlates with HBV replication; high-titer HBV in serum signifies high infectivity; persistence for 6–8 weeks suggests a chronic carrier state
Anti-HBe	Presence in carrier of HBsAg suggests a lower titer of HBV and resolution of infection
HBcAg	No commercial test available; found only in liver tissue
Anti-HBc	High titer indicates active HBV infection; low titer presents in chronic infection
Anti-HBc-IgM	Recent infection with HBV positive for 4–6 months after infection; detectable in "window" period after surface antigen disappears
Anti-HBc-IgG	Appears later and may persist for years if viral replication continues
HVC	Etiologic agent of hepatitis C
Anti-HCV	Serologic determinant of hepatitis C infection

IgM and IgG, Immunoglobulins M and G; HAV, hepatitis A virus; anti-HAV, antibody to HAV (IgM and IgG subclasses); anti-HAV-IgM, IgM class antibody to HAV; anti-HAV-IgG, IgG class antibody to HAV; HBV, hepatitis B virus; HBsAg, hepatitis B surface antigen; anti-HBs, antibody to HBsAg; HBeAg, hepatitis B e antigen; anti-HBe, antibody to HBeAg; HBcAg, hepatitis B core antigen; anti-HBc, antibody to HBcAg; anti-HBc-IgM, IGM class antibody to HBcAg; anti-HBc-IgG, IgG class antibody to HBcAg; HVC, hepatitis C virus; anti-HCV, antibody to hepatitis C.

ceases before the onset of jaundice); it has not been found in urine or other body fluids. It causes the short-incubation form of viral hepatitis (15–50 days). There is no chronic carrier state.

II. **Pathophysiology.** Although it appears to be a very rare occurrence, one case report documented intrauterine transmission of hepatitis A. The risk of transmission is limited because the period of viremia is short and fecal contamination does not occur at the time of delivery.

III. **Clinical presentation.** Most infants are asymptomatic, with mild abnormalities of liver function.

IV. **Diagnosis**

A. **IgM antibody to hepatitis A virus (anti-HAV-IgM)** is present during the acute or early convalescent phase of disease. In most cases it becomes detectable 5–10 days after exposure and can persist for up to 6 months after infection. **Anti-HAV-IgG** appears in the convalescent phase, remains detectable, and confers immunity.

B. **LFTs.** Characteristically, the transaminases (aspartate transaminase [AST, or serum glutamic oxaloacetic transaminase or SGOT] and alanine transaminase [ALT, or serum glutamic pyruvic transaminase or SGPT]) and serum bilirubin levels (total and direct) are elevated, whereas the alkaline phosphatase level is normal.

V. **Management**

A. **Immune globulin,** 0.02 mL/kg IM, should be given to the newborn whose mother's symptoms began between 2 weeks before and 1 week after delivery. Hepatitis A vaccines are now available; however, effectiveness in postexposure prophylaxis is unknown; therefore, they are currently not recommended.

B. **Isolation.** The infant should be isolated with enteric precautions.

C. **Breast-feeding** is not contraindicated.

HEPATITIS B

I. **Definition.** Hepatitis B (**serum hepatitis**) is caused by a double-shelled DNA virus. It has a long incubation period (45–160 days) after exposure.

II. **Pathophysiology.** Each year in the United States approximately 20,000 infants are born to HBV-infected pregnant women, and without immunoprophylaxis approximately 5500 would become chronically infected. In the fetus and neonate, transmission has been suggested by the following mechanisms:

A. **Transplacental transmission** either during pregnancy or at the time of delivery secondary to placental leaks.

B. **Natal transmission** by exposure to hepatitis B surface antigen (HBsAg) in amniotic fluid, vaginal secretions, or maternal blood. This accounts for 90% of neonatal infections. The role of the mode of delivery in the transmission of HBV from mother to infant has not been fully determined.

C. **Postnatal transmission** by fecal-oral spread, blood transfusion, or other mechanisms.

III. **Risk factors**

A. **Factors associated with higher rates of HBV transmission** to neonates include the following:

1. The presence of HBe antigen and absence of anti-HBe in maternal serum: attack rates of 70–90%, with up to 90% of these infants being chronic carriers, compared with 15% of infants of anti-HBe-positive mothers.

2. Asian racial origin, particularly Chinese, with attack rates of 40–70%.

3. Maternal acute hepatitis in the third trimester or immediately postpartum (70% attack rate).

4. Higher-titer HBsAg in maternal serum (attack rates parallel the titer).

5. Antigenemia present in older siblings.

B. **Factors not related to transmission** include the following:

1. The particular HBV subtype in the mother.

2. The presence or absence of HBsAg in amniotic fluid.

3. The presence or titer of anti-HBc in cord blood.
IV. Clinical presentation. Maternal hepatitis B infection has not been associated with abortion, stillbirth, or congenital malformations. Prematurity has occurred, especially with acute hepatitis during pregnancy. Fetuses or newborns exposed to HBV present a wide spectrum of disease. The infants are rarely ill and usually asymptomatic; jaundice appears <3% of the time. Various clinical presentations include the following:
A. **Mild transient acute infection.**
B. **Chronic active hepatitis with or without cirrhosis.**
C. **Chronic persistent hepatitis.**
D. **Chronic asymptomatic HBsAg carriage.**
E. **Fulminant fatal hepatitis B (rare).**
V. Diagnosis
A. **Differential diagnosis.** Major diseases to consider include biliary atresia and acute hepatitis secondary to other viruses (eg, hepatitis A, CMV, rubella, and HSV).
B. **Transaminases.** AST (SGOT) and ALT (SGPT) levels may be markedly increased before the rise in bilirubin levels.
C. **Bilirubin** (direct and indirect) levels may be elevated. The rise in direct bilirubin will occur later.
D. **Liver biopsy** is occasionally indicated to differentiate biliary atresia from neonatal hepatitis.
E. **Hepatitis panel testing (see Table 68–1)**
   1. **Mother.** Test for HBsAg, HBeAg, anti-HBe, and anti-HBc.
   2. **Infant.** Test for HBsAg and anti-HBc-IgM. Most infants demonstrate antigenemia by 6 months of age, with peak acquisition at 3–4 months. Cord blood is not a reliable indicator of neonatal infection (1) because contamination could have occurred with antigen-positive maternal blood or vaginal secretions and (2) because of the possibility of noninfectious antigenemia from the mother.
VI. Management
A. **HBsAg-positive mother.** If the mother is HBsAg-positive, regardless of the status of her HBe antigen or antibody, the infant should be given hepatitis B immune globulin (HBIG), 0.5 mL IM, within 12 h after delivery. Additionally, hepatitis B vaccine, Recombivax (5 mcg [1.0 mL]) or Engerix (10 mcg [0.5 mL]) IM (in the anterolateral thigh), is given at birth and at 1 month and 6 months of age. If the first dose is given simultaneously with HBIG, it should be administered at a separate site, preferably in the opposite leg. For preterm infants weighing <2 kg, this initial dose of vaccine should not be counted in the required 3-dose schedule, and the subsequent 3 doses should be initiated when the infant weighs ≥2 kg. HBIG and HBV vaccinations do not interfere with routine childhood immunizations.
B. **Infant born to mother whose HBsAg status is unknown.** Test the mother as soon as possible. While awaiting the results, give the infant hepatitis B vaccine within 12 h of birth in the dose used for infants born to HBsAg-positive mothers. If the mother is found to be HBsAg-positive, the infant should receive HBIG (0.5 mL) within 7 days of birth. If the infant is preterm and the maternal HBsAg status cannot be determined within the initial 12 h after birth, HBIG should be given as well as hepatitis vaccine.
C. **Isolation.** Precautions are needed in handling blood and secretions.
D. **Breast-feeding.** HBsAg has been detected in breast milk of HBsAg-positive mothers but only with special concentrating techniques. One Taiwan study showed no difference in infection rates between bottle- and breast-fed infants. Given the efficacy of HBV vaccine with HBIG, even the theoretical risk for transmission through breast-feeding is of little concern, and breast-feeding can be encouraged.
E. **Vaccine efficacy.** The overall protective efficiency rate in neonates given HBV vaccine and HBIG exceeds 93%. The HBV-infected neonate is usually

asymptomatic but may develop mild clinical hepatitis and usually becomes a chronic carrier.
  F. **Immunization program.** The World Health Organization recommended that all countries add HBV vaccine to their routine childhood immunization program by 1997. Two dose schedules have been proposed; each includes 3 separate doses. In option 1, these are at birth, 1–2 months, and at 6–18 months; in option 2, doses should be given at 1–2 months, 4 months, and 6–18 months.

HEPATITIS C

  I. **Definition.** Hepatitis C virus (HCV) is a single-stranded RNA virus that accounts for 20% of all cases of acute hepatitis.
 II. **Pathophysiology.** Hepatitis C is transmitted primarily by parenteral and percutaneous means (eg, tattooing). Historically, exposure to blood and blood products was the most common source of infection; however, because of screening tests to exclude infectious donors, the risk of HCV is <0.01% per unit transfused. Vertical perinatal transmission of HCV ranges from 0–6%. In women coinfected with HCV and HIV, the transmission rate is higher (5–36%), most likely related to these women having higher titers of HCV RNA than do the HIV-negative women.
III. **Clinical presentation.** The average incubation period is generally 6–7 weeks, with a range of 2–26 weeks. Infants with acute hepatitis C typically are asymptomatic or have a mild clinical illness. Approximately 65–70% of patients experience chronic hepatitis, 20% cirrhosis, and 1–5% hepatocellular carcinoma.
 IV. **Diagnosis.** Detection of antibody to HCV (**anti-HCV**) in serum using second-generation EIAs with a recombinant immunoblot assay (**RIBA**) used as a confirmation test of positives (with both these tests having a 95% sensitivity and specificity). Highly sensitive reverse transcriptase (RT) **PCR tests** are available for detection and quantification of HCV RNA. LFTs may be elevated and fluctuate widely over time. The interval between exposure to HCV or onset of illness and detection of anti-HCV may be 5–6 weeks.
  V. **Management**
     A. **If the mother was infected during the last trimester,** the risk of transmission to the infant is highest. Immune globulin prophylaxis is not recommended. It does not appear that a vaccine against hepatitis C will be available for at least another several years.
     B. **Serologic testing** for anti-HCV in children born to HCV-infected women should not be done sooner than 2 years of age, when maternal anti-HCV will have decreased below detectable levels and endogenous anti-HCV is detectable in infected infants. RT-PCR for HCV RNA can be done at 1–2 months of age.
     C. **Breast-feeding.** Advise mothers that transmission of virus is possible; however, currently it is not believed to be a contraindication to breast-feeding.
 VI. **Treatment.** Interferon-α is the only treatment currently available for chronic HCV; however, it is not approved for use in patients <18 years old.

HEPATITIS D

Hepatitis D, also known as *delta hepatitis,* is a defective RNA virus that cannot survive independently and requires the helper function of DNA virus hepatitis B. Therefore, it occurs either as coinfection with hepatitis B or as superinfection of a hepatitis B carrier. It has been reportedly transmitted from mother to infant. Prevention of hepatitis B infection will prevent hepatitis D. There are, however, no available treatments to prevent it in HBsAg carriers before or after exposure. Management should be similar to that for hepatitis B infection (see prior discussion). Diagnosis of HDV is based on the detection of HDV antigen and IgM and IgG antibodies. It should be assessed in known carriers of hepatitis B because coinfection may lead to acute or fulminant hepatitis or a more rapid progression of chronic hepatitis.

HEPATITIS E

Hepatitis E was formerly known as enterically transmitted non-A, non-B hepatitis. It is rarely symptomatic in children <15 years old. There is a very high mortality rate (20%) when acquired in third-trimester pregnant women. Fetal loss usually occurs. Commercial kits are now available to detect anti-HEV. There is an ~1–2% prevalence of anti-HEV in the North American population. The only treatment is supportive.

VARICELLA-ZOSTER INFECTIONS

Varicella-zoster virus (VZV) is a member of the herpesvirus family. There are three forms of varicella-zoster infections that involve the neonate: fetal, congenital, and postnatal. In the mother, infection is usually manifested as typical chickenpox or occasionally as herpes zoster or shingles (intrauterine infection is less common than with maternal varicella).

FETAL VARICELLA-ZOSTER SYNDROME

I. **Definition.** This form occurs when the mother has her first exposure to VZV during pregnancy.
II. **Incidence.** This form is fortunately rare; the incidence of varicella during pregnancy is 1–7 per 10,000 pregnancies. The incidence of embryopathy and fetopathy after maternal varicella infection in the first 20 weeks is ~2%.
III. **Pathophysiology.** Transmission of the virus probably occurs via respiratory droplets. The virus replicates in the oropharynx, and viremia results, before the onset of rash, with transplacental passage to the fetus. Almost all cases reported have involved exposure between the 8th and 20th weeks of pregnancy, except for three reported cases of maternal varicella between 25 and 28 weeks. The defects are the result of viral replication and destruction of developing fetal ectodermal tissue.
IV. **Clinical presentation.** Clinical examination may disclose defects in a number of organ systems, as outlined next.
  A. **Limbs.** Hypoplasia or atrophy of an extremity, paralysis with muscular atrophy, and hypoplastic or missing fingers are frequent findings. This is caused by invasion of the brachial and lumbar plexus. Equinovarus is also seen.
  B. **Eyes.** Microphthalmos, chorioretinitis, cataracts, optic atrophy, and Horner's syndrome (ptosis, miosis, and enophthalmos).
  C. **Skin.** Findings are cicatricial skin lesions and the residua of infected bullous skin lesions.
  D. **CNS.** Microcephaly, seizures, encephalitis, cortical atrophy, and mental retardation in about one half of the patients. Calcifications frequently present.
V. **Diagnosis**
  A. **PCR and nucleic acid hybridization assays** can detect VZV DNA in fresh and formalin-fixed tissue samples of infants with signs of infection.
  B. **Serum VZV-specific IgM antibody.** This documents infection in the infant.
VI. **Management**
  A. **Mother.** If the mother is exposed to VZV infection in the first or second trimester, treat with **varicella-zoster immune globulin (VZIG)** if the history of varicella is negative or uncertain. (For dosage, see Chapter 80.) If chickenpox is diagnosed during pregnancy, antiviral therapy with acyclovir should be considered. This therapy has not been associated with congenital abnormalities, although the information is limited.
  B. **Infant.** Supportive care of the infant is required because there is usually profound neurologic impairment. The infant often dies because of secondary infections. Survivors usually suffer profound mental retardation and major neu-

rologic handicaps. Acyclovir therapy may be helpful to stop the progression of eye disease.

C. **Isolation.** Isolation is not necessary.

CONGENITAL VARICELLA-ZOSTER INFECTION

I. **Definition.** This is the form of the disease that occurs when a pregnant woman suffers chickenpox during the last 14–21 days of pregnancy or within the first few days postpartum. Disease begins in the neonate within the first 10 days of life.

II. **Incidence.** Although the congenital form is more common than the teratogenic form, it is still rare: Only 0.1 per 1000 pregnant women develop chickenpox.

III. **Pathophysiology.** There is an attack rate of 24–50% for the infant experiencing chickenpox within the first 10 days of life when maternal varicella occurs during the last 3 weeks of pregnancy. If the infant is born within 5 days of the onset of rash in the mother, the disease will be more severe because there is insufficient time for maternal antibody formation; the resulting death rate is 30% in untreated affected infants. If the onset of maternal disease is >5 days before delivery or infant disease onset is within the first 4 days of life, transplacental antibody transmission occurs and generally results in a milder case of chickenpox and deaths are infrequent.

IV. **Clinical presentation.** There may be only mild involvement of the infant, with vesicles on the skin, or the following may be seen:

A. **Skin.** A centripetal rash (beginning on the trunk and spreading to the face and scalp, sparing the extremities) begins as red macules and progresses to vesicles and encrustation. Lesions are more common in the diaper area and skinfolds. There may be 2 or 3 lesions or thousands of them. The differential diagnosis includes HSV and enterovirus. The main complication is staphylococcal and streptococcal secondary skin infections. Septicemia was seen in <0.5% of patients in one study.

B. **Lungs.** Lung involvement is seen in all fatal cases. It usually appears 2–4 days after the onset of the rash but may be seen up to 10 days after. Signs include fever, cyanosis, rales, and hemoptysis. Chest x-ray film shows a diffuse nodular-miliary pattern, especially in the perihilar region.

C. **Other organs.** Focal necrosis may be seen in the liver, adrenals, intestines, kidneys, and thymus. Glomerulonephritis, myocarditis, encephalitis, and cerebellar ataxia are sometimes seen.

V. **Diagnosis**

A. **PCR** is the most sensitive and specific method for detection of VZV DNA in clinical specimens. This is the method of choice for investigation of skin swabs, biopsies, and amniotic fluid for diagnosis of infections.

B. **Cultures.** VZV can be isolated from cultures of vesicular lesions during the first 3 days of the rash.

C. **Serum testing of VZV antibody.** Detection of IgM/IgA class antibodies is the most convincing for active infection. Testing during the acute and convalescent periods will document resolution.

VI. **Management**

A. **VZIG**

1. **Perinatal infection.** Infants of mothers who develop VZV infection within 5–7 days before or 48–72 h after delivery should receive 125 units of VZIG as soon as possible and not later than 96 h (see Chapter 80). These infants treated with VZIG should be placed in strict respiratory isolation for 28 days after receiving VZIG because treatment will prolong the incubation period. VZIG does not reduce the clinical attack rate in treated newborns; however, they tend to develop milder infections than the untreated neonates.

2. **Maternal rash occurring >7 days before delivery.** These infants do not need VZIG. It is believed that infants will have received antibodies via the placenta.

B. **Acyclovir** therapy at a dose of 10–15 mg/kg every 8 h should be considered in symptomatic neonates.
C. **Use antibiotics** if secondary bacterial skin infections occur.
D. **Serum test for VZV antibodies.** Performance of this test during the acute and convalescent periods documents resolution of the infection.

POSTNATAL VARICELLA-ZOSTER INFECTION

I. **Definition.** This form of the disease presents on days 10–28 of life. It does not represent transplacental infection from the mother.
II. **Pathophysiology.** Postnatal VZV infection occurs by droplet transmission. It is more common than congenital chickenpox. This disease is usually mild because of passive protection from maternal antibodies.
III. **Clinical presentation.** The typical chickenpox rash is seen with centripetal spread, beginning on the trunk and spreading to the face and scalp and sparing the extremities. All stages of the rash may appear at the same time, from red macules to clear vesicles to crusting lesions. Complications of this form of the disease are rare but may include secondary infections and varicella pneumonia.
IV. **Diagnosis.** Same as for congenital varicella-zoster (see the previous section).
V. **Management.** This form of the disease is usually mild, and death is extremely rare. Acyclovir therapy is *controversial*.
VI. **Nosocomial chickenpox in the neonatal nursery.**
  A. **VZIG** is recommended for infants of <28 weeks' gestational age or weighing ≤1000 g regardless of the maternal history. It is also recommended in premature infants whose mothers do not have a history of chickenpox.
  B. **Infants of >28 weeks' gestation** should have sufficient transplacental antibodies, if the mother is immune, to protect them from the risk of complications.
  C. **Isolation.** Exposed infants should be placed in strict isolation for 10–21 days after the onset of the rash in the index case. Exposed infants who receive VZIG should be in strict respiratory isolation for 28 days.

SYPHILIS

I. **Definition.** Syphilis is a sexually transmitted disease caused by *Treponema pallidum*. **Early congenital syphilis** is when clinical manifestations occur before 2 years of age; **late congenital syphilis** is when manifestations occur at >2 years of age. In 1990, a new surveillance case definition for congenital syphilis was adopted by the CDC to improve reporting of congenital syphilis by public health agencies. It calls for reporting all infants (and stillbirths) born to women with untreated or inadequately treated syphilis at delivery, regardless of neonatal symptoms or findings.
II. **Incidence.** Primary and secondary syphilis in the general population has increased in the late 1980s and early 1990s; however, it has subsequently declined (rates decreased 84% from 1990–1997) in all but large urban areas and the rural South. A major contributor to the increase had been the use of crack cocaine and the exchange of drugs for sex and multiple partners. The more recent downward trend is partly because of awareness of the syphilis epidemic with wider screening practices. An estimated 2–5 infants are affected with congenital syphilis for every 100 women diagnosed with primary or secondary syphilis.
III. **Pathophysiology.** Treponemas appear able to cross the placenta at any time during pregnancy, thereby infecting the fetus. Syphilis can cause preterm delivery, stillbirth (30–40% of fetuses with congenital syphilis are stillborn), congenital infection, or neonatal death, depending on the stage of maternal infection and duration of fetal infection before delivery. Untreated infection in the first and second trimesters often leads to significant fetal morbidity, whereas with third-trimester infection many infants are asymptomatic. Infection can also be acquired by the

neonate via contact of infectious lesions during passage through the birth canal. Virtually all infants born to untreated women with primary and secondary syphilis have congenital infection; 50% are clinically symptomatic. The infection rate is only 40% with early latent disease and 6–14% with late latent stages. The mortality rate may be as high as 54% in infected infants.

IV. Clinical presentation. Generally, neonates do not have signs of primary syphilis from in utero-acquired infection. Two thirds show no clinical signs of infection at birth and are identified by routine prenatal screening. Their manifestations are systemic and similar to those of adults with secondary syphilis. There is an additional 40–60% chance of CNS involvement. The most common findings in the neonatal period include hepatosplenomegaly, jaundice, and osteochondritis. Other signs include generalized lymphadenopathy, pneumonitis, myocarditis, nephrosis, pseudoparalysis (atypical Erb's palsy), rash (vesicobullous, especially on the palms and soles), hemolytic anemia (normocytic or normochromic), leukemoid reaction, and hemorrhagic rhinitis (snuffles). Late congenital syphilis manifests by Hutchinson's teeth, healed retinitis, eighth nerve deafness, saddle nose, mental retardation, arrested hydrocephalus, and saber shins. Other clues to the diagnosis of congenital syphilis include placentomegaly and congenital hydrops.

V. Diagnosis

  A. Laboratory studies. Patients with congenital or acquired syphilis produce several different antibodies, which are grouped as nonspecific, nontreponemal antibody (NTA) tests and specific antitreponemal antibody (STA) tests. NTA tests are inexpensive, rapid, and convenient screening tests that may indicate disease activity. They test a patient's serum or CSF for its ability to flocculate a suspension of a cardiolipin-cholesterol lecithin antigen. They are used as initial screening tests and quantitatively to monitor a patient's response to treatment and to detect reinfection and relapse. False-positive reactions can be secondary to autoimmune disease, IV drug addiction, aging, pregnancy, and many infections, such as hepatitis, mononucleosis, measles, and endocarditis. The interpretation of NTA and STA tests can be confounded by maternal IgG antibodies that are passed transplacentally to the fetus.

    1. Nonspecific reagin antibody tests. The two most often used of those nonspecific reagin antibody tests include the following.

      a. Venereal Disease Research Laboratory (VDRL) slide test. A VDRL titer at least 2 dilutions (4-fold) higher in the infant than in the mother signifies probable active infection. Titers should be monitored and repeated. If titers decrease in the first 8 months of life, the infant is probably not infected.

      b. Rapid plasma reagin test. This is an NTA test that detects antibodies to cardiolipin and is a screening test for syphilis. It should not be used on spinal fluid. A normal test result is negative, and any positive test should be followed up with a specific treponemal test. Titers can also be reported as for the VDRL test.

    2. Specific treponemal tests. Specific STA tests verify a diagnosis of current or past infection. These tests should be performed if NTA test results are positive. These antibody tests do not correlate with disease activity and are not quantified. They are useful for diagnosing a first episode of syphilis and for distinguishing a false-positive result of NTA tests. However, they have limited use for evaluating response to therapy and possible reinfections.

      a. FTA-ABS test. This test may be positive in the infant secondary to maternal transfer of IgG. If positivity persists after 6–12 months, the infant is probably infected.

      b. Microhemagglutination test for _T. pallidum_ (MHTPA). This test uses less serum and is easier than FTA to perform.

      c. IgM FTA-ABS. This test measures antibody to the treponeme developed by the infant. It is not as specific as initially thought because false positive results may occur. The test must be done at the CDC.

    d. Newer serologic assays. Direct antigen tests for *T. pallidum,* including an ELISA that uses monoclonal antibody to the organism's surface proteins, as well as a PCR test that can detect the organism in CSF, amniotic fluid, and other specimens, are being tested and could become commercially available, obviating diagnosis of syphilis based on indirect evidence of antibody response.

  3. Microscopic dark-field examination should be performed on appropriate lesions for spirochetes.

  4. Complete blood cell count with differential. Monocytosis is typically seen; look for hemolytic anemia or a leukemoid reaction.

  5. Lumbar puncture. CNS disease may be detected by positive serologic tests, dark-field examination positive for spirochetes, elevated monocyte count, or elevated spinal fluid protein levels. FTA on CSF is not reliable. The VDRL test is the only one approved for use on CSF. PCRs on CSF may prove useful.

  B. Radiologic studies. X-ray studies of the long bones may show sclerotic changes of the metaphysis and diaphysis, with widespread osteitis and periostitis.

VI. Management

  A. Treated mother. Infants born to mothers who received adequate penicillin treatment for syphilis during pregnancy are at minimal risk. The infant should be treated if maternal treatment was inadequate, unknown, or given during the last 4 weeks of pregnancy or if a drug other than penicillin (eg, erythromycin) was used. In a pregnant woman who has been treated for syphilis, quantitative NTA tests should be done monthly for the duration of the pregnancy. Appropriate treatment should result in a progressive decrease in titer.

  B. VDRL-positive infant. Infants with positive VDRL tests, even if this is only an indication of maternal transfer of IgG, should be treated if adequate follow-up cannot be obtained.

  C. Definitive treatment. (For drug dosages, see Chapter 80.) Because of reported treatment failures with penicillin G benzathine, current treatment guidelines recommend treating all infants with congenital syphilis with aqueous crystalline penicillin G, 100,000–150,000 units/kg/24 h IV, or alternately 50,000 units/kg/day of procaine penicillin IM; the duration of therapy should be 10–14 days in both instances. Asymptomatic infants born to mothers whose treatment for syphilis may have been inadequate should be fully evaluated, including CSF examination. Some experts would treat with aqueous crystalline or procaine penicillin G. However, if CSF is normal, as well as normal x-ray films of long bones, platelet count, and liver functions, many experts would treat with a single IM dose of 50,000 units/kg of penicillin G benzathine. However, if the mother is infected with HIV-1, a complete 10- to 14-day course of therapy is recommended.

  D. Isolation procedures. Precautions regarding drainage, secretions, and blood and body fluids are indicated for all infants with suspected or proven congenital syphilis until therapy has been given for 24 h.

  E. Follow-up care. The infant should have repeated quantitative NTA tests at 3, 6, and 12 months. Most infants will have a negative titer with adequate treatment. A rising titer requires further investigation and retreatment.

GONORRHEA

  I. Definition. Infection with *Neisseria gonorrhoeae* **(a Gram-negative diplococcus)** is a reproductive tract infection that is an important infection in pregnancy because of transmission to the fetus or neonate.

II. Incidence. The prevalence of gonococcus infection among pregnant women is ~1–2%. If routine ophthalmic prophylaxis was not used, ~50% of colonized mothers would acquire gonorrhea infections.

III. Pathophysiology. *N. gonorrhoeae* primarily affects the endocervical canal. The infant may become infected during passage through an infected cervical canal or by contact with contaminated amniotic fluid if rupture of membranes has occurred.

IV. Clinical presentations

A. Ophthalmia neonatorum. The most common clinical manifestation is gonococcal ophthalmia neonatorum. This occurs in <2% of cases of positive maternal gonococcal infection if appropriate eye prophylaxis is given. For a description of this disease, see Chapter 35.

B. Gonococcal arthritis. The onset of gonococcal arthritis can be at any time from 1 to 4 weeks after delivery. It is secondary to gonococcemia. The source of bacteremia has been attributed to infection of the mouth, nares, and umbilicus. The most common sites are the knees and ankles, but any joint may be affected. The infant may present with mild or moderate symptoms. Drainage of affected joint and antibiotics are necessary.

C. Amniotic infection syndrome. This occurs when there is premature rupture of membranes, with inflammation of the placenta and umbilical cord. The infant may have clinical evidence of sepsis. This infection is associated with a high infant mortality rate.

D. Meningitis.

E. Scalp abscess. This is usually secondary to intrauterine fetal monitoring.

F. Stomatitis.

V. Diagnosis

A. Mother. Endocervical scrapings should be obtained for culture.

B. Infant

1. Gram's stain of any exudate, if present, should be obtained.

2. Culture. Material may be obtained by swabbing the eye or nasopharynx or the orogastric or anorectal areas. Blood should be obtained for culture. Cultures for concomitant infection with *Chlamydia trachomatis* should also be done. Gonococcal cultures from nonsterile sites (eg, the pharynx, rectum, and vagina) should be done using selective media.

3. Spinal fluid studies. Cell count, protein, culture, Gram's stain, and others should be ordered.

4. Ligase chain reaction (LCR) has been studied and may be a superior alternative to culture for identification of *N. gonorrhoeae*.

VI. Management

A. Antibiotic therapy

1. Maternal infection. Most infants born to mothers with gonococcal infection do not experience infection. However, because there have been some reported cases, it is recommended that full-term infants receive a single injection of ceftriaxone (125 mg IV or IM) and that premature infants receive 25–50 mg/kg (maximum, 125 mg).

2. Nondisseminated infection, including ophthalmia neonatorum, treatment is ceftriaxone (25–50 mg/kg/day IV or IM, not to exceed 125 mg) given once. Alternative treatment for ophthalmia is cefotaxime (100 mg/kg IV or IM) as a single dose. Infants with ophthalmia should have their eyes irrigated with saline immediately and at frequent intervals until the discharge is eliminated. Topical antibiotics are inadequate and unnecessary with systemic therapy.

3. Disseminated infection (eg, arthritis and septicemia) treatment is ceftriaxone (25–50 mg/kg IV or IM once a day for 7 days) or cefotaxime (50–100 mg/kg/day IV or IM in 2 divided doses for 7 days). For **meningitis,** continue treatment for 10–14 days.

B. Isolation. All infants with gonococcal infection should be placed in contact isolation until effective parenteral antimicrobial therapy has been given for 24 h.

CHLAMYDIAL INFECTION

I. **Definition.** *C. trachomatis* is a highly specialized gram-negative bacterium that possesses a cell wall, contains DNA and RNA, and can be inactivated by several antimicrobial agents. However, because of its inability to generate adenosine triphosphate, it is an obligate intracellular parasite. It may cause urethritis, cervicitis, urethral symptoms, and salpingitis in the mother. In the infant, it may cause conjunctivitis and pneumonia.

II. **Incidence.** It is the second most common sexually transmitted disease after trichomoniasis. The risk of infection to infants born to infected mothers is between 50% and 75%; conjunctivitis occurs in 20–50%, and pneumonia in about 30%. Cervical chlamydial infection varies widely, dependent on the population, with significant increases in young, low socioeconomic, and nonwhite populations (median of 15%).

III. **Pathophysiology.** *C. trachomatis* subtypes B–K cause the sexually transmitted form of the disease and the associated neonatal infection. They frequently cause a benign subclinical infection. The infant acquires infection during vaginal delivery through an infected cervix. Infection after C-section is very rare and usually occurs only with early rupture of amniotic membranes.

IV. **Clinical presentation**
   A. **Conjunctivitis.** See Chapter 35.
   B. **Pneumonia.** This is one of the most common forms of pneumonia in the first 3 months of life. The respiratory tract may be directly infected during delivery. Approximately one half of infants presenting with pneumonia will have concurrent or previous conjunctivitis. Pneumonia usually presents at 3–11 weeks of life. The infants experience a gradual increase in symptoms over several weeks. Initially, there is often 1–2 weeks of mucoid rhinorrhea followed by cough and increasing respiratory rate. More than 95% of cases are afebrile. The cough is characteristic, paroxysmal, and staccato, and it interferes with sleeping and eating. These infants may also have pulmonary congestion, and apnea may be present; however, this tends to be associated with secondary infection occurring together with chlamydia. Approximately one third have otitis media.

V. **Diagnosis**
   A. **Laboratory studies**
      1. **Tissue culture.** Because chlamydia are obligate intracellular organisms, culture specimens must contain epithelial cells.
      2. **Direct fluorescent antibody (DFA)** staining for elementary bodies in clinical specimens using monoclonal antibody.
      3. **EIA.**
      4. **DNA probe.** Positive DFA, EIA, or DNA probe should be verified by culture or by a second nonculture test different from the first.
      5. **PCR.** Nucleic acid amplification as well as LCRs.
      6. **IgM antibody to *C. trachomatis* (pneumonia).** Either a significant rise in titer or high levels of the titer (1:32) indicate infection.
      7. **Culture of the respiratory tract.** Material should be obtained for culture via nasopharyngeal aspiration or deep suctioning of the trachea and placed in special transport medium.
      8. **Gram's stain of eye discharge (see Chapter 35).**
      9. **Other tests.** In cases of pneumonia, the white blood cell count is normal, but there is eosinophilia in 70% of cases. Blood gas measurements show mild to moderate hypoxia.
   B. **Radiologic studies.** In cases of pneumonia, the chest x-ray film may reveal hyperexpansion of the lungs, with bilateral diffuse interstitial or alveolar infiltrates.

VI. **Management**
   A. **Prevention.** In high-risk mothers, material should be obtained for culture and treatment should be given before delivery. Infants born to mothers known to

have untreated chlamydial infection should be evaluated and treated with oral erythromycin for 14 days.
B. **Conjunctivitis.** See Chapter 35.
C. **Pneumonia.** Give erythromycin, 50 mg/kg/day in 4 divided doses for 14 days. This will not only shorten the clinical course but will decrease the duration of nacopharyngeal shedding. No isolation measures are necessary. For more details on dosing and pharmacologic information, see Chapter 80.

HUMAN IMMUNODEFICIENCY VIRUS

I. **Definition.** HIV is an enveloped RNA virus that is a member of the lentivirus subfamily of retroviruses. Infection is most commonly secondary to HIV-1. HIV-2 is very uncommon in the United States. HIV results in a broad spectrum of disease, with AIDS representing the most severe end of the clinical spectrum.

II. **Incidence.** The Joint United Nations Program on HIV/AIDS approximated that 34.7 million people worldwide were infected with HIV-1 at the end of 2000. More than 95% of the total live in developing countries. Young women represent the fastest growing group that has AIDS, accounting for 41% of adults aged 13–24 years in 1999. An estimated 2.4 million infected women give birth annually, 600,000 children acquired HIV infection during 2000, primarily through mother-to-child transmission. The transmission rate of HIV-1 from mother to child (vertical transmission) has been reduced significantly over the past number of years by an extended regimen of zidovudine (ZDV) given to mothers during pregnancy and labor and to the neonate postdelivery.

III. **Pathophysiology.** HIV-1 is particularly tropic for CD4+ T cells and cells of monocyte or macrophage lineage. After infection of the cell, viral RNA is uncoated and a double-strand DNA transcript is made. This DNA is transported to the nucleuc and integrated into the host genome DNA. There is eventual destruction of both the cellular and humoral arms of the immune system. As well, HIV-1 gene products or cytokines elaborated by infected cells may affect macrophage, B lymphocyte, and T-lymphocyte function. Hypergammaglobulinemia caused by polyclonal B-cell activation by HIV-1 is often detected in early infancy. Disruption of B-cell function results in poor secondary antibody synthesis and response to vaccination. As well, profound defects in cell-mediated immunity occur, allowing a predisposition to opportunistic infections such as fungus, *Pneumocystis carinii* pneumonia (PCP), and chronic diarrhea. The virus can also invade the CNS and produce psychosis and brain atrophy.

IV. **Risk factors**
A. **High-risk mother.** Any infant born to a high-risk mother is at risk. High-risk mothers include IV drug users, hemophiliacs, spouses of bisexual males, women from areas where the disease is more prevalent in heterosexuals, and spouses of hemophiliacs. Several mechanisms for viral transmission exist, including maternal disease state, fetal exposure to infected maternal body fluids, depressed maternal immune response, and breast-feeding. The risk of transmission appears to be greater if the mother's disease is advanced, her CD4 count is reduced, or there is increased viral burden (P24 antigenemia) or positive HIV blood cultures. The amount of maternal virus (viral load) may predict transmission better than clinical or immunologic indicators. Transplacental infection has been proven by evidence of infection in aborted first-trimester fetal tissues as well as isolation of HIV-1 in blood samples obtained at birth. Potential routes of infection include mixture of maternal and fetal blood and infection across the placenta when its integrity is compromised (eg, placentitis [syphilitic] and chorioamnionitis). Increased risk of vertical transmission has been correlated with rupture of membranes for more than 4 h, vaginal delivery, chorioamnionitis, and invasive obstetric procedures.
B. **Blood transfusion.** Screening of blood donors has reduced but has not totally eliminated the risk because some newly infected persons are viremic but

seronegative for 2–4 months and because some infected persons (5–15%) are seronegative. The current risk of transmission of HIV per unit transfused is less than 1 in 225,000.

C. **Breast milk.** Breast-feeding is the predominant means of postnatal HIV transmission to infants and accounts for approximately an additional 14% transmission risk among breast-feeding populations. HIV-1 RNA and proviral DNA have been detected in both the cell-free and cellular portions of breast milk. Colostrum viral load appears to be particularly high. Risk from breast milk is highest when maternal primary infection occurs within the first few months after delivery. Current guidelines recommend that women infected or at risk of infection with HIV-1 abstain from breast-feeding if local sanitary conditions and access to infant formulas are good. This may not be true in developing countries.

V. **Clinical presentation.** Disease progression after vertical HIV-1 infection is highly variable.

A. **Age.** Vertically infected children experience more rapid disease progression than those infected at an older age or adults. More than 80% of vertically infected children manifest HIV-1-related symptoms or CD4 T-cell depletion by 2 years of age. An AIDS-defining condition developed in ~23% by 1 year and in ~40% by 4 years of age in vertically infected infants.

B. **Signs and symptoms.** The newborn may be asymptomatic or may have low birth weight, weight loss, or failure to thrive. Recurrent upper respiratory tract infections, otitis media, sinusitis, and invasive bacterial infections are common. Recurrent oral thrush is common, and candida esophagitis may become particularly troublesome. There is a high risk for acquiring PCP. Other infections that increase in frequency and difficulty to control include acute and recurrent VZV infections, measles, CMV, and gastrointestinal infections (eg, *Salmonella, Giardia, Campylobacter,* rotavirus, and *Cryptosporidium*). Nonspecific features of infection can include hepatosplenomegaly, lymphadenopathy, and fever. Neurologic disease may be either static (delayed attainment of milestones) or progressive, with impaired brain growth, failure to reach milestones, and progressive motor deficits. Common CT scan findings include basal ganglia calcification and cortical atrophy. Cardiac abnormalities, pericardial disease, myocardial dysfunction, dysrhythmias, and cardiomyopathies are common, particularly in advanced disease.

VI. **Diagnosis.** Diagnosis is based on (1) suspicion of infection because of epidemiologic risk or clinical presentation and (2) confirmation by different virologic assays in infants <18 months old or serologic tests if the infant is >18 months old.

A. **All other causes of immunodeficiency must be excluded.** These include both primary and secondary immunodeficiency states. Primary immunodeficiency diseases include DiGeorge syndrome, Wiskott-Aldrich syndrome, ataxia-telangiectasia, agammaglobulinemia, severe combined immunodeficiency, and neutrophil function abnormality. Secondary immunodeficiency states include those caused by immunosuppressive therapy, starvation, and lymphoreticular cancer.

B. **Laboratory studies**
1. **Virologic assays.** With the use of current virologic assays, HIV infection may be diagnosed as early as the first day after birth in some infants and by 1 month of age in most infected infants. The HIV DNA PCR assay is the preferred diagnostic tool. Estimated sensitivity of HIV DNA PCR is ~38% at birth, 93% at 14 days, and 96% at 28 days of age. HIV RNA PCR may have even superior sensitivity and specificity for early diagnosis of HIV; however, data are limited. ZDV prophylaxis does not appear to alter the diagnostic sensitivity of either HIV DNA PCR or RNA assays. The effect of combination antiretroviral maternal and infant treatment on sensitivity of viral diagnostic testing is unknown. A perinatally HIV exposed infant is determined to be infected with the presence of two positive results of HIV virologic assays performed on the infant's blood obtained at two different oc-

casions. (Do not use cord blood.) Virologic assays should be performed: within the first 48 h after birth, at 14 days, between 1–2 months, and at 3–6 months of age. A positive test confirmed at 2 weeks of age warrants a change in the recommended ZDV prophylactic monotherapy. Infection with HIV can be reasonably excluded with two or more negative virologic assays, at least one of which is performed after 1 month and another performed after 4 months in the absence of breast-feeding. In the absence of hypogammaglobulinemia, two or more negative HIV-specific antibody tests performed beyond 6 months of age in a child without clinical evidence of HIV disease can reasonably exclude HIV infection. Follow-up tests should include either two negative ELISA tests between 6 and 18 months or one negative ELISA at 18–24 months. P$_{24}$ antigen assay is less sensitive than viral culture or PCR and should be used only if the other tests are unavailable. A seropositive child of an HIV-infected mother who is repeatedly HIV antibody–negative by 18 months of age and has never had a positive HIV culture, PCR, or P24 antigen is considered a seroconverter.
2. **Surrogate markers for disease.** Immunologic abnormalities, including hypergammaglobulinemia, a low CD4$^+$ T-lymphocyte count, or a decreased CD4$^+$ percentage.
C. **Presence of a "marker" disease** that indicates cellular immunodeficiency. Marker diseases include candidiasis, cryptococcosis, *Mycobacterium avium* infection, Epstein-Barr virus infection, PCP, strongyloidiasis, and Kaposi's sarcoma. CMV infection and toxoplasmosis are included if toxoplasmosis occurs >1 month after birth and CMV infection presents >6 months after birth.
VII. **Management**
   A. **Prevention**
   1. **Prenatal.** Barriers to prevention of perinatal HIV-1 infection include continued increase in HIV-1 infection among women of childbearing age, unplanned pregnancy, delayed or lack of prenatal care, and lack of offer or acceptance of prenatal HIV-1 testing. Routine voluntary prenatal HIV testing allows for educating patients about HIV infection, discussion regarding modes of transmission, encouraging notification of sexual and needle-sharing partners, and discussion about interaction of HIV infection and pregnancy and possible intervention strategies as well as contraception provision. Further interventions can be made by complete evaluation of HIV-infected pregnant women, including a complete history and physical examination, lymphocyte profile, complete blood cell count, hepatitis B serology, sexually transmitted disease (STD) workup, urine toxicology, and purified protein derivative (PPD). With this information, patients can be referred to drug treatment programs, treated for STDs, given prophylaxis for PCP, and treated for tuberculosis or with isoniazid if positive on PPD and negative on the chest x-ray film. These measures will help improve the outcome for newborns and help decrease transmission.
   2. **Perinatal.** Mother-to-child transmission rates in the United States have declined significantly to 3–6% after rapid implementation of the Pediatric Aids Clinical Trials Group (PACTG) 076 regimen. Transmission rates of 2% or less have been reported among women receiving prophylactic ZDV and having an elective cesarean section and those treated with highly active antiretroviral therapy that results in an undetectable viral load. The current recommended protocol is ZDV (also known as AZT or Retrovir), 100 mg orally 5 times/day starting at 14 weeks' gestation for the duration of the pregnancy; intrapartum 2 mg/kg IV over 1 h, followed by 1 mg/kg/h for the duration of labor; and newborn zidovudine syrup, 2 mg/kg of body weight orally every 6 h, started at 8–12 h after birth and continued for the first 6 weeks of life. The only observed short-term toxicity in ZDV-treated infants was anemia, which was not clinically significant. More recently, highly active antiretroviral therapy (HAART) consisting of a combination of two nucleosides and a protease inhibitor has become the standard of care for

nonpregnant as well as pregnant HIV-infected patients. Perinatal antiretroviral therapy is very costly and logistically very difficult; therefore, a safe and effective vaccine regimen begun at birth would be a much more attractive strategy and might provide lifetime protection. Phase I studies evaluating potential HIV-1 vaccines are under way in neonates.

3. **Delivery.** Recent data from individual patient meta-analysis and a randomized control trial confirmed that C-section performed before labor and rupture of membranes reduces mother-to-child viral transmission by 50% to 8%, independent of the use of antiretroviral therapy or ZDV prophylaxis. This may not be applicable in developing nations because of increased risks of postpartum morbidity and operative mortality. The use of invasive procedures in labor (eg, fetal scalp electrodes, operative vaginal delivery, and episiotomy) should be avoided because of the potential risk for enhanced transmission.

4. **Postdelivery.** Thoroughly clean off amniotic fluid and blood. Isolate the infant with the same precautions as for hepatitis B (blood and secretion precautions). Initiate antiretroviral treatment per the regimen described in Human Immunodeficiency Virus, section VII,A,2. Obtain serial laboratory evaluation as discussed. Ensure that the infant has the best possible follow-up care.

B. **General supportive care**
1. **IVIG.** HIV-infected infants are appropriate candidates for routine IVIG prophylaxis (400 mg/kg/dose every 28 days).
2. **Vaccines.** Routine immunization schedules should be followed for DTP (diphtheria-tetanus-pertussis), MMR (measles-mumps-rubella), HBV, and Hib (*H. influenzae* type b). Routine polio schedule is administered as IM inactivated polio vaccine (Salk). Pneumococcal vaccine is given at 2 years of age, and influenza vaccine is given annually.
3. **Nutrition.** Close nutritional monitoring should be part of the routine care of these children.
4. **Prophylaxis.** It has become clear that very aggressive prophylaxis of these children will significantly improve their morbidity and mortality. CDC guidelines state that all infants born to HIV-infected women receive prophylaxis beginning at 4–6 weeks regardless of CD4+ lymphocyte count. The drug of choice for this is trimethoprim-sulfamethoxazole (TMP/SMX). Alternates include daily oral dapsone and monthly IV pentamidine. Prophylaxis is continued until HIV infection has been reasonably excluded. All HIV-infected infants or infants whose status is indeterminate should continue prophylaxis until 12 months of age. Thereafter, prophylaxis is based on CD4+ lymphocyte count or percentage. Prophylaxis should be given as needed for exposure to tuberculosis and VZV (see Chapter 80).
5. **Other aspects of supportive care.** Neurodevelopmental supportive services include preschool early intervention programs and school-based developmental disability programs. Aggressive management and protocols for pharmacologic and nonpharmacologic pain management should be used.

RESPIRATORY SYNCYTIAL VIRUS

I. **Definition.** Respiratory syncytial virus (RSV) is a large, enveloped RNA virus–paramyxovirus.

II. **Incidence.** It infects essentially all children during the first 3 years of life. Initial infection occurs most commonly during the child's first year. Reinfection throughout life is common. RSV causes epidemics between October and April. It is a common cause of nosocomial infection. It can survive up to 6 h on nonporous surfaces. Hospitalization for respiratory illness is more common for infants who were born at <32 weeks' gestation.

III. Clinical presentation. RSV usually begins in the nasopharynx with coryza and congestion. Low-grade fever often is associated initially. During the first 2–5 days, it may progress to the lower respiratory tract with development of cough, dyspnea, and wheezing. Severe lower respiratory tract infections are most often seen in patients with congenital heart disease or bronchopulmonary dysplasia.

IV. Diagnosis

A. **ELISA and DFA** have sencitivity and specificity of between 90–100%. These rapid tests detect RSV antigen in epithelial cells obtained by nasopharyngeal washings.

B. **Chest x-ray film** usually reveals infiltrates or hyperinflation.

C. **Blood gas.** Hypoxemia with arterial saturations of 85–90%, usually there is no evidence of CO_2 retention.

V. Management

A. **Immunization**

1. **Passive.** Palivizumab (Synagis) was licensed by the Food and Drug Administration in 1999 for the prevention of RSV by providing passive immunity. It is a humanized RSV monoclonal antibody. It is administered as an intramuscular injection (15 mg/kg) monthly during RSV season. It is well tolerated with infrequent, minimal side effects. However, because it is an RSV-specific antibody, it has no effect on preventing any other respiratory infections. Severely compromised children may be better protected with RSV-IGIV, which is a polyclonal antibody enriched for neutralizing antibodies to RSV. Its drawback compared with palivizumab is that it must be administered as a monthly IV infusion.

2. **Active.** A trial of formalin-inactivated vaccine failed. A live attenuated vaccine is a possible solution; however, the failure of natural RSV infection to protect fully against subsequent infection makes development of successful active immunization more difficult. It will probably be at least another 5–10 years before routine immunization against RSV becomes available.

B. **Ribavirin.** The most recent AAP guideline states that "ribavirin may be considered" in patients with congenital heart disease, bronchopulmonary dysplasia, or cystic fibrosis or in patients who are "severely ill."

C. **Bronchodilators.** A clinical trial is warranted, and such treatment should continue only if improvement is noted.

D. **Antibiotics, theophylline, and corticosteroids** have been shown not to be indicated as treatments for RSV.

E. **Isolation.** Exercise contact precautions for the duration of the illness. Infected secretions remain viable for up to 6 h on countertops. Gowns, gloves, and scrupulous hand-washing practices are required. Wear masks and goggles for close contact (eg, with suctioning).

LYME DISEASE

I. Definition. Lyme disease is caused by the spirochete *Borrelia burgdorferi* and is transmitted by the bite of a deer tick.

II. Incidence. Transplacental transmission has been reported, but no causal relationship between maternal Lyme disease and abnormalities of pregnancy has been documented. More than 90% of cases have been reported in the northeastern coastal states.

III. Clinical presentation. Several studies of treated and untreated Lyme disease in pregnancy found no increased risk to the fetus that could be ascribed to *B. burgdorferi* infection. One blood serologic study suggested an increased rate of cardiac malformation; however, studies have shown no such association.

IV. Diagnosis. Diagnosis in the adult is made on clinical findings (flu-like symptoms, erythema chronicum migrans skin lesions, and joint pain and swelling) because many diagnostic tests are often negative or falsely positive.

V. Management. Although prevention of maternal exposure is the best cure, treatment of pregnant women is the same as it is for nonpregnant women, except that tetracyclines are contraindicated. In the case of a infant born to a mother not treated for Lyme disease during pregnancy, a serologic evaluation for postnatal production of antibodies is advisable. Empiric treatment is not indicated. If Lyme disease is diagnosed, treatment should include penicillin or ceftriaxone for 21 days after cultures from the blood and CSF have been obtained.

ANTHRAX BACTERIA (*Bacillus anthracis*)

  I. Definition. This is historically a zoonotic infection in humans acquired by transfer of organisms from sick animals or their products. Currently, the means of infection is restricted to undeveloped countries.
 II. Incidence. In developed nations, the risk of infection is related primarily to terrorist biologic warfare.
III. Pathophysiology. There has been no evidence for human-to-human transmission. Three forms of the disease occur: inhalation or pulmonary anthrax, cutaneous anthrax, and gastrointestinal anthrax. The form of the disease is determined by the type of exposure to the organism.
 IV. Clinical presentation. This is dependent on the route of entry of the anthrax into the body.
  V. Diagnosis. Contact local public health authorities if suspicion of exposure or disease is high. Nasal swab cultures have been used as an epidemiologic tool; however, their value in diagnosis is limited. A negative swab does not rule out exposure. In symptomatic cases, obtain specimens from affected tissue or site for culture, PCR, and immunohistochemical staining procedures.
 VI. Prophylaxis and treatment. Base treatment on advice of public health officials. Penicillins, including amoxicillin, are not recommended for initial treatment of clinical disease. Nevertheless, penicillins, including amoxicillin, are likely effective for postexposure prophylaxis. For clinical disease, treat with ciprofloxacin or doxycycline pending susceptibility testing. If penicillin susceptibility is confirmed, change to oral amoxicillin. Treat for 60 days to ensure that spores have had time to germinate and be eradicated.

REFERENCES

Ahmed A et al: Cerebrospinal fluid values in the term neonate. *Pediatr Dis J* 1996;15:298.
American Academy of Pediatrics: *Red Book: Report of the Committee on Infectious Diseases,* 25th ed. American Academy of Pediatrics, 2000.
American Academy of Pediatrics Committee on Infectious Diseases: Reassessment of the indications for ribavirin therapy in respiratory syncytial virus infections. *Pediatrics* 1996;97:137.
American Academy of Pediatrics Committees on Infectious Diseases and on Fetus and Newborn: Revised guidelines for prevention of early onset group B streptococcal (GBS) infection. *Pediatrics* 1997;99:489.
Andres J: Neonatal hepatobiliary disorders. *Clin Perinatol* 1996;23:321.
Babl F et al: Neonatal gonococcal arthritis after negative prenatal screening and despite conjunctival prophylaxis. *Pediatr Dis J 2000;19:346.*
Bale J, Murph J: Infections of the central nervous system in the newborn. *Clin Perinatol* 1997; 24:787.
Benitz W et al: Serial serum C-reactive protein levels in the diagnosis of neonatal infection. *Pediatrics* 1998;102: e41.
Bernstein HM et al: Use of myeloid colony-stimulating factors in neonates with septicemia. *Curr Opin Pediatr* 2002;14:91.
Bomela HN et al: Use of C-reactive protein to guide duration of empiric antibiotic therapy in suspected early neonatal sepsis. *Pediatr Infect Dis J* 2000;19:531.
Boyer K: Congenital toxoplasmosis: current status of diagnosis, treatment and prevention. *Pediatr Infect Dis* 2000;11:165.

Fowler K et al: Progressive and fluctuating sensorineural hearing loss in children with asymptomatic congenital cytomegalovirus infection. *J Pediatr* 1997;130:624.

Franz A et al: Reduction of unnecessary antibiotic therapy in newborn infants using interleukin-8 and C-reactive protein as markers of bacterial infections. *Pediatrics* 1999;104:447.

Garcia-Prats J et al: The critically ill neonate with infection: management considerations in the term and preterm infant. *Pediatr Infect Dis* 2000;11:4.

Garcia-Prats J et al: Rapid detection of microorganisms in blood cultures of newborn infants utilizing an automated blood culture system. *Pediatrics* 2000;105:523.

Gervacio C et al: Early-onset neonatal group B streptococcal sepsis: intrapartum antibiotic prophylaxis in the clinical setting. *J Perinatol* 2001;21:9.

Girardet R et al: Comparison of the urine-based ligase chain reaction test to culture for detection of *Chlamydia trachomatis* and *Neisseria gonorrhoeae* in pediatric sexual abuse victims. *Pediatr Infect Dis* 2001;20:144.

Goldenberg R et al: Sexually transmitted disease and adverse outcomes of pregnancy. *Clin Perinatol* 1997;24:23.

Hammerschlag M: Chlamydial infections. *J Pediatr* 1989;114:727.

Harris N et al: Zidovudine and perinatal human immunodeficiency virus type 1 transmission: a population-based approach. *Pediatrics* 2002;109:e60.

Jenson H: Congenital syphilis. *Pediatr Infect Dis* 1999;10:183.

Kane M: Hepatitic viruses and the neonate. *Clin Perinatol* 1997;24:181.

Keyserling H: Other viral agents of perinatal importance. *Clin Perinatol* 1997;24:193.

Klein JO (eds): *Infectious Diseases of the Fetus and Newborn Infant*, 3rd ed. Saunders, 1990.

Kline M: Vertically acquired human immunodeficiency virus infection. *Pediatr Infect Dis* 1999;10:147.

Kneyber M et al: Current concepts on active immunization against respiratory syncytial virus for infants and young children. *Pediatr Infect Dis* 2002;21:685.

Kohl S: Herpes simplex infections in newborn infants. *Pediatr Infect Dis* 1999;10:154.

Lindsay M, Nesheim S: Human immunodeficiency virus infection in pregnant women and their newborns. *Clin Perinatol* 1997;24:161.

Litwin C, Hill H: Serologic and DNA-based testing for congenital and perinatal infections. *Pediatr Infect Dis* 1997;16:1166.

Luzuriaga K, Sullivan J: Viral and immunopathogenesis of vertical HIV-1 infection. *Pediatr Clin North Am* 2000;47:65.

Manroe BL et al: The neonatal blood count in health and disease. Reference values for neutrophilic cells. *J Pediatr* 1997;95:85.

Mast E, Alter M: Hepatitis C. *Semin Pediatr Infect Dis* 1997;8:17.

Mast E, Alter M: Viral hepatitis A,B, and C in the newborn infant. *Semin Pediatr Infect Dis* 1999; 10:201.

McGann K: Herpes virus infections in the fetus and neonate. Epidemiology and clinical manifestations. *Semin Pediatr Infect Dis* 1997;8:136.

Meissner HC et al: Immunoprophylaxis with palivizumab, a humanized respiratory syncytial virus monoclonal antibody, for prevention of respiratory syncytial virus infection in high risk infants: a consensus opinion. *Pediatr Infect Dis* 1999;18:223.

Mofenson L et al: Technical report: perinatal human immunodeficiency virus testing and prevention of transmission. *Pediatrics* 2000;106:E88.

Mustonen K et al: Congenital varicella-zoster virus infection after maternal subclinical infection: clinical and neuropathological findings. *J Perinatol* 2001;21:141.

Nelson C, Demmler G: Cytomegalovirus infection in the pregnant mother, fetus and newborn infant. *Clin Perinatol* 1997;24:151.

Nielsen N, Bryson Y: Diagnosis of HIV infection in children. *Pediatr Clin North America* 2000; 47:39.

Nissen, M, Sloots T: Rapid diagnosis in pediatric infectious diseases: the past, the present and the future. *Pediatr Infect Dis J* 2002;21:605.

Nupponen I et al: Neutrophil CD11b expression and circulating interleukin-8 as diagnostic markers for early-onset neonatal sepsis. *Pediatrics* 2001;108:e12.

Pass R: Cytomegalovirus infection. *Pediatr in Rev* 2002;23:163.

Patt H, Feigin R: Diagnosis and management of suspected cases of bioterrorism: a pediatric perspective. *Pediatrics* 2002;109:685.

Risser W, Hwang L: Problems in the current case definitions of congenital syphilis. *J Pediatr* 1996;129:499.

Rodriguez W: Respiratory syncytial virus infections in infants. *Semin Pediatr Infect Dis* 1999; 10:161.

Rosenthal P, Lightdale J: Laboratory evaluation of hepatitis. *Pediatr Rev* 2000;21:178.

Royce R et al: Sexual transmission of HIV. *N Engl J Med* 1997;336:1072.

Rudnick C: Neonatal herpes simplex virus infections. *Am Fam Physician* 2002;65:1138.

Sanchez P: Laboratory tests for congenital syphilis. *Pediatr Infect Dis J* 1998;17:70.
Sauerbrei A, Wutzler P: The congenital varicella syndrome. *J Perinatol* 2000;20:548.
Sauerbrei A, Wutzler P: Neonatal varicella. *J Perinatol* 2001;21:545.
Shetty A: Preventing mother-to-child transmission of HIV-1: an international perspective. *NeoReviews* 2001;2:e75.
Skidmore S: Hepatitis C-Z: recent advances. *Arch Dis Child* 2002;86:339.
Solder B et al: Effect of antiretroviral combination therapy on quantitative plasma human immunodeficiency virus-ribonucleic acid in children and adolescents infected with human immunodeficiency virus. *J Pediatr* 1997;130:293.
Sood S: Lyme disease. *Pediatr Infect Dis J* 1999;18:913.
Tajiri H et al: Prospective study of mother-to-infant transmission of hepatitis C virus. *Pediatr Infect Dis J* 2001;20:10.
US Department of Health and Human Services: Prevention of perinatal group B streptococcal disease: a public health perspective. *MMWR Morb Mortal Wkly Rep* 1996;45:1.
Whitley R: Herpes simplex virus infection. *Semin Pediatr Infect Dis* 2002;13:6.
Whitley R, Kimberlin D: Treatment of viral infections during pregnancy and the neonatal period. *Clin Perinatol* 1997;24:267.

69 Intrauterine Growth Retardation (Small for Gestational Age Infant)

I. **Definition.** In the past, the terms **intrauterine growth retardation (IUGR)** and **small for gestational age (SGA)** were used interchangeably. Although related, they are not synonymous. **IUGR is failure of normal fetal growth caused by multiple adverse effects on the fetus, whereas SGA describes an infant whose weight is lower than population norms or lower than a predetermined cutoff weight.** SGA infants are defined as having a birth weight **below the 10th percentile** for gestational age or **>2 standard deviations below the mean** for gestational age. The **ponderal index**, arrived at by the following formula, can be used to identify infants whose soft tissue mass is below normal for the stage of skeletal development (Battaglia & Lubchenco, 1967). Thus, a ponderal index below the 10th percentile may be used to identify IUGR infants. Thus, all IUGR infants may not be SGA, and all SGA infants may not be small as a result of a growth-restrictive process.

$$\text{Ponderal index} = \frac{\text{Birth weight} \times 100}{\text{Crown-heel length}^3}$$

II. **Incidence.** About 3–10% of all pregnancies are associated with IUGR, and 20% of stillborn infants are growth retarded. The perinatal mortality rate is *5–20* times higher for growth-retarded fetuses, and serious short- or long-term morbidity is noted in half of the affected surviving infants. IUGR is estimated to be the predominant cause for low birth weight in developing countries. It is estimated that one third of infants with birth weights <2500 g are in fact growth retarded and not premature. Term infants with birth weights below the 3rd percentile have higher morbidity and 10 times higher mortality than appropriate for gestational age infants. In the United States, uteroplacental insufficiency is the leading cause of IUGR. An estimated 10% of cases are secondary to congenital infection. Chromosomal and other genetic disorders are reported in 5–15% of IUGR infants.

III. **Pathophysiology.** Fetal growth is influenced by fetal, maternal, and placental factors.

A. **Fetal factors** (Table 69–1)

1. **Genetic factors.** Approximately 20% of birth weight variability in a given population is determined by fetal genotype. Genetic determinants of fetal growth have their greatest impact in early gestation during the period of rapid cell development. Racial and ethnic backgrounds influence size at birth irrespective of socioeconomic status. Males weigh an average of 150–200 g more than females at birth. This weight increase occurs late in gestation. Birth order affects fetal size; infants born to primiparous women weigh less than subsequent siblings. Genetic disorders such as achondroplasia, Russell-Silver syndrome, and leprechaunism also present with IUGR.

2. **Chromosomal anomalies.** Chromosomal deletions or imbalances result in diminished fetal growth. Growth retardation is observed as a major feature of short-arm deletion of chromosome 4, long-arm deletion of chromosome 13, and trisomies 13, 18, and 21. Additional X chromosomes beyond norm are associated with diminished birth weight (eg, XXY, XXXY).

TABLE 69-1. FETAL FACTORS IN INTRAUTERINE GROWTH RETARDATION

Genetic factors
Racial, ethnic, and population differences
Genetic disorders
Chromosomal disorders
Female sex
Congenital anomalies
Congenital infections
Inborn errors of metabolism

3. **Congenital malformations.** Anencephaly, gastrointestinal atresia, Potter's syndrome, and pancreatic agenesis are examples of congenital anomalies associated with IUGR. Frequency of IUGR increases as the number of congenital defects increases.
4. **Fetal cardiovascular anomalies** (with the possible exception of transposition of the great vessels and tetralogy of Fallot). Abnormal hemodynamics are thought to be the basis of IUGR.
5. **Congenital infection.** TORCH infections (*t*oxoplasmosis, *o*ther, *r*ubella, *c*ytomegalovirus, and *h*erpes simplex virus) are often associated with IUGR (see Chapter 68). Cytomegalovirus and rubella are associated with severe IUGR. The incidence of IUGR is highest when infection occurs in the first trimester. The clinical findings in different congenital infections are nonspecific and overlap considerably. IUGR with rubella causes damage during organogenesis and results in a decreased number of cells, whereas cytomegalovirus infection results in cytolysis and localized necrosis within the fetus.
6. **Inborn errors of metabolism.** Transient neonatal diabetes, galactosemia, and phenylketonuria are other disorders associated with IUGR. Single-gene defects associated with impaired insulin secretion or action are associated with impaired fetal growth (ie, leprechaun syndrome).
B. **Maternal factors** (Table 69-2)
1. **Reduced uteroplacental blood flow.** Maternal disorders such as preeclampsia-eclampsia, chronic renovascular disease, and chronic hypertensive vascular disease often result in decreased uteroplacental blood flow and associated IUGR. Impaired delivery of oxygen and other

TABLE 69-2. MATERNAL FACTORS IN INTRAUTERINE GROWTH RETARDATION (IUGR)

Pregnancy-induced hypertension (>140/90 mm Hg)
Weight gain (<0.9 kg/every 4 weeks)
Fundal lag (<4 cm for gestational age)
Cyanotic heart disease
Heavy smoking
Residing at high altitude
Substance abuse and drugs
Short stature
Low socioeconomic class
Anemia (hematocrit <30%)
Prepregnancy weight (<50 kg)
Prior history of IUGR
Chronic hypertension
Renal disease
Severe maternal malnutrition
Multiple pregnancy
Low maternal age

essential nutrients is thought to limit organ growth and musculoskeletal maturation.

2. **Maternal malnutrition.** The major risk factors for IUGR include small maternal size (height and prepregnancy weight) and low maternal weight gain. Low body mass index, defined as (weight [kg]/height [m^2])/100, is a major predictor of IUGR. Maternal malnutrition leads to deficient substrate supply to the fetus. Total caloric consumption rather than protein or fat consumption appears to be the principal nutritional influence on birth weight. Famine causes a modest decline in birth weight, and in third-world countries, severe maternal malnutrition is the leading cause of IUGR. Negative effects on birth weight are most pronounced when starvation occurs in the last trimester.

3. **Multiple pregnancy.** Impaired growth results from failure to provide optimal nutrition for more than one fetus in utero. There is a progressive decrease in weight of singletons, twins, and triplets. In parabiotic twins, the smaller twin has decreased nutrient delivery secondary to abnormal placental blood flow resulting from arteriovenous communication in the chorionic plate.

4. **Drugs** (see also Chapter 67)
   a. **Cigarettes and alcohol.** Chronic abuse of cigarettes or alcohol is demonstrably associated with IUGR. The effects of alcohol and tobacco seem to be dose-dependent, with IUGR becoming more serious and predictable with heavy abuse.
   b. **Heroin.** Maternal heroin addiction is also often associated with IUGR.
   c. **Cocaine.** Cocaine use in pregnancy is associated with increased rates of IUGR (Orro & Dixon, 1987). The cause of IUGR may be mediated by placental insufficiency or direct toxic effect on the fetus.
   d. **Others.** Other drugs and chemical agents causing IUGR include known teratogens, antimetabolites, and therapeutic agents such as trimethadione, warfarin, and phenytoin. Each of these agents causes characteristic malformation syndromes. Repeated use of antenatal steroids and lithium use are also associated with low birth weight.

5. **Maternal hypoxemia.** Mothers with hemoglobinopathies, especially sickle cell disease, often have IUGR infants. Infants born at high altitudes tend to have lower mean birth weights for gestational age.

6. **Other maternal factors.** Maternal short stature, young maternal age, short interpregnancy interval, *uterine anomalies,* low socioeconomic class, primiparity, grand multiparity, and low prepregnancy weight are associated with subnormal birth weight.

C. **Placental factors** (Table 69–3)
   1. **Placental insufficiency.** In the first and second trimesters, fetal growth is determined mostly by inherent fetal growth potential. By the third trimester, placental factors (ie, an adequate supply of nutrients) assume major importance for fetal growth. When the duration of pregnancy exceeds the capacity of the placenta to nurture, placental insufficiency results, with subsequent impaired fetal growth. This phenomenon occurs mostly in postterm gestations but may occur at any time during gestation.

TABLE 69–3. PLACENTAL FACTORS IN INTRAUTERINE GROWTH RETARDATION

Abruptio placentae
Hemangioma
Single umbilical artery
Infarction
Aberrant cord insertion
Umbilical vessel thrombosis

2. **Anatomic problems.** Various anatomic factors, such as multiple infarcts, aberrant cord insertions, umbilical vascular thrombosis, and hemangiomas, are described in IUGR placentas. Premature placental separation may reduce the surface area exchange, resulting in impaired fetal growth. An adverse intrauterine environment is apt to affect both placental and fetal development; hence, IUGR infants usually have small placentas.

IV. **Classification**
   A. **Symmetric IUGR** (HC = Ht = Wt, all <10%). The head circumference (HC), length (Ht), and weight (Wt) are all proportionately reduced for gestational age. Symmetric IUGR is due to either decreased growth potential of the fetus (congenital infection or genetic disorder) or extrinsic conditions that are active early in pregnancy.
   B. **Asymmetric IUGR** (HC = Ht < Wt, all <10%). Fetal weight is reduced out of proportion to length and head circumference. The head circumference and length are closer to the expected percentiles for gestational age than is the weight. In these infants, brain growth is usually spared. The usual causes are uteroplacental insufficiency, maternal malnutrition, or extrinsic conditions appearing late in pregnancy.

V. **Diagnosis**
   A. **Establishing gestational age.** Determining the correct gestational age is imperative. The last menstrual period, size of the uterus, time of quickening (fluttering movements in the abdomen caused by fetal activity, appreciated by the mother for the first time), and early ultrasound measurements are used to determine gestational age.
   B. **Fetal assessment**
      1. **Clinical diagnosis.** The patient's history will raise the index of suspicion regarding suboptimal growth. Manual estimations of weight, serial fundal height measurements, and maternal estimates of fetal activity are simple clinical measures. Imprecision and inconsistency have prevented widespread confidence in these clinical methods.
      2. **Hormonal evaluation.** Hormonal assays were at one time popular for assessment of IUGR but are rarely used today. Maternal urinary estriol and human placental lactogen levels tend to be low or falling in pregnancies with IUGR, although there is marked individual variation.
      3. **Ultrasonography.** Because of its reliability of dating pregnancy, ability to detect impaired fetal growth by anthropomorphic measurements, and ability to detect fetal anomalies, ultrasonography currently offers the greatest promise for diagnosis. The following anthropomorphic measurements are used in combination to predict growth impairment with a high degree of accuracy.
         a. **Biparietal diameter (BPD).** When serial measurements of BPD are less than optimal, 50–80% of infants will have subnormal birth weights.
         b. **Abdominal circumference.** The liver is the first organ to suffer the effects of growth retardation. Reduced abdominal circumference is the earliest sign of asymmetric growth retardation and diminished glycogen storage.
         c. **Ratio of head circumference to abdominal circumference.** This ratio normally changes as pregnancy progresses. In the second trimester, the head circumference is greater than the abdominal circumference. At about 32–36 weeks' gestation, the ratio is 1:1, and after 36 weeks the abdominal measurements become larger. Persistence of a head-abdomen ratio <1 late in gestation is predictive of asymmetric IUGR.
         d. **Femur length.** Femur length appears to correlate well with crownheel length and provides an early and reproducible measurement of length. Serial measurements of femur length are as effective as head measurements for detecting symmetric IUGR.

e. **Placental morphology and amniotic fluid assessment** may help in distinguishing a constitutionally small fetus from a growth-retarded fetus. For example, placental aging with oligohydramnios suggests IUGR and fetal jeopardy, whereas normal placental morphology with a normal amount of amniotic fluid suggests a constitutionally small fetus.

4. **Doppler velocity waveform** assessed in maternal and fetal circulations may detect IUGR. Decreased maternal arcuate arterial waveform velocities indicate decreased uteroplacental perfusion. Fetal Doppler arterial waveform velocities indicate chronic fetal distress and hypoxia. Greatest risk is associated with absent or reversed diastolic flow in umbilical arteries.

C. **Neonatal assessment.** See also Chapter 3.

1. **Reduced birth weight** for gestational age is the simplest method of diagnosing IUGR. However, this method tends to misdiagnose constitutionally small infants and miss appropriate-sized growth-retarded infants.

2. **Physical appearance.** When infants with congenital malformation syndromes and infections are excluded, the remaining group of IUGR infants have characteristic physical appearance. These infants in general are thin, with loose, peeling skin because of loss of subcutaneous tissue, a scaphoid abdomen, and a disproportionately large head.

3. **Lubchenco charts** (see Figure 3–2) may underestimate IUGR because they are based on observations made well above sea level.

4. **A ponderal index** below the 10th percentile helps to identify neonates with IUGR, especially those with birth weight <2500 g.

5. **Ballard score.** Gestational age can also be assessed by means of the Ballard scoring system. This examination is accurate within 2 weeks of gestation in infants weighing <999 g at birth and is most accurate at 30–42 h of age. Plotting of individual growth parameter alone may not show IUGR. Use the ponderal index as shown in section I. IUGR infants have a higher rating on this scale than premature infants with similar weights. See Chapter 3 for Ballard examination and scoring.

VI. **Complications** (Table 69–4)

A. **Hypoxia**

1. **Perinatal asphyxia.** IUGR infants frequently have birth asphyxia because they tolerate the stress of labor poorly. IUGR accounts for a large proportion of stillborn infants with hypoxia in utero.

2. **Persistent pulmonary hypertension (persistent fetal circulation).** Many IUGR infants are subjected to chronic intrauterine hypoxia, which results in abnormal thickening of the smooth muscles of the small pulmonary arterioles. This, in turn, reduces pulmonary blood flow and results in varying degrees of pulmonary artery hypertension. Because of this, IUGR infants are at risk for persistent pulmonary hypertension. Hyaline membrane disease is less frequently seen in IUGR because these infants tend to manifest advanced pulmonary maturity secondary to chronic intrauterine stress.

3. **Respiratory distress syndrome.** Several reports suggest accelerated fetal pulmonary maturation in association with IUGR secondary to

---

TABLE 69–4. NEONATAL COMPLICATIONS OF INTRAUTERINE GROWTH RETARDATION

Metabolic disorders: hypoglycemia, hypocalcemia
Hypothermia
Hematologic disorders: polycythemia
Hypoxia: birth asphyxia, meconium aspiration, persistent fetal circulation
Congenital malformation

chronic intrauterine stress. One (McIntire 1999) suggests that the incidence of respiratory distress syndrome was inversely proportional to the gestational age and birth weight percentile.
   4. **Meconium aspiration.** Postterm IUGR infants are at risk for meconium aspiration.
B. **Hypothermia.** Thermoregulation is compromised in IUGR infants because of diminished subcutaneous fat insulation. Infants with IUGR secondary to fetal malnutrition late in gestation tend to be scrawny as a result of loss of subcutaneous fat. They tend to be more alert than their premature counterparts.
C. **Metabolic**
   1. **Hypoglycemia.** Carbohydrate metabolism is seriously disturbed, and IUGR infants are highly susceptible to hypoglycemia as a consequence of diminished glycogen reserves and decreased capacity for gluconeogenesis. Oxidation of free fatty acids and triglycerides is reduced in IUGR infants, which limits alternate fuel sources. Hyperinsulinism, excess sensitivity to insulin, and deficient catecholamine release during hypoglycemia suggest abnormality of counterregulatory hormone mechanisms during periods of hypoglycemia in IUGR infants. Hypothermia may potentiate the problem of hypoglycemia.
   2. **Hyperglycemia.** Very low birth weight infants have low insulin secretion, resulting in hyperglycemia.
   3. **Hypocalcemia.** Hypocalcemia may occur in IUGR infants after asphyxia.
D. **Hematologic disorders.** Hyperviscosity and polycythemia may result from increased erythropoietin levels secondary to fetal hypoxia associated with IUGR. *Thrombocytopenia, neutropenia, and altered coagulation profile are also seen in IUGR infants.* Polycythemia may also contribute to hypoglycemia and lead to cerebral injury.
E. **Altered immunity.** IUGR infants have decreased IgG levels. In addition, the thymus is reduced in size by 50% and peripheral blood lymphocytes are decreased.
VII. **Management.** Antenatal diagnosis is the key to proper management of IUGR.
A. **History of risk factors.** The presence of maternal risk factors should alert the obstetrician to the likelihood of fetal growth retardation. Ultrasonography confirms the diagnosis. Correctable causes of impaired fetal growth warrant immediate attention.
B. **Delivery and resuscitation.** Appropriate timing of delivery is important. Delivery is usually undertaken when the lungs are mature or when biophysical data obtained by monitoring reveal fetal distress. Labor is particularly stressful to IUGR fetuses. Skilled resuscitation should be available because birth asphyxia is common.
C. **Prevention of heat loss.** Meticulous care should be taken to prevent heat loss (see Chapter 5).
D. **Hypoglycemia.** Close monitoring of blood glucose levels is essential for all IUGR infants. Hypoglycemia should be treated promptly with parenteral dextrose and early feeding, as outlined in Chapter 43.
E. **Hematologic disorders.** A central hematocrit reading should be obtained to detect polycythemia.
F. **Congenital infection.** IUGR infants should be examined for congenital malformations or signs of congenital infections. Many intrauterine infections are clinically silent, and screening for these should be done routinely in IUGR infants. (See the discussion of TORCH infections in Chapter 68.)
G. **Genetic anomalies.** Screening for genetic anomalies should be done as indicated by the physical examination.
VIII. **Outcome.** *Neurodevelopmental morbidities are seen 5–10 times more often in IUGR infants compared with AGA infants.* Neurodevelopmental outcome depends not only on the cause of IUGR but also on the adverse events in the neonatal course (eg, perinatal asphyxia or hypoglycemia). Many studies reveal

evidence of minimal brain dysfunction, including hyperactivity, short attention span, and learning problems.

A. **Symmetric versus asymmetric IUGR.** Infants with symmetric IUGR caused by decreased growth potential generally have a poor outcome, whereas those with asymmetric IUGR in which brain growth is spared usually have a good outcome.

B. **Preterm IUGR** infants have a higher incidence of abnormalities than the general population because they are subjected to the risks of prematurity in addition to the risks of IUGR. Outcomes are significantly poorer for children whose brain growth failure occurred before 26 weeks' gestation.

C. **Chromosomal disorders.** IUGR infants with major chromosomal disorders have a 100% incidence of handicap.

D. **Congenital infections.** Infants with congenital rubella or cytomegalovirus infection with microcephaly have a poor outcome, with a handicap rate >50%.

E. **Learning ability.** The school performance of IUGR infants is significantly influenced by social class; children from higher social classes score better on achievement tests.

F. **Adult disorders.** Epidemiologic evidence indicates that obesity, insulin-resistant diabetes, and cardiovascular diseases are more common among adults who were IUGR at birth.

REFERENCES

Allen MC. Developmental outcome and follow-up of the small for gestational age infant. *Semin Perinatol* 1984;8:123.

Anderson MS, Hay WW: IUGR and small for gestation age infant. *Pathophysiology and Management of Newborn* 1999;25:411.

Ballard JL et al: A simplified score for assessment of fetal maturation of newly born infants. *J Pediatr* 1979;95:769.

Banks BA ot al: Multiple courses of antenatal corticosteroids and outcome of premature infants. *Am J Obstet Gynecol* 1999;181:709.

Barker DJP: Fetal and infant origin of adult disease. *BMJ* 1993;301:1111.

Battaglia FC, Lubchenco LO: A practical classification of newborn infants by weight and gestational age. *J Pediatr* 1967;17:159.

Blair E: Intrauterine growth and spastic cerebral palsy. *Am J Obstet Gynecol* 1990;162:229.

Cunningham GF et al: Fetal growth disorders. *Obstetrics* 2001;29:743.

Hay WW: Fetal growth: its regulation and disorders. *Pediatrics* 1997;99:585.

Kleigman RM, Das UG: Intrauterine growth retardation. *Neonatal-Perinatal Med* 2002;13:229.

Lubchenco LO et al: Intrauterine growth estimated from live born birthweight data. *Pediatrics* 1963;32:793.

McIntire DD et al: Birth weight in relation to morbidity and mortality among newborn infants. *N Engl J Med* 1999;340:1234.

Orro AS, Dixon SD: Perinatal cocaine and methamphetamine exposure. *J Pediatr* 1987;111:571.

Warshaw JB: Intrauterine growth retardation. *Pediatr Rev* 1986;8:107.

Williams RL et al: Fetal growth and perinatal viability in California. *Obstet Gynecol* 1982;52:624.

70 Multiple Gestation

I. **Incidence.** The incidence of multiple gestation is probably underestimated. Fewer than half of twin pregnancies diagnosed with ultrasonography during the first trimester are finally delivered as twins, a phenomenon that has been termed *vanishing twin*. Twins occur in 1–2% of deliveries after 20 weeks, and the triplet rate is ~0.1%. Two gestational sacs can be identified with ultrasonography by 6 weeks' gestation. In addition, routine screening for maternal alpha-fetoprotein will identify about half of the pregnancies with multiple gestations at an early gestational age. About 12–20% of twins are identified after the onset of labor.

The incidence of monozygotic twinning is remarkably constant at 3–5 per 1000 pregnancies, whereas the rate for dizygotic twinning varies from 4–50 per 1000 pregnancies. About one third of twins in the United States are monozygotic. The rate of monozygotic twinning is considered a chance phenomenon, whereas dizygotic twinning results from multiple ovulation, shows wide ethnic variability, and may have a familial tendency.

II. **Risk factors.** The incidence of dizygotic twinning increases with a family history of twins, maternal age (peak at 35–39 years), previous twin gestation, increasing parity, maternal height, fecundity, social class, frequency of coitus, and exposure to exogenous gonadotropins (20–40% incidence) and clomiphene (6–8% incidence).

The risk of twinning decreases with undernourishment. Ethnic background (African Americans > Caucasians > Asians) is a preconception risk factor for multiple gestation.

Over the last two decades, there has been a striking increase in the frequency of pleural births. Between 1980 and 1994, there was a 42% increase in the number of twin births, and the twin birth rate (ie, the number of twin births to total live births) increased 30% from 18.9 to 24.6 per 1000 live births (*MMWR*, 1997). The rate of triplet births has escalated more rapidly, increasing 100% between 1980 and 1989. White women, especially those >30 years of age, accounted for the bulk of this increase. It is likely that much of this increase stems from the use of ovulation-inducing drugs for the treatment of infertility (Kiely et al, 1992). By 1997, the use of assisted reproductive technology accounted for more than 40% of triplets born in the United States (Schieve et al, 2002).

III. **Placentation**
   A. **Classification.** Placental examination affords a unique opportunity to identify two thirds to three fourths of monozygotic twins at birth.
      1. **Twin placentation is classified according to the placental disk** (single, fused, or separate), number of chorions (monochorionic or dichorionic), and number of amnions (monoamniotic or diamniotic) (Figure 70–1).
      2. **Heterosexual (assuredly dizygotic) twins** always have a dichorionic placenta.
      3. **Monochorionic twins** are always of the same sex. All monochorionic twins are believed to be monozygotic. In 70% of monozygotic twin pregnancies, the placentas are monochorionic, and the possibility exists for commingling of the fetal circulations. Fewer than 1% of twin pregnancies are monoamniotic.
   B. **Complications.** Twin gestations are associated with an increased frequency of anomalies of the placenta and adnexa; for example, a single umbilical artery or velamentous or marginal cord insertion (6–9 times more common with twin gestation). The cord is more susceptible to trauma from

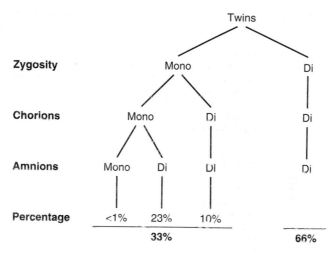

FIGURE 70–1. Percentage distribution of twins according to placental type, Mono, Monoamniotic; Di, diamniotic.

twisting. The vessels near the insertion are often unprotected by Wharton's jelly and are especially prone to thrombosis when compression or twisting occurs. Intrapartum fetal distress from cord compression and fetal hemorrhage from associated vasa previa are potential problems with velamentous insertion of the cord.

C. **Determination of zygosity.** The most efficient way to identify zygosity is as follows:
   1. **Gender examination.** Male-female pairs are dizygotic. The dichorionic placenta may be separate or fused.
   2. **Placental examination.** Twins with a monochorionic placenta (monoamniotic or diamniotic) are monozygotic. Care should be taken not to confuse apposed fused placentas for a single chorion. If doubt exists on gross inspection of the dividing membranes, a transverse section should be studied. The zygosity of twins of the same sex with dichorionic membranes cannot be immediately known. Genetic studies are needed (eg, blood typing, human leukocyte antigen [HLA] typing, DNA markers, and chromosome marking) to determine zygosity.

IV. **Mortality rates.** Although perinatal mortality rates for singleton pregnancies have continued to fall during the last decade, there has been little change in mortality rates for multiple pregnancies.
   A. **Twins.** For twin gestations, the fetal mortality rate is 4%, the neonatal mortality rate 7.6% (1.2% for singletons), and the perinatal mortality rate 11.6% (2.2% for singletons). The perinatal death rate for twins is 9 times the rate for first-born singletons and 11 times the rate for second-born singletons.
   1. **Monoamniotic twins.** The mortality rate for monoamniotic twins is highest (50–60%), largely because of cord entanglement.
   2. **Monozygotic twins.** Monozygotic twins have a perinatal mortality and morbidity rate that is 2–3 times that of dizygotic twins. Diamniotic monochorionic twins have a mortality rate of 25%, and dichorionic twins, a mortality rate of 8.9%.
   3. **Prematurity in twins.** Approximately 10% of preterm deliveries are twin gestations, and they account for 25% of perinatal deaths in preterm deliveries.

4. Fetal death. Death of one fetus may affect the outcome of the survivor profoundly or minimally (Dudley & Dalton, 1986). When the cause of death is intrinsic to one dichorionic fetus and does not threaten the other fetus, complications are rare. Hazardous intrauterine environments threaten both twins, whether monochorionic or dichorionic. With monochorionic placentas, the incidence of major complications or death in the surviving twin is ~50%.

B. Triplets. The neonatal mortality rate for triplets is 18.8%, and the perinatal mortality rate is 25.5%.

V. Morbidity

A. Prematurity. Prematurity and uteroplacental insufficiency are the major contributors to perinatal complications. The average twin delivery occurs at 37 weeks, and multiple gestation is complicated by preterm delivery (<35 weeks) in 21.5% of patients. The incidence of premature rupture of membranes is doubled in multiple gestations (Merenstein & Weisman, 1996).

B. Intrauterine growth retardation. The incidence of low birth weight in twins is ~50–60%, a figure that is 5–7 times higher than the incidence of low birth weight in singletons. In general, the more fetuses in a gestation, the smaller is their weight for gestational age (Figure 70–2). Twins tend to grow at normal rates up to about 30–34 weeks' gestation, when they reach a combined weight of 4 kg. Thereafter, they grow more slowly. Two thirds of twins show some signs of growth retardation at birth.

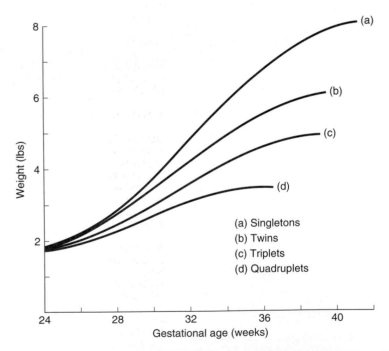

FIGURE 70–2. Growth curve showing the mean weights of infants from single and multiple pregnancies by gestational age. *(From Phelan MC: Twins. In Stevenson RE et al [editors]:* Human Malformations and Related Anomalies. *Oxford University Press, 1993. Modified from McKeown T, Record RG: Observations of foetal growth in multiple pregnancy in man.* J Endocrinol *1952;8:386.)* Reproduced by permission of the Society for Endocrinology.

C. **Uteroplacental insufficiency.** The incidence of acute and chronic uteroplacental insufficiency is increased in multiple gestations. Five-minute Apgar scores of 0–3 are reported for 5–10% of twin gestations. These low scores may relate to acute stresses of labor, cord prolapse (1–5%), or trauma during delivery superimposed on chronic uteroplacental insufficiency.

VI. **Congenital anomalies.** Birth defects are 2–3 times more common in monozygotic twins than in singletons or dizygotic twins, who have a 2–3% incidence of major defects diagnosed at birth. Three mechanisms are postulated for the increased frequency of structural defects in monozygotic twins: (1) deformations caused by intrauterine space constraint, (2) disruption of normal blood flow secondary to placental vascular anastomoses, and (3) defects in morphogenesis. Such defects are usually discordant in monozygotic twins; however, in purely genetic conditions (eg, chromosomal abnormalities or single-gene defects), concordance would be the rule.

A. **Anomalies unique to multiple pregnancies.** Certain anomalies, such as conjoined twins and acardia, are unique to multiple pregnancies.

B. **Deformations.** Twins are more likely to suffer from intrauterine crowding and restriction of movement, leading to synostosis, torticollis, facial palsy, positional foot defects, and other defects (MacLennan, 1984).

C. **Vascular disruptions.** Disruptions related to monozygotic vascular shunts may result in birth defects. Acardia occurs from an artery-to-artery placental shunt, in which reverse flow leads to the development of an amorphous recipient twin. In utero death of a cotwin may result in thromboembolic phenomena, including disseminated intravascular coagulation, cutis aplasia, porencephaly or hydranencephaly, limb reduction defects, intestinal atresias, or gastroschisis.

D. **Malformations.** Monozygotic twinning results in increased frequency of the following specific malformations: (1) sacrococcygeal teratoma, (2) sirenomelia sequence, including VACTERL association (vertebral abnormalities, anal atresia, cardiac abnormalities, tracheoesophageal fistula, renal dysplasia, and limb deformities), (3) cloacal exstrophy sequence, (4) holoprosencephaly sequence, and (5) anencephaly.

VII. **Twin-twin transfusion syndrome (see also discussion of anemia in Chapter 61)**

A. **Vascular anastomoses.** The chorionic vascular bed of monozygotic (and usually monochorionic) twins seems to have limitless variations. However, almost all monochorionic placentas demonstrate vascular anastomoses, whereas dichorionic placentas rarely do. Vascular anastomoses may be superficial direct communications easily visible on inspection between arteries (most common) or veins (uncommon), deep connections from arteries to veins via villi, or combinations of superficial and deep connections. This commonality of chorionic vasculature sets the stage for twin-twin transfusion syndrome.

B. **Incidence.** Despite the high frequency of vascular anastomosis in monochorionic placentation, the twin-twin transfusion syndrome is relatively uncommon (~15% of monochorionic gestations).

C. **Clinical manifestations.** Clinically, the twin-twin transfusion syndrome is diagnosed when twins have a hemoglobin difference of >5 g/dL and is due to artery-to-vein anastomoses.

1. **The donor twin** tends to be pale and have a low birth weight, oligohydramnios, anemia, hypoglycemia, decreased organ mass, hypovolemia, and amnion nodosum. Donor twins often require volume expansion, red blood cell transfusion, or both.

2. **The recipient twin** is frequently plethoric and has a high birth weight, polyhydramnios, polycythemia or hyperviscosity, increased organ mass, hypervolemia, and hyperbilirubinemia. Recipient twins often require partial exchange transfusion with fresh-frozen plasma.

3. Rarely, either or both of the twins involved in a fetofetal transfusion may present with hydrops fetalis.

VIII. Neonatal implications and management

A. **Site of delivery.** When a complicated twin gestation has been identified, delivery should ideally be conducted at a high-risk perinatal center with two experienced pediatric delivery teams in attendance.

B. **Placental examination.** Examination of placenta(s) in the delivery room provides an early opportunity to determine zygosity and anticipate certain problems.

C. **Physical examination.** Infants should be examined for evidence of intrauterine growth retardation, congenital anomalies, and twin-twin transfusion syndrome. Central hematocrits should be obtained in both infants to look for anemia or polycythemia. When one of the infants has a congenital anomaly, the normal twin is at increased risk for complications of pregnancy and growth retardation. In particular, death of one fetus puts the others at risk for fetal disseminated intravascular coagulation. Resulting cystic encephalomalacia is estimated to occur in 12% of monochorionic twin gestations (D'Alton & Simpson, 1995).

D. **Complications in newborn period.** The second-born twin is 2–4 times as likely to develop respiratory distress syndrome (Rokos et al, 1968), probably secondary to perinatal stress; however, the first-born twin may be at risk for necrotizing enterocolitis (Samm et al, 1986).

E. **Cobedding of multiples.** Coincident with the rise in multiple births has been an interest in cobedding of multiples (DellaPorta et al, 1998). Although specific risks and benefits have yet to be determined, it is the policy at Northside Hospital in Atlanta, Georgia to allow cobedding of multiples with a physician's order. Among other criteria, eligible multiples need to be free of infection, have stable temperature in an open crib, have no indwelling catheters, and be on room air or nasal cannula. Color coding of all equipment and monitors is used to ensure proper identification, and the parents are required to sign a consent form.

F. **Economic considerations.** It has been estimated that the perinatal health care costs associated with pleural births were 4 times higher for twins and 11 times higher for triplets than those of a singleton birth (Callahan et al, 1994). The increasing rate of pleural births and the concordant decline in mortality risk has more than doubled the need for medical and social services for these children and their families (Kiely et al, 1992).

IX. Risks beyond the neonatal period

A. **Catch-up growth.** In monozygotic twins, birth weight differences may be as much as 20%, but the lighter twin has a remarkable ability to make up intrauterine growth deficits. However, if the birth weight of the lighter twin is less than the 10th percentile, the prognosis is guarded. With such marked discordance, the undersized twin often continues to be inferior in growth and intelligence into adult life.

B. **Acquired illnesses.** Illness in one twin increases the risk of illness in the other (Seigle & Seigle, 1982). Epilepsy has an 85% concordance rate in identical twins. With acute lymphocytic leukemia or juvenile diabetes mellitus of one twin, the incidence in the other twin is 20% and 50%, respectively.

C. **Social problems.** Inadequate nurturing and child abuse are more likely with twins. Counseling for parents of twins may be invaluable (Seigle & Seigle, 1982).

REFERENCES

Babson SG, Phillips DS: Growth and development of twins dissimilar in size at birth. *N Engl J Med* 1973;289:937.

Benirschke K: Multiple gestation: incidence, etiology, and inheritance. In Creasy RK, Resnik R (eds): *Maternal-Fetal Medicine*. Saunders, 1984.

Callahan TL et al: The economic impact of multiple-gestation pregnancies and the contribution of assisted-reproduction techniques to their incidence. *N Engl J Med* 1994;331:244.

D'Alton ME, Simpson LL: Syndromes in twins. *Semin Perinatol* 1995;19:375.

DellaPorta K et al: Co-bedding of twins in the neonatal intensive care unit. *Pediatr Nurs* 1998;24:6.

Dudley DKL, Dalton ME: Single fetal death in twin gestation. *Semin Perinatol* 1986;10:65.

Hecht F, Hecht BK: Genetic and related biomedical aspects of twinning. *Pediatr Rev* 1983;5:179.

Johnson SF, Driscoll SG: Twin placentation and its complications. *Semin Perinatol* 1986;10:9.

Koet MP et al: Follow-up study of physical growth of monozygous twins with discordant within-pair birth weights. *Pediatrics* 1986;77:336.

Kiely JL et al: Triplets and higher-order multiple births: time trends and infant mortality. *Am J Dis Child* 1992;146:862.

Little J, Bryan E: Congenital anomalies in twins. *Semin Perinatol* 1986;10:50

Macgillivray I: Epidemiology of twin pregnancy. *Semin Perinatol* 1986;10:4.

MacLennan AH: Multiple gestation: clinical characteristics and management. In Creasy RK, Resnik R (eds): *Maternal-Fetal Medicine*. Saunders, 1984.

Merenstein GB, Weisman LE: Premature rupture of the membranes: neonatal consequences. *Semin Perinatol* 1996;20:375.

Newton ER: Antepartum care in multiple gestation. *Semin Perinatol* 1986;10:19.

Rokos J et al: Hyaline membrane disease in twins. *Pediatrics* 1968;42:204.

Samm M et al: Necrotizing enterocolitis in infants of multiple gestation. *Am J Dis Child* 1986;140:937.

Schieve LA et al: Low and very low birth weight in infants conceived with the use of assisted reproductive technology *N Engl J Med* 2002;346:731.

Seigle SJ, Seigle MM: Practical aspects of pediatric management of families of twins. *Pediatr Rev* 1982;4:8.

Smith DW: *Recognizable Patterns of Human Malformation*, 3rd ed. Saunders, 1982.

State specific variation in rates of twin births -United States, 1992 -1994. *MMWR Morb Mortal Wkly Rep* 1997;46:121.

Wenstrom KD, Gall SA: Incidence, morbidity and mortality, and diagnosis of twin gestations. *Clin Perinatol* 1988;15:1.

71 Necrotizing Enterocolitis and Spontaneous Intestinal Perforation

I. **Definitions**
   A. **Necrotizing enterocolitis** (NEC) is an acquired neonatal disorder representing an end expression of serious intestinal injury after a combination of vascular, mucosal, and metabolic (and other unidentified) insults to a relatively immature gut.
   B. **Spontaneous intestinal perforation** is a clinical syndrome of undetermined cause resembling NEC with less systemic involvement and a less severe clinical course. It may represent a variant of classic NEC.

II. **Incidence**
   A. **NEC is predominantly a disorder of preterm infants,** with an incidence of 6–10% in infants weighing <1.5 kg. The incidence increases with decreasing gestational age. Seventy to 90% of cases occur in high-risk low birth weight infants, whereas 10–25% occur in full-term newborns. Infants with NEC represent 2–5% of neonatal intensive care unit (NICU) admissions.
   B. **NEC occurs sporadically or in epidemic clusters.**

III. **Pathophysiology.** Currently, there is no single unifying theory for the pathogenesis of NEC that satisfactorily explains all of the clinical observations associated with this disorder. The generally accepted pathophysiologic sequence of events resulting in overt clinical disease is thought to involve an initial ischemic or toxic mucosal damage resulting in a loss of mucosal integrity. Then, with the availability of suitable substrate provided by enteral feedings, there is bacterial proliferation followed by invasion of the damaged intestinal mucosa by gas-producing (methane and hydrogen) organisms that cause intramural bowel gas (pneumatosis intestinalis). This sequence of events may then progress to transmural necrosis or gangrene of the bowel and finally to perforation and peritonitis.

IV. **Risk factors**
   A. **Prematurity.** There is an inverse relationship between risk and gestational age. The lower the gestational age, the greater is the risk because of the immaturity of the circulatory, gastrointestinal, and immune systems.
   B. **Asphyxia and acute cardiopulmonary disease** lead to low cardiac output and diminished perfusion states, resulting in redistribution of cardiac output away from the mesenteric circulation and causing episodic intestinal ischemia.
   C. **Enteral feedings.** NEC is rare in unfed infants. About 90–95% of infants with NEC have received at least one enteral feeding. The explanations for this include the following:
      1. **Enteral feeding** provides necessary substrate for proliferation of enteric pathogens.
      2. **Hyperosmolar formula or medications** cause altered mucosal permeability and direct mucosal damage.
      3. **There is a loss or lack of immunoprotective factors** in commercially prepared formulas and in stored breast milk.
      4. **Breast-feeding** significantly lowers the risk of NEC.
   D. **Polycythemia and hyperviscosity syndromes.** These have been shown to be definite risk factors clinically and experimentally probably because of diminished perfusion and intestinal ischemia in watershed areas of the GI tract.
   E. **Exchange transfusions.** There has been a clinically observed association between NEC and exchange transfusions. This is probably due to intestinal ischemia resulting from wide variations in venous or arterial perfusion pressures.

F. Feeding volumes, timing of enteral feeding, and rapid advancement in enteral feedings. These appear to play a role, but clinical evidence remains controversial.

G. Enteric pathogenic microorganisms. Bacterial and viral pathogens, including *Escherichia coli, Klebsiella, Enterobacter, Pseudomonas, Salmonella, Staphylococcus epidermidis, Clostridium* sp, coronaviruses, rotaviruses, and enteroviruses, have been implicated, either directly or indirectly, by blood, stool, or peritoneal space cultures.

V. Clinical presentation. The time of NEC onset varies inversely with gestational age. In the very low birth weight (VLBW) group, onset invariably follows initiation of enteral feedings and is usually diagnosed between 14 and 20 days of age. In full-term infants, age of onset is within the first week of life. During epidemic clustering of cases, age of onset is variable. The presentation may vary from abdominal distention (the most frequent early sign, noted in 70% of cases), ileus, and increased volume of gastric aspirate or bilious aspirate (two thirds of cases) to frank signs of shock, bloody stools, peritonitis, and perforation. NEC may also present insidiously with nonspecific signs such as labile temperature, apnea, bradycardia, or other signs of suspect sepsis.

The clinical syndrome has been classified into stages by Walsh and Kliegman (1986) to include systemic, intestinal, and radiographic findings.

A. Stage I: suspected NEC
   1. **Systemic** signs are nonspecific, including apnea, bradycardia, lethargy, and temperature instability.
   2. **Intestinal** findings include feeding intolerance, recurrent gastric residuals, and guaiac-positive stools.
   3. **Radiographic** findings are normal or nonspecific.

B. Stage IIA: mild NEC
   1. **Systemic** signs are similar to those in stage I.
   2. **Intestinal** findings include prominent abdominal distention with or without tenderness, absent bowel sounds, and gross blood in the stools.
   3. **Radiographic** findings include ileus, with dilated loops with focal areas of pneumatosis intestinalis.

C. Stage IIB: moderate NEC
   1. **Systemic** signs include stage 1 signs plus mild acidosis and thrombocytopenia.
   2. **Intestinal** findings include increasing distention, abdominal wall edema, and tenderness with or without a palpable mass.
   3. **Radiographic** findings include extensive pneumatosis and early ascites. Intrahepatic portal venous gas may be present.

D. Stage IIIA: advanced NEC
   1. **Systemic** findings include respiratory and metabolic acidosis, assisted ventilation for apnea, decreasing blood pressure and urine output, neutropenia, and coagulopathy.
   2. **Intestinal** findings include spreading edema, erythema or discoloration, and induration of the abdominal wall.
   3. **Radiographic** findings include prominent ascites, paucity of bowel gas, and possibly a persistent sentinel loop.

E. Stage IIIB: advanced NEC
   1. **Systemic** findings reveal generalized edema, deteriorating vital signs and laboratory indices, refractory hypotension, shock syndrome, disseminated intravascular coagulation (DIC), and electrolyte imbalance.
   2. **Intestinal** findings reveal a tense, discolored abdomen and ascites.
   3. **Radiographic findings** commonly show absent bowel gas and often evidence of intraperitoneal free air.

VI. Diagnosis. A high index of suspicion should be entertained for any infant with a history of a combination of the risk factors enumerated under section IV.
   A. Clinical diagnosis. NEC is a tentative diagnosis in any infant presenting with the triad of feeding intolerance, abdominal distention, and grossly

bloody stools (hematochezia) or acute change in stool character. Alternatively, the earliest signs may be identical to those of neonatal sepsis.
B. Laboratory studies. The following should be performed as baseline studies. If there is clinical progression of disease or if these laboratory tests are abnormal, the tests should be repeated every 8–12 h.

1. **Complete blood cell count (CBC) with differential.** The white blood cell (WBC) may be normal but is more frequently either elevated, with a shift to the left, or low (leukopenia).
2. **Platelet count.** Thrombocytopenia is seen. Fifty percent of patients with proven NEC have platelet counts <50,000/µL.
3. **Blood culture** for aerobes, anaerobes, and fungi (*Candida* sp).
4. **Stool screening** for occult blood. Routine testing of stools for occult blood does not identify a population at greater risk for NEC. In suspect patients, the presence of occult blood may influence management but may not be helpful in making a diagnosis of NEC.
5. **Arterial blood gas measurements.** Metabolic or combined acidosis or hypoxia may be seen.
6. **Electrolyte panel.** Electrolyte imbalances, particularly hypo- or hypernatremia, and hyperkalemia are common.
7. **Stool cultures for rotaviruses and enteroviruses** should be obtained if diarrhea is an epidemic in the nursery.

C. Radiologic studies
1. **Flat plate x-ray studies of the abdomen**
   a. **Supportive for NEC.** Look for abnormal bowel gas patterns, ileus, a fixed sentinel loop of bowel, or areas suspicious for pneumatosis intestinalis.
   b. **Confirmatory of NEC.** Look for (1) intramural bowel gas (pneumatosis intestinalis) and (2) intrahepatic portal venous gas (in the absence of an umbilical venous catheter).
2. **Lateral decubitus and cross-table lateral studies of the abdomen.** These studies are more likely to demonstrate a pneumoperitoneum.
   Note: Perforation commonly occurs within 48–72 h after pneumatosis or portal venous gas. In the presence of pneumatosis intestinalis or portal venous gas, flat plate and left lateral decubitus or cross-table lateral x-ray studies of the abdomen should be obtained every 6–8 h to check for the development of pneumoperitoneum, signaling intestinal perforation. Serial x-ray studies may be discontinued with clinical improvement, usually after 48–72 h.

VII. Management. The main principle of management for confirmed NEC is to treat it as an acute abdomen with impending or septic peritonitis. The goal is to prevent progression of disease, intestinal perforation, and shock. If NEC occurs in epidemic clusters, cohort isolation has been shown to limit transmission. Signs to watch closely for include progressive distention and discoloration of the abdomen, refractory metabolic acidosis, falling platelet counts, and shock.
A. Basic NEC protocol. Any infant with suspected NEC should be managed according to the following protocol:
1. **Nothing by mouth** to allow gastrointestinal rest. Initiate or advance peripheral or central total parenteral nutrition (TPN) to maintain basal nutritional needs.
2. **Use of a nasogastric tube** (on low intermittent suction) to keep the bowel decompressed.
3. **Close monitoring of vital signs and abdominal circumference.**
4. **Removal of the umbilical catheter** and placement of peripheral venous and arterial catheters, depending on severity of illness (*controversial*).
5. **Antibiotics.** Start ampicillin and gentamicin or cefotaxime intravenously. Add anaerobic coverage (clindamycin or metronidazole [Flagyl]) if peritonitis or perforation is suspected. (For dosages, see Chapter 80.)

6. **Monitoring for gastrointestinal bleeding.** Check all gastric aspirates and stools for blood.
7. **Strict monitoring of fluid intake and output.** Try to maintain urine output of 1–3 mL/kg/h.
8. **Removal of potassium from intravenous fluids** in the presence of hyperkalomia or anuria.
9. **Laboratory monitoring.** Check CBC, platelet count, and electrolyte panel every 12–24 h until stablo.
10. **Septic workup.** As a part of tho workup, some institutions routinely perform lumbar puncture for culture of cerebrospinal fluid before starting antibiotics (*controversial*).
11. **Radiologic studies.** Perform abdominal flat plate x-ray studies with lateral decubitus or cross-table studies every 6–8 h in the acute phase to detect bowel perforation.

B. **Management of stage I.** Start the basic NEC protocol described in section VII,A. If all cultures are negative and the infant has improved clinically, antibiotics can be stopped after 3 days. The infant may also be fed after 3 days if clinically improved.

C. **Management of stages IIA and B**
1. **Basic NEC protocol,** including antibiotics for 10 days (see section VII,A,5).
2. **NPO for 2 weeks.** Oral feedings may be started 7–10 days after radiographic resolution of pneumatosis.
3. **Continue and advance TPN** to achieve a caloric intake of ≥90–110 cal/kg/day.
4. **Respiratory support.** Appropriate level of ventilatory support to correct hypoxia and respiratory and metabolic acidosis and maintain acceptable arterial blood gas parameters. Progressive abdominal distention causing loss of lung volume may increase the need for positive-pressure ventilation.
5. **Fluid and electrolyte management.** Adjust total fluid intake, making allowance for third space losses, transfusion of blood and blood products, and prerenal and renal failure. Hyperglycemia resulting from glucose intolerance frequently complicates fluid and electrolyte management of the extremely low birth weight (ELBW) infant with NEC.
6. **Surgical consultation** is required.
7. **Low-dose dopamine infusion.** Low-dose dopamine infusion (2–4 mg/kg/min) to improve intestinal blood and renal perfusion in low-flow states. (This practice varies among institutions.)

D. **Management of stages IIIA and IIIB**
1. **Basic NEC protocol,** as described in section VII,A.
2. **Plus stage II management,** as described in section VII,C.
3. **Blood pressure support.** Refractory hypotension is common and multifactorial in origin. Treatment includes replacement of ongoing fluid losses, volume expansion with colloids (see Chapter 46), and vasopressors such as dopamine (for dosage, see Chapter 80). The goal is to maintain adequate mean blood pressure (see Appendix C) and urine output (1–3 mL/kg/h).
4. **Progressive leukopenia, granulocytopenia, and thrombocytopenia** usually parallel a deteriorating clinical status. Granulocyte transfusion and granulocyte colony-stimulating factor (G-CSF) are not routinely indicated. Blood and platelet transfusions are frequently needed.

E. **Surgical management (see also Chapter 78)**
1. **Exploratory laparotomy** is indicated if there is evidence of intestinal perforation. The procedure includes resection of the diseased segment and exteriorization of a functioning loop. Occasionally, a "second-look" laparotomy is needed.

2. **Peritoneal drainage.** In selected cases in unstable (or ELBW) infants, some centers place a drain in one or both lower quadrants of the abdomen, followed by conservative supportive care. A delayed laparotomy is undertaken if there is continued lack of improvement over the next 24–48 h.

   Other indications (relative and not absolute) for surgical intervention in the absence of free intraperitoneal air include the following:
3. **Deteriorating clinical condition** with failure to respond to appropriate medical management.
   a. **Evidence of a persistent, fixed sentinel loop over 24 h,** suggesting a segment of gangrenous bowel. In these instances, a diagnostic paracentesis to obtain peritoneal fluid for visual examination, Gram's stain, WBC, and culture may be helpful. The presence of brown or particulate peritoneal fluid and bacteria on Gram's stain, a WBC of >300/mm^3, and positive culture results are strongly suggestive of gangrenous bowel or a silent perforation. Introduction of air may confound later diagnosis of perforation. (This approach is not a uniform practice.)
   b. **Metrizamide,** a water-soluble contrast agent, has been used for the diagnosis of a silent perforation in selected cases.
4. **Right lower quadrant mass.**
5. **Abdominal wall erythema** suggests peritonitis and may also be an indication for operative intervention.
6. **Spontaneous intestinal perforation** in the VLBW infant. As a recently recognized entity, it is also a cause of intestinal perforation in VLBW infants and appears to have several clinical features that distinguish it from classic NEC. The clinical course is of insidious onset without the usual gastrointestinal signs of NEC (feeding intolerance, abdominal distention, and bloody stools). Instead, a bluish discoloration of the lower abdomen is often the only presenting early sign. Radiographic findings are limited to intraperitoneal air with no evidence of pneumatosis intestinalis, portal venous gas, or a sentinel loop. The perforations almost always are in the distal ileum, well demarcated, and discrete. Management and treatment are standard for perforated bowel. Outcome and prognosis are better than for NEC with perforation. In some centers the incidence of spontaneous bowel perforations exceeds the number of cases of NEC with perforation.
VIII. **Prevention.** Breast milk has been shown to decrease the risk and incidence of NEC. Studies with the use of immunoglobulins and prophylactic enteral antibiotics to prevent NEC remain largely experimental.
IX. **Prognosis**
   A. **NEC with perforation** is associated with a mortality of 20–40%.
   B. **Recurrent NEC** is a rare complication.
   C. **Subacute or intermittent symptoms of bowel obstruction** resulting from stenosis or strictures of the colon and, less commonly, of the small bowel are seen in ~10–20% of cases. A barium enema is usually confirmatory.
   D. **Infants undergoing extensive surgical resection** require long-term parenteral nutrition, enterostomy care, and management of short-gut syndrome. Chronic electrolyte imbalance and failure to thrive are common.
   E. **In the absence of short-gut syndrome,** growth, nutrition, and gastrointestinal function appear to catch up and are normal by the end of the first year.

REFERENCES

Buonomo C: The radiology of necrotizing enterocolitis. *Radiol Clin North Am* 1999;37:1187.
Bury RG, Tudehope D: Enteral antibiotics for preventing necrotizing enterocolitis in low birthweight or preterm infants. *Cochrane Database Syst Rev* 2001;1:CD000405.

Chandler JC, Hebra A: Necrotizing enterocolitis in infants with very low birth weight. *Semin Pediatr Surg* 2000;9:63.

Foster J, Cole M: Oral immunoglobulin for preventing necrotizing enterocolitis in preterm and low birth-weight neonates. *Cochrane Database Syst Rev* 2001;3:CD001816.

McKeon RE et al: Role of delayed feeding and of feeding increments in necrotizing enterocolitis. *J Pediatr* 1992;124:764.

Moss RL et al: A meta-analysis of peritoneal drainage versus laparotomy for perforated necrotizing enterocolitis. *J Pediatr Surg* 2001;36:1210.

Stoll BJ, Kliegman RM: Necrotizing enterocolitis. *Clin Perinatol* 1994;21.

Uceda JE et al: Intestinal perforations in infants with a very low birth weight: a disease of increasing survival? *J Pediatr Surg* 1995;30:1314.

Walsh MC, Kliegman RM: Necrotizing enterocolitis: treatment based on staging criteria. *Pediatr Clin North Am* 1986;33:179.

72 Neurologic Diseases

HYDROCEPHALUS

I. Definitions
A. **Hydrocephalus** is dilation of the cerebral ventricular system secondary to a disturbance in cerebrospinal fluid (CSF) dynamics. It is usually associated with increased intracranial pressure (ICP) and a large head circumference (HC); however, ventricular dilation commonly precedes head growth, and the HC may be normal initially.

B. **Noncommunicating hydrocephalus** results from obstruction anywhere along the CSF pathway from the third ventricle to the cisterna magna.

C. **Communicating hydrocephalus** results when CSF is able to pass through the foramen at the base of the brain but is improperly drained by the cerebral and cerebellar subarachnoid spaces.

D. **Congenital hydrocephalus** refers to a state of progressive ventricular enlargement apparent from the first days of life and, by implication, with onset in utero.

E. **Macrocephaly** is present when the HC is ≥2 SD above the mean. Macrocephaly is not always associated with hydrocephalus. Macrocephaly without hydrocephalus is usually familial and benign, but it may be associated with neurocutaneous diseases (eg, neurofibromatosis or Sturge-Weber syndrome), metabolic storage diseases (eg, Hunter's or Hurler's syndrome), Beckwith-Wiedemann syndrome, or achondroplasia.

F. **Hydrocephalus ex vacuo** is ventriculomegaly that is not caused by impaired CSF dynamics, but rather is the result of a destructive or atrophic process involving the periventricular white matter. It is *not* associated with increased ICP and is *not* accompanied by rapid head growth.

II. Pathophysiology
A. **Congenital hydrocephalus** results from developmental malformations of the CSF pathway occurring between 6 and 17 weeks' gestation.

B. **Obstruction of CSF flow or derangement in CSF absorption.** The currently accepted belief is that CSF flows through the aqueduct, fourth ventricle, and foramina of Luschka and Magendie to the cisterna magna. From there, the CSF flows over the surface of the hemispheres to be reabsorbed into the bloodstream via the arachnoid granulations, which contain the arachnoid villi. Hydrocephalus can result from obstruction anywhere along the pathway from the third ventricle to the cisterna magna. Greitz et al (1997) proposed a new theory that the main absorption of CSF occurs through the brain capillaries and that hydrocephalus results from *hemodynamic* disturbances. With this new theory, "communicating" hydrocephalus may be caused by any process that restricts cerebral arterial pulsations (restricted arterial pulsation hydrocephalus), and "obstructive" hydrocephalus is the result of ventricular dilatation and compression of the cortical veins (venous congestion hydrocephalus).

C. **Increased CSF production.** Rarely, hydrocephalus results from excessive production of CSF (eg, from papilloma of the choroid plexus).

III. Causes of ventricular dilation
A. **Common causes**
   1. Congenital aqueductal stenosis (X-linked recessive or, rarely, autosomal recessive) accounts for approximately one third of neonatal hydrocephalus.
   2. Neural tube defects (NTDs) with Arnold-Chiari malformation.

3. Posthemorrhagic obstruction (see the following section on intraventricular hemorrhage).
4. Loss of periventricular white matter as a result of periventricular leukomalacia (PVL) or periventricular hemorrhagic infarction (PHI). This is the most common cause of hydrocephalus ex vacuo.

B. **Less common causes**
1. Postinfectious.
2. Dandy-Walker malformation.
3. Other syndromes of vermian agenesis.
4. Aneurysm of the vein of Galen.
5. Severe fetomaternal alloimmune thrombocytopenia.
6. Tumors.
7. Arachnoidal cyst.
8. Achondroplasia.
9. Osteopetrosis.
10. Fetal intraventricular hemorrhage.

IV. **Clinical presentation**
A. **Fetal hydrocephalus**
1. Usually more severe and accompanied by serious anomalies of the central nervous system (CNS) (eg, holoprosencephaly or encephalocele, major extraneural anomalies, or both).
2. Polyhydramnios (10%).
3. Breech presentation (30%).
4. Increased incidence of prematurity, postmaturity, and stillbirths.

B. **NTDs**
1. Eighty percent of infants with NTDs have hydrocephalus.
2. The HC may be normal or nearly normal at birth.

C. **Posthemorrhagic hydrocephalus (PHH)**
1. Approximately 35% of infants with intraventricular hemorrhage (IVH) develop PHH.
   a. Approximately two thirds will have spontaneous arrest or resolution of ventriculomegaly within 4 weeks of progressive ventricular dilation.
   b. Thirty percent will have persistent ventricular dilation beyond 4 weeks.
   c. Five percent will experience rapid ventricular dilation before 4 weeks.
2. In infants who have exhibited arrest or resolution of ventriculomegaly spontaneously or with treatment, ~5% will experience late progressive ventricular dilation and require ventriculoperitoneal (VP) shunt placement.

D. **Signs of hydrocephalus** include apnea, bradycardia, irritability, lethargy, vomiting, a tense fontanelle, widely split sutures, cerebral bruit, dilated scalp veins, and rapid head growth. Sclerae may be visible above the irises ("setting-sun sign"). Papilledema is rarely observed in neonates.

V. **Diagnosis**
A. **Antenatal diagnosis.** Fetal hydrocephalus may be detected as early as 15–18 weeks' gestation. Amniocentesis is advisable to evaluate chromosomal abnormalities associated with hydrocephalus (trisomies 13 and 18), fetal gender (X-linked aqueductal stenosis), and alpha-fetoprotein (AFP) levels. Maternal serology may establish intrauterine infection.
B. **Physical examination.** The occipitofrontal HC is carefully measured. A rate of head growth >2 cm/week usually signals the rapid progression of ventricular dilation.
1. Parents of infants with macrocephaly may also have increased HCs (normal ±2 SD is 54 ±3 cm for women and 55 ±3 cm for men). No further evaluation is required unless there are signs of increased ICP.
2. Fifty percent of infants with X-linked aqueductal stenosis have a characteristic flexion deformity of the thumb.
3. Infants with Dandy-Walker malformation have occipital cranial prominence.

4. Chorioretinitis may be evident after intrauterine infection.
5. A cerebral bruit may signal the presence of an arteriovenous malformation (AVM) of the vein of Galen.
C. **Cranial ultrasonography** is the most important screening tool for premature infants.
   1. **Indications**
      a. Birth weight <1500 g.
      b. Larger, sick premature infants.
      c. Rapidly enlarging HC.
      d. Signs of increased ICP.
   2. **Yield.** Screening at 2 weeks of age will detect 98% of cases of PHH and possibly early PVL.
   3. **Serial ultrasound** scans at 1- to 2-week intervals are necessary to monitor the progression of ventricular dilation until there is stabilization or regression of the ventriculomegaly.
   4. **Ventricular dilation may be sonographically detected days to weeks** *before* **the appearance of traditional clinical signs** (ie, rapid head growth, a full anterior fontanelle, and separated cranial sutures).
D. **Computed tomography (CT) scan or magnetic resonance imaging (MRI) of the head**
   1. Ventricular dilation is estimated from the ventricular-biparietal ratio.
   2. Determination of the size of the cerebral mantle.
   3. Detection of associated CNS anomalies (eg, disorder of neuronal migration).
   4. Detection of parenchymal destruction (eg, calcification or cysts).
   5. Determination of the likely site of disturbance of CSF dynamics.
E. **Proton magnetic resonance spectroscopy** can help differentiate between cortical atrophy with hydrocephalus ex vacuo and hydrocephalus.

VI. **Management**
A. **In the presence of significant fetal hydrocephalus**
   1. **With pulmonary maturity.** Prompt delivery by cesarean section.
   2. **If the lungs are immature,** there are three options.
      a. Immediate delivery (with the risks of prematurity).
      b. Delayed delivery (with the risks of persistently increased ICP) until the lungs are mature. Administer antenatal steroids for induction of lung maturity, and deliver the infant as soon as lung maturity is established.
      c. In utero ventricular drainage with a ventriculoamniotic shunt or transabdominal external drainage.
   3. **Consultation.** Ideal management calls for a team approach with the obstetrician, neonatologist, neurosurgeon, ultrasonographer, geneticist, ethicist, and family members.
B. **Of hydrocephalus associated with congenital aqueductal stenosis or NTDs.** Decompress by prompt placement of a ventricular bypass shunt into an intracranial or extracranial compartment.
C. **Of PHH.** Ventriculomegaly should not be equated with hydrocephalus. Distinction between hydrocephalus ex vacuo and PHH has major clinical and therapeutic implications. Infants with cortical atrophy and hydrocephalus ex vacuo will not benefit from CSF diversion.
   1. **Mild hydrocephalus** usually arrests within 4 weeks of progressive ventricular dilation or returns to normal within the first few months of life.
   2. **Temporizing measures**
      a. **Serial lumbar punctures** (LPs) may be instituted if there is communicating hydrocephalus. Removal of 10–15 mL/kg CSF is frequently necessary. Approximately two thirds of this group of infants will undergo arrest with partial or total resolution, and one third will still require VP shunting. The risk of meningitis is ~1%.
      b. **Drugs to decrease CSF production.** Acetazolamide may be administered with or without furosemide (see Chapter 80). Complications in-

clude significant metabolic acidosis, hypercalciuria, and nephrocalcinosis.

c. **Ventricular drainage** can be done by direct or tunneled external ventricular drain or by a subcutaneous ventricular catheter that drains to a reservoir or to subgaleal or supraclavicular spaces. This is indicated for infants who have not responded adequately to LPs and who are not good candidates for placement of a VP shunt. The incidence of infection with these devices is ~5%.

3. **Permanent management.** The method of choice is placement of **VP shunts.** The outcome is better with "early" shunting. It remains *controversial* whether an elevated CSF protein level increases the risk of shunt complications and whether shunting should be delayed in patients with a high CSF protein content. VP shunt placement is indicated in nearly all cases to facilitate nursing care and comfort, possibly except for those infants with severe or lethal birth defects.

   Long-term complications of shunts include scalp ulceration, infection (usually staphylococcal), arachnoiditis, occlusion, development or clinical worsening of an inguinal hernia or hydrocele, organ perforation (secondary to intraperitoneal contact of a catheter with a hollow viscus), slit ventricle syndrome (symptoms of raised ICP in the presence of slit ventricles), blindness, endocarditis, and renal and heart failure. Age of <6 months appears to be a major risk factor for shunt infection in infants.

VII. **Prognosis**
   A. **Outcomes have significantly improved** with modern neurosurgical techniques. Long-term survival now approaches 90%, and approximately two thirds of survivors have normal or near-normal intellectual capabilities.
   B. **Predictors of unfavorable outcome**
      1. Cerebral mantle width <1 cm before shunt placement.
      2. Cause of the hydrocephalus, for example, mean IQ score, decreases in the following order: communicating hydrocephalus and myelomeningocele > aqueductal stenosis > Dandy-Walker malformation.
      3. Reduced size of the corpus callosum is associated with decreased nonverbal cognitive skills and motor abilities.
      4. In preterm infants with PHH, poor long-term outcome is strongly correlated with the severity of IVH, the presence of PHI or cystic PVL, the need for VP shunt, shunt infections, and a high number of shunt revisions. Resch et al (1996) showed that 23% of 299 preterm infants with IVH and PVH developed PHH. A third of those infants with PHH died. Neurodevelopmental assessment of the PHH survivors at 5 years of age revealed that 25% were developing normally, 25% showed mild neurologic symptoms or slight developmental delay, 28% had handicaps or moderate mental retardation, and 22% had severe handicaps or severe mental retardation.

INTRAVENTRICULAR HEMORRHAGE

I. **Definition.** IVH is an intracranial hemorrhage that originates in the periventricular subependymal germinal matrix with subsequent entrance of blood into the ventricular system. It is predominantly a disorder of preterm infants. **"Early" IVH** is defined as IVH diagnosed at <72 h after birth, and the term **"late" IVH** is used for IVH diagnosed after 72 h of life.

II. **Incidence.** The overall incidence of IVH has decreased in recent years from 40–60% to ~20% or less in infants weighing <1500 g at birth. The incidence and severity of IVH are inversely proportional to gestational age. Batton et al (1994) showed that the incidence of major IVH (large IVH or any intraparenchymal hemorrhage) was 5.2% (vs 13–28% in earlier studies) in their cohort of infants of <1500 g who did not receive any prenatal or postnatal pharmacotherapy for the prevention of IVH other than antenatal steroids administered to accelerate pulmonary maturity. Major IVH occurred in 16% of infants born at ≤25 weeks and in only 2.1% of infants born at >25 weeks' gestation. However, despite the decline in its incidence, IVH remains a major problem because the survival rates for infants <1000 g continue to increase. Although cases of prenatal IVH have been reported, the **"risk period"** is during the first 3–4 postnatal days: ~50% of IVH occurs in the first 6–12 h of life, 75% by the second day, and 90% by the third day. Ten to 65% of infants with early IVH have progression of the hemorrhage, with maximal extent occurring within 3–5 days of the initial diagnosis.

III. **Pathogenesis**
   A. The **germinal matrix (GM)** is a **weakly supported** and **highly vascularized** area that is located between the caudate nucleus and the thalamus at the level of, or slightly posterior to, the foramen of Monro. The blood vessels (not readily distinguishable as arterioles, venules, or capillaries) in these areas represent the **"watershed" zone** of the ventriculofugal and ventriculopedal vessels of the immature cerebrum and are **prone to hypoxic-ischemic injury.** These vessels are irregular, with large luminal areas, and are **prone to rupture.** The GM begins to involute after 34 weeks' postconceptional age (PCA).
   B. **Fluctuations in cerebral blood flow (CBF)** play an extremely important role because sick premature infants have **pressure-passive cerebral circulation.** A sudden rise in systemic blood pressure can result in an increase in CBF with subsequent rupture of the GM vessels. Decreases in CBF can result in ischemic injury to the GM vessels, which rupture on reperfusion.
   C. **The deep venous circulation takes a U-turn in the subependymal region at the level of the foramen of Monro.** This unique venous anatomy and the open communication between the GM vessels and the venous circulation contribute to the importance of increased cerebral venous pressure.
   D. **Rupture** through the GM ependymal layer results in entrance of blood into the lateral ventricles. Eighty percent of IVH cases are accompanied by the spread of blood throughout the ventricular system.

IV. **Neuropathologic consequences and accompaniment of IVH**
   A. **GM is the site of production of neurons and glial cells of the cerebral cortex and basal ganglia.** GM destruction may result in impairment of myelinization, brain growth, and subsequent cortical development.
   B. **Periventricular hemorrhagic infarction** is a **venous infarction** that is associated with severe and usually asymmetric IVH in ~85% of cases and invariably occurs on the side with the larger amount of intraventricular blood. A probable mechanism is that the intraventricular and GM blood clot results in obstruction of the medullary and terminal veins, followed by periventricular ischemia, with subsequent hemorrhagic infarction. It is often mistakenly described as an "extension" of IVH. Periventricular hemorrhagic infarction is neuropathologically distinct from periventricular leukomalacia (PVL).
   C. **PHH** is more common in those infants with the highest grade of hemorrhage. It is most frequently attributable to obliterative arachnoiditis either over the convexities of the cerebral hemispheres with occlusion of the arachnoid villi or in the posterior fossa with obstruction of outflow of the fourth ventricle. Rarely, aqueductal stenosis is caused by an acute clot or reactive gliosis.
   D. **PVL** is a frequent accompaniment of IVH but apparently is not caused by IVH itself. PVL is the ischemic, usually nonhemorrhagic, and symmetric lesion of periventricular white matter resulting from hypotension, apnea, and other ischemic events known to decrease CBF. Preterm infants born to mothers with prolonged rupture of membranes or chorioamnionitis seem to be at an increased risk for PVL.

V. **Risk factors**
   A. **Strong risk factors**
      1. Extreme prematurity.

2. Presence of labor (early IVH).
3. Birth asphyxia (early IVH).
4. The need for vigorous resuscitation at birth (early IVH).
5. Pneumothorax.
6. Ventilated preterm infants, especially those who breathe out of synchrony with the ventilator.
7. Seizures.
8. Sudden elevation in arterial blood pressure as in rapid volume expansion and administration of hypertonic sodium bicarbonate.
B. **Other antenatal risk factors** include heavy cigarette smoking and alcohol consumption, chorioamnionitis, use of indomethacin for tocolysis, and ominous fetal heart rate tracing.
C. **Other neonatal risk factors** include hypothermia, hypotension, hypercarbia, acidosis, exchange transfusion, elevated central venous pressure, "restlessness," patent ductus arteriosus (PDA), PDA ligation, decreased hematocrit resulting in decreased arterial oxygen content, hypoglycemia, heparin use, and disturbances of hemostasis. Even those procedures that we perceive as routine in the care of premature infants may also be contributory: tracheal suctioning, abdominal examination, handling, and instillation of mydriatics.
D. Studies suggest that high-frequency ventilation is *not* associated with an increased risk of IVH.

VI. **Classification.** Numerous systems have been proposed, but the one developed by Papile is most often used. Although it was developed for CT scanning, it has been applied to ultrasonography.

- **Grade I:** GM hemorrhage.
- **Grade II:** IVH without ventricular dilatation.
- **Grade III:** IVH with ventricular dilatation.
- **Grade IV:** GM hemorrhage or IVH with parenchymal involvement.

VII. **Clinical presentation.** The clinical presentation is extremely diverse, and diagnosis requires neuroimaging confirmation. Symptoms and signs may mimic those of other common neonatal disorders, such as metabolic disturbances, asphyxia, sepsis, or meningitis. IVH may be totally asymptomatic, or there may be subtle symptoms (eg, a bulging fontanelle, a sudden drop in hematocrit, apnea, bradycardia, acidosis, seizures, and changes in muscle tone or level of consciousness). A **catastrophic syndrome** is characterized by rapid onset of stupor or coma, respiratory abnormalities, seizures, decerebrate posturing, pupils fixed to light, eyes fixed to vestibular stimulation, and flaccid quadriparesis.

VIII. **Diagnosis**
A. **Ultrasonography is the procedure of choice** for screening and diagnosis. Sonograms are usually obtained via the anterior fontanelle. In the presence of normally sized ventricles, scanning through the posterior fontanelle may increase the rate of detection of IVH. Although CT scanning and MRI are acceptable alternatives, they are more expensive and require transport from the intensive care unit to the imaging device.
1. **Indications**
a. All infants with birth weight <1500 g.
b. Larger infants, if risk factors are present or if there is evidence of increased ICP or hydrocephalus.
2. **Sonograms** should be obtained on the first day of life in selected infants with risk factors for early IVH because 50% of cases of IVH occur during the first 6–12 h of life.
3. **A scan obtained at 4–7 days of life** will detect 90–100% of all hemorrhages.
4. **Periventricular white matter injury** (detected as intraparenchymal echodensities [IPEs]) and PHH may be detected on scans obtained at 2 weeks of life.

5. **Some clinicians** find it helpful to also obtain a sonogram, CT, or MRI before discharge or at 36 weeks' PCA.
B. **Laboratory studies**
   1. **LP.** Examination of CSF is normal in up to 20% of infants with IVH. CSF initially shows elevated red and white blood cells, with elevated protein concentration. The degree of elevation of CSF protein correlates approximately with the severity of the hemorrhage. It is frequently difficult to distinguish IVH from a "traumatic tap." Within a few days after hemorrhage, the CSF becomes xanthochromic, with a decreased glucose concentration. Often, the CSF shows a persistent increase in white blood cells and protein and a decreased glucose level, making it difficult to rule out meningitis except by negative cultures.
   2. **Elevated counts of absolute nucleated erythrocytes** beyond day 1 of life may be a marker for impending or existing severe IVH.
IX. **Management**
   A. **Prenatal prevention**
      1. Avoidance of premature delivery.
      2. Transportation in utero.
      3. Data suggest that active labor may be a risk factor for early IVH and that there may be a protective role for cesarean (C-) section. Anderson et al (1992) showed that C-section before the active phase of labor resulted in a lower frequency of severe IVH and of progression to severe IVH, although it did not affect the overall incidence of IVH.
      4. Tocolysis using indomethacin probably should be avoided because it has been associated with an increased rate of necrotizing enterocolitis, IVH, PDA, respiratory distress syndrome (RDS), and bronchopulmonary dysplasia.
      5. **Antenatal pharmacologic interventions**
         a. **Antenatal steroids.** Several large, multicenter trials have shown a clear efficacy of antenatal steroids in reducing IVH. In a seminal study by Leviton et al (1993), the incidence of GM hemorrhage or IVH was 2- to 3-fold lower in infants whose mothers received a complete course of antenatal steroids compared with those whose mothers received no steroids or an incomplete course (<48 h). Moreover, this beneficial effect appears to be independent of the improvement in pulmonary function in RDS. The prevention of IVH may be a composite effect of enhanced vascular integrity, decreased hyaline membrane disease, and possibly altered cytokine production (Perlman et al, 1996).
         b. **Phenobarbital.** Clinical trials from the early 1990s strongly suggested an overall reduction in the total incidence of IVH in preterm infants. Later a large collaborative study (Shankaran, 1997) of 344 infants whose mothers received antenatal phenobarbital (within 24 h before delivery) failed to demonstrate a protective effect against IVH for preterm infants. Currently, antenatal phenobarbital is not recommended for prevention of IVH.
   B. **Postnatal prevention**
      1. Avoid birth asphyxia.
      2. Avoid large fluctuations in blood pressure.
      3. Avoid overly rapid infusion of volume expanders or hypertonic solutions.
      4. Use prompt but cautious cardiovascular support to prevent hypotension.
      5. Correct acid-base abnormalities.
      6. Correct abnormalities of coagulation.
      7. Avoid poorly synchronized mechanical ventilation.
      8. Blood sampling from umbilical arterial catheters (UACs) produces fluctuations in CBF velocity and may contribute to IVH. A study by Lott et al (1996) showed smaller CBF velocity changes with low-positioned UACs.
      9. Available data suggest that **surfactant therapy** may cause a transient increase in CBF velocity and cerebral blood volume as well as electroen-

cephalographic depression, but the effects are generally not marked. In the majority of the studies published to date, surfactant appears to have a beneficial effect in the prevention of IVH. The combined use of antenatal steroids and postnatal surfactant therapy may have added benefits.
10. **Postnatal pharmacologic interventions** may be considered. None of the following regimens have been definitively proven to be safe and effective.
   a. **Indomethacin.** Ment et al (1994a, 1994b) reported that low-dose prophylactic indomethacin significantly lowered the incidence and severity of IVH but did not appear to be of benefit in the prevention or extension of early IVH. Subsequent reviews and reports have rendered indomethacin prophylaxis for IVH highly *controversial*. There are reports of reduced cerebral blood flow after indomethacin as well as no difference in long-term neurologic outcome for treated versus nontreated infants (Shalak & Perlman, 2002).
   b. **Pancuronium** is not currently recommended for the prevention of IVH.
   c. **Vitamin E.** The timing, dosage, and route remain *controversial*.
C. **Management of acute hemorrhage**
  1. **General supportive care** to maintain a normal blood volume and a stable acid-base status.
  2. **Avoid fluctuations** of arterial and venous blood pressures.
  3. **Follow-up serial imaging** (ultrasonography or CT scanning) to detect progressive hydrocephalus. See the previous section on hydrocephalus.
D. **Prevention of PHH**
  1. **LPs.** Several randomized controlled trials of infants with IVH failed to show a difference between infants undergoing LPs with supportive care and those receiving supportive care only.
  2. **Intraventricular fibrinolytic therapy** (tissue-type plasminogen activator, urokinase, and streptokinase). Data from preliminary studies are encouraging, but further studies are needed. The CSF plasminogen level is lower in neonates with IVH than in those without hemorrhage, and the potential for intraventricular fibrinolytic treatment may be limited by low concentrations of plasminogen.
E. **For treatment and outcome of moderate or severe PHH,** see the previous section on hydrocephalus.
X. **Prognosis and outcome**
A. **Short-term outcome** is related to the severity of IVH, with a mortality rate and PHH rate of 5–10% and 5–20%, respectively, for infants with mild to moderate IVH; 20% and 55%, respectively, for infants with severe IVH (blood filling the ventricles); and ~50% and ~80%, respectively, for those with severe IVH and parenchymal involvement.
B. **Long-term major neurologic sequelae depend primarily on the extent of associated parenchymal injury,** ranging from 5–15% in infants with minor degrees of hemorrhage (slightly higher than in infants without hemorrhage) to 30–40% in infants with severe hemorrhage, and as high as 100% in those infants with parenchymal involvement.
  1. **Markers for poor prognosis** include severe IVH, persistent or transient cerebral ventriculomegaly, persistent or transient IPEs, cystic PVL, and cranial midline shift. Triple lesions of IVH, persistent or transient ventriculomegaly, and persistent or transient IPEs have an approximate odds ratio for disability of 65, compared with 4.6 in the presence of isolated GM hemorrhage or IVH (Whitaker et al, 1996).
  2. **The incidence of major motor and cognitive deficits** is markedly increased in infants with extensive IPEs compared with that in infants with localized IPEs. Cognitive function may be impaired because of injuries to pathways associated with integration, fine motor coordination, and processing skills.

3. **Resulting motor deficits** correlate with the topography of the IPEs and usually manifest as either spastic hemiparesis or asymmetric spastic quadriparesis. Longitudinal studies have shown that there can be significant motor recovery in the first 2 years of life, especially in infants with grades III–IV IVH.
4. **Visual impairment** can result from ventriculomegaly or from extensive periventricular white matter loss with involvement of the striate and parastriate cortex.
5. **Hearing impairment** can result from injury to the auditory radiations.
6. Children who were at high risk for IVH should be assessed periodically until school age because some studies have shown an increased risk of disability at 5–8 years of age in children who had no hemorrhage or minor hemorrhage.
7. **Markers for fair or good prognosis**
   a. A less severe grade of IVH.
   b. A normal sonogram at discharge from the neonatal intensive care unit (NICU).
   c. Absence of ventricular dilation.
   d. Absence of periventricular white matter injury.
   e. Shorter neonatal hospitalization.
   f. Higher social and environmental status.

NEONATAL SEIZURES

I. **Definition.** A seizure is defined clinically as a paroxysmal alteration in neurologic function (ie, behavioral, motor, or autonomic function) (Volpe, 2001).
II. **Incidence.** Neonatal seizures are not uncommon. The incidence ranges from 1.5 in 1000 to 14 in 1000 live births.
III. **Pathophysiology.** The neurons within the CNS undergo depolarization as a result of inward migration of sodium. Repolarization occurs via efflux of potassium. A seizure occurs when there is excessive depolarization, resulting in excessive synchronous electrical discharge. Volpe (2001) proposed the following four possible reasons for excessive depolarization: (1) failure of the sodium-potassium pump because of a disturbance in energy production, (2) a relative excess of excitatory versus inhibitory neurotransmitter, (3) a relative deficiency of inhibitory versus excitatory neurotransmitter, and (4) alteration in the neuronal membrane, causing inhibition of sodium movement. The basic mechanisms of neonatal seizures, however, are unknown.

There are numerous causes of neonatal seizures, but relatively few account for most cases (Table 72–1). Therefore, only common causes of seizures are discussed here.

A. **Perinatal asphyxia** is the most common cause of neonatal seizures. These occur within the first 24 h of life in most cases and may progress to overt status epilepticus. In premature infants, seizures are of the generalized tonic type, whereas in full-term infants they are of the multifocal clonic type. Accompanying subtle seizures are usually present in both types.
B. **Intracranial hemorrhage,** whether subarachnoid, periventricular, or intraventricular, may occur as a result of hypoxic insults that can lead to neonatal seizures. Subdural hemorrhage, usually a result of trauma, can cause seizures.
   1. **Subarachnoid hemorrhage.** In primary subarachnoid hemorrhage, convulsions often occur on the second postnatal day, and the infant appears quite well during the interictal period.
   2. **Periventricular or intraventricular hemorrhage** arising from the subependymal germinal matrix is accompanied by subtle seizures, decerebrate posturing, or generalized tonic seizures, depending on the severity of the hemorrhage.

TABLE 72–1. CAUSES OF NEONATAL SEIZURES

Perinatal asphyxia
Intracranial hemorrhage
  Subarachnoid hemorrhage
  Periventricular or intraventricular hemorrhage
  Subdural hemorrhage
Metabolic abnormalities
  Hypoglycemia
  Hypocalcemia
  Electrolyte disturbances: hypo- and hypernatremia
Amino acid disorders
Congenital malformations
Infections
  Meningitis
  Encephalitis
  Syphilis, cytomegalovirus infections, toxoplasmosis
  Cerebral abscess
Drug withdrawal
Toxin exposure (particular local anesthetics)
Inherited seizure disorders
  Benign familial epilepsy
  Tuberous sclorosis
  Zellweger syndrome
  Pyridoxine dependency

3. **Subdural hemorrhage** over the cerebral convexities leads to focal seizures and focal cerebral signs.
C. **Metabolic disturbances**
   1. **Hypoglycemia** is frequently seen in infants with intrauterine growth retardation and in infants of diabetic mothers (IDMs). The duration of hypoglycemia and the time lapse before initiation of treatment determine the occurrence of seizures. Seizures are less frequent in IDMs, perhaps because of the short duration of hypoglycemia.
   2. **Hypocalcemia** has been noted in low birth weight infants, IDMs, asphyxiated infants, infants with DiGeorge syndrome, and infants born to mothers with hyperparathyroidism. Hypomagnesemia is a frequent accompanying problem.
   3. **Hyponatremia** occurs because of improper fluid management or as a result of the syndrome of inappropriate antidiuretic hormone (SIADH).
   4. **Hypernatremia** is seen with dehydration as a result of inadequate intake in breast-fed infants, excessive use of sodium bicarbonate, or incorrect dilution of concentrated formula.
   5. **Other metabolic disorders**
      a. **Pyridoxine dependency** leads to seizures resistant to anticonvulsants. Infants with this disorder experience intrauterine convulsions and are born with meconium staining. They resemble asphyxiated infants.
      b. **Amino acid disorders.** Seizures in infants with amino acid disturbances are invariably accompanied by other neurologic manifestations. Hyperammonemia and acidosis are commonly present in amino acid disorders.
D. **Infections.** Intracranial infection secondary to bacterial or nonbacterial agents may be acquired by the neonate in utero, during delivery, or in the immediate perinatal period.
   1. **Bacterial infection.** Meningitis resulting from **group B streptococcus, Escherichia coli**, or **Listeria monocytogenes** infection is accompanied by seizures during the first week of life.

2. Nonbacterial infection. Nonbacterial causes such as toxoplasmosis and infection with herpes simplex, cytomegalovirus, rubella, and coxsackie B viruses lead to intracranial infection and seizures.

E. Drug withdrawal. Three categories of drugs used by the mother lead to passive addiction and drug withdrawal (sometimes accompanied by seizures) in the infant. These are **analgesics** such as heroin, methadone, and propoxyphene (Darvon); **sedative-hypnotics** such as secobarbital; and **alcohol.**

F. Toxins. Inadvertent injection of local anesthetics into the fetus at the time of delivery (paracervical, pudendal, or saddle block anesthesia) may cause generalized tonic-clonic seizures. Mothers often notice the absence of pain relief during delivery.

IV. Clinical presentation. It is important to understand that **seizures in the neonate are different from those seen in older children.** The differences are perhaps due to the neuroanatomic and neurophysiologic developmental status of the newborn infant. In the neonatal brain, glial proliferation, neuronal migration, establishment of axonal and dendritic contacts, and myelin deposition are incomplete. **Four types of seizures,** based on clinical presentation, are recognized: **subtle, clonic, tonic, and myoclonic.**

A. Subtle seizures. These seizures are not clearly clonic, tonic, or myoclonic and are more common in premature than in full-term infants. Subtle seizures are more commonly associated with an electroencephalographic seizure in premature infants than in full-term infants. They consist of tonic horizontal deviation of the eyes with or without jerking; eyelid blinking or fluttering; sucking, smacking, or drooling; "swimming," "rowing," or "pedaling" movements; and apneic spells. Apnea accompanied by electroencephalographic abnormalities has been called **convulsive apnea.** It is differentiated from nonconvulsive apnea (which is due to sepsis, lung disease, or metabolic abnormalities) by the absence of electroencephalographic abnormalities. Apnea as a manifestation of seizures is usually accompanied or preceded by other subtle manifestations. In premature infants, apnea is less likely to be a manifestation of seizures.

B. Clonic seizures are more common in full-term infants than in premature infants and are commonly associated with an electroencephalographic seizure. There are two types of clonic seizures.

1. Focal seizures. Well-localized, rhythmic, slow, jerking movements involving the face and upper or lower extremities on one side of the body or the neck or trunk on one side of the body. Infants are usually not unconscious during or after the seizures.

2. Multifocal seizures. Several body parts seize in a sequential, nonjacksonian fashion (eg, left arm jerking followed by right leg jerking).

C. Tonic seizures occur primarily in premature infants. Two types of tonic seizures are seen.

1. Focal seizures. Sustained posturing of a limb, asymmetric posturing of the trunk or neck, or both. These are commonly associated with an electroencephalographic seizure.

2. Generalized seizures. Most commonly, these occur with a tonic extension of both upper and lower extremities (as in decerebrate posturing) but may also present with tonic flexion of the upper extremities with extension of the lower extremities (as in decorticate posturing). It is uncommon to see electroencephalographic seizure disorders.

D. Myoclonic seizures are seen in both full-term and premature infants and are characterized by single or multiple synchronous jerks. Three types of myoclonic seizures are seen.

1. Focal seizures typically involve the flexor muscles of an upper extremity and are not commonly associated with electroencephalographic seizure activity.

2. **Multifocal seizures** exhibit asynchronous twitching of several parts of the body and are not commonly associated with electroencephalographic seizure activity.

3. **Generalized seizures** present with bilateral jerks of flexion of the upper and sometimes the lower extremities. They are more commonly associated with electroencephalographic seizure activity.

   Note: It is important to distinguish jitteriness from seizures. Jitteriness is not accompanied by abnormal eye movements, and movements cease on application of passive flexion. In jitteriness, movements are stimulus sensitive and are not jerky.

V. Diagnosis

A. **History.** Although it is often difficult to obtain a thorough history in infants transported to tertiary care facilities from other hospitals, the physician must make a concerted effort to elicit pertinent historical data.

   1. **Family history.** A positive family history of neonatal seizures is usually obtained in cases of metabolic errors and benign familial neonatal convulsions.

   2. **Maternal drug history** is critical in cases of narcotic withdrawal syndrome.

   3. **Delivery.** Details of the delivery provide information regarding maternal analgesia, the mode and nature of delivery, the fetal intrapartum status, and the resuscitative measures used. Information regarding maternal infections during pregnancy points toward an infectious basis for seizures in an infant.

B. **Physical examination**

   1. **A thorough general physical examination** should precede a well-planned neurologic examination. Determine the following:
      a. **Gestational age.**
      b. **Blood pressure.**
      c. **Presence of skin lesions.**
      d. **Presence of hepatosplenomegaly.**

   2. **Neurologic evaluation** should include assessment of the level of alertness, cranial nerves, motor function, primary neonatal reflexes, and sensory function. Some of the specific features to look for are the size and "feel" of the fontanelle, retinal hemorrhages, chorioretinitis, pupillary size and reaction to light, extraocular movements, changes in muscle tone, and status of primary reflexes.

   3. **Notation of the seizure pattern.** When seizures are noted, they should be described in detail, including the site of onset, spread, nature, duration, and level of consciousness. Recognition of subtle seizures requires special attention.

C. **Laboratory studies.** In selecting and prioritizing laboratory tests, one must use the information obtained by history taking and physical examination and look for common and treatable causes.

   1. **Serum chemistries.** Estimations of serum glucose, calcium, sodium, blood urea nitrogen, and magnesium and blood gas levels must be performed. They may reveal the abnormality causing the seizures.

   2. **Spinal fluid examination.** Evaluation of the CSF is essential because the consequences of delayed treatment or nontreatment of bacterial meningitis are grave.

   3. **Metabolic disorders.** (See also Chapter 65.) With a family history of neonatal convulsions, a peculiar odor about the infant, milk intolerance, acidosis, alkalosis, or seizures not responsive to anticonvulsants, other metabolic causes should be investigated.
      a. **Blood ammonia levels** should be checked.
      b. **Amino acids** should be measured in urine and plasma. The urine should be tested for reducing substances.

     i. Urea cycle disorders. Respiratory alkalosis is seen as a result of direct stimulation of the respiratory center by ammonia.

     ii. Maple syrup urine disease. With 2,4-dinitrophenylhydrazine (2,4-DNPH) testing of urine, a fluffy yellow precipitate will be seen in cases of maple syrup urine disease.

D. Radiologic studies

    1. Ultrasonography of the head is performed to rule out IVH or periventricular hemorrhage.

    2. CT scanning of the head provides detailed information regarding intracranial disease. CT scanning is helpful in looking for evidence of infarction, hemorrhage, calcification, and cerebral malformations. Experience with this technique suggests that valuable information is obtained in term infants with seizures, especially when seizures are asymmetric.

E. Other studies

    1. Electroencephalography. Electroencephalograms (EEGs) obtained during a seizure will be abnormal. Interictal EEGs may be normal. However, an order to obtain an ictal EEG should not delay other diagnostic and therapeutic steps. The diagnostic value of an EEG is greater when it is obtained in the first few days because diagnostic patterns indicative of unfavorable prognosis disappear thereafter. Electroencephalography is valuable in confirming the presence of seizures when manifestations are subtle or when neuromuscular paralyzing agents have been given. EEGs are of prognostic significance in full-term infants with recognized seizures. For proper interpretation of EEGs, it is important to know the clinical status of the infant (including the sleep state) and any medications given.

VI. Management. Because repeated seizures may lead to brain injury, **urgent treatment is indicated. The method of treatment depends on the cause.**

A. Hypoglycemia. Hypoglycemic infants with seizures should receive 10% dextrose in water, 2–4 mL/kg intravenously, followed by 6–8 mg/kg/min by continuous intravenous infusion.

B. Hypocalcemia is treated with slow intravenous infusion of calcium gluconate (for dosage and other pharmacologic information, see Chapter 80). If serum magnesium levels are low (<1.52 mEq/L), magnesium should be given.

C. Anticonvulsant therapy. Conventional anticonvulsant treatment is used when no underlying metabolic cause is found. Loading doses of phenobarbital and phenytoin control 70% of neonatal seizures.

    1. Phenobarbital is usually given first (for dosage and other pharmacologic information, see Chapter 80). Neither gestational age nor birth weight seems to influence the loading or maintenance dose of phenobarbital. When phenobarbital alone fails to control seizures, another agent is used. Gilman et al (1989) found that sequentially administered phenobarbital controlled seizures in term and preterm newborns in 77% of cases. If seizures are not controlled at a serum phenobarbital level of 40 mcg/mL, Gilman et al recommend administering a second agent (eg, phenytoin [Dilantin]).

    2. Phenytoin (Dilantin) is used next by many practitioners. Fosphenytoin may be a preferred form. (For dosage and other pharmacologic information, see Chapter 80).

    3. Pyridoxine trial with EEG monitoring is recommended (for dosage information, see Chapter 80).

    4. Diazepam (Valium) has not been used extensively in the control of neonatal seizures. When used as a third agent, it did not improve seizure control. However, when used as a continuous intravenous infusion, 0.3 mg/kg/h, it was quite effective in controlling seizures in eight neonates, all of whom became somnolent but did not require artificial ventilation.

5. **Lorazepam (Ativan),** given intravenously, has been quite effective and safe, even when repeated 4–6 times in a 24-h period (for dosage and other pharmacologic information, see Chapter 80).
6. **Intravenous midazolam and oral carbamazepine** have been found to be effective (for dosage information, see Chapter 80).
7. **Paraldehyde,** given rectally, has been used as an effective anticonvulsant (for dosage and other pharmacologic information, see Chapter 80).

D. **Duration of anticonvulsant therapy.** The optimal duration of anticonvulsant therapy has not been established. Although some clinicians recommend continuation of phenobarbital for a prolonged period, others recommend stopping it after seizures have been absent for 2 weeks.

VII. **Prognosis.** As a result of improved obstetric management and modern neonatal intensive care, the outcome of infants experiencing seizures has improved. The mortality rate has decreased from 40 to 20% (Volpe, 1995), but neurologic sequelae are still seen in 25–35% of cases. As would be expected, the prognosis varies with the cause. Infants with hypocalcemic convulsions have an excellent prognosis, whereas those with seizures secondary to congenital malformations have a poor prognosis. Symptomatic hypoglycemia has a 50% risk of death or complications, whereas CNS infection carries a risk of 70%. Asphyxiated infants with seizures have a 50% chance of a poor outcome. Seventeen percent of patients with neonatal seizures have recurrent seizures later in life.

NEURAL TUBE DEFECTS

I. **Definitions.** NTDs are malformations of the developing brain and spinal cord. In normal development, the closure of the neural tube occurs at about the 29th day postconception. Most current hypotheses consider NTDs to be defects from failure of neural tube closure rather than other theories describing the reopening of a previously closed tube. Most likely, the closure starts at several distinct sites rather than as one continuous process. The nomenclature for NTDs is not standardized and is thus often confusing. Frequently used terms are as follows:

A. **Anencephaly** is defective closure of the upper or rostral end of the anterior neural tube. Hemorrhagic and degenerated neural tissue is exposed through an uncovered cranial opening extending from the lamina terminalis to the foramen magnum. Infants with anencephaly have a typical appearance with prominent eyes when viewed face on. **Craniorachischisis totalis** (a neural plate–like structure without skeletal or dermal covering resulting from complete failure of neural tube closure) and **myeloschisis** or **rachischisis** (in which the spinal cord is exposed posteriorly without skeletal or dermal covering because of failure of posterior neural tube closure) are other, less frequent open lesions.

B. **Encephalocele** (herniation of brain tissue outside the cranial cavity resulting from a mesodermal defect occurring at or shortly after anterior neural tube closure) is usually a closed lesion. Approximately 80% of encephaloceles occur in the occipital region.

C. **Myelomeningocele** is often also referred to as **spina bifida** (protrusion of the spinal cord into a sac on the back through deficient axial skeleton with variable dermal covering). More than 80% occur in the lumbar region, and ~80% are not covered by skin. In contrast to myelomeningoceles, **meningoceles** (closed lesions involving the meninges only) usually do not result in neurologic deficits.

D. **Spina bifida occulta and occult spinal dysraphism** are disorders of the caudal neural tube that are covered by skin (skin dimples or only very small skin lesions are present). These dysraphic disturbances range from cystic dilation of the central canal (**myelocystocele**), over bifid spinal cords with or without a separating bony, cartilaginous, or fibrous septum (**diastemato-**

myelia or **diplomyelia**), to a **tethered cord with a dermal sinus** or other visible changes such as hair tufts, lipomas, or hemangiomas. The term *spina bifida occulta* is used incorrectly when it is applied to an incomplete ossification of the posterior vertebral arch, a frequent and insignificant finding that is neither clinically nor genetically related to NTDs.

II. **Incidence, occurrence, and recurrence risks.** Statistics related to NTDs have likely been affected by folate prevention measures. The effects of folate on most of the confounding variables leading to NTDs listed next have not been reevaluated at this time.

A. **Incidence**
  1. The overall worldwide incidence is ~1 in 1000 live births.
  2. Spina bifida occulta, anencephaly, and myelomeningocele are the more frequently encountered NTDs.
  3. At early embryonic stages, the incidence of NTDs is as high as 2.5%; many abort spontaneously.
  4. The California Birth Defects Monitoring Program reported the following frequencies of NTDs in live-born infants for 11 California counties for 1990–1992: all NTDs, 0.6 per 1000 live births; anencephaly, 0.2 per 1000 live births. The National Center for Health Statistics (Centers for Disease Control [CDC]) reported a downward trend for NTDs. Spina bifida cases (for the United States) decreased from a high of 0.28 per 1000 live birth in 1995 to about 0.2 in 2001. The frequency of anencephaly changed from a high of 0.13 in 1997 to about 0.09 in 2001.
  5. In the early 1990s the annual medical costs of NTDs for the United States were estimated to be $200 million.

B. **Geographic variation, sex, race, and social class**
  1. The incidence is higher in females versus males.
  2. The risk is approximately doubled for infants born to Hispanic women compared with white women. The risk seems lower in Ashkenazi Jews than in whites of European descent.
  3. Some populations with frequent consanguineous matings (eg, Indian Sikhs or Palestinian Muslim Arabs) have an increased risk.
  4. The risk for African-Americans and Asians is lowest (but the incidence in northern China is higher: 6 in 1000 births).
  5. The risk is increased in infants of particularly young or particularly old mothers of lower socioeconomic class. This increase may be related to nutritional factors considering the observation by the March of Dimes that, among women surveyed in 2001, those least likely to consume a vitamin preparation containing folic acid were women 18–24 years old, those who did not attend college, and those with annual incomes <$25,000.

C. **Ninety-five percent of children with NTDs are born to couples with no family history of such defects.**

D. **Risk modifiers for NTDs.** The occurrence of NTDs appears higher in:
  1. Women with insulin-dependent diabetes mellitus (the risk appears to be influenced by the level of control).
  2. Women with seizure disorders who are being treated with valproic acid or carbamazepine.
  3. Women with a family history of NTDs.

E. **Recurrence risk** is as follows:
  1. Two to 3% with one affected sibling. Some types of NTDs may be folic acid resistant, and with folic acid treatment a residual risk of ~1% remains.
  2. Approximately 4–6% with two affected siblings.

III. **The causes of NTDs** seem to be multifactorial in most cases of anencephaly, encephalocele, myelomeningocele, and meningocele. Interactions between genetic and environmental factors result in disturbance of normal development. Recognized causes or contributing factors include the following:

A. **Nutritional and vitamin deficiencies**
  1. Folic acid.

   2. Vitamin B$_{12}$.
   3. Zinc.
   B. Chromosome abnormalities, including trisomies 13 and 18, triploidy, un-
   balanced translocations, and ring chromosomes.
   C. Genetic syndromes. NTDs have been observed as part of a variety of syndromes, some with mendelian inheritance patterns. A typical example is
   Meckel-Gruber syndrome (autosomal recessive), which presents with encephalocele, microcephaly, polydactyly, cystic dysplastic kidneys, and other
   anomalies of the urogenital system. Some genetic publications list up to 50
   syndromes associated with NTDs in the differential diagnosis.
   D. Teratogens
   1. Nitrates (cured meat, blighted potatoes, salicylates, and hard water).
   2. Antifolates (aminopterin, methotrexate, phenytoin, phenobarbital, primi-
   done, carbamazepine, and valproic acid).
   3. Thalidomide.
   4. Hyperglycemia in infants of diabetic mothers.
   5. The question of whether fertility drugs such as clomiphene are associated with NTDs remains *controversial.* **Lead** and **glycol ethers** have
   also been suspected to be associated with NTDs.
   6. Data from the California Birth Defects Monitoring Program indicate a
   possible increase in NTDs in mothers who lived within ¼ mile of hazardous waste sites included in the list of "superfund" sites of the Environmental Protection Agency. A study on the effect of parental occupation
   found that Mexican-American women with NTD-affected pregnancies
   were more likely to have had occupational exposure to solvents, but associations were not believed to be compelling.
   E. Maternal hyperthermia. The potential of hyperthermia to result in NTDs remains *controversial.*
   F. Other causes. An overall increase in birth defects has been reported in infants of **teenage mothers** (<20 years old) compared with those whose
   mothers are in the 25- to 29-year age range. The relative risk of nervous
   system defects in infants of teen mothers is 3.4 times that for children of 25-
   to 29-year-old mothers. Although a low body mass index does not increase
   the risk for NTDs, **obesity** does. The parents' ages are not related to the occurrence of NTDs per se; the risk for **twins** seems higher (a 2- to 5-time increase).
IV. Prevention of NTDs
   A. The **British Medical Research Council (MRC)** demonstrated in 1991 that
   high-dose folate (4 mg/day), but not multivitamin without folate, reduced the
   recurrence risk of NTDs by 72%.
   B. Based on results from the MRC, the **U.S. National Institute of Child Health
   and Human Development (NICHD)** and **CDC** recommend the following:
   **1. Women who have had 1 or more affected offspring with NTDs
   should consume 4.0 mg of folic acid per day,** from at least 1 month
   before conception through the first 3 months of pregnancy.
   2. Multivitamins should not be used because excessive amounts of vitamins A and D would be ingested to reach an intake of 4 mg of folic acid.
   3. Consumption of high-dose folic acid must be under a physician's supervision because there is still little information regarding its long-term effects and symptoms of pernicious anemia may be obscured, with the potential to result in serious neurologic damage.
   4. Because 4 mg of folic acid did not prevent all NTDs in the MRC study,
   patients should be cautioned that folic acid supplementation does not
   preclude the need for counseling or consideration of prenatal testing for
   NTDs.
   C. The **American Academy of Pediatrics** Committee on Genetics has en-
   dorsed the **U.S. Department of Health and Human Services** (1992) recommendation, as follows:

1. **All women of childbearing age (15–44 years) in the United States who are capable of becoming pregnant should consume 0.4 mg of folic acid per day** for the purpose of reducing their risk of having a pregnancy affected by spina bifida or other NTDs. This amount of folic acid is estimated to reduce the NTD risk by 50–70%. This amount (0.4 mg) is also the US Recommended Daily Allowance of folic acid.
2. An intake of >1 mg is not generally recommended.
3. Folic acid should ideally be taken at least 1 month before conception and at least through the first month of gestation.

D. **Sources of folic acid**
1. **Dietary.** The average diet in the United States contains 0.2 mg of folate, which is less bioavailable than folic acid. Folate intake of 0.4 mg/day can be achieved through careful selection of folate-rich foods (spinach and other leafy green vegetables, dried beans, peas, liver, and citrus fruits). Some breakfast cereals are fortified with folic acid. **Since January 1998, enriched foods (including flour, cornmeal, pasta, and rice) are fortified in folic acid by order of the US Food and Drug Administration.**
2. **Supplementation.** Folic acid is available over the counter in dosages up to 0.8 mg. Folic acid is also available by prescription in 1-mg tablets. Prenatal vitamins contain 0.8 or 1 mg of folic acid. A survey by the March of Dimes revealed that only 27% of nonpregnant women 18–45 years of age took a vitamin preparation containing folic acid in 2001. Awareness of the U.S. Public Health Service recommendation regarding folic acid did more than double from 1995 to 2002 (from 15 to 32%) for the same group. Multiple sources are available to provide educational material to the public (March of Dimes: 1-888-MODIMES or www.marchofdimes.org, www.cdc.gov, www.aap.org, www.acog.org).

E. **Current epidemiologic and biochemical evidence** suggests that NTDs are not primarily due to folate insufficiency but rather arise from changes in the metabolism of folate and possibly B_{12} in predisposed women. The mechanisms may also involve homocysteine metabolism. Polymorphisms of methylene tetrahydrofolate reductase and other genes encoding proteins involved in folate metabolism may be associated with an increased frequency of NTDs. Of further interest is that the homocysteine-lowering effect of folic acid supplementation may also reduce the risk for cardiovascular disease.

F. **Intestinal hydrolysis of dietary folate** is not impaired in mothers who have had infants with NTDs, although the response curve to a folate-enriched meal appears to differ significantly from that of mothers who have not had infants with NTDs.

V. **Prenatal detection of NTDs**
A. **Prenatal screen using maternal serum AFP** at 14–16 weeks' gestation. Elevated levels (>2.5 multiples of the mean, which are adjusted to gestational age) are indicative of open NTDs at a sensitivity of 90–100%, a specificity of 96%, and a negative predictive value of 99–100% but a low positive predictive value.
B. **Prenatal diagnosis.** Documentation of an elevated maternal serum AFP is followed by:
1. **Genetic counseling.** The physician needs to make sure that the patient receives information regarding her risk for NTDs and other conditions with elevated AFP (gastroschisis or other conditions leading to fetal skin defects), to evaluate causes of possible false-positive results (imprecise dates or twin pregnancies), to learn about options regarding further evaluation (see later discussion), and to provide nondirective counseling regarding treatment options.
2. **Detailed fetal ultrasonography with anomaly screening.** In skilled hands, a detailed ultrasonogram can be extremely sensitive and specific for detection of NTDs. Sonographic determination of the level of the le-

sion has been shown to be useful in predicting the ambulatory potential of fetuses with NTDs. Ultrasonography is also done to rule out other major congenital defects.

3. **Measurement of the amniotic fluid AFP and acetylcholinesterase.** Amniocentesis is usually done between 16 and 18 weeks' gestation, although it can technically be done as early as 14 weeks' gestation. If indicated, karyotype can also be obtained. The detection rate for anencephaly and open spina bifida is 100% when results of amniotic fluid acotylcholinesterase and AFP are combined, with a false-positive rate of only 0.04%.

VI. **Management: anencephaly**

A. Approximately 75% are stillborn, and most live-born infants with anencephaly die within the first 2 weeks of birth.

B. Considering the 100% lethality of anencephaly, usually only **supportive care** is given: warmth, comfort, and enteral nutrition. Support services for the family, including social work and genetic and general counseling, are essential. There are some ethically *controversial* issues regarding the extent of care and other issues (eg, organ donation), and it may be advisable to involve other support systems (eg, ethics committees, support groups, or religious guidance [if desired by the family]).

VII. **Management: encephalocele**

A. **Physical examination and initial management.** In addition to the general principles of neonatal resuscitation, an especially careful physical examination is indicated. Look for **associated malformations.** As mentioned in Neural Tube Defects, section III,C, some genetic publications list up to 50 syndromes associated with NTDs. We recommend that the child be given nothing by mouth until the **consultations** by subspecialties such as neurosurgery and, if indicated, genetic tests are done and the need for immediate treatment (perhaps surgery) is assessed. **Imaging studies** (ultrasonography, CT, and MRI) should be arranged.

B. **Neurosurgical intervention** may be indicated to prevent ulceration and infection, except in those cases with massive lesions and marked microcephaly. The encephalocele and its contents are often excised because the brain tissue within is frequently infarcted and distorted. Surgery may be deferred, depending on the size, skin coverage, and location. **Ventriculoperitoneal shunt (VP)** placement may be required because as many as 50% of cases have secondary hydrocephalus.

C. **Counseling and long-term outcome.** A multidisciplinary approach is necessary to counsel the family regarding recurrence risk, long-term outcome, and follow-up. The family should be informed about the availability of **support groups** (March of Dimes and others; March of Dimes Birth Defect Foundation can be reached at 1-888-MODIMES). The degree of **developmental deficits** is determined mainly by the extent of herniation and location; cerebral hemispheres from both sides or one side, the cerebellum, and even the brainstem can be involved. **Visual deficits** are common with occipital encephaloceles. **Motor and intellectual deficits** are found in ~50% of patients.

VIII. **Management: myelomeningocele.** Although fetal surgery for NTDs remains *controversial*, many maternal-fetal specialists believe that this option should be mentioned to parents. After birth, a multidisciplinary team approach, including the primary care physician, geneticist, genetic counselor, neonatologist, urologist, neurosurgeon, orthopedic surgeon, and social worker, is necessary.

A. **Physical examination** should include careful evaluation for other malformations (see section VII,A). In addition, special efforts should be made to correlate motor, sensory, and sphincter function and reflexes to the functional level of lesion (Table 72–2).

1. **Extent of neurologic dysfunction** correlates with the level of the spinal cord lesion.

TABLE 72-2. CORRELATION AMONG LEVEL OF MYELOMENINGOCELE, LEVEL OF CUTANEOUS
SENSATION, SPHINCTER FUNCTION, REFLEXES, AND POTENTIAL FOR AMBULATION

Level of lesion	Innervation	Cutaneous sensation (pinprick)	Sphincter function	Reflexes	Ambulation potential
Thoracolumbar	T12–L2	Groin (L1) Anterior upper thigh (L2)	—	—	Full braces Wheelchair bound
Lumbar	L3–L4	Anterior lower thigh and knee (L3) Medial leg (L4)	—	Knee jerk	May ambulate with braces and crutches
Lumbosacral	L5–S1	Lateral leg and medial foot (L5) Sole of foot (S1)	—	Ankle jerk	May ambulate with or without short leg braces
Sacral	S2–S4	Posterior leg and thigh (S2) Middle of buttock (S3) Medial buttock (S4)	Bladder and rectal function	Anal wink	May ambulate without braces

Voluntary muscle movements are difficult to elicit in newborns with myelomeningocele and are, therefore, not helpful during initial evaluation. Furthermore, motor examination may be distorted initially by reversible spinal cord dysfunction above the level of the actual defect induced by exposure of the open cord.

2. **Paraplegia** below the level of the defect.
3. The presence of the **anal wink and anal sphincter tone** suggests functioning sacral spinal segments and is prognostically important. In one study, 90% of patients with a positive anocutaneous reflex were determined to be "dry" on a regimen of intermittent catheterization as opposed to 50% of those with a negative reflex.
B. **Initial management.** In addition to following the general principles of neonatal resuscitation and newborn care, appropriate management of the spinal lesion is essential.
   1. There are institutional differences in the specifics of how to cover the lesion, and provision of a **sterile cover** can be achieved by several means. Some surgeons do prefer to have only a sterile plastic material or wrap applied to the lesion and ask to avoid contact with gauze or other material that could adhere to the tissue and result in mechanical damage when removed. It is advisable to try to keep the defective area moist while avoiding bacterial contamination. If tolerated, the patient should be positioned on the side.
   2. Be aware that a high rate of **latex allergies** has been reported in patients with NTDs. In some centers, all patients with myelodysplasia are, therefore, considered at risk for anaphylaxis and other allergic complications, and latex avoidance is practiced as a preventive protocol. One study showed that after 6 years of a latex-free environment the prevalence of latex sensitization fell from 26.7% to 4.5% of children with spina bifida.
   3. In most centers, patients are started on **antibiotics** (ampicillin and gentamicin) and are given nothing by mouth.
   4. Arrange for **imaging studies** to evaluate for hydrocephalus or other malformations detected or suspected on physical examination.
C. **Surgical management.** Usually, closure of the back lesion is done within 24 or 48 h to prevent infection and further loss of function.
D. **Hydrocephalus** is common and often **noncommunicative** secondary to **Arnold-Chiari malformation** of the foramen magnum and upper cervical canal (usually type II), with resultant downward displacement of the medulla, pons, and cerebellum and obstruction of CSF flow.

1. The risk of hydrocephalus is 95% for infants with thoracolumbar, lumbar, and lumbosacral lesions and 63% for those with occipital, cervical, thoracic, or sacral lesions.
2. In most cases, hydrocephalus is not evident until after closure of the myelomeningocele, and placement of a **VP shunt** may be required at a later date.
3. Aggressive treatment with early VP shunt placement may improve cognitive function.
4. **Serial ultrasound scans** are necessary to monitor progression of hydrocephalus because ventricular dilation may occur without rapid head growth or signs of increased ICP. The hydrocephalus usually becomes clinically overt 2–3 weeks after birth.
5. Despite treatment of the myelomeningocele and hydrocephalus, ~50% of these infants may still succumb to death from aspiration, laryngeal stridor, and apnea attributable to the hindbrain anomaly.
E. **Urinary tract dysfunction** is one of the major causes of morbidity and mortality after the first year of life.
   1. More than 85% of myelomeningoceles located above S2 are associated with neurogenic bladder dysfunction, with urinary incontinence and ureteral reflux. Poor bladder emptying immediately after NTD closure may be temporary ("spinal shock"), and improvement of bladder function may be observed up to 6 weeks after repair.
   2. Without proper management, **hydronephrosis** develops with progressive scarring and destruction of the kidneys. Many of these infants succumb to urosepsis.
   3. Renal ultrasonography and a voiding cystourethrogram may identify patients who could benefit from anticholinergic medication, clean and intermittent catheterization, prophylactic antibiotics, or early surgical intervention of the urinary tract.
   4. Other associated renal anomalies include renal agenesis, horseshoe kidney, and ureteral duplications.
F. **Orthopedic complications**
   1. The lower extremities lack innervation and become atrophied.
   2. **Deformities** of the foot, knee, hip, and spine are common as a result of muscle imbalance, abnormal in utero positioning, or teratologic factors.
   3. **Hip dislocation** or subluxation is usually evident within the first year of life, especially in patients with midlumbar myelomeningocele.
   4. Treatment of orthopedic abnormalities be instituted as soon as there is sufficient healing of the back wound.
   5. Physical therapists assist with proper positioning of the extremities to minimize contractures and to maximize function.
G. **Outcome of aggressive therapy**
   1. The overall **mortality** rate is now <15% by 3–7 years of age. One study revealed a survival rate of infants with spina bifida of 87.2% for the first year. In multivariable analysis, factors associated with increased mortality were low birth weight and high lesions.
   2. Infants with sacral lesions have essentially no mortality.
   3. The outcome in regard to the highest potential for ambulation depends largely on the level of the original lesion (see Table 72–2) and is modified by the orthopedic treatment and complications (see section VIII,F).
   4. The majority of children with lumbar myelomeningocele score within the normal range on **intelligence** and achievement tests, with the greatest and possibly progressive deficits on performance IQ, arithmetic achievement, and visuomotor integration, while keeping pace on reading and spelling.
   5. An IQ >80 is found in essentially all patients with lesions below S1.
   6. Approximately 50% of survivors with thoracolumbar lesions have IQ >80.
   7. Cognitive function is improved in the presence of favorable socioeconomic and environmental factors.

IX. Management: spina bifida occulta
  A. **Neonatal features.** The presence of spina bifida occulta is suggested by overlying abnormal collections of hair, hemangioma, pigmented macule, aplasia cutis congenita, skin tag, subcutaneous mass, cutaneous dimples, or tracts.
  B. If undetected in the neonatal period, **clinical presentation later in infancy** includes the following:
    1. Delay in development of sphincter control.
    2. Delay in walking.
    3. Development of a foot deformity.
    4. Recurrent meningitis.
    5. A sudden deterioration may represent vascular insufficiency produced by tension on a tethered cord, angulation of the cord around fibrous or related structures, or cord compression from a tumor or cyst.
  C. **Diagnosis**
    1. **Ultrasonography** is useful for screening.
    2. **MRI** provides superior anatomic details. The advantages of MRI are that contrast is not needed and the infants are not exposed to radiation.
  D. **Surgical correction** may be necessary in the newborn period to avoid the onset of symptoms. Surgical release of a tethered cord or decompression of the spinal cord within 48 h of sudden deterioration may completely or partially reverse recently acquired deficits.

REFERENCES

Agarwal SK et al: Outcome analysis of vesicoureteral reflux in children with myelodysplasia. *J Urol* 1997;157:980.

Anderson GD et al: The effect of cesarean section on intraventricular hemorrhage in the preterm infant. *Am J Obstet Gynecol* 1992;166:1091.

Aziz K et al: Province-based study of neurologic disability of children weighing 500 through 1249 grams at birth in relation to neonatal cerebral ultrasound findings. *Pediatrics* 1995;95:837.

Batton DG et al: Current gestational age–related incidence of major intraventricular hemorrhage. *J Pediatr* 1994;125:623.

Bender J: Parental occupation and neural tube defect-affected pregnancies among Mexican Americans. *J Occup Environ Med* 2002;44:650.

Bernes SM, Kaplan AM: Evolution of neonatal seizures. *Pediatr Clin North Am* 1994;41:1069.

Biggio et al: Can prenatal ultrasound findings predict the ambulatory status in fetuses with open spina bifida? *Am J Obstet Gynecol* 2001;185:1016.

Birmingham PK et al: Do latex precautions in children with myelodysplasia reduce intraoperative allergic reactions? *J Pediatr Orthop* 1996;16:799.

Bluml S et al: Differentiation between cortical atrophy and hydrocephalus using ^{1}H MRS. *Magn Reson Med* 1997;37:395.

Bower C et al: Absorption of pteroylpolyglutamates in mothers of infants with neural tube defects. *Br J Nutr* 1993a;69:827.

Bower C et al: Maternal folate status and the risk for neural tube defects. The role of dietary folate. *Ann NY Acad Sci* 1993b;678:146.

Brock DJH et al: Prenatal diagnosis of neural tube defects with monoclonal antibody specific for acetylcholinesterase. *Lancet* 1985;21:5.

Centers for Disease Control and Prevention: Economic costs of birth defects and cerebral palsy—United States, 1992. *MMWR Morb Mortal Wkly Rep* 1995;44:694.

Centers for Disease Control and Prevention: Knowledge and use of folic acid by women of childbearing age—United States, 1997. *MMWR Morb Mortal Wkly Rep* 1997;46:721.

Clark RH et al: Intraventricular hemorrhage and high-frequency ventilation: a meta-analysis of prospective clinical trials. *Pediatrics* 1996;98:1058.

Committee on Genetics: Folic acid for the prevention of neural tube defects. *Pediatrics* 1993;92:493.

Dansky LV et al: Mechanisms of teratogenesis: folic acid and antiepileptic therapy. *Neurology* 1992;42(suppl 5):32.

Dimmick JE, Kalousek DK: *Developmental Pathology of the Embryo & Fetus.* Lippincott, 1992.

Donn SM et al: Prevention of intraventricular hemorrhage with phenobarbital therapy: Now what? *Pediatrics* 1986;77:779.

Dykes FD et al: Intraventricular hemorrhage: a prospective evaluation of etiopathogenesis. *Pediatrics* 1980;66:42.

Dykes FD et al: Posthemorrhagic hydrocephalus in high-risk preterm infants: natural history, management and long-term outcome. *J Pediatr* 1989;114:611.

Fohr IP et al: 5,10-Methylentetrahydrofolate reductase genotype determines the plasma homocysteine lowering effect of supplementation with 5-methyltetrahydrofolate or folic acid in healthy young women. *Am J Clin Nutr* 2002;75:275.

Fraser RK et al: The unstable hip and mid-lumbar myelomeningocele. *J Bone Joint Surg* 1992; 74:143.

Garland JS et al: Effect of maternal glucocorticoid exposure on risk of severe intraventricular hemorrhage in surfactant-treated preterm infants. *J Pediatr* 1995;126:272.

Gilman JT et al: Rapid sequential phenobarbital treatment of neonatal seizures. *Pediatrics* 1989; 83:674.

Glick PL et al: Management of ventriculomegaly in the fetus. *J Pediatr* 1984;105:97.

Goh D, Minns RA: Intracranial pressure and cerebral arterial flow velocity indices in childhood hydrocephalus: current review. *Child Nerv Syst* 1991;7:392.

Green DW et al: Nucleated erythrocytes and intraventricular hemorrhage in preterm neonates. *Pediatrics* 1995;96:475.

Greitz D et al: A new view on the CSF-circulation with the potential for pharmacological treatment of childhood hydrocephalus. *Acta Paediatr* 1997;86:125.

Hanlo PW et al: Relationship between anterior fontanelle pressure measurements and clinical signs in infantile hydrocephalus. *Child Nerv Syst* 1996;12:200.

Horbar JD: Prevention of periventricular-intraventricular hemorrhage. In Sinclair J, Bracken MB (eds): *Effective Care of the Newborn Infant*. Oxford University Press, 1992.

Hudgins RJ et al: Natural history of fetal ventriculomegaly. *Pediatrics* 1988;82:692.

Hudgins RJ et al: Treatment of intraventricular hemorrhage in the premature infant with urokinase. *Pediatr Neurosurg* 1994;20:190.

Kaempf JW et al: Antenatal phenobarbital for the prevention of periventricular and intraventricular hemorrhage: a double-blind, randomized, placebo-controlled, multihospital trial. *J Pediatr* 1990;117:933.

Laurence KM et al: Double blind randomized controlled trial of folate treatment before conception to prevent recurrence of neural tube defects. *BMJ* 1981;282:1509.

Lazzara A et al: Clinical predictability of intraventricular hemorrhage in preterm infants. *Pediatrics* 1980;65:30.

Lemire RJ: Neural tube defects: clinical correlations. *Clin Neurosurg* 1983;30:165.

Lemire RJ et al: Neural tube defects. *JAMA* 1988;259:558.

Leviton A, Gilles F: Ventriculomegaly, delayed myelination, white matter hypoplasia, and "periventricular" leukomalacia: how are they related? *Pediatr Neurol* 1996;15:127.

Leviton A et al: Antenatal corticosteroids appear to reduce the risk of postnatal germinal matrix hemorrhage in intubated low birth weight newborns. *Pediatrics* 1993;91:1083.

Lott JW et al: Umbilical artery catheter blood sampling alters cerebral blood flow velocity in preterm infants. *J Perinatol* 1996;15:341.

Main DM, Mennuti MT: Neural tube defects: issues in prenatal diagnosis and counseling. *Obstet Gynecol* 1986;67:1.

March of Dimes and the Gallop Organization: *Folic Acid and the Prevention of Birth Defects. A National Survey of Pre-pregnancy Awareness and Behavior Among Women of Childbearing Age 1995–2001*. March of Dimes, 2001.

Massager N et al: Anterior fontanelle pressure monitoring for the evaluation of asymptomatic infants with increased head growth rate. *Child Nerv Syst* 1996;12:38.

McCullough DC, Balzer-Martin LA: Current prognosis in overt neonatal hydrocephalus. *J Neurosurg* 1982;57:378.

Medical Research Council Vitamin Study Research Group: Prevention of neural tube defects: results of the Medical Research Council Vitamin Study. *Lancet* 1991;338:131.

Meeropol E et al: Allergic reaction to rubber in patients with myelodysplasia. *N Engl J Med* 1990;323:1072.

Ment LR et al: Antenatal steroids, delivery mode, and intraventricular hemorrhage in preterm infants. *Am J Obstet Gynecol* 1995;172:795.

Ment LR et al: Low-dose indomethacin and prevention of intraventricular hemorrhage: a multicenter randomized trial. *Pediatrics* 1994a;93:543.

Ment LR et al: Low-dose indomethacin therapy and extension of intraventricular hemorrhage: a multicenter randomized trial. *J Pediatr* 1994b;124:951.

Ment LR et al: Neurodevelopmental outcome at 36 months' corrected age of preterm infants in the multicenter indomethacin intraventricular hemorrhage prevention trial. *Pediatrics* 1996; 98:714.

Michejda M et al: Present status of intrauterine treatment of hydrocephalus and its future. *Am J Obstet Gynecol* 1986;155:873.

Mills JL, Raymond E: Effects of recent research on recommendations for periconceptional folate supplement use. Ann NY Acad Sci 1993;678:137.

Morrow JD, Wachs TD: Infants with myelomeningocele: visual recognition memory and sensorimotor abilities. Dev Med Child Neurol 1992;34:488.

Myianthopoulos NC, Melnick M: Studies in neural tube defects: epidemiologic and etiologic aspects. Am J Med Genet 1987;26:783.

National Center for Health Statistics: Trends in Spina Bifida and Anencephalus in the United States, 1991–2001. Available from www.cdc.gov/nchs.

Nelson KB, Grether JK: Can magnesium sulfate reduce the risk of cerebral palsy in very low birthweight infants? Pediatrics 1995;95:263.

Nieto A et al: Efficacy of latex avoidance for primary prevention of latex sensitization in children with spina bifida. J Pediatr 2002;140:370.

Noetzel MJ: Myelomeningocele: current concepts of management. Clin Perinatol 1989;16:311.

Papile LS et al: Incidence and evolution of the subependymal intraventricular hemorrhage: a study of infants with weights less than 1500 g. J Pediatr 1978;92:529.

Perlman JM et al: Bilateral cystic periventricular leukomalacia in the premature infant: associated risk factors. Pediatrics 1996;97:822.

Philip AGS et al: Intraventricular hemorrhage in preterm infants: declining incidence in the 1980s. Pediatrics 1989;84:797.

Poland RL: Vitamin E for prevention of perinatal intracranial hemorrhage. Pediatrics 1990;85:865.

Rasmussen AG et al: A comparison of amniotic fluid alpha-fetoprotein and acetylcholinesterase in the prenatal diagnosis of open neural tube defects and anterior abdominal wall defects. Prenat Diagn 1993;13:93.

Recommendations for the use of folic acid to reduce the number of cases of spina bifida and other neural tube defects. MMWR Morb Mortal Wkly Rep 1992;41(RR-14):1.

Resch B et al: Neurodevelopmental outcome of hydrocephalus following intra-/periventricular hemorrhage in preterm infants: short- and long-term results. Child Nerv Syst 1996;12:27.

Robbin M et al: Elevated levels of amniotic fluid α-fetoprotein: sonographic evaluation. Radiology 1993;188:165.

Rodgers WB et al: Surgery of the spine in myelodysplasia. Clin Orthop Rel Res 1997;338:1.

Salafia CM et al: Maternal, placental, and neonatal associations with early germinal matrix/intraventricular hemorrhage in infants born before 32 weeks' gestation. Am J Perinatol 1995;12:429.

Sanders et al: The anocutaneous reflex and urinary continence in children with myelomeningocele. Br J Urol 2002;89:720.

Sandovnick AD et al: Use of genetic counseling services for neural tube defects. Am J Med Genet 1987;26:811.

Schorah CJ et al: Possible abnormalities of folate and vitamin B_{12} metabolism associated with neural tube defects. Ann NY Acad Sci 1993;678:81.

Sgouros S et al: Long-term complications of hydrocephalus. Pediatr Neurosurg 1995;23:127.

Shalak L, Perlman JM: Hemorrhagic-ischemic cerebral injury in the preterm infant: current concepts. Clin Perinatol 2002;29:745.

Shankaran S et al: Antenatal phenobarbital therapy and neonatal outcome: I. Effect on intracranial hemorrhage. Pediatrics 1996a;97:644.

Shankaran S et al: Antenatal phenobarbital therapy and neonatal outcome: II. Neurodevelopmental outcome at 36 months. Pediatrics 1996b;97:649.

Shankaran S et al: The effect of antenatal phenobarbital therapy on neonatal intracranial hemorrhage in preterm infants. N Engl J Med 1997;337:466.

Shaw GM et al: Epidemiological characteristics of phenotypically distinct neural tube defects among 0.7 million California births, 1983–1987. Teratology 1994;49:143.

Shaw GM et al: Maternal periconceptional vitamin use, genetic variation of infant reduced folate carrier (A80G), and risk of spina bifida. Am J Med Genet 2002;108:1.

Shaw GM et al: Risk of neural tube defect–affected pregnancies among obese women. JAMA 1996;275:1093.

Smithells RW et al: Further experience of vitamin supplementation for the prevention of neural tube defect recurrences. Lancet 1983;1:1027.

Stafstrom CE: Neonatal seizures. Pediatr Rev 1995;16:248.

Stoneking et al: Early evolution of bladder emptying after meningomyelocele closure. Urology 2001;58:767.

U.S. Department of Health and Human Services: Recommendations for the use of folic acid to reduce the number of cases of spina bifida and other neural tube defects. MMWR Morb Mortal Wkly Rep 1992;41:1.

Varvarigou A et al: Early ibuprofen administration to prevent patent ductus arteriosus in premature newborn infants. JAMA 1996;275:539.

Verget RG et al: Primary prevention of neural tube defects with folic acid supplementation: Cuban experience. *Prenat Diagn* 1990;10:149.

Verma U et al: Obstetric antecedents of intraventricular hemorrhage and periventricular leukomalacia in the low-birth-weight neonate. *Am J Obstet Gynecol* 1997;176:275.

Vintzileos AM et al: Congenital hydrocephalus: review and protocol for perinatal management. *Obstet Gynecol* 1983;62:539.

Vohr B, Ment LR: Intraventricular hemorrhage in the preterm infant. *Early Hum Dev* 1996;44:1.

Volpe JJ: Intraventricular hemorrhage and brain injury in the premature infant. *Pediatr Clin North Am* 1989a;2:361.

Volpe JJ: Neonatal seizures: current concepts and revised classification. *Pediatrics* 1989b;84: 422.

Volpe JJ: *Neurology of the Newborn*, 3rd ed. Saunders, 1995.

Volpe JJ: *Neurology of the Newborn*, 4th ed. Saunders, 2001.

Warkany J: Hydrocephalus. In Warkany J (ed). *Congenital Malformations*. Year Book, 1971.

Weekes EW et al: Nutrient levels in amniotic fluid from women with normal and neural tube defect pregnancies. *Biol Neonate* 1992;61:226.

Wells JT, Ment LR: Prevention of intraventricular hemorrhage in preterm infants. *Early Hum Dev* 1995;42:209.

Whitaker AH et al: Neonatal cranial ultrasound abnormalities in low birth weight infants: relation to cognitive outcomes at six years of age. *Pediatrics* 1996;98:719.

Whitelaw A et al: Phase I study of intraventricular recombinant tissue plasminogen activator for treatment of posthaemorrhagic hydrocephalus. *Arch Dis Child* 1996;75:F20.

Wills KE et al: Intelligence and achievement in children with myelomeningocele. *J Pediatr Psychol* 1990;15:161.

Wong LY, Paulozzi LJ: Survival of infants with spina bifida: a population study, 1979–94. *Paediatr Perinat Epidemiol* 2001;15:374.

73 Perinatal Asphyxia

I. **Definition.**
A. **Perinatal asphyxia** (from the Greek term *sphyzein* meaning **"a stopping of the pulse"**) is a condition caused by a lack of oxygen in respired air, resulting in impending or actual cessation of apparent life.
B. **Perinatal asphyxia** is a condition of impaired blood gas exchange that, if it persists, leads to progressive hypoxemia and hypercapnia with a metabolic acidosis.
C. **Essential characteristics** defined jointly by the American Academy of Pediatrics (AAP) and the American College of Obstetricians and Gynecologists (ACOG) *should* be present: (1) profound metabolic or mixed acidemia (pH <7.00) on umbilical cord arterial blood sample, if obtained; (2) persistence of an Apgar score of 0–3 for >5 min; (3) neurologic manifestations in the immediate neonatal period to include seizures, hypotonia, coma, or hypoxic-ischemic encephalopathy (HIE); and (4) evidence of multiorgan system dysfunction in the immediate neonatal period.
D. **Biochemical indices.** There is no specific blood test to diagnose perinatal asphyxia.
   1. The normal umbilical arterial base excess is a negative 6 mEq/L with −10 to −12 mEq/L as the upper statistical limit of normal. Base excess > −20 mEq/L is required to show neurologic damage associated with metabolic acidosis.
   2. The precise value that is required to define damaging acidemia is not known. A pH <7.0 realistically represents clinically significant acidosis. Acidemia alone does not establish that hypoxic injury has occurred.
E. **Apgar score**
   1. Conceived to report on the state of the newborn and effectiveness of resuscitation. It is a poor tool for assessing asphyxia. Low Apgar scores are unlikely to be the cause of morbidity but rather the results of prior causes.
   2. An infant with an Apgar score of 0–3 at 5 min, improving to ≥4 by 10 min, has >99% chance of not having cerebral palsy (CP) at 7 years of age; 75% of children who develop CP have normal Apgar scores at birth.
   3. A 1996 revised AAP/ACOG statement again emphasized that the Apgar score *alone* should not be used as evidence that neurologic damage was caused by hypoxia resulting in neurologic injury or by inappropriate intrapartum management.

II. **Incidence of asphyxia and its relationship to CP.** The incidence of HIE is 2–9 in 1000 live term births. The incidence of CP has not fallen despite improved obstetric and neonatal interventions and remains at 1–2 in 1000 live term births. Only 8–17% of CP in term infants is associated with adverse perinatal events suggestive of asphyxia; the cause of ≥90% of cases remains unknown. **One cannot state with a reasonable degree of medical certainty that CP in a given child was due to intrapartum asphyxia merely because the physician can find no other explanation.** The death rate in term infants with HIE is ~11% and ~0.3 in 1000 live term births are severely affected. The incidence of HIE, deaths, and handicap rates are all significantly higher for premature infants.

III. **Mechanisms of asphyxia during labor, delivery, and the immediate postpartum period.**
A. **Interruption of the umbilical circulation** (cord compression).
B. **Inadequate perfusion of the maternal side of the placenta** (maternal hypotension, hypertension, abnormal uterine contractions).

    C. **Impaired maternal oxygenation** (cardiopulmonary disease, anemia).
    D. **Altered placental gas exchange** (placental abruption, previa, insufficiency).
    E. **Failure of the neonate to accomplish lung inflation** and successful transition from fetal to neonatal cardiopulmonary circulation.
IV. **Pathophysiology.** Figure 73–1 shows the corresponding respiratory and cardiovascular effects during prolonged asphyxia.
    A. **Adaptive responses of the fetus or newborn to asphyxia.** The fetus and neonate are much more resistant to asphyxia than adults. In response to asphyxia, the mature fetus redistributes the blood flow to the heart, brain, and adrenals to ensure adequate oxygen and substrate delivery to these vital organs.
    B. **Impairment of cerebrovascular autoregulation** results from direct cellular injury and cellular necrosis from prolonged acidosis and hypercarbia.
    C. **The majority of neuronal disintegration occurs *after* termination of the asphyxial insult** because of persistence of abnormal energy metabolism

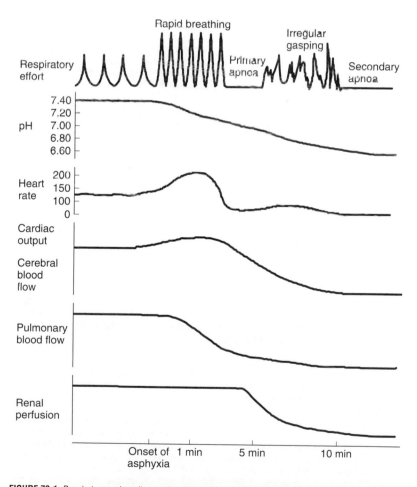

FIGURE 73-1. Respiratory and cardiovascular effects during prolonged asphyxia.

and low adenosine triphosphate (ATP) levels. A cascade of deleterious events is triggered, resulting in formation of free radicals, increased extracellular glutamate, increased cytosolic Ca^{2+}, and delayed cell death.

1. **Effects of increased cytosolic Ca^{2+}**
   a. **Degradation of cellular lipids, proteins, and DNA via activation of phospholipases, proteases, and nucleases.**
   b. **Uncoupling of oxidative phosphorylation.**
   c. **Increased release of glutamate.**
   d. **Production of free radicals** as the result of oxygenation of arachidonic acid and hypoxanthine and accumulation of nitric oxide via **activation of nitric oxide synthetase.**

2. **Effects of increased extracellular glutamate.** Immediate neuronal death (in minutes) as a result of osmolar lysis from influx of Na^+, Cl^-, and H_2O; delayed neuronal death (in hours) from activation of glutamate receptors, Ca^{2+} influx, and the effects of increased cytosolic Ca^{2+}.

D. **Major circulatory changes** *during* **asphyxia**
   1. **Loss of cerebrovascular autoregulation** under conditions of hypercapnia, hypoxemia, or acidosis. Cerebral blood flow (CBF) becomes "pressure passive," leaving the infant at risk for cerebral ischemia with systemic hypotension and cerebral hemorrhage with systemic hypertension.
   2. **Increase in CBF** secondary to redistribution of cardiac output, initial systemic hypertension, loss of cerebrovascular autoregulation, and local accumulation of vasodilator factors (H^+, K^+, adenosine, and prostaglandins).
   3. **With prolonged asphyxia,** there is a decrease in cardiac output, hypotension, and a corresponding fall in CBF. In general, brain injury occurs only when the asphyxia is severe enough to impair CBF.

E. **The postasphyxial human newborn is in a persistent state of vasoparalysis and cerebral hyperemia,** the severity of which is correlated with the severity of the asphyxial insult. Cerebrovascular hemorrhage may occur on reperfusion of the ischemic areas of the brain. However, when there has been prolonged and severe asphyxia, local tissue recirculation may not be restored because of collapsed capillaries in the presence of severe cytotoxic edema.

F. **Cerebral edema** is a *consequence* of extensive cerebral necrosis rather than a cause of ischemic cerebral injury.

G. **Regional vulnerability** changes with postconceptional age (PCA) and as the infant matures.
   1. Periventricular white matter is most severely affected in infants <34 weeks' PCA. The "watershed" areas between the anterior and middle cerebral arteries and between the middle and posterior cerebral arteries are predominantly involved in term infants.
   2. Areas of brain injury in profound asphyxia correlate temporally and topographically with the progression of myelinization and of metabolic activity within the brain at the time of the injury. White matter is, therefore, more susceptible to hypoxic injury.
   3. The topography of brain injury observed in vivo corresponds closely to the topography of glutamate receptors.
   4. When CBF is increased in response to asphyxia, regional differences exist such that there is relatively more blood flow to the brainstem than to higher cerebral structures.

V. **Neuropathologic findings**
   A. **Cortical changes.** Cortical edema, with flattening of cerebral convolutions, is followed by cortical necrosis until finally a healing phase results in gradual cortical atrophy. Cortical atrophy, if severe, may result in **microcephaly.**
   B. **Selective neuronal necrosis** is the most common type of injury observed in neonatal HIE.
   C. **Other findings seen in term infants** include status marmoratus of the basal ganglia and thalamus (the marbled appearance is a result of the char-

acteristic feature of hypermyelinization) and parasagittal cerebral injury (bilateral and usually symmetric, with the parieto-occipital regions affected more often than those regions anteriorly).

D. **Periventricular leukomalacia (PVL)** is hypoxic-ischemic necrosis of periventricular white matter resulting from cerebral hypoperfusion and the vulnerability of the oligodendrocyte within the white matter to free radicals, excitotoxin neurotransmitters, and cytokines. Injury to the periventricular white matter is the must significant problem contributing to long-term neurologic deficit in the premature infant, although it does occur in sick full-term infants as well. The incidence of PVL increases with the length of survival and the severity of postnatal cardiorespiratory disturbances. PVL involving the pyramidal tracts usually results in spastic diplegic or quadriplegic CP. Visuoperception deficits may result from involvement of the optic radiation.

E. **Porencephaly, hydrocephalus, hydranencephaly, and multicystic encephalomalacia** may follow focal and multifocal ischemic cortical necrosis, PVL, or intraparenchymal hemorrhage.

F. **Brainstem damage** is seen in the most severe cases of hypoxic-ischemic brain injury and results in permanent respiratory impairment.

VI. **Clinical presentation**

A. The *majority* of infants who experience intrauterine hypoxic-ischemic insults do *not* exhibit overt neonatal neurologic features or subsequent neurologic evidence of brain injury. It is generally accepted that after acute perinatal asphyxia there should be an acute encephalopathy, often accompanied by multiorgan malfunction.

B. **Occurrence of neonatal neurologic syndrome** shortly after birth is a sine qua non for recent (ie, intrapartum) insult. Prenatal insult *may* also have occurred. The primary signs of central nervous system (CNS) injury in the term infant include seizures, abnormal respiratory patterns (apnea), posturing and movement disorders, impaired suck, and jitteriness. The absence of this neonatal neurologic syndrome rules out intrapartum insult as the cause of major brain injury.

C. **The severity of HIE** correlates with the duration and severity of the asphyxial insult. A constellation of neurologic signs evolves over the first 72 h of life best characterized by Sarnat and Sarnat in 1976: stage I (hyperalert, awake state), stage 2 (lethargic, obtunded, hypotonic, seizures), and stage 3 (stuporous, comatose, flaccid, posturing). Moderately to severely affected infants are usually obtunded if not comatose, with generalized hypotonia and paucity of spontaneous movements. Depressed reflexes and cranial nerve palsies are common findings. Presentation of hypertonicity and irritability generally are not noted until the second week of life.

D. **Occurrence of seizures within the first 12–24 h after birth** is indicative of intrapartum insult until proven otherwise. Seizures may also be secondary to hypoglycemia. Perlman and Risser (1996) showed that the combination of a 5-min Apgar score of ≤5 and the need for intubation in the delivery room in association with an umbilical cord arterial pH ≤7.00 has an odds ratio of 340 for the development of seizures in the first 24 h of life.

E. **Hypoxic-ischemic spinal cord injury.** Ischemic injury to anterior horn cells within the spinal cord gray matter is relatively common among hypotonic and hyporeflexic neonates after severe perinatal hypoxia-ischemia. Electromyographic examinations show injury to the lower motor neuron above the level of the dorsal root ganglion (Clancy et al, 1989).

F. **Clinical presentation** may be further obscured by the coexistence of skull fracture, subdural hematoma, or subarachnoid hemorrhage resulting from traumatic delivery.

G. **Multiple organ involvement.** A prospective study by Martin-Ancel et al (1995) showed that involvement of 1 or more organs occurred in 82% of infants with perinatal asphyxia. The central nervous system (CNS) was the organ most frequently involved (72%). Severe CNS injury always occurred with involvement of other organs, although moderate CNS involvement was isolated in 20% of the infants. Renal involvement occurred in 42% of the infants, pulmonary involvement in 26%, cardiac involvement in 29%, and gastrointestinal involvement in 29%. Fifteen percent of neonates experienced renal failure, and 19% had respiratory failure. All of the infants in this study with an Apgar score <5 at 5 min had severe involvement of at least 1 organ, whereas 90% of the infants with an Apgar score ≥5 at 5 min did not have severe involvement of any organ.

1. **Cardiovascular system.** Shock, hypotension, tricuspid insufficiency, myocardial necrosis, congestive heart failure, and ventricular dysfunction.
2. **Renal function.** Oliguria-anuria, acute tubular or cortical necrosis (hematuria, proteinuria), and renal failure.
3. **Hepatic function.** Elevated serum γ-glutamyl transpeptidase activity, ammonia and indirect bilirubin, and decreased clotting factors at 3–4 days' postnatal age in moderate to severe asphyxia.
4. **Gastrointestinal tract.** Paralytic ileus or delayed (5–7 days) necrotizing enterocolitis.
5. **Lungs.** **Respiratory distress syndrome** (see Chapter 74) from surfactant deficiency or dysfunction, pulmonary hemorrhage (shock lung), and persistent pulmonary hypertension (see Chapter 62).
6. **Hematologic system.** Thrombocytopenia can result from shortened platelet survival or disseminated intravascular coagulopathy. Increased numbers of nucleated red blood cells have been reported (see later discussion).
7. **Metabolic.** Acidosis, hypoglycemia (hyperinsulinism), hypocalcemia (increased phosphate load, correction of metabolic acidosis), and hyponatremia/syndrome of inappropriate antidiuretic hormone secretion (SIADH).
8. **Acute Perinatal Asphyxia Scoring System.** A simple scoring system can be used to identify those newborns depressed at birth who are at greatest risk for multiple organ system sequelae. The scoring system is composed of the 5-min Apgar, umbilical artery base deficit, and fetal heart rate (FHR) monitor tracing (Carter et al, 1998). Multiple organ system morbidity was more likely to occur when the score exceeds 6.

VII. **Diagnosis.** Recognition of neonatal HIE depends principally on information gained from a careful history and a thorough physical examination with appropriate laboratory studies as outlined previously. Neurodiagnostic and neuroimaging studies can help determine the extent of the injury and may also be of value prognostically.

A. **Antenatal indicators of uteroplacental insufficiency or fetal compromise** (see also Chapter 1) may include the following:

1. **Reactive FHR and subsequent prolonged FHR deceleration** suggestive of a sudden catastrophic event (pattern of acute asphyxia).
2. **Reactive FHR, which, during labor, becomes nonreactive, associated with rising FHR baseline and repetitive late decelerations** (pattern of intrapartum asphyxia).
3. **A persistent nonreactive FHR tracing with a fixed baseline rate, from admit until delivery,** is suggestive of prior neurologic injury. This FHR pattern is often associated with reduced fetal movement, old passage of meconium, oligohydramnios, and abnormal fetal pulmonary vasculature (persistent pulmonary hypertension).
4. **FHR patterns are not always specific,** with a substantial false-positive rate. Improving the predictive value of FHR pattern in detecting intrapartum asphyxia may require supplementary tests:
   a. **Fetal vibroacoustic stimulation**
   b. **Fetal pulse oximetry**
   c. **A decreased biophysical profile score**

    d. An amniotic fluid index ≤5.

    e. An increased pulsatility index in the umbilical artery or decreased fetal cerebral resistance on Doppler ultrasonography.

  5. ACOG cautions against using terms such as asphyxia, hypoxia, and fetal distress when applied to continuous electronic fetal monitoring or auscultation.

B. EEG. Evolution of EEG changes may provide information on the severity of the asphyxial injury, and the type of EEG abnormality may be indicative of a specific pathologic variety. Identification of EEG abnormalities within the first hours after delivery may be helpful in selecting infants for treatment with neuroprotective agents.

C. Computed tomography (CT) scan. The value of CT in the assessment of diffuse cortical neuronal injury is most apparent *several weeks* after severe asphyxial insults. It is of particular value in the identification of focal and multiple ischemic brain injury. During the first week after an insult, the striking, bilateral, diffuse hypodensity reflects marked cortical neuronal injury, with associated edema corresponding closely to the occurrence of maximum intracranial pressure.

D. Ultrasonography is the method of choice for routine screening of the premature brain. It is of major value in the identification of intraventricular hemorrhage and necrosis of basal ganglia and thalamus. It is superior to CT in identifying both the acute and subacute-chronic manifestations of periventricular white matter injury. Its limitations in the first weeks of life include its inability to reliably identify mild injury, to visualize lesions that are peripherally located, and to distinguish between hemorrhagic and ischemic lesions in the cerebral parenchyma.

E. Magnetic resonance imaging (MRI) is the technique of choice for evaluation of hypoxic-ischemic cerebral injury in term and premature newborns. The advantages of MRI include the following:

  1. It does not expose the neonate to radiation.

  2. It demonstrates better anatomic imaging detail and resolution than CT, especially of the deep cortical structures (eg, the basal ganglia and thalamus) and corticospinal tracts.

  3. It clearly demonstrates the myelinization delay that almost invariably accompanies asphyxial brain injury. MRI may provide insight into the timing and duration of the asphyxial injury. Delayed myelinization is a negative predictor of long-term neurodevelopmental outcome.

  4. MRI is probably the best method available to diagnose hypoxic brain injuries in *mildly to moderately* affected patients and to detect discrete lesions of the cerebellum and brainstem.

  5. It may provide clues to other disorders (eg, metabolic or neurodegenerative disorders) that may also present as obtundation or coma in the newborn period.

  6. In experienced hands, ischemic lesions can be identified as early as 24 h after the insult.

  7. MRI can help differentiate between partial asphyxia and anoxia.

    a. Partial asphyxia. Injury is caused primarily by mild or moderate hypoxia or hypotension. Regions of the brain with the most tenuous perfusion are affected, and susceptibility varies as the infant matures (ie, periventricular white matter in premature infants and "watershed" areas in term infants). Deep gray matter structures of the cerebrum are typically spared.

    b. Anoxia. Injury is the result of a cardiorespiratory arrest or profound hypotension. The volume of damaged brain varies with the duration of the injury. An arrest of long duration (≥25 min) damages nearly the entire brain. Arrests of shorter duration show specific patterns that vary with PCA: at 26–32 weeks, the lateral thalami are primarily affected; at 34–36 weeks, the lentiform nucleus and hippocampus and

the perirolandic cortex are affected; and by 40 weeks, the corticospinal tracts from the internal capsule to the perirolandic cortex are affected. More severe or prolonged events result in injury to the optic
radiations.
   8. MRI demonstrates the structural sequelae of asphyxial injury on follow-
      up and has prognostic value. Repeat MRI at 3 months of age will usually
      show the full extent of brain injury.
F. **Evoked electrical potentials** (auditory, visual, or somatosensory) performed within the first hours of life may help to select infants for treatment
   with neuroprotective agents. They also have prognostic value in defining
   areas of CNS damage. Persistence of deficits beyond the neonatal period
   correlates with persistence of other signs of brain injury.
G. **Potentially useful techniques**
   1. **Magnetic resonance spectroscopy (MRS)** provides a measure of "en-
      ergy reserve." Using phosphorus-/(^{31}P) MRS, it has been shown that as-
      phyxiated newborns tend to have lower phosphocreatine/inorganic phos-
      phate ratios (impaired brain oxidative phosphorylation) and lower
      ATP/total phosphorus ratios than normal patients.
   2. **Proton MRS** allows noninvasive observations to be made of the de-
      rangement of cerebral metabolites (N-acetylaspartate (NAA) and lactic
      acid) when oxidative phosphorylation is impaired. The normalization of
      phosphorous metabolite ratios with time may reflect loss of severely af-
      fected neurons. Neuronal loss, gliosis, and delay in myelination would be
      reflected by a relative loss of NAA.
   3. **Near-infrared spectroscopy** on the first day after injury may demon-
      strate increased cerebral venous oxygen saturation and decreased cere-
      bral oxygen extraction, despite increased cerebral oxygen delivery, sug-
      gestive of a postasphyxial decrease in oxygen utilization.
VIII. **Management**
   A. **Optimal management is prevention.** The first goal is to identify the fetus
      being subjected to or likely to experience hypoxic-ischemic insults with labor
      and delivery.
   B. **Immediate resuscitation.** Any newborn that is apneic at birth must be
      promptly resuscitated because it cannot be determined whether the infant is
      in primary or secondary apnea.
      1. **Maintenance of adequate ventilation.** Use an assisted ventilatory rate
         to maintain physiologic levels of P_{CO_2}. Hypercarbia can further increase
         cerebral intracellular acidosis and impair cerebrovascular autoregulation,
         whereas hypocarbia (Pa_{CO_2} <20–25 mm Hg) has been associated with
         PVL in preterm infants and late-onset sensorineural hearing loss in full-
         term infants.
      2. **Maintenance of adequate oxygenation** (Pa_{O_2} >40 in premature infants
         and Pa_{O_2} >50 in term infants). Avoid hyperoxia (see later discussion),
         which may lead to additional brain injury from possible reduction in CBF
         and vaso-obliterative changes.
      3. **Maintenance of adequate perfusion.** Maintain arterial blood pressure
         in the "normal" range for gestational age and weight. Volume expanders
         and inotropic support are often required. With the loss of cerebrovascular
         autoregulation, it is important to avoid systemic hypotension and hyper-
         tension.
      4. **Correct metabolic acidosis** with cautious use of volume expanders.
         The primary objective is to sustain tissue perfusion. *Perfuse or lose!* Use
         bicarbonate only when cardiopulmonary resuscitation (CPR) is prolonged
         and the infant remains unresponsive. Bicarbonate administration may
         lead to hypercarbia and intracellular acidosis and increase lactate.
      5. **Maintain a normal serum glucose level** (~75–100 mg/dL) to provide
         adequate substrate for brain metabolism. Avoid hyperglycemia to pre-
         vent hyperosmolality and a possible increase in brain lactate levels.

6. **Control of seizures**
   a. **Phenobarbital is the drug of choice.** It is usually continued until the EEG is normal and there are no clinical seizures for ≥2 months. The benefit of prophylactic therapy remains *controversial*. High-dose phenobarbital (40 mg/kg) reduced the incidence of seizures and improved neurologic outcome at 3 years in term asphyxiated newborns (Hall et al, 1998).
   b. If seizures persist despite therapeutic phenobarbital levels, diazepam, lorazepam, and phenytoin may be used (for dosages and other pharmacologic information, see Chapter 80).
7. **Prevention of cerebral edema. The cornerstone of prevention of serious brain swelling is avoidance of fluid overload.** Maintain slight to moderate fluid restriction (eg, 60 mL/kg). If cerebral edema is severe, further restriction of fluid intake to 50 mL/kg is imposed. Observe the infant for SIADH. Glucocorticoids and osmotic agents are not recommended.
C. **Potential new therapies should aim at preventing delayed neuronal death once an asphyxial insult has occurred.** It is estimated that there is a 6- to 12-h window of opportunity after acute asphyxia whereby administration of a neuroprotective agent could reduce or prevent brain damage. Protecting the brain from injury would depend on the baseline fetal brain status.
   1. **Magnesium** has an inhibitory effect on excitation of the *N*-methyl-D-aspartate type of glutamate receptors and competitively blocks Ca^{2+} entry through voltage-dependent Ca^{2+} channels during hypoxia. Apnea may occur, and higher doses carry a significant risk of hypotension. Use of magnesium sulfate ($MgSO_4$) remains *controversial*.
   2. **Prevention of free radical formation**
      a. **Xanthine oxidase inhibitor.** In a pilot study (Van Bel et al, 1998), allopurinol reduced free radical formation and enhanced electrical brain activity in severely asphyxiated newborns. In addition, allopurinol reduced nonprotein iron (a prooxidant).
      b. **Resuscitation with room air.** In the Resair 2 trial (Saugstad 2001), room air–resuscitated infants recovered more quickly as assessed by time to first cry, 5-min Apgar score, and sustained pattern of respiration. Neonates resuscitated with 100% oxygen manifest biochemical changes indicative of prolonged oxidative stress at 4 weeks of age (Vento et al, 2001).
   3. **Excitatory amino acid antagonists.**
   4. **Calcium channel blockers.**
   5. **Inhibition of nitric oxide production.** Increased plasma nitric oxide levels has been shown as a marker for severity of brain injury and poor neurologic outcome (Shi et al, 2000).
   6. **Selective head cooling.** Hypothermia is thought to protect the brain from injury by preventing the decline in high-energy phosphates. Phosphocreatine and adenosine triphosphate are maintained while cerebral lactate levels are reduced. Selective head cooling coupled with mild systemic hypothermia was found to be safe in a group of asphyxiated term infants (Gunn et al, 1998).
   7. Any multicentered trial testing a new therapy to prevent or limit brain injury will require early enrollment soon after birth in infants at greatest risk of developing the sequelae of HIE.
IX. **Prognosis.** *Most survivors of perinatal asphyxia do not have major sequelae.* Peliowski and Finer (1992) showed that the overall risk of death for children with all stages of HIE combined was 12.5%, 14.3% for neurologic handicap, and 25% for death plus handicap. Depressed FHR, meconium-stained amniotic fluid, low "extended" Apgar scores, low scalp and cord pH, or clinical signs of neurologic depression soon after birth signify the acute clinical condition of the newborn. However, their predictive value for later neurodevelopmental outcome is less than satisfactory, especially when taken individually. Furthermore, envi-

ronmental, psychosocial, behavioral, and developmental influences may significantly affect long-term outcome.

A. **Findings associated with increased risk of neurologic sequelae**
   1. **Apgar score of 0–3 at 20 min of age.**
   2. **Presence of multiorgan failure,** particularly oliguria persisting beyond 24 h of life.
   3. **Severity of the neonatal neurologic syndrome.** Severe HIE (Sarnat stage 3) carries a mortality rate of ~80%, and survivors often have multiple disabilities, including spastic CP, severe or profound mental retardation, cortical blindness, or seizure disorder (Robertson & Finer, 1993). There is no permanent sequelae for mild HIE (Sarnat stage 1). Moderately affected (stage 2) patients have outcomes that vary with their overall clinical course and duration of their neurologic condition. Stage 2 beyond 5 days is a poorer prognostic sign.
   4. **Duration of neonatal neurologic abnormalities.** Disappearance of neurologic abnormalities by 1–2 weeks and the ability to nipple feed normally is an excellent prognostic sign.
   5. **Presence of neonatal seizures,** especially if they occur within the first 12 h after birth and are difficult to control.
   6. **An abnormal MRI** obtained in the first 24–72 h is associated with a poor outcome, irrespective of birth variables. On the other hand, a normal MRI obtained in the first 24–72 h almost always predicts a favorable outcome, even in a severely asphyxiated infant (Martin & Barkovich, 1995). An abnormal signal in the posterior limb of the internal capsule predicted an unfavorable outcome in 33 of 36 infants with Sarnat stage 2 HIE (Rutherford et al, 1998). The prognostic value is improved by repeating the study after several months, when delayed myelinization and structural damage are better appreciated.
   7. **Severity and duration of EEG abnormalities.** Normal to mildly abnormal EEG patterns within the first days after delivery are significantly correlated with normal outcomes, and moderately to severely abnormal EEG patterns are significantly related to abnormal outcomes (van Lieshout et al, 1995). A burst-suppression or isoelectric pattern on any day and prolonged EEG depression after day 12 are associated with a poor outcome. Recovery of normal EEG background by day 7 is associated with a normal outcome. The early presence (within the first days after birth) of a normal or near-normal EEG, even in a "comatose" child, is a strong predictor of a good neurologic outcome.
   8. **Persistent abnormalities of brainstem function** are generally incompatible with long-term survival.
   9. **Abnormal visual, auditory, or somatosensory evoked potentials** persisting beyond day 7 of life. Normal somatosensory evoked potentials (SSEPs) are highly predictive of a normal outcome. Eken et al (1995) showed that SSEPs performed within 6 h after delivery had a positive predictive value of 82% for moderate to severe HIE and a negative predictive value of 92%. Abnormal visual evoked potential (VEP) throughout the first week of life or an absent VEP at anytime guaranteed an abnormal outcome in asphyxiated full-term infants (Muttitt et al, 1991).
   10. **Subsequent hearing is normal in most children who have suffered perinatal or postnatal asphyxia.** Children with residual neurodevelopmental deficits have more frequent peripheral hearing loss and more abnormalities of the central components of auditory evoked potentials than those who do not have neurodevelopmental deficits, suggestive of residual dysfunction in the rostral brainstem (Jiang, 1995; Jiang & Tierney, 1996).
   11. **Microcephaly** at 3 months of age is predictive of poor neurodevelopmental outcome (Shankaran et al, 1991). A decrease in head circumference (HC) ratios (actual HC/mean HC for age × 100%) of >3.1% between birth and 4 months of age is highly predictive of the eventual

development of microcephaly before 18 months of age (Cordes et al, 1994). Suboptimal rate of head growth associated with moderate cerebral white matter changes on MRI may be a better predictor of poor neurodevelopmental outcome (Mercuri et al, 2000).

12. **Decreased cerebral concentrations of phosphocreatine or ATP at birth on quantitative** ^{31}**P MRI** (Martin et al, 1996).

13. **Elevated brain lactate levels** (Leth et al, 1996), **elevated ratio of lactate to N-acetylaspartate**(Penrice et al, 1996) **and lactate to choline** (Barkovich et al, 1999) on **proton MRS, and low CSF cyclic adenosine monophosphate (cAMP) levels** (Pourcyrous et al, 1999).

14. **Increased CBF** on Doppler sonography in the first 3 days after birth (Leth et al, 1996).

15. **Decreased cerebral resistive index** on Doppler sonography (Gonzalez de Dios et al, 1995).

16. The presence of **optic atrophy** is an indicator of poor visual outcome (Luna et al, 1995). Many children with postasphyxial CNS abnormalities have lower visual acuity scores and smaller visual fields.

B. Nondisabled survivors of moderate HIE have delayed skills in reading, spelling, or arithmetic and have more difficulties with attention and short-term recall than survivors of mild HIE and normal individuals.

X. **Ethics.** Decision making is often difficult, but it is easier if the medical team and families communicate openly and clearly. (See also Chapters 15 and 32.) Shared decision making creates a partnership between parents and the physician and potentially reduces conflicts. Discussing best- and worst-case outcomes may help to define the range of potential outcome.

XI. **Medicolegal issues**

A. **Fetal monitoring.** In the presence of a reactive FHR pattern and normal fetal movement, the key is to monitor the baseline rate (Phelan & Kim, 2000). A rise or fall in FHR baseline should alert the labor and delivery team to impending fetal asphyxia.

B. **Timing of asphyxia to the intrapartum period** may be the cause of CP if there is no evidence of an antenatal injury (clinically or neuroimaging study) and there is classic criteria of severe asphyxia (ACOG) while excluding other causes of neonatal encephalopathy.

C. **Nucleated red blood cells (nRBCs).** Phelan et al (1998) attempted to time asphyxia to the magnitude of nRBC count. They showed that preadmission asphyxia resulted in a higher nRBC count than acute asphyxia. Adopting nRBC count to time asphyxia may be misleading because the magnitude of elevation not only relates to the duration of the asphyxia but to the severity of the asphyxia as well. Increased nRBC count may also be seen in prematurity, intrauterine growth retardation (IUGR), chorioamnionitis, and diabetes.

D. **When asked whether an identified event led to a subsequent adverse outcome, it is important to realize that the baseline fetal brain status is unknown.**

REFERENCES

American Academy of Pediatrics Committee on Fetus and Newborn and American College of Obstetrics and Gynecologists Committee on Obstetric Practice: Use and abuse of the Apgar score. *Pediatrics* 1996;98:141.

American College of Obstetricians and Gynecologists: *ACOG Technical Bulletin: Fetal and Neonatal Neurologic Injury.* American College of Obstetricians and Gynecologists, 1992.

Barkovich AJ et al: Perinatal asphyxia: MR findings in the first 10 days. *Am J Neuroradiol* 1995;16:427.

Barkovich AJ et al: Proton MR spectroscopy for the evaluation of brain injury in asphyxiated, term neonates. *Am J Neuroradiol* 1999;20:1399.

Carter BS et al: Prospective validation of a scoring system for predicting neonatal morbidity after acute perinatal asphyxia. *J Pediatr* 1998;132:619.

Clancy RR et al: Hypoxic-ischemic spinal cord injury following perinatal asphyxia. *Ann Neurol* 1989;25:185.

Cordes I et al: Early prediction of the development of microcephaly after hypoxic-ischemic encephalopathy in the full-term newborn. *Pediatrics* 1994;93:703.

Eken P et al: Predictive value of early neuroimaging, pulsed Doppler and neurophysiology in full term infants with hypoxic-ischaemic encephalopathy. *Arch Dis Child* 1995;73:F75.

Gonzalez de Dios J et al: Variations in cerebral blood flow in various states of severe neonatal hypoxic-ischemic encephalopathy. *Rev Neurol* 1995;23:639.

Graf H et al: Evidence for a detrimental effect of bicarbonate therapy in hypoxic lactic acidosis. *Science* 1984;227:754.

Gressens P et al: The germinative zone produces the most crucial cortical astrocytes after neuronal migration in the developing mammalian brain. *Biol Neonate* 1992;61:4.

Gunn AJ et al: Selective head cooling in newborn infants after perinatal asphyxia: a safety study. *Pediatrics* 1998;102:885.

Hall RT et al: High-dose phenobarbital therapy in term newborn infants with severe perinatal asphyxia: a randomized prospective study with three-year follow-up. *J Pediatr* 1998;132:345.

Harbord MG, Weston PF: Somatosensory evoked potentials predict neurologic outcome in full-term neonates with asphyxia. *J Paediatr Child Health* 1995;31:148.

Hull J, Dodd KL: Falling incidence of hypoxic-ischemic encephalopathy in term infants. *Br J Obstet Gynaecol* 1992;99:386.

Ikeda T et al: Fetal heart rate patterns in postasphyxial fetal lambs with brain damage. *Am J Obstet Gynecol* 1998;179:1329.

Jiang ZD: Long-term effect of perinatal and postnatal asphyxia on developing human auditory brainstem responses: peripheral hearing loss. *Int Pediatr Otorhinolaryngol* 1995;33:225.

Jiang ZD, Tierney TS: Long-term effect of perinatal and postnatal asphyxia on developing human auditory brainstem responses: brainstem impairment. *Int Pediatr Otorhinolaryngol* 1996;34:111.

Leth H et al: Use of brain lactate levels to predict outcome after perinatal asphyxia. *Acta Paediatr* 1996;85:859.

Levene M et al: Acute effects of two different doses of magnesium sulfate in infants with birth asphyxia. *Arch Dis Child* 1995;73:F174.

Leviton A, Gilles F: Ventriculomegaly, delayed myelination, white matter hypoplasia, and "periventricular" leukomalacia: how are they related? *Pediatr Neurol* 1996;15:127.

Low JA: Intrapartum fetal asphyxia: definition, diagnosis and classification. *Am J Obstet Gynecol* 1997;176:957.

Luna B et al: Grating acuity and visual field development in infants following perinatal asphyxia. *Dev Med Child Neurol* 1995;37:330.

Martin E, Barkovich AJ: Magnetic resonance imaging in perinatal asphyxia. *Arch Dis Child* 1995;72:F62.

Martin E et al: Diagnostic and prognostic value of cerebral ^{31}P magnetic resonance spectroscopy in neonates with perinatal asphyxia. *Pediatr Res* 1996;40:749.

Martin-Ancel A et al: Multiple organ involvement in perinatal asphyxia. *J Pediatr* 1995;127:786.

Mercuri E et al: Head growth in infants with hypoxic-ischemic encephalopathy: correlation with neonatal magnetic resonance imaging. *Pediatrics* 2000;106:235.

Muttitt SC et al: Serial visual evoked potentials and outcome in term birth asphyxia. *Pediatr Neurol* 1991;7:86.

Naqeeb NA et al: Assessment of neonatal encephalopathy by amplitude-integrated electroencephalography. *Pediatrics* 1999;103:1263

Peliowski A, Finer NN: Hypoxic-ischemic encephalopathy in the term infant. In Sinclair J, Lucey J (eds): *Effective Care of Newborn Infant*. Oxford University Press, 1992.

Penrice J et al: Proton magnetic resonance spectroscopy of the brain in normal preterm and term infants, and early changes after perinatal hypoxia-ischemia. *Pediatr Res* 1996;40:6.

Perlman JM: Intrapartum hypoxic-ischemic cerebral injury and subsequent cerebral palsy: medicolegal issues. *Pediatrics* 1997;99:851.

Perlman JM: Markers of asphyxia and neonatal brain injury. *N Engl J Med* 1999;341:364.

Perlman JM, Risser R: Can asphyxiated infants at risk for neonatal seizures be rapidly identified by current high-risk markers? *Pediatrics* 1996;97:456.

Phelan JP, Kim JO: Fetal heart rate observations in the brain-damaged infant. *Semin Perinatol* 2000;24:221.

Phelan JP et al: Neonatal nucleated red blood cells and lymphocyte counts in fetal brain injury. *Obstet Gynecol* 1998;91:485.

Pourcyrous M et al: Prognostic significance of cerebrospinal fluid cyclic adenosine monophosphate in neonatal asphyxia. *J Pediatr* 1999;134:90.

Robertson CMT, Finer NN: Long-term follow-up of term neonates with perinatal asphyxia. *Clin Perinatol* 1993;20:483.

Rutherford MA et al: Abnormal magnetic resonance signal in the internal capsule predicts poor neurodevelopmental outcome in infants with hypoxic-ischemic encephalopathy. *Pediatrics* 1998;102:323.

Sarnat HB, Sarnat MS: Neonatal encephalopathy following fetal distress. *Arch Neurol* 1976; 33:696.

Saugstad OD: Resuscitation of newborn infants with room air or oxygen. *Semin Neonatol* 2001; 6:233.

Sexson WR, Overall SW: Ethical decision making in perinatal asphyxia. *Clin Perinatol* 1996; 23:509.

Shankaran S et al: Acute neonatal morbidity and long-term central nervous system sequelae of perinatal asphyxia in term infants. *Early Hum Dev* 1991;25:135.

Shi Y et al: Role of carbon monoxide and nitric oxide in newborn infants with postasphyxial hypoxic-ischemic encephalopathy *Pediatrics* 2000;106.1447.

Van Bel F et al: Effect of allopurinol on postasphyxial tree radical formation, cerebral hemodynamics, and electrical brain activity. *Pediatrics* 1998;101:185.

Van Lieshout HBM et al: The prognostic value of the EEG in asphyxiated newborns. *Acta Neurol Scand* 1995;91:203.

Vento M et al: Resuscitation with room air instead of 100% oxygen prevents oxidative stress in moderately asphyxiated term neonates. *Pediatrics* 2001;107:642.

Volpe JJ: *Neurology of the Newborn*, 4th ed. Saunders, 2001.

74 Pulmonary Diseases

AIR LEAK SYNDROMES

I. **Definition.** The pulmonary air leak syndromes (pneumomediastinum, pneumothorax, pulmonary interstitial emphysema [PIE], pneumopericardium, pneumoperitoneum, and pneumoretroperitoneum) comprise a spectrum of disease with the same underlying pathophysiology. Overdistention of alveolar sacs or terminal airways leads to disruption of airway integrity, resulting in dissection of air into surrounding spaces.

II. **Incidence.** Although the exact incidence of the air leak syndromes is hard to determine, they are most commonly seen in infants with underlying lung disease (such as respiratory distress syndrome [RDS], meconium aspiration, and pulmonary hypoplasia) who are on ventilatory support in the neonatal intensive care unit (NICU). In general, the more severe the lung disease, the higher is the incidence of pulmonary air leak. Whereas air leak syndromes are seen most commonly in infants on ventilatory support, they all have been reported to occur spontaneously.

III. **Pathophysiology.** Overdistention of terminal air spaces or airways—the common denominator in all the pulmonary air leaks—can result from uneven alveolar ventilation, air trapping, or injudicious use of alveolar distending pressure in infants on ventilatory support. As lung volume exceeds physiologic limits, mechanical stresses occur in all planes of the alveolar or respiratory bronchial wall, with eventual tissue rupture. Air can track through the perivascular adventitia, causing PIE, or dissect along vascular sheaths toward the hilum, causing pneumomediastinum. Rupture of the mediastinal pleura results in pneumothorax. Pneumoretroperitoneum and pneumoperitoneum may occur when mediastinal air tracks downward to the extraperitoneal fascial planes of the abdominal wall, mesentery, and retroperitoneum and eventually ruptures into the peritoneal cavity.

A. **Barotrauma.** The common denominator of the air leak syndromes is barotrauma. Barotrauma results whenever positive pressure is applied to the lung; it cannot be avoided in the ill newborn infant needing ventilatory support, but its effects should be minimized.

1. **Peak inspiratory pressure (PIP), positive end-expiratory pressure (PEEP), inspiratory time (IT), respiratory rate, and the inspiratory waveform** play important roles in the development of barotrauma. It is difficult to determine which of these parameters is the most damaging and which plays the largest role in the development of the air leaks.

2. **Inadvertent PEEP** secondary to a very rapid rate and a short expiratory time may also be important.

B. **Other causes of lung overdistention.** Barotrauma is not the only cause of lung overdistention. Atelectatic alveoli in RDS may cause uneven ventilation and subject the more distensible areas of the lung to receive high pressures, placing them at risk for rupture. Small mucous plugs in the airway in meconium aspiration may cause gas trapping secondary to a ball-valve effect. Other events, such as inappropriate intubation of the right main stem bronchus, failure to wean after surfactant replacement therapy, and vigorous resuscitation or the development of high opening pressures with the onset of air breathing, can also lead to overdistention, with rupture of airway integrity at birth.

C. **Lung injury**

1. **Large tidal volume.** It has long been considered that lung injury is primarily a result of high-pressure ventilation (barotrauma). Although re-

ports show variable relationships between airway pressures and lung injury, more recent studies support the concept that lung overdistention resulting from high maximal lung volume ("volutrauma") and transalveolar pressure, rather than high airway pressure, is the harmful factor. In infants with low lung compliance, a high PIP may cause only small alveolar distention that may not be associated with significant injury.

2. **Atelectasis.** The alveolar units in patients with RDS are subjected to a cycle of recruitment and derecruitment. Strategies to decrease this mechanism of atelectatic trauma—optimizing lung recruitment and decreasing lung injury and severity of lung disease—will lessen the risk for pulmonary air leak.

IV. Risk factors

   A. Ventilatory support. The infant on ventilatory support has an increased risk of developing one of the air leak syndromes. Some investigators report an incidence as high as 12% in infants on any type of ventilatory support.

   B. Meconium staining. Other infants at risk include those who are meconium stained at birth. In these infants, meconium may be plugged in the airways, with resultant air trapping. During inspiration, the airway expands, allowing air to enter. However, during exhalation, there is airway collapse with resultant trapping of air behind meconium plugs.

   C. Failure to wean after surfactant therapy. Studies have shown that prophylactic use of surfactant therapy in infants at risk for RDS is associated with a decrease in the incidence of pneumothorax and PIE. Similar findings were noted in treating premature newborns with established RDS. With the return of pulmonary compliance after receiving surfactant, appropriate decreases in pressure support and more cautious ventilatory management of these infants is necessary immediately after therapy. The clinician must closely watch for improvement in the infant's arterial blood gas levels and must wean ventilatory support as required.

V. Clinical presentation. Air leak syndromes are potentially lethal, and a high index of suspicion is necessary for the diagnosis of air leak syndromes. On clinical grounds, respiratory distress or a deteriorating clinical course strongly suggests air leak. See section IX: Specific Air Leak Syndromes.

VI. Diagnosis. The definitive diagnosis of all of these syndromes is made radiographically. An anteroposterior (AP) chest x-ray film along with a cross-table lateral film is essential in diagnosing an air leak.

VII. Prevention. The best mode of treatment for all of the air leak syndromes is prevention and judicious use of ventilatory support, with close attention to distending pressure, PEEP, and IT. Despite the availability of surfactant and high-frequency ventilators and advancements in respiratory monitoring, air leak syndromes continue to be a problem in neonatal care. Barotrauma remains a prominent disadvantage to ventilatory support. The judicious use of ventilatory pressures and the adjustment of ventilator settings to provide a minimum of barotrauma are extremely important in the NICU. The use of surfactant therapy for RDS has been shown to substantially decrease the incidence of pneumothorax and PIE. Although studies report that high-frequency ventilation (HFV) reduced the incidence of air leaks, the use of this strategy in infants exposed to antenatal steroids and postnatal surfactant remains to be confirmed.

VIII. Prognosis. The prognosis for the infant in whom an air leak develops depends on the underlying condition. In general, if the air leak is treated rapidly and effectively, the long-term outcome should not change. However, it must be remembered that early-onset PIE (>24 h of age) is associated with a high mortality rate. Chronic lung disease (CLD) of the newborn, or bronchopulmonary dysplasia (BPD), is also associated with severe pulmonary air leak syndromes.

IX. Specific air leak syndromes

   A. Pneumomediastinum

      1. Definition. Pneumomediastinum is air in the mediastinum from ruptured alveolar air that has traversed fascial planes.

2. **Incidence.** The incidence of pneumomediastinum before the era of neonatal intensive care was approximately 2 in 1000 live births. The exact incidence is related to the degree of ventilatory support and is clearly higher today. It has been reported to occur in at least 25% of patients with coexisting pneumothorax.

3. **Pathophysiology.** Pneumomediastinum is preceded by PIE in almost every instance. After alveolar rupture, air traverses fascial planes and passes into the mediastinum.

4. **Risk factors.** See section IV: Risk Factors.

5. **Clinical presentation.** Unless accompanied by pneumothorax, a pneumomediastinum may be totally asymptomatic. Spontaneous pneumomediastinum may develop in term infants not on ventilatory support and may be accompanied by mild respiratory distress. Physical findings in addition to respiratory distress may include an increase in AP diameter of the chest and difficulty in auscultating heart sounds.

6. **Diagnosis.** On the radiograph, pneumomediastinum may present in several ways. The classic description is that of a "wind-blown spinnaker sail" (a lobe or lobes of the thymus being elevated off the heart). In other cases, a halo may be seen around the heart in the AP projection, or evidence on this projection may be completely absent. The cross-table lateral projection will show an anterior collection of air that may be difficult to distinguish from a pneumothorax.

7. **Management.** There is no definitive treatment for pneumomediastinum. One should resist the temptation to insert a drain into the mediastinum because it will not be beneficial and may cause more problems than it will solve. An oxygen-rich environment can be used in the term infant to attempt nitrogen washout if the pneumomediastinum is believed to be clinically significant.

8. **Prognosis.** The prognosis is good because recovery is frequently spontaneous without treatment.

B. **Pneumothorax**

1. **Definition.** Pneumothorax is air between the visceral and parietal pleural surfaces.

2. **Incidence.** The incidence of pneumothorax varies between units. Before the modern era of neonatal intensive care, the incidence of pneumothorax was 1–2%. With the advent of neonatal ventilator care, however, the incidence has risen dramatically. Although the exact incidence is difficult to determine, it is directly related to the degree of ventilatory support delivered.

3. **Pathophysiology**
   a. **The term infant not on ventilatory support.** Pneumothorax may develop spontaneously. It usually occurs at delivery, when a large initial opening pressure is necessary to inflate collapsed alveolar sacs. The overall frequency based on radiographic surveys is approximately 1% of all live births.
   b. **The infant on ventilatory support** will have alveolar overdistention secondary to either injudicious use of distending pressure or failure to wean ventilatory pressure when compliance begins to return. Pneumothorax is usually preceded by rupture of the alveoli, with the interstitial air then traversing via fascial planes to the mediastinum. The air breaks through the mediastinal pleura to form a pneumothorax.

4. **Risk factors.** See section IV: Risk Factors.

5. **Clinical presentation.** The clinical presentation of the neonate with pneumothorax depends on the setting in which it develops.
   a. **Term infants with a spontaneous pneumothorax** may be asymptomatic or only mildly symptomatic. These infants usually have tachypnea and mild oxygen needs early but may progress to the classic signs of respiratory distress (grunting, flaring, retractions, and tachypnea).

b. The infant on ventilatory support will generally have a sudden, rapid clinical deterioration characterized by cyanosis, hypoxemia, hypercarbia, and respiratory acidosis. The most common time for the development of this complication is either immediately after the initiation of ventilatory support or when the infant begins to improve and compliance returns (eg, after surfactant therapy). In either case, other clinical signs may include decreased breath sounds on the involved side, shifted heart sounds, and asynchrony of the chest. When compression of major veins and decreased cardiac output occur because of downward displacement of the diaphragm, signs of shock may be evident.

6. **Diagnosis.** A high index of suspicion is necessary for the diagnosis of pneumothorax.

   a. **Transillumination of the chest.** With the aid of transillumination, the diagnosis of pneumothorax may be made without a chest x-ray film. A fiberoptic light probe placed on the infant's chest wall will illuminate the involved hemithorax. Although this technique is beneficial in an emergency, it should not replace a chest x-ray film as the means of diagnosis.

   b. **Chest x-ray films.** Radiographically, pneumothorax is diagnosed on the basis of the following characteristics:

      i. **Presence of air in the pleural cavity** separating the parietal and visceral pleura. The area appears hyperlucent with absence of pulmonary markings.

      ii. **Collapse** of the ipsilateral lobes.

      iii. **Displacement of the mediastinum** to the contralateral side.

      iv. **Downward displacement of the diaphragm.** In infants with RDS, the compliance may be so poor that the lung may not collapse, with only minimal shift of the mediastinal structures. The anteroposterior x-ray film may not demonstrate the classic radiographic appearance if a large amount of the intrapleural air is situated just anterior to the sternum. In these situations, the cross-table lateral x-ray film will show a large lucent area immediately below the sternum, or the lateral decubitus x-ray film (with the suspected side up) will show free air.

   c. **Transcutaneous carbon dioxide (tcPco$_2$).** Reference percentiles for tcPco$_2$ level and slope of the trended tcPco$_2$ over various time intervals have been used to detect the occurrence of pneumothorax preclinically. The area under the curve (AUC) for 5 consecutive minutes with a 5-min tcPco$_2$ slope more than the 90th percentile shows good discrimination for a pneumothorax. However, false-positive results such as presence of a blocked or misplaced endotracheal tube may be encountered. If the problem with tcPco$_2$ persists after appropriately suctioning the endotracheal tube, then a confirmatory x-ray film should be ordered.

7. **Management.** Treatment of pneumothorax depends on the clinical status of the infant.

   a. **Oxygen supplementation.** In the term infant who is mildly symptomatic, an oxygen-rich environment is often all that is necessary. The inspired oxygen facilitates nitrogen washout of the blood and tissues and thus establishes a difference in the gas tensions between the loculated gases in the chest and those in the blood. This diffusion gradient results in rapid resorption of the loculated gas, with resolution of the pneumothorax. This mode of therapy is not appropriate in the preterm infant because of the high oxygen levels needed for washout and resulting increase in oxygen saturation. This makes it unsuitable for premature infants with risk for retinopathy of prematurity (ROP).

   b. **Decompression.** In the symptomatic neonate or the neonate on mechanical ventilatory support, immediate evacuation of air is necessary. The technique is described in Chapter 51, p 293, section V,A. Placement of a chest tube of appropriate size will eventually be necessary (see Chapter 19).

C. PIE
1. **Definition.** PIE is dissection of air into the perivascular tissues of the lung from alveolar overdistention or overdistention of the smaller airways.
2. **Incidence.** This disorder arises almost exclusively in the very low birth weight infant on ventilatory support. It may also emerge in the extremely low birth weight infant without mechanical ventilation but receiving ventilatory support by continuous positive airway pressure (CPAP). It has been reported to occur in at least one third of infants <1000 g who have RDS on the first day of life. If seen within the first 24 h of life, it generally is associated with a poor prognosis. As time passes, its occurrence is less common, but it may be seen at any time during ventilatory management.
3. **Pathophysiology.** PIE may be the precursor of all other types of pulmonary air leaks. With overdistention of the alveoli or conducting airways, or both, rupture may occur, and there may be dissection of the air into the perivascular tissue of the lung. The interstitial air moves in the connective tissue planes and around the vascular axis, particularly the venous ones. Once in the interstitial space, the air moves along bronchioles, lymphatics, and vascular sheaths or directly through the lung interstitium to the pleural surface. The extrapulmonary air is trapped in the interstitium (PIE), or it may extend and cause pneumomediastinum, pneumopericardium, or pneumothorax. PIE may exist in two forms: localized (which involves one or more lobes) or diffuse (bilateral).
4. **Risk factors.** See section IV: Risk Factors.
5. **Clinical presentation.** The patient in whom PIE develops may have sudden deterioration. More commonly, however, the onset of PIE will be heralded by a slow, progressive deterioration of arterial blood gas levels and the apparent need for increasing ventilatory support. Invariably, a diffusion block develops in these patients, with the alveolar membrane becoming separated from the capillary bed by the interstitial air. The response to increased ventilatory support in the face of poor arterial blood gas levels may lead to worsening of PIE and sudden clinical deterioration. However, some infants with severe PIE may actually improve if the PIE progresses to pneumothorax.
6. **Diagnosis.** In infants with PIE, the chest x-ray film will generally reveal radiolucencies that are either linear or cyst-like in nature. The linear radiolucencies vary in length and do not branch; they are seen in the periphery of the lung as well as medially and may be mistaken for air bronchograms. The cyst-like lucencies vary from 1.0–4.0 mm in diameter and can be lobulated.
7. **Management**
   a. **Lessening lung injury.** In general, once PIE is diagnosed, an attempt should be made to decrease ventilatory support and lessen lung trauma. Decreasing the PIP, decreasing the PEEP, or shortening the IT may be required. All of these maneuvers will decrease injury and possibly improve PIE. During this time, some degree of hypercarbia and hypoxia may have to be accepted.
   b. **Positioning of the infant** with the involved side down has also proved beneficial in some cases of unilateral PIE.
   c. **Other treatments.** More invasive measures include selective collapse of the involved lung on the side with the worse involvement, with selective intubation or even the insertion of chest tubes before the development of pneumothorax. In cases of severe PIE, surgical resection of the affected lobe may be considered.
   d. **HFV** has proved useful in infants with severe PIE and with other types of pulmonary air leak. Both high-frequency oscillatory ventilation

(HFOV) and high-frequency jet ventilation (HFJV) have been used effectively in the treatment of PIE and other types of air leak syndromes. Although these treatment modalities may improve survival of the infant with PIE, the long-term pulmonary outcome remains uncertain; however, randomized controlled trials have been completed and have revealed good results. The earlier that HFV is initiated after the onset of PIE or pulmonary air leak, the greater are the chances for survival.

8. **Prognosis.** See section VIII: Prognosis.

D. **Pneumopericardium**

1. **Definition.** Pneumopericardium is air in the pericardial sac, which is usually secondary to passage of air along vascular sheaths. It is always a complication of mechanical ventilatory support.

2. **Incidence.** Pneumopericardium is a rare occurrence. In a study of extremely low birth weight infants who were ventilated and 41% having pulmonary air leak, 2% were found to have pneumopericardium.

3. **Pathophysiology.** It is often said that pneumopericardium is always preceded by pneumomediastinum, but this is not universally true. The mechanism by which pneumopericardium develops is not well understood, but it is probably due to passage of air along vascular sheaths. From the mediastinum, air can travel along the fascial planes in the subcutaneous tissues of the neck, chest wall, and anterior abdominal wall and into the pericardial space, causing pneumopericardium.

4. **Risk factors.** See section IV: Risk Factors.

5. **Clinical presentation.** The clinical signs of pneumopericardium range from asymptomatic to the full picture of cardiac tamponade. The first sign of pneumopericardium may be a decrease in blood pressure or a decrease in pulse pressure. There may also be an increase in heart rate with distant heart sounds.

6. **Diagnosis.** Pneumopericardium has the most classic radiographic appearance of all the air leaks. A broad radiolucent halo completely surrounds the heart, including the diaphragmatic surface. This picture is easily distinguished from all the other air leaks by its extension completely around the heart in all projections.

7. **Treatment.** Treatment of pneumopericardium is essential and requires the placement of a pericardial drain or repeated pericardial taps. The procedure is described in Chapter 26.

E. **Pneumoperitoneum**

1. **Definition.** Pneumoperitoneum is air in the peritoneal cavity that is usually caused by gastrointestinal perforation, but it can also be caused by air that has ruptured from the mediastinum into the peritoneum.

2. **Incidence.** Pneumoperitoneum from passage of air into the chest is rare.

3. **Pathophysiology.** Pneumoperitoneum in the newborn most commonly arises from a perforated hollow viscus or a preceding abdominal operation. It can also be secondary to ventilator-assisted pulmonary air leakage. Air from the ruptured alveoli can flow transdiaphragmatically along the great vessels and esophagus into the retroperitoneum. When air accumulates in the retroperitoneum, rupture into the peritoneal cavity can occur.

4. **Risk factors.** See section IV: Risk Factors.

5. **Clinical presentation.** Depending on the cause and severity, pneumoperitoneum can present with or without associated abdominal findings. Because pneumoperitoneum can occur as a result of pneumothorax, pneumomediastinum, and pulmonary interstitial air, infants can present with signs of respiratory distress, as mentioned earlier.

6. **Diagnosis.** Pneumoperitoneum can be detected in radiographic films as free air under the diaphragm. Pneumothorax, pneumomediastinum, PIE, and pneumopericardium may precede its occurrence if the pneumomedi-

astinum is caused by pulmonary air leak. However, the absence of these air leaks cannot be considered proof that gastrointestinal perforation is the cause. The presence of an intra-abdominal air-fluid level, leakage of radiographic isotonic contrast agents, analysis of oxygen saturation levels or P_{O_2} in intraperitoneal air can be used to distinguish whether the air leak is pulmonary or gastrointestinal in origin.

7. **Treatment.** Conservative management may be strongly considered if evidence of pulmonary air leak precedes or simultaneously appears with pneumoperitoneum. In cases of bowel perforation, laparotomy is usually required.

APNEA AND PERIODIC BREATHING

I. **Definitions.** Simply defined, apnea is the absence of respiratory gas flow for a period of 20 s or greater or of shorter duration if associated with bradycardia or significant desaturation.

    A. **Central apnea** is of central nervous system (CNS) origin and is characterized by the absence of gas flow with no respiratory effort.

    B. **Obstructive apnea** is continued respiratory effort not resulting in gas flow.

    C. **Mixed apnea** is a combination of the central and obstructive types.

    D. **Periodic breathing,** defined as three or more periods of apnea lasting 3 s or more within a 20-s period of otherwise normal respiration, is also common in the newborn period. Currently, it is not known whether there is an association between apnea and periodic breathing.

II. **Incidence.** The incidence of apnea and periodic breathing in the term infant has not been adequately determined. More than 50% of infants weighing <1500 g and 90% of infants weighing <1000 g will have apnea. Mixed apnea is the most common type, followed by central and obstructive. Another 30% will have periodic breathing.

III. **Pathophysiology.** Apnea and periodic breathing probably have a common pathophysiologic origin, apnea being a step further along the continuum than periodic breathing. Although the exact pathophysiology of these events has not yet been elucidated, there are many theories.

    A. **Immaturity of respiratory control.** Because apnea is seen most commonly in the premature infant, some type of immaturity of the respiratory control mechanism is thought to play a role in most cases of apnea.

        1. **Hypoxic response.** The preterm infant is known to have an abnormal biphasic response to hypoxia: a brief period of tachypnea followed by apnea. This response is unlike that seen in the adult or older child in whom hypoxia produces a state of prolonged tachypnea.

        2. **Carbon dioxide response.** The carbon dioxide response curve is shifted in the preterm infant; higher levels of carbon dioxide are required before respiration is stimulated.

    B. **Sleep-related response.** Sleep states may also play an important role in the development of apnea in the preterm infant. A shift from one sleep state to another is often characterized by instability of respiratory activity in the adult. The preterm infant is sleeping approximately 80% of the time and has difficulty making the transition between the sleeping and waking states. This may be associated with an increased risk for apnea.

    C. **Protective reflexes** such as the apneic response to noxious substances in the airway may also play a role in apneic episodes in the newborn infant.

    D. **Muscle weakness.** Overall muscle weakness (of both the muscles of respiration and the muscles that maintain airway patency) also plays an important role in pathophysiology.

    E. **All of these factors point to an immature respiratory control mechanism in the preterm infant.** Whether the immaturity is operational at the level of the brainstem, the peripheral chemoreceptors, or the central receptors has yet to be determined. What is likely is that apnea results from a combination of immature afferent impulses to the respiratory control centers along with immature efferents from these receptor sites, giving rise to poor ventilatory control.

F. **Pathologic states** can also lead to apnea in the infant. The following disorders have all been associated with apnea in the neonatal period.
   1. **Hypothermia and hyperthermia.**
   2. **Metabolic disturbances** such as hypoglycemia and hyponatremia.
   3. **Sepsis.**
   4. **Anemia.**
   5. **Hypoxemia.**
   6. **CNS abnormalities** such as intraventricular hemorrhage (IVH) or stroke.
   7. **Necrotizing enterocolitis (NEC).**
   8. **Drug withdrawal and drug effects** (eg, maternal antepartum magnesium therapy).
   9. **Gastroesophageal reflux.**

IV. **Risk factors**
   A. **Preterm infants.** The preterm infant is at the greatest risk for apnea. Because apnea is believed to develop secondary to an immature or poorly developed respiratory control mechanism, this association is especially noted in extremely low birth weight infants.
   B. **Sleep positioning.** The "back to sleep" campaign, which was initiated in 1992, has led to a 40% reduction in the incidence of sudden infant death syndrome (SIDS).
   C. **Neurologic disorders.** Because respiration depends on the integration of numerous CNS functions, the child with certain neurologic diseases may be at increased risk for apnea. Examples of central neurologic disorders include CNS infection and structural abnormalities (eg, holoprosencephaly), and peripheral disorders include Werdnig-Hoffman in Dorland's and myasthenia gravis.
   D. **Sibling with SIDS.** The Collaborative Home Infant Monitoring Evaluation (CHIME) study showed that the incidence of apnea was the same in siblings of SIDS and normal term infants. Evidence supports an increased chance of obstructive sleep apnea (OSA) in infants with a family history of OSA, SIDS, and apparent life-threatening event.
   E. **Gastroesophageal reflux.** Its relationship to apnea has been the source of much debate; some studies show no temporal relationship to apnea of prematurity, but it is a cause of apnea in the term infant.

V. **Clinical presentation**
   A. **Apnea within 24 h after delivery.** Although apnea may be present at any time during the neonatal period, if it presents within the first 24 h of life, it is usually not simple apnea of prematurity. Apnea during this period must be suspected as being associated with infant or maternal conditions (eg, neonatal sepsis, hypoglycemia, intracranial hemorrhage, maternal antepartum magnesium treatment, or maternal exposure to narcotics).
   B. **Apnea after the first 24 h of life.** When apnea occurs after the first 24 h of life and is not associated with any other pathologic condition, it may be classified as apnea of prematurity. Apnea may also occur after weaning from prolonged ventilatory support and may be associated with intermittent hypoxia secondary to hypoventilation or atelectasis.

VI. **Diagnosis.** A high index of suspicion is necessary to diagnose apnea. If significant apnea is detected, an extensive workup is required to make an accurate diagnosis and develop a logical treatment plan.
   A. **Monitoring of infants at risk.** All preterm infants should be closely monitored for the development of this often life-threatening condition. Close attention should be paid to the type of monitoring that is given to infants in intensive care units. Preterm infants are commonly on heart rate monitors only, and they will be identified as having apnea only if the heart rate drops below the monitor alarm limit (usually set at 80 beats/min). In this case,

these infants may suffer profound hypoxia before bradycardia develops, or they may have apnea with significant hypoxemia but without a drop in heart rate. In order to detect apnea, these infants should have continuous monitoring of respiratory activity or monitoring of oxygenation, or both, using either transcutaneous oximetry or pulse oximetry.

B. History. A thorough review of maternal septic risk factors, medications, and birth history are required. Additional history of feeding intolerance along with abdominal distention might suggest NEC.

C. Physical examination. Specific attention should be paid to physical findings such as lethargy, hypothermia or hyperthermia, cyanosis, and respiratory effort. A thorough physical examination, including neurologic exam, should also be performed.

D. Laboratory studies
1. **Sepsis screen,** including complete blood cell count with differential, platelet count, and serial C-reactive proteins, will help to rule out sepsis and anemia.
2. **Pulse oximetry** will screen for hypoxia, with arterial blood gas when indicated.
3. **Serum glucose, electrolyte, and calcium levels** will aid in the diagnosis of metabolic disturbances.

E. Radiographic studies
1. **Chest x-ray** study to detect evidence of pathologic lung changes (eg, atelectasis, pneumonia, or air leak).
2. **Abdominal x-ray** study to detect signs of NEC (see Chapter 71).
3. **Ultrasonography of the head** to detect IVH or other CNS abnormality.
4. **Computed tomography (CT) scan of the head** may also be appropriate in infants with definite signs of neurologic disease.

F. Other studies
1. **Electroencephalography.** An electroencephalogram (EEG) may be necessary to complete the workup if there is any question about the neurologic status of the infant. Apnea as the sole presentation of seizures is uncommon.
2. **Pneumography.** A pneumogram is another tool in the diagnosis of apnea. Pneumography is especially useful in the infant whose cause of apnea has not yet been identified. Chest leads provide a tracing that gives a continuous recording of heart rate, chest wall movement, pulse oximetry, and airflow via a nasal thermistor. With the addition of a thermistor, central apnea can easily be distinguished from obstructive apnea. The addition of the pulse oximeter helps in determining whether there are oxygen desaturations during periods of apnea or heart rate drops. This distinction is important for the treatment of the disorder and should be directed specifically to the type of apnea that is detected. A pH probe for the detection of gastroesophageal reflux is also important for completion of an overall evaluation for apnea.
3. **Polysomnography.** This is a rarely used test. In research-oriented centers, a polysomnogram (a study that monitors specific EEG leads and muscle movement) can be used for a more thorough workup of apnea. This study not only will determine the type of apnea that occurs but can also relate it to the sleep stage of the infant.

VII. Management. Treatment for apnea must be individualized.

A. Specific therapy. If an identifiable cause of apnea is determined, it should be treated accordingly. For example, sepsis should be treated with antibiotics (see Chapter 80); hypoglycemia, with glucose infusion; electrolyte abnormalities (see the specific abnormality in On-Call Problems) and anemia should be corrected.

B. General therapy. If a cause cannot be identified or if one can be identified but is not amenable to treatment (eg, IVH), several approaches to treatment exist.

1. **Supplemental oxygen.** Merely increasing the ambient oxygen concentration will often alleviate apneic spells. The mechanism of action is probably secondary to decreasing the number of unidentified hypoxic spells. Concern about worsening ROP is warranted, and oxygenation should, therefore, be monitored.

2. **CPAP** is used with some success, probably acting by the same mechanism as supplemental oxygen. This method is an invasive therapeutic modality and should be used only when other methods have failed.

3. **Pharmacologic therapy.** If the just-mentioned methods fail, the next line of approach is to begin administration of respiratory stimulants.

   a. **Theophylline** is commonly used in the treatment of apnea. The exact mechanism of action is open to debate, but it probably works through a variety of mechanisms, including an effect on the adenosine tissue receptors, direct stimulation of the respiratory centers, and lowering of the threshold to carbon dioxide. Some clinicians think it may act by direct stimulation of the diaphragm. (For dosage and other pharmacologic information, see Chapter 80.)

   b. **Caffeine** can also be used in the treatment of apnea. Because caffeine has fewer side effects, has a greater gap between therapeutic and toxic levels, does not alter cerebral blood flow, and has a longer half-life than theophylline, it is the preferred agent. If the intravenous preparation is not available, theophylline is still an effective drug. Caffeine levels are no longer considered absolutely necessary in the management of most infants with apnea. (For dosage, see Chapter 80.)

   c. **Doxapram.** Doxapram, a potent respiratory stimulant, has been shown to be effective when theophylline and caffeine have failed. The duration of treatment with doxapram has been limited to 5 days, but the drug may be used longer if indicated. Benzyl alcohol is the preservative used in doxapram. The duration of therapy depends on the cumulative dose of benzyl alcohol, and there have been concerns about long-term neurodevelopmental outcome.

4. **Mechanical ventilation.** Some infants continue to have apneic spells despite pharmacologic treatment. If the apnea is severe and is associated with hypoxia or significant bradycardia, intubation and mechanical ventilation may be indicated.

C. **Discharge planning and follow-up.** A major issue in the management of infants with apnea is deciding when to stop administration of methylxanthines and whether or not the infant needs to be discharged on methylxanthines, a home monitor, or both.

1. **Discontinuing medications.** Consider stopping methylxanthine therapy when the apnea has resolved and the infant weighs between 1800 and 2000 g. A more aggressive approach is to stop therapy when the infant has been apnea free for a period of 7 days regardless of age. If the infant remains asymptomatic after discontinuation of methylxanthine therapy, the child may be discharged without further therapy.

2. **Reinstituting medications.** If symptomatic apnea recurs after discontinuing therapy, methylxanthine therapy should be reinstituted and a decision made to discharge the infant on this medication or to keep the infant hospitalized longer. Earlier discharge with monitoring is acceptable in an attempt to shorten the length of hospital stay. The use of home monitors in addition to methylxanthine therapy is *controversial.* Therapeutic methylxanthine levels are maintained until the child reaches 52 weeks' postconceptional age; then methylxanthine therapy is discontinued and the recording checked. If the recording is normal, therapy can be stopped. If the recording is abnormal, the infant may need to be restarted on methylxanthines and monitoring continued. Another attempt can be made to discontinue methylxanthines in 4 weeks.

3. **Home apnea monitoring.** Use of home apnea monitors continues to be *controversial.* The CHIME study showed that after 43 weeks' postconceptional age (PCA) cardiorespiratory events occurred no more frequently in preterm infants than term infants. No study has shown an improved morbidity and mortality with home infant monitoring for apnea. Currently, no standard of care exist among neonatologists, but reasonable indications for home apnea monitor use include the following:

a. Significant event not associated with feeds
b. Home methylxanthine therapy for apnea
c. Presence of a tracheostomy
d. Home oxygen therapy. If home monitoring is to be used, the most appropriate type of monitor is one that has the ability to store and record waveforms. These monitors allow for continued evaluation and management of the infant at risk. Waveform monitors measure transthoracic impedance and electrocardiograms (ECGs) and will document captured waveform data, alarms, and physiologic events, which should give clinicians a better understanding of the patient's symptoms.

VIII. **Prognosis.** The best indicator of prognosis in apnea is cause. Apnea of prematurity has an excellent prognosis, whereas that associated with IVH has a poorer prognosis. In most infants, apnea resolves without the occurrence of long-term deficiencies.

BRONCHOPULMONARY DYSPLASIA

I. **Definition.** Classic BPD is a neonatal form of CLD that follows a primary course of respiratory failure (eg, RDS, meconium aspiration syndrome) in the first days of life. A "new" form of BPD has been described in extremely low birth weight infants. It occurs in infants who initially had minimal or no lung disease.

BPD is defined as an oxygen dependency for >28 days after birth. The severity of pulmonary dysfunction in early childhood is more accurately predicted by an oxygen dependence at 36 weeks' PCA in infants < 32 weeks' gestational age (GA) and at 56 days of age in infants with older GA.

II. **Incidence.** The incidence of BPD is influenced by many risk factors, the most important of which is lung maturity. The incidence of BPD increases from 7 to 70% with a decrease in birth weight from a range of 1001–1250 g to 500–750 g.

III. **Pathophysiology.** A primary lung injury is not always evident at birth. The secondary development of a persistent lung injury is associated with an abnormal repair process and will lead to structural changes such as defective alveolarization and pulmonary vascular dysgenesis. Although classic BPD is mainly the result of exposure to high oxygen concentration and mechanical ventilation, the new BPD is mainly due to extreme prematurity, sepsis, and PDA.

A. **The major factors contributing to BPD are as follows:**
1. **Oxygen exposure.** Prolonged exposure to high concentrations of oxygen will decrease alveolar septation, decrease alveolar vascularization, increase terminal air space size, increase lung fibrosis, and inhibit lung growth.
2. **Mechanical ventilation.** Positive distending pressure (barotrauma) and the presence of an endotracheal tube (bacterial colonization) may lead to lung injury.
3. **Inflammation.** Inflammation is central to the development of BPD. An exaggerated inflammatory response (alveolar influx of numerous proinflammatory cytokines as well as macrophages and leukocytes) occurs in the first few days of life in infants in whom BPD subsequently develops.
B. **Pathologic changes.** Compared with the presurfactant era, lungs of infants currently dying from BPD have normal-appearing airways, less fibrosis, and more uniform inflation. However, these lungs have fewer and larger alveoli, indicating an interference with septation.

IV. **Risk factors.** Major risk factors are prematurity, white race, male gender, chorioamnionitis, tracheal colonization with ureaplasma, and the increased survival of the extremely low birth weight infant. Other risk factors are RDS, symptomatic PDA, sepsis, oxygen therapy, vitamin A deficiency, and a family history of atopic disease.

V. **Diagnosis**
   A. **General presentation.** BPD is usually suspected in infants with progressive and idiopathic deterioration of pulmonary function. Infants in whom BPD develops often require oxygen therapy or mechanical ventilation beyond the first week of life. Severe cases of BPD are usually associated with poor growth, pulmonary edema, and a hyperreactive airway.
   B. **Physical examination**
      1. **General signs.** Worsening respiratory status is manifested by an increase in the work of breathing, an increase in oxygen requirement, or an increase in apnea-bradycardia, or a combination of these.
      2. **Pulmonary examination.** Retractions and diffuse rales are common. Wheezing or prolongation of expiration may also be noted.
      3. **Cardiovascular examination.** A right ventricular heave, single S_2, or prominent P_2 may accompany cor pulmonale.
      4. **Abdominal examination.** The liver may be enlarged secondary to right-sided heart failure or may be displaced downward into the abdomen secondary to pulmonary hyperinflation.
   C. **Laboratory and radiologic studies.** Those studies are intended to rule out differential diagnosis such as sepsis or PDA during the acute nature of the disease and to detect problems related to CLD or its therapy.
      1. **Arterial blood gas levels** frequently reveal carbon dioxide retention. However, if the respiratory difficulties are chronic and stable, the pH is usually subnormal (pH ≥7.25).
      2. **Electrolytes.** Abnormalities of electrolytes may result from chronic carbon dioxide retention (elevated serum bicarbonate), diuretic therapy (hyponatremia, hypokalemia, or hypochloremia), or fluid restriction (elevated urea nitrogen and creatinine), or all three.
      3. **Urinalysis.** Microscopic examination may reveal the presence of red blood cells, indicating a possible nephrocalcinosis as a result of prolonged diuretic treatment.
      4. **Chest x-ray study.** Radiographic findings may be quite variable. Most frequently, BPD appears as diffuse haziness and lung hypoinflation in infants who were very immature at birth and have persistent oxygen requirements. In other infants, a different picture will be seen reminiscent of that originally described by Northway: streaky interstitial markings, patchy atelectasis intermingled with cystic area, and severe overall lung hyperinflation. Because those findings persist for a prolonged period, new changes (such a secondary infection) are difficult to detect without the benefit of comparison to previous x-ray films.
      5. **Renal ultrasonography.** Radiologic studies of the abdomen should be considered during diuretic therapy to detect the presence of nephrocalcinosis. It should be performed when red blood cells are present in the urine.
      6. **Other studies. Electrocardiography** and **echocardiography** are indicated in nonimproving or worsening BPD. ECGs and echocardiograms could detect cor pulmonale, manifested by right ventricular hypertrophy and elevation of pulmonary artery pressure with right axis deviation, increased right systolic time intervals, thickening of the right ventricular wall, and abnormal right ventricular geometry.

VI. **Management**
   A. **Prevention of BPD**
      1. **Prevention of prematurity and RDS.** Therapies directed toward decreasing the risk of prematurity and the incidence of RDS include improving prenatal care and antenatal corticosteroids.

2. **Reducing exposure to risk factors**
   a. **Successful measures should include** minimizing exposure to oxygen, ventilation strategies that minimize the use of excessive tidal volume (above 4–6 mL/kg), prudent administration of fluids, aggressive closure of PDA, and adequate nutrition. Early surfactant replacement therapy may be beneficial, but the avoidance of intubation and mechanical ventilation with the initiation of CPAP shortly after birth may prove to be the most effective preventive strategy.
   b. **Nonproven measures.**
      i. **Although infants colonized with _Ureaplasma urealyticum_ are at the highest risk for BPD,** the routine use of antibiotic therapy for its eradication has not been shown to be beneficial.
      ii. **Vitamin A** is known to be important in epithelial cell differentiation and repair and extremely low birth weight infant have low blood level. Vitamin A supplementation in those infants decreases the incidence of BPD, but the magnitude of this effect is fairly small.

B. **Treatment of BPD.** Once BPD is present, the goal of management is to prevent further injury by minimizing respiratory support, improving pulmonary function, preventing cor pulmonale, and emphasizing growth and nutrition.
   1. **Respiratory support**
      a. **Supplemental oxygen.** Maintaining adequate oxygenation is important in the infant with BPD to prevent hypoxia-induced pulmonary hypertension, bronchospasm, cor pulmonale, and growth failure. However, the least required oxygen should be delivered to minimize oxygen toxicity. Arterial oxygen saturation (Sao_2) should be monitored during the infant's various activities, including rest, sleep, and feeding. The optimal oxygen saturation level has not been established, and whether the level should exceed the range between 90 and 94% is _controversial._ Nonfrequent blood gas measurements are important for the assessment of trends in pH, $Paco_2$, and serum bicarbonate but are of limited use in monitoring oxygenation because they provide information about only one point in time.
      b. **Positive-pressure ventilation.** Mechanical ventilation should be used only when clearly indicated. Problems with air trapping can be significant; thus, a ventilatory strategy using a slower rate with longer inspiration and expiration times than when ventilated for RDS should be implemented. Similarly inspiratory pressure needs to be limited at the expense of tolerating $Paco_2$ in excess of 50–60 mm Hg. Nasal CPAP can be useful as an adjunctive therapy after extubation.
   2. **Improving lung function**
      a. **Fluid restriction.** Restricting fluid to 130 mL/kg/day or less is often required. It can be accomplished by concentrating proprietary formulas to 24 cal/oz. Increasing the caloric density further, to 27–30 cal/oz, requires the addition of fat (eg, medium-chain triglyceride oil or corn oil) and carbohydrate (eg, Polycose) to avoid excessive protein intake.
      b. **Diuretic therapy**
         i. **Chlorothiazide and spironolactone.** This combination is ideal for chronic management. It has been shown to improve lung function and has relatively few side effects. When used in doses of 20 mg/kg/day (chlorothiazide) and 2 mg/kg/day (spironolactone), a good diuretic response can often be achieved.
         ii. **Furosemide.** Furosemide (1–2 mg/kg every 12 h, orally or intravenously) is a more potent diuretic than chlorothiazide and spironolactone and is particularly useful for rapid diuresis. It is associated with side effects such as electrolyte abnormalities, interference with bilirubin-albumin binding capacity, calciuria with bone

demineralization and renal stone formation, and ototoxicity, thereby limiting its usefulness as a chronic medication. In infants with less acute CLD, an every-other-day furosemide regimen could be used to lessen its side effects.

iii. **Bumetanide** (0.015–0.1 mg/kg daily or every other day, orally or intravenously). When administered orally, 1 mg of bumetanide (Bumex) has a diuretic effect similar to that of 40 mg of furosemide. Whereas furosemide's bioavailability is 30–70%, bumetanide's bioavailability is >90%. Bumetanide produces side effects similar to those of furosemide, except that it may produce less ototoxicity and less interference with bilirubin-albumin binding.

c. **Bronchodilators**

i. **β_2-Agonists.** Inhaled β_2-agonists have been shown to produce measurable improvements in lung mechanics and gas exchange in infants with BPD. Their effect is usually time limited. Because of their side effects (eg, tachycardia, hypertension, hyperglycemia, and possible arrhythmia), their use (**albuterol** [0.2 mg/kg/dose nebulized as needed every 2–8 h]) should be limited to the management of acute exacerbations of BPD. Xopenex (levalbuterol, 0.1 mg/kg/dose nebulized as needed every 8 h) is a nonracemic form of albuterol recently introduced in pediatric and adult population. Its experience in newborns is limited. Its potential advantages are better and longer efficacy; hence, lower doses have a therapeutic effect enabling a significant reduction in the adverse effects associated with racemic albuterol. If bronchodilators are being used long-term, a frequent reevaluation of their benefit is essential.

ii. **Theophylline.** The beneficial actions of theophylline include smooth airway muscle dilation, improved diaphragmatic contractility, central respiratory stimulation, and mild diuretic effects. It appears to improve lung function in BPD when levels are maintained at >10 mcg/mL. Side effects are fairly common and may include CNS irritability, gastroesophageal reflux, and gastrointestinal irritation.

iii. **Anticholinergic agents.** The best studied and most available inhaled quaternary anticholinergic is ipratropium bromide (nebulized Atrovent [175 mcg, diluted in 3 mL of normal saline over 10 min every 8 h]). Its bronchodilatory effect is more potent than that of atropine and similar to that of albuterol. Combined albuterol and ipratropium therapy has a larger effect than either agent alone. Unlike atropine, systemic effects do not occur because of its poor systemic absorption.

d. **Corticosteroids.** The use of postnatal steroids should be limited to severe cases of BPD with a low chance of survival because of impaired gas exchange. Parents should be informed that the use of postnatal steroids could be associated with impaired brain and somatic growth and increased incidence of cerebral palsy. The initiation of steroid therapy in the first day increases death rate and the incidence of gastrointestinal perforation. Other side effects include infection, hypertension, gastric ulcer, hyperglycemia, adrenocortical suppression, lung growth suppression, and hypertrophic cardiomyopathy. Because of the central role of inflammation in the pathogenesis of BPD, steroid treatment can be very effective, especially in severe cases. Various steroid regimens have been proposed.

i. **Dexamethasone (DXM)**, 0.25 mg/kg twice daily for 3 days and then gradually tapered by a 10% dose decrease every 3 days for a total course of 42 days, is one of the original regimens that has proven efficacious in the treatment of BPD. Because of the concern about the possible neurologic adverse effect, many other regimens of shorter duration or dosage have been used and no standards have been accepted.

    ii. Methylprednisolone (Solu-Medrol), a corticosteroid with much weaker genomic activity than DXM, has almost similar nongenomic activity and thus possibly fewer CNS and somatic side effects. In a pilot study, methylprednisolone, 0.6, 0.4, 0.2 mg/kg/dose every 6 h for 3 days, followed by betamethasone, 0.1 mg/kg orally every other day for a total of 21 days, was found to have similar beneficial effects and fewer side effects (eg, periventricular leukomalacia, hyperglycemia) than DXM. These findings still need to be confirmed by large randomized controlled trials.

    iii. Nebulized corticosteroids (beclomethasone [100–200 mcg 4 times/day]) produced fewer side effects than oral or parenteral forms but seems to be much less efficacious in the treatment of BPD.

  3. Growth and nutrition. Because growth is essential for recovery from BPD, adequate nutritional intake is crucial. Infants with BPD frequently have high caloric needs (120–150 kcal/kg/day or more) because of increased metabolic expenditures. Concentrated formula is often necessary to provide sufficient calories and prevent pulmonary edema. In addition, specific micronutrient supplementation, such as antioxidant therapy, may also enhance pulmonary and nutritional status.

  C. Discharge planning. Oxygen can often be discontinued before NICU discharge. However, home oxygen therapy can be a safe alternative to long-term hospitalization. The need for home respiratory, heart rate, and oxygen monitoring must be decided on an individual basis but is generally recommended for infants discharged home on oxygen. Synagis (palivizumab, humanized monoclonal antibodies against respiratory syncytial virus [RSV]) should be given monthly (15 mg/kg intramuscularly) throughout the RSV season. All parents should be instructed in cardiopulmonary resuscitation (CPR).

  D. General care. Care plans for older infants with BPD should include adapting their routine for home life and involving the parents in their care. Immunizations should be given at the appropriate chronologic age. Periodic screening for chemical evidence of rickets and echocardiographic evidence of right ventricular hypertrophy is recommended. Assessment by a developmental specialist and occupational or physical therapist, or both, can be useful for prognostic and therapeutic purposes.

VII. Prognosis. The prognosis for infants with BPD depends on the degree of pulmonary dysfunction and the presence of other medical conditions. Most deaths occur in the first year of life as a result of cardiorespiratory failure, sepsis, or respiratory infection or as sudden, unexplained death.

  A. Pulmonary outcome. The short-term outcome of infants with BPD, including those requiring oxygen at home, is surprisingly good. Weaning from oxygen is usually possible before their first birthday, and they demonstrate catch-up growth as their pulmonary status improves. However, in the first year of life, rehospitalization is necessary for ~30% of patients for treatment of wheezing, respiratory infections, or both. Although upper respiratory tract infections are probably no more common in infants with BPD than in normal infants, they are more likely to be associated with significant respiratory symptoms. Most adolescents and young adults who had moderate to severe BPD in infancy have some degree of pulmonary dysfunction, consisting of airway obstruction, airway hyperreactivity, and hyperinflation.

  B. Neurodevelopmental outcome. Children with BPD appear to be at increased risk for adverse neurodevelopmental outcome compared with comparable infants without BPD. Neuromotor and cognitive dysfunction appears to be more common. In addition, children with BPD may be at higher risk for significant hearing impairment and ROP. They are also at risk for later problems, including learning disabilities, attention deficits, and behavior problems.

HYALINE MEMBRANE DISEASE (RESPIRATORY DISTRESS SYNDROME)

I. **Definition.** Hyaline membrane disease (HMD) is another name for RDS. This clinical diagnosis is warranted in a preterm newborn with respiratory difficulty, including tachypnea (>60 breaths/min), chest retractions, and cyanosis in room air that persists or progresses over the first 48–96 h of life, and a characteristic chest x-ray appearance (uniform reticulogranular pattern and peripheral air bronchograms). The clinical course of the disease varies with the size of the infant, severity of disease, use of surfactant replacement therapy, presence of infection, degree of shunting of blood through the patent ductus arteriosus (PDA), and whether or not assisted ventilation was initiated.

II. **Incidence.** HMD occurs in 60% of infants with birth weight between 501 and 1500 g (Lemons et al, 2001). The incidence is inversely proportional to the gestational age and birth weight. The incidence and severity of HMD are expected to decrease after the increase in use of antenatal steroids in recent years. Survival has improved significantly, especially after the introduction of exogenous surfactant (Malloy & Freeman, 2000) and is now at >90%. Currently, HMD accounts for <6% of all neonatal deaths.

III. **Pathophysiology.** Surfactant deficiency is the primary cause of HMD, often complicated by an overly compliant chest wall. Both factors lead to progressive atelectasis and failure to develop an effective functional residual capacity (FRC). Surfactant is a surface-active material produced by airway epithelial cells called type II pneumocytes. This cell line differentiates, and surfactant synthesis begins at 24–28 weeks' gestation. Type II cells are sensitive to and decreased by asphyxial insults in the perinatal period. The maturation of this cell line is delayed in the presence of fetal hyperinsulinemia. The maturity of type II cells is enhanced by the administration of antenatal corticosteroids and by chronic intrauterine stress such as pregnancy-induced hypertension, intrauterine growth retardation, and twin gestation. Surfactant, composed chiefly of phospholipid (75%) and protein (10%), is produced and stored in the characteristic lamellar bodies of type II pneumocytes. This lipoprotein is released into the airways, where it functions to decrease surface tension and maintain alveolar expansion at physiologic pressures.

A. **Lack of surfactant.** In the absence of surfactant, the small air spaces collapse; each expiration results in progressive atelectasis. Exudative proteinaceous material and epithelial debris, resulting from progressive cellular damage, collect in the airway and directly decrease total lung capacity. In pathologic specimens, this material stains typically as eosinophilic hyaline membranes lining the alveolar spaces and extending into small airways.

B. **Presence of an overly compliant chest wall.** In the presence of a chest wall with weak structural support secondary to prematurity, the large negative pressures generated to open the collapsed airways cause retraction and deformation of the chest wall instead of inflation of the poorly compliant lungs.

C. **Decreased intrathoracic pressure.** The infant with HMD who is <30 weeks' gestational age often has immediate respiratory failure because of an inability to generate the intrathoracic pressure necessary to inflate the lungs without surfactant.

D. **Shunting.** The presence or absence of a cardiovascular shunt through a PDA or foramen ovale, or both, may change the presentation or course of the disease process. Shortly after birth, the predominant shunting is right to left across the foramen ovale into the left atrium, which may result in venous admixture and worsening hypoxemia. After 18–24 h, left-to-right shunting through the PDA may become predominant as a result of falling pulmonary vascular resistance, leading to pulmonary edema and impaired alveolar gas exchange. Unfortunately, this usually occurs when the infant is starting to recover from HMD and can be aggravated by surfactant replacement therapy.

IV. Risk factors. Factors that increase or decrease the risk of HMD are listed in Table 74–1.

V. Clinical presentation

    A. History. The infant is often preterm, either by dates or by gestational examination, or has a history of asphyxia in the perinatal period. Infants have some respiratory difficulty at birth, which becomes progressively more severe. The classic worsening of the atelectasis seen on chest x-ray film and increasing oxygen requirement for these infants have been greatly modified by the availability of exogenous surfactant therapy and our increased ability to provide effective mechanical ventilatory support.

    B. Physical examination. The infant with HMD exhibits tachypnea, grunting, nasal flaring, and retractions of the chest wall. The infant may have cyanosis in room air. Grunting occurs when the infant partially closes the vocal cords to prolong expiration and develop or maintain some FRC. This mechanism actually improves alveolar ventilation. The retractions occur and increase as the infant is forced to develop high transpulmonary pressure to reinflate atelectatic air spaces.

VI. Diagnosis

    A. Chest x-ray study. An AP chest x-ray film should be obtained for all infants with respiratory distress of any duration. The typical radiographic finding of HMD is a uniform reticulogranular pattern, referred to as a ground-glass appearance, accompanied by peripheral air bronchograms. During the clinical course, sequential x-ray films may reveal air leaks secondary to mechanical ventilatory intervention as well as the onset of changes compatible with BPD.

    B. Laboratory studies

        1. Blood gas sampling is essential in the management of HMD. Usually, intermittent arterial sampling is performed. Although there is no consensus, most neonatologists agree that arterial oxygen tensions of 50–70 mm Hg and arterial carbon dioxide tensions of 45–60 mm Hg are acceptable. Most would maintain the pH at or above 7.25 and the arterial oxygen saturation at 88–95%. In addition, continuous transcutaneous oxygen and carbon dioxide monitors or oxygen saturation monitors, or both, are proving invaluable in the minute-to-minute monitoring of these infants.

TABLE 74–1. RISK FACTORS THAT INCREASE OR DECREASE THE RISK OF HYALINE MEMBRANE DISEASE

Increased risk	Decreased risk
Prematurity	Chronic intrauterine stress
Male sex	Prolonged ruptured membranes
Familial predisposition	Maternal hypertension
Cesarean section without labor	Narcotic/cocaine use
Perinatal asphyxia	IUGR or SGA
Chorioamnionitis	Corticosteroids
Hydrops	Thyroid hormone
Maternal diabetes	Tocolytic agents

IUGR, intrauterine growth retardation; SGA, small for gestational age.

2. **Sepsis workup.** A partial sepsis workup, including complete blood cell count and blood culture, should be considered for each infant with a diagnosis of HMD, because early-onset sepsis (eg, infection with group B streptococcus or *Haemophilus influenzae*) can be indistinguishable from HMD on clinical grounds alone.

3. **Serum glucose levels** may be high or low initially and must be monitored closely to assess the adequacy of dextrose infusion. Hypoglycemia alone can lead to tachypnea and respiratory distress.

4. **Serum electrolyte levels including calcium** should be monitored every 12–24 h for management of parenteral fluids. Hypocalcemia can contribute to more respiratory symptoms and is common in sick, nonfed, preterm, or asphyxiated infants.

C. **Echocardiography** is a valuable diagnostic tool in the evaluation of an infant with hypoxemia and respiratory distress. It is used to confirm the diagnosis of PDA as well as to document response to therapy. Significant congenital heart disease can be excluded by this technique as well.

VII. **Management**

A. **Prevention.**

1. **Antenatal corticosteroids.** The 1994 National Institutes of Health Consensus Development Conference on the effect of corticosteroids for fetal maturation on perinatal outcomes concluded that antenatal corticosteroids reduce the risk of death, HMD, and IVH. Use of antenatal betamethasone to enhance fetal pulmonary maturity is now established and generally considered to be standard of care. The recommended glucocorticoid regimen consists of the administration to the mother of two 12-mg doses of betamethasone given intramuscularly 24 h apart. Dexamethasone is no longer recommended because of increased risk for cystic periventricular leukomalacia among very premature infants exposed to the drug prenatally (Baud et al, 1999).

2. Several preventive measures may improve the survival of infants at risk for HMD and include **antenatal ultrasonography** for more accurate assessment of gestational age and fetal well-being, **continuous fetal monitoring** to document fetal well-being during labor or to signal the need for intervention when fetal distress is discovered, **tocolytic agents** that prevent and treat preterm labor, and **assessment of fetal lung maturity** before delivery (lecithin-sphingomyelin [L-S] ratio and phosphatidylglycerol; see Chapter 1) to prevent iatrogenic prematurity.

B. **Surfactant replacement** (see also Chapter 6) is now considered a standard of care in the treatment of intubated infants with HMD. Since the late 1980s, more than 30 randomized clinical trials involving >6000 infants have been conducted. The systematic review of these trials (Soll & Andruscavage, 1999) demonstrates that surfactant, whether used prophylactically in the delivery room to prevent HMD or in the treatment of the established disease, leads to a significant decrease in the risk of pneumothorax and the risk of death. These benefits were observed in both the trials of natural surfactant extracts and synthetic surfactants. Surfactant replacement, although proved to be immediately effective in reducing the severity of HMD, has not clearly been shown to decrease the long-term oxygen requirements or the development of chronic lung changes. Currently, long-term follow-up studies have not shown significant differences between surfactant-treated patients and nontreated control groups with regard to PDA, IVH, ROP, NEC, and BPD. Evidence exists that the length of stay on mechanical ventilation and total ventilator days have been reduced with the use of surfactant at all gestational age levels, even with the increase of extremely low birth weight infants. A dramatic fall in deaths from HMD began in 1991. This probably reflected the introduction across the nation of surfactant replacement therapy. In long-term follow-up studies, no adverse effects attributable to surfactant therapy have been identified.

C. Respiratory support

1. **Endotracheal intubation and mechanical ventilation** are the mainstays of therapy for infants with HMD in whom apnea or hypoxemia with respiratory acidosis develops. Mechanical ventilation usually begins with rates of 30–60 breaths/min and inspiratory-expiratory ratios of 1:2. An initial PIP of 18–30 cm H_2O is used, depending on the size of the infant and the severity of the disease. A PEEP of 4–5 cm H_2O results in improved oxygenation, presumably because it assists in the maintenance of an effective FRC. The lowest possible pressures and inspired oxygen concentrations are maintained in an attempt to minimize damage to parenchymal tissue. Ventilators with the capacity to synchronize respiratory effort may generate less inadvertent airway pressure and lessen barotrauma. The early use of HFOV has become an increasingly popular and frequently used ventilator mode for low birth weight infants (Gerstmann et al, 1996; Plavka et al, 1999).

2. **CPAP and nasal synchronized intermittent mandatory ventilation (SIMV).** Nasal CPAP (NCPAP) or nasopharyngeal CPAP (NPCPAP) may be used early to delay or prevent the need for endotracheal intubation. To minimize lung injury associated with intubation and mechanical ventilation, there has been a recent interest in using CPAP as an initial treatment strategy to treat HMD even in very low and extremely low birth weight infants. In some centers, this practice has been used successfully and resulted in decreased incidence of BPD (Aly, 2001; De Klerk & De Klerk, 2001; Van Marter et al, 2000). In addition, early treatment with surfactant, administered during a short period of intubation followed by extubation and application of NCPAP is increasingly being used in Europe. This approach has been used in premature infants <30 weeks' gestation and significantly reduces the subsequent need for mechanical ventilation (Kamper, 1999; Verder et al, 1999). NCPAP and NPCPAP may be used on extubation and may decrease the chance of reintubation. **Nasal SIMV** is potentially useful way of augmenting NCPAP. The relatively recent ability to synchronize the ventilator breaths with the infant's own respiratory cycle has made this mode of ventilation feasible. In three trials, nasal SIMV has been shown to reduce the incidence of symptoms of extubation failure when compared with NCPAP (Davis et al, 2001).

3. **Complications.** Pulmonary air leaks, such as pneumothorax, pneumomediastinum, pneumopericardium, and PIE, may occur. Chronic complications include respiratory problems such as BPD and tracheal stenosis.

D. Fluid and nutritional support. In the very ill infant, it is now possible to maintain nutritional support with parenteral nutrition for an extended period. The specific needs of preterm and term infants are becoming better understood, and the nutrient preparations available reflect this understanding (see Chapter 8).

E. Antibiotic therapy. Antibiotics that cover the most common neonatal infections are usually begun initially. Aminoglycoside dosing intervals are increased for the premature infant.

F. Sedation is commonly used to control ventilation in these sick infants. **Phenobarbital** is often used to decrease the infant's activity level. **Morphine, fentanyl,** or **lorazepam** may be used for analgesia as well as sedation. Muscle paralysis with **pancuronium** for infants with HMD remains *controversial*. Sedation might be indicated for infants who "fight" the ventilator and exhale during the inspiratory cycle of mechanical ventilation. This respiratory pattern may increase the likelihood of complication such as air leak and, therefore, should be avoided. Sedation of infants with fluctuating cerebral blood flow velocity theoretically decreases the risk of IVH.

VIII. Prognosis. Although the survival of infants with HMD has improved greatly, the prognosis for survival with or without respiratory and neurologic sequelae are highly dependent on birth weight (Table 74–2) and gestational age. Major morbidity (BPD, NEC, and severe IVH) and poor postnatal growth remain high for the smallest infants.

TABLE 74-2. PROGNOSIS AND OUTCOMES IN PATIENTS WITH HYALINE MEMBRANE DISEASE BASED ON BIRTH WEIGHT

Birth weight (g)	Survival rate (%)	Risk of BPD[a]	Risk of stage III/IV ROP
<501	10	All	Very high
501–750	75	Most	Moderate
751–1000	85	Half	Present
1001–1500	96	Few	Low

BPD, bronchopulmonary dysplasia; ROP, retinopathy of prematurity.
[a]Patients on oxygen at 28 days.

MECONIUM ASPIRATION

I. **Definition.** Meconium is the first intestinal discharge of the newborn infant and is composed of epithelial cells, fetal hair, mucus, and bile. Intrauterine stress may cause in utero passage of meconium into the amniotic fluid. The meconium-stained amniotic fluid may be aspirated by the fetus when fetal gasping or deep breathing movements are stimulated by hypoxia and hypercapnia. The presence of meconium in the trachea may cause airway obstruction as well as an inflammatory response, resulting in severe respiratory distress. The presence of meconium in amniotic fluid can be a **warning sign of fetal distress** but is not a sensitive independent marker of fetal distress. Mothers with meconium-stained amniotic fluid should be carefully monitored during labor.

II. **Incidence.** The incidence of meconium-stained amniotic fluid varies from 8 to 20% of all deliveries. Meconium aspiration primarily affects **term and postmature infants.** The passage of meconium in an asphyxiated infant <34 weeks' gestation is unusual and may represent bilious reflux secondary to intestinal obstruction.

III. **Pathophysiology**
   A. **In utero passage of meconium.** Control of fetal meconium passage is dependent on hormonal and parasympathetic neural maturation. After 34 weeks' gestation, the incidence of meconium-stained amniotic fluid increases from 1.6% between 34 and 37 weeks' gestation to 30% at 42 weeks or more. The exact mechanisms for in utero passage of meconium remain unclear, but fetal distress and vagal stimulation are two probable factors.
   B. **Aspiration of meconium.** After intrauterine passage of meconium, deep irregular respiration or gasping, either in utero or during labor and delivery, can cause aspiration of the meconium-stained amniotic fluid. Before delivery, the progression of the aspirated meconium is, as a rule, impeded by the presence of the viscous liquid that normally fills the fetal lung and airways. Therefore, the distal progression occurs mostly after birth in conjunction with the reabsorption of lung fluid. Early consequences of meconium aspiration include airway obstruction, decreased lung compliance, and increased expiratory large airway resistance.
      1. **Airway obstruction.** Thick, meconium-stained amniotic fluid can result in acute upper airway obstruction. As the aspirated meconium progresses distally, total or partial airway obstruction may occur. In areas of total obstruction atelectasis develops, but in areas of partial obstruction a ball-valve phenomenon occurs, resulting in air trapping and alveolar hyperexpansion. Air trapping increases the risk of air leak to 21–50%.

2. **Chemical pneumonitis.** With distal progression of meconium, chemical pneumonitis develops, with resulting bronchiolar edema and narrowing of the small airways. Meconium at the alveolar level may inactivate existing surfactant. Uneven ventilation resulting from areas of partial obstruction, atelectasis, and superimposed pneumonitis causes carbon dioxide retention and hypoxemia. Pulmonary vascular resistance increases as a direct result of alveolar hypoxia, acidosis, and hyperinflation of the lungs. The increase in pulmonary vascular resistance may lead to atrial and ductal right-to-left shunting and further hypoxemia.

IV. **Risk factors.** The following factors have been associated with an increased risk of meconium passage and subsequent tracheal aspiration:
  A. **Postterm pregnancy.**
  B. **Preeclampsia-eclampsia.**
  C. **Maternal hypertension.**
  D. **Maternal diabetes mellitus.**
  E. **Abnormal fetal heart rate.**
  F. **Intrauterine growth retardation.**
  G. **Abnormal biophysical profile.**
  H. **Oligohydramnios.**
  I. **Maternal heavy smoking, chronic respiratory or cardiovascular disease.**

V. **Clinical presentation.** The presentation of an infant who has aspirated meconium-stained amniotic fluid is variable. Symptoms depend on the severity of the hypoxic insult and the amount and viscosity of the meconium aspirated.
  A. **General features**
    1. **The infant.** Infants with meconium aspiration syndrome often exhibit signs of postmaturity: They are small for gestational age with long nails and peeling yellow- or green-stained skin. These infants may have respiratory distress at birth or in the transition period. If there has been significant perinatal asphyxia, they may have respiratory depression with poor respiratory effort and decreased muscle tone.
    2. **The amniotic fluid.** The meconium present in amniotic fluid varies in appearance and viscosity, ranging from thin, green-stained fluid to a thick, "pea soup" consistency. Although meconium aspiration syndrome can occur in the presence of thin, stained amniotic fluid, the majority of infants who become ill have a history of thick, meconium-stained fluid.
  B. **Airway obstruction.** Early meconium aspiration syndrome is characterized by airway obstruction. Large amounts of thick meconium, if not removed, can result in an acute large airway obstruction. These infants may be apneic or have gasping respirations, cyanosis, and poor air exchange. The airway must be rapidly cleared by endotracheal suctioning. Later, as the meconium is driven down to more distal airways, the smaller airways are affected, resulting in air trapping and scattered atelectasis.
  C. **Respiratory distress.** The infant who has aspirated meconium into the distal airways but does not have total airway obstruction manifests signs of respiratory distress secondary to increased airway resistance, decreased compliance, and air trapping (ie, **tachypnea, nasal flaring, intercostal retractions, increased AP diameter of the chest,** and **cyanosis**). Some infants **may have a delayed presentation,** with only mild initial respiratory distress, which becomes more severe hours after delivery as atelectasis and chemical pneumonitis develop.
    Note: Many infants with meconium-stained amniotic fluid appear normal at birth and exhibit no signs of respiratory distress.
  D. **Other pulmonary abnormalities.** If air trapping develops, there may be a noticeable increase in AP diameter of the chest. Auscultation often reveals decreased air exchange, rales, rhonchi, or wheezing.

VI. **Diagnosis**
  A. **Laboratory studies. Arterial blood gas levels** characteristically reveal hypoxemia. Hyperventilation may result in respiratory alkalosis in mild

cases, but infants with severe disease usually manifest respiratory acidosis as a result of airway obstruction, atelectasis, and pneumonitis. If the patient has suffered perinatal asphyxia, combined respiratory and metabolic acidosis are present.
  B. **Radiologic studies.** A chest radiograph typically reveals hyperinflation of the lung fields and flattened diaphragms. There are coarse, irregular patchy infiltrates. Pneumothorax or pneumomediastinum may be present. The severity of x-ray findings may not always correlate with the clinical disease.
  C. **Cardiac echocardiogram.** Pulmonary hypertension with the resultant hypoxemia from right-to-left atrial and ductal shunt is a frequently associated finding in infants with meconium aspiration pneumonia.
VII. **Management**
  A. **Prenatal management.** The key to management of meconium aspiration lies in prevention during the prenatal period.
    1. **Identification of high-risk pregnancies.** The approach to prevention begins with recognition of predisposing maternal factors that may cause uteroplacental insufficiency and subsequent fetal hypoxia during labor (see section IV: Risk Factors).
    2. **Monitoring.** During labor, careful observation and fetal monitoring should be performed. Any signs of fetal distress (eg, appearance of meconium-stained fluid with membrane rupture, loss of beat-to-beat variability, fetal tachycardia, or deceleration patterns) warrant assessment of fetal well-being by scrutiny of fetal heart tracings and fetal scalp pH. If the assessment identifies a compromised fetus, corrective measures should be undertaken or the infant should be delivered in a timely manner.
    3. **Amnioinfusion.** In mothers with moderate or thick, meconium-stained amniotic fluid, amnioinfusion decreases the incidence and severity of meconium aspiration syndrome.
  B. **Delivery room management.** Delivery room management of the meconium-stained infant is discussed in Chapter 2. The severity of meconium aspiration can be markedly decreased by early removal of aspirated tracheal meconium. Those infants who are depressed or have thick, meconium-stained fluid should be intubated and their trachea suctioned using a meconium trap aspirator. The approach to infants who are vigorous or who have thin or moderately stained amniotic fluid remains *controversial.*
  C. **Management of the newborn with meconium aspiration.** Infants with meconium below their trachea are at risk for pulmonary hypertension, air leak syndromes, and pneumonitis and must be observed closely for signs of respiratory distress.
    1. **Respiratory management**
      a. **Pulmonary toilet.** If suctioning the trachea does not result in clearing of secretions, it may be advisable to leave an endotracheal tube in place in symptomatic infants for pulmonary toilet. Chest physiotherapy every 30 min to 1 h, as tolerated, will aid in clearing the airway. Chest physiotherapy may be contraindicated in labile infants with significant persistent pulmonary hypertension.
      b. **Arterial blood gas levels.** On admission to the NICU, arterial blood gas measurements to assess ventilatory compromise and supplemental oxygen requirements should be obtained. If the patient requires >0.4 FIO_2 or demonstrates pronounced lability, an arterial catheter for frequent sampling should be inserted.
      c. **Oxygen monitoring.** A pulse oximeter will provide important information regarding the severity of the child's respiratory status and will also assist in preventing hypoxemia. Comparing oxygen saturation values from a probe placed on the right arm to those from a probe placed on the lower extremities may help to identify those infants with right-to-left ductal shunting secondary to pulmonary hypertension.

d. Chest x-ray films should be obtained after delivery if the infant is in distress. A chest radiograph may also help determine which patients will experience respiratory distress. However, the radiograph often poorly correlates with the clinical presentation.

e. Antibiotic coverage. Meconium inhibits the normally bacteriostatic quality of amniotic fluid. Because it is difficult to differentiate meconium aspiration from pneumonia radiographically, infants with infiltrates on chest x-ray film should be started on broad-spectrum antibiotics (ampicillin and gentamicin; for dosages, see Chapter 80) after appropriate cultures have been obtained.

f. Supplemental oxygen. A major goal is to prevent episodes of alveolar hypoxia leading to hypoxic pulmonary vasoconstriction and the development of persistent pulmonary hypertension of the newborn. For that purpose, supplemental oxygen is provided "generously," such that arterial oxygen tension is maintained at least in the range of 80–90 mm Hg. Some clinicians may elect to maintain Pao_2 at a higher level because the risk of retinopathy should be negligible among full-term infants. The same goal of preventing alveolar hypoxia requires cautious weaning from oxygen therapy. Many of the patients are very labile, and weaning from oxygen should be made slowly, sometimes at a pace of 1% at a time. The prevention of alveolar hypoxia includes a high index of suspicion for the diagnosis of air leak as well as efforts to minimize handling of the child.

g. Mechanical ventilation. Patients with severe disease who are in impending respiratory failure with hypercapnia and persistent hypoxemia require mechanical ventilation. Those infants who do not respond to conventional ventilation should be given a trial HFV.

   i. Rate settings. Ventilation must be tailored to the individual patient. These patients typically require higher inspiratory pressures and faster rates than those with HMD. Relatively short inspiratory time allows for adequate expiration in patients with preexisting air trapping.

   ii. Complications. The clinician must maintain a high index of suspicion for air leak. For any unexplained deterioration of clinical status, the possibility of a pneumothorax should be considered and appropriate evaluation undertaken. With the development of atelectasis, air trapping, and decreased lung compliance, high mean airway pressures may be required in a patient who is at risk for air leak. The approach to ventilation must be directed at preventing hypoxemia and providing adequate ventilation at the lowest mean airway pressure possible to reduce the risk of catastrophic air leak.

h. HFV. Both HFJV and HFOV have been shown to be efficacious in infants in whom adequate ventilation cannot be maintained on conventional ventilation without using excessive ventilatory pressures. It has also been used to maximize the beneficial effects of inhaled nitric oxide.

i. Surfactant. Infants with severe meconium aspiration syndrome who require mechanical ventilation and have radiologic evidence of parenchymal lung disease are likely to benefit from early surfactant therapy. Because of the frequently associated pulmonary hypertension, close monitoring at the time of the surfactant therapy will be required to prevent the consequences of transient airway obstruction that may develop during the tracheal instillation of surfactant.

j. Extracorporeal membrane oxygenation (ECMO). Patients who cannot be ventilated by the just-mentioned therapies may be candidates for ECMO (see Chapter 11). Oxygenation index (FIO_2 × mean airway pressure [$\overline{Paw}$] × 100 ÷ Pao_2) >40 in association with a $\overline{Paw}$ ≥20 cm H_2O may predict infants who will require ECMO.

2. **Cardiovascular management.** Persistent pulmonary hypertension is frequently associated with meconium aspiration. The development of pulmonary hypertension may be a result of hypoxic pulmonary vasoconstriction, abnormal muscularization of the pulmonary microcirculation, or both. To minimize the risk of persistent pulmonary hypertension, aggressive resuscitation and stabilization are essential. Consider nitric oxide therapy if pulmonary hypertension is associated with meconium aspiration. In such event the use of high-frequency oscillation may further optimize the response to nitric oxide.

3. **General management.** Infants who have aspirated meconium and require resuscitation often develop metabolic abnormalities such as hypoxia, acidosis, hypoglycemia, and hypocalcemia. Because these patients may have suffered perinatal asphyxia, surveillance for any end-organ damage is essential (see Chapter 73).

VIII. **Prognosis.** Complications are common and are associated with significant mortality. New modalities of therapy such as administration of exogenous surfactant, high-frequency ventilation, inhaled nitric oxide, and ECMO have reduced the mortality to <5%. In patients surviving severe meconium aspiration, BPD or CLD may result from prolonged mechanical ventilation. Those with a significant asphyxial insult may demonstrate neurologic sequelae.

TRANSIENT TACHYPNEA OF THE NEWBORN

I. **Definition.** Transient tachypnea of the newborn (TTN) is also known as wet lung or type II RDS. It is a benign disease of near-term, term, or large premature infants who have respiratory distress shortly after delivery that usually resolves within 3–5 days.

II. **Incidence.** The incidence of TTN is estimated at 1–2% of all newborns.

III. **Pathophysiology. Its true cause is unknown** but three factors are involved.
   A. **Delayed resorption of fetal lung fluid.** TTN is thought to occur because of delayed resorption of fetal lung fluid from the pulmonary lymphatic system. The increased fluid volume causes a reduction in lung compliance and increased airway resistance. This results in tachypnea and retractions. Infants delivered by elective cesarean section are at risk because of lack of the normal vaginal thoracic squeeze, which forces lung fluid out.
   B. **Pulmonary immaturity.** One study noted that a mild degree of pulmonary immaturity is a central factor in the cause of TTN. The authors found a mature L-S ratio but negative phosphatidylglycerol (the presence of phosphatidylglycerol indicates completed lung maturation). Infants who were closer to 36 weeks' gestation than to 38 weeks had an increased risk of TTN.
   C. **Mild surfactant deficiency.** One hypothesis is that TTN may represent a mild surfactant deficiency in these infants.

IV. **Risk factors**
   A. **Elective cesarean section delivery.**
   B. **Male sex.**
   C. **Macrosomia.**
   D. **Excessive maternal sedation.**
   E. **Prolonged labor.**
   F. **Negative amniotic fluid phosphatidylglycerol.**
   G. **Birth asphyxia.**
   H. **Fluid overload to the mother, especially with oxytocin infusion.**
   I. **Maternal asthma.**
   J. **Delayed clamping of the umbilical cord.** Optimal time is 45 s.
   K. **Breech delivery.**
   L. **Fetal polycythemia.**
   M. **Infant of a diabetic mother.**

N. Prematurity (can occur but is less frequent).
O. Infant of drug-dependent mother (narcotics).
P. Very low birth weight neonates.
Q. Exposure to B-mimetic agents.
V. Clinical presentation. The infant is usually near term, term, or large and premature and shortly after delivery has tachypnea (>60 breaths/min and can be up to 100–120 breaths/min). The infant may also have grunting, nasal flaring, rib retraction, and varying degrees of cyanosis. The infant often appears to have the classic "barrel chest" secondary to the increased AP diameter. There are usually no signs of sepsis. Some infants may have edema and a mild ileus on physical examination. One can also see tachycardia with usually a normal blood pressure.

VI. Diagnosis
  A. Laboratory studies
   1. Prenatal testing. A mature L-S ratio with the presence of phosphatidyl-glycerol in the amniotic fluid may help to rule out HMD.
   2. Postnatal testing
     a. Arterial blood gas on room air will show some degree of mild hypoxia. Hypocarbia is usually present. Hypercarbia, if it exists, is usually mild (Pco_2 >55 mm Hg). Extreme hypercarbia is rare and, if present, another diagnosis should be considered.
     b. Complete blood cell count with differential is normal in TTN but should be obtained if one is considering an infectious process. The hematocrit will also rule out polycythemia.
     c. Urine and serum antigen test may help to rule out certain bacterial infections.
     d. Plasma endothelin-1 levels (ET-1). One study revealed that plasma ET-1 levels were higher in RDS patients compared with those with TTN. This test may prove useful in differentiating RDS from TTN.
  B. Radiologic studies
   1. Chest x-ray study. The typical findings in TTN are as follows:
     a. Hyperexpansion of the lungs, a hallmark of TTN.
     b. Prominent perihilar streaking (secondary to engorgement of periar-terial lymphatics).
     c. Mild to moderately enlarged heart.
     d. Depression (flattening) of the diaphragm, best seen on a lateral view of the chest.
     e. Fluid in the minor fissure and perhaps fluid in the pleural space.
     f. Prominent pulmonary vascular markings.
  C. Other tests. Any infant who is hypoxic on room air must have a **100% oxygen test** to rule out heart disease. (This test is described on p 354.)

VII. Management
  A. General
   1. Oxygenation. Initial management consists of providing adequate oxygenation. Start with hood oxygen and deliver enough to maintain normal arterial saturation. These infants typically require only hood oxygen, usually <60%. If the oxygen needs to be increased and 100% hood oxygenation does not work, change to NCPAP. If these maneuvers are not effective, intubate the infant and proceed with mechanical ventilation. If the infant requires 100% oxygen or endotracheal intubation with ventilator support, another disease process should be suspected.
   2. Antibiotics. Most infants are initially treated with broad-spectrum antibiotics until the diagnosis of sepsis or pneumonia is excluded.
   3. Feeding. Because of the risk of aspiration, an infant should not be fed by mouth if the respiratory rate is >60 breaths/min. If the respiratory rate is <60 breaths/min, oral feeding is permissible. If the rate is 60–80 breaths/min, feeding should be by nasogastric tube. If the rate is >80 breaths/min, intravenous nutrition is indicated.

4. **Fluid and electrolytes.** Fluid status should be monitored and hydration maintained.
5. **Diuretics.** Two randomized trials using furosemide showed an increase in weight loss in the treated group but no difference in decrease or duration of respiratory symptoms or length of hospital stay.

B. **Confirm the diagnosis.** TTN is often a diagnosis of exclusion, and other causes of tachypnea should be excluded first. The usual causes of tachypnea include the following:

1. **Pneumonia/sepsis.** If the infant has pneumonia/sepsis, the prenatal history will usually suggest infection. There may be maternal chorioamnionitis, premature rupture of membranes, and fever. The blood cell count may show evidence of infection (neutropenia or leukocytosis with abnormal numbers of immature cells). The urine antigen test may be positive if the infant has group B streptococcal infection. Remember that it is best to give broad-spectrum antibiotics if there is any suspicion or evidence of infection. The antibiotics can always be discontinued if the cultures are negative in 3 days.
2. **Heart disease.** The 100% oxygen test should be done to rule out heart disease (see p 354). Cardiomegaly may be seen.
3. **HMD.** The infant will normally be premature or have some reason for delayed lung maturation, such as maternal diabetes. The chest x-ray film is helpful because it shows the typical HMD reticulogranular pattern with air bronchograms and underexpansion (atelectasis) of the lungs.
4. **Cerebral hyperventilation.** This disorder is seen when CNS lesions cause overstimulation of the respiratory center, resulting in tachypnea. The CNS lesions can include meningitis or hypoxic-ischemic insult. Arterial blood gas measurements show respiratory alkalosis.
5. **Metabolic disorders.** Infants with hypothermia, hyperthermia, or hypoglycemia may have tachypnea.
6. **Polycythemia and hyperviscosity.** This syndrome may present with tachypnea with or without cyanosis.

VIII. **Prognosis.** TTN is self-limited and usually lasts only 2–5 days with no risk of further pulmonary dysfunction.

REFERENCES

Allen RW et al: Effectiveness of chest tube evacuation of pneumothorax in neonates. *J Pediatr* 1981;99:629.

Alpan G et al: Doxapram in the treatment of idiopathic apnea on prematurity unresponsive to aminophylline. *J Pediatr* 1984;104:634.

Aly H: Nasal prongs continuous positive airway pressure: a simple yet powerful tool. *Pediatrics* 2001;108:759.

American Academy of Pediatrics Committee on Fetus and Newborn: Postnatal corticosteroids to treat or prevent chronic lung disease in preterm infants. *Pediatrics* 2002;109:330.

Behrman RE et al: *Nelson Textbook of Pediatrics,* 16th ed. Saunders, 2002.

Ballard J et al: Hazards of delivery room resuscitation using oral methods of endotracheal suctioning. *Pediatr Infect Dis* 1986;5:198.

Bancalari E, Gerhardt T: Bronchopulmonary dysplasia. *Pediatr Clin North Am* 1986;33:1.

Baud O et al: Antenatal glucocorticoid treatment and cystic periventricular leukomalacia in very premature infants. *N Engl J Med* 1999;341:1190.

Bednarek FJ, Roloff DW: Treatment of apnea of prematurity with aminophylline. *Pediatrics* 1973;55:335.

Bhakoo ON et al: Spectrum of respiratory distress in very low birthweight neonates. *Ind J Pediatr* 2000;67:803.

Bhuta T, Henderson-Smart D: *Rescue High-Frequency Oscillatory Ventilation Versus Conventional Ventilation for Pulmonary Dysfunction in Preterm Infants.* The Cochrane Library, 2000.

Blanchard PW et al: Pharmacotherapy in bronchopulmonary dysplasia. *Clin Perinatol* 1987;14:881.

Brooks JG et al: Selective bronchial intubation for the treatment of severe localized pulmonary emphysema in newborn infants. *J Pediatr* 1977;91:648.

Carson BS: Prevention of meconium aspiration syndrome. *Neonatal Grand Rounds* 1986;3:3.

Cotton R: Hyaline membrane disease: from tragedy to triumph. *Perspect Neonatol* 1999;1:4.

Creasy RK, Resnik R: *Maternal-Fetal Medicine: Principles and Practice.* Saunders, 1984.

Croswell HE, Stewart DL: Pulmonary interstitial emphysema in a nonventilated preterm infant. *Arch Pediatr Adolesc Med* 2001;155:615.

Cummings J et al: A controlled trial of dexamethasone therapy in preterm infants at high risk of bronchopulmonary dysplasia. *N Engl J Med* 1989;320:1505.

Davis P et al: Nasal intermittent positive pressure ventilation (NIPPV) versus nasal continuous positive airway pressure (NCPAP) for preterm neonates after extubation. *Cochrane Database Syst Rev* 2001;3:CD002272.

De Klerk A, De Klerk R: Nasal continuous positive airway pressure and outcomes of preterm infants. *J Paediatr Child Health* 2001;37:161

deRoux SJ, Prendergast NC: Large sub-pleural air cysts: an extreme form of pulmonary interstitial emphysema. *Pediatr Radiol* 1998;28:981.

Donn SM, Nicks JJ: Special ventilatory techniques and modalities. In Goldsmith JP et al (eds): *Assisted Ventilation of the Neonate,* 3rd ed. Saunders, 1996.

Durand M et al: Oxygenation index in patients with meconium aspiration: conventional and extracorporeal membrane oxygenation therapy. *Crit Care Med* 1990;18:373.

Dye T et al: Amnioinfusion and the intrauterine prevention of meconium aspiration. *Am J Obstet Gynecol* 1994;171:1601.

Escobedo MB, Gonzales A: Bronchopulmonary dysplasia in the tiny infant. *Clin Perinatol* 1986; 13:315.

Fanaroff AA, Martin RJ (eds): *Neonatal-Perinatal Medicine—Diseases of the Fetus and Infant,* 6th ed. Mosby, 2002.

Fiascone JM et al: Bronchopulmonary dysplasia: review for the pediatrician. *Curr Probl Pediatr* 1989;19:169.

Ficheux H et al: Simultaneous determination of hemoglobin and coproporphyrin by second derivative differential spectrophotometry: application to the diagnosis of meconium aspiration. *Clin Chim Acta* 1989;189:53.

Findlay RD et al: Surfactant replacement therapy for meconium aspiration syndrome. *Pediatrics* 1996;97:48.

Gannon CM et al: Volutrauma, $Paco_2$ levels, and neurodevelopmental sequelae following assisted ventilation. *Clin Perinatol* 1998;25:159.

Gerstmann DR et al: The Provo multicenter early high-frequency oscillatory ventilation trial: improved pulmonary and clinical outcome in respiratory distress syndrome. *Pediatrics* 1996: 98:1044.

Gessler P et al: Lobar pulmonary interstitial emphysema in a premature infant on continuous positive airway pressure using nasal prongs. *Eur J Pediatr* 2002;160:263.

Goetzman BW: Understanding bronchopulmonary dysplasia. *Am J Dis Child* 1986;140:332.

Greenough A et al: Synchronized mechanical ventilation for respiratory support in newborn infants. *Cochrane Database Syst Rev* 2001;1:CD000456.

Hacking D, Stewart M: Neonatal pneumomediastinum. *N Engl J Med* 2001;344:1839.

Heneghan MA et al: Early pulmonary interstitial emphysema in the newborn: a grave prognostic sign. *Clin Pediatr* 1987;26:361.

Hensley M et al: *Lung Volume Reduction Surgery for Diffuse Emphysema.* The Cochrane Library, 2001.

Ho JJ et al: *Continuous Distending Pressure for Respiratory Distress Syndrome in Preterm Infants.* The Cochrane Library, 2000.

Houlihan CM, Knuppel RA: Meconium-stained amniotic fluid: current controversies. *J Reprod Med* 1994;39:888.

Jobe AH: Glucocorticoids in perinatal medicine: misguided rockets? *J Pediatr* 2000;137:1.

Kamper J: Early nasal continuous positive airway pressure and minimal handling in the treatment of very-low-birth-weight infants. *Biol Neonate* 1999;76(suppl 1):22.

Kattwinkel J: Neonatal apnea: pathogenesis and therapy. *J Pediatr* 1977;90:342.

Kattwinkel J et al: Apnea of prematurity. *J Pediatr* 1985;86:588.

Keszler M et al: Combined high-frequency jet ventilation in a meconium aspiration model. *Crit Care Med* 1986;14:34.

Kuo CY et al: Study of plasma endothelin-1 concentrations in Taiwanese neonates with respiratory distress. *Chang Gung Med J* 2001;24:239.

Lemons J et al: Very low birth weight outcomes of the National Institute of Child Health and Human Development Neonatal Research Network, January 1995 through December 1996. *Pediatrics* 2001;107:e1.

Levine EM et al: Mode of delivery and risk of respiratory diseases in newborns. *Obstet Gynecol* 2001;97:439.

Linder N et al: Need for endotracheal intubation and suction in meconium-stained neonates. *J Pediatr* 1988;112:613.

Lotze A et al: Multicenter study of surfactant (beractant) use in the treatment of term infants with severe respiratory failure. *J Pediatr* 1998;132:40.

Malloy MH, Freeman DH: Respiratory distress syndrome mortality in the United States, 1987 to 1995. *J Perinatol* 2000;20:414.

Mansfield PB et al: Pneumopericardium and pneumomediastinum in infants and children. *J Pediatr Surg* 1973;8:691.

McIntosh N et al: Clinical diagnosis of pneumothorax is late: use of trend data and decision support might allow preclinical detection. *Pediatr Res* 2002;48:408.

McNamara F et al: Obstructive sleep apnea in infants: relation to family history of sudden infant death syndrome, apparent life-threatening events, and obstructive sleep apnea. *J Pediatr* 2000;136:318.

Merritt TA et al: Contemporary issues in fetal and neonatal medicine. In Merritt TA et al (eds): *Bronchopulmonary Dysplasia*. Blackwell, 1988.

Merritt TA et al: Immunologic consequences of exogenous surfactant administration. *Semin Perinatol* 1988;12:221.

Messineo A et al: Lung volume reduction in lieu of pneumonectomy in an infant with severe unilateral pulmonary interstitial emphysema. *Pediatr Pulmonol* 2001;31:389.

Miller MJ et al: Continuous positive airway pressure selectively reduces obstructive apnea in preterm infants. *J Pediatr* 1985;106:91.

Miller MJ et al: Respiratory disorders in preterm and term infants. In Fanaroff AA, Martin RJ (eds): *Neonatal-Perinatal Medicine: Diseases of the Fetus and Infant*, 7th ed. Mosby, 2002.

Moriette G et al: Prospective randomized multicenter comparison of high-frequency oscillatory ventilation and conventional ventilation in preterm infants of less than 30 weeks with respiratory distress syndrome. *Pediatrics* 2001;107:363.

Moses D et al: Inhibition of pulmonary surfactant function by meconium. *Am J Obstet Gynecol* 1991;164:477.

Murphy JD et al: Pulmonary vascular disease in fatal meconium aspiration. *J Pediatr* 1984; 104:758.

National Center for Health Statistics: *LCWK3 Deaths, Percent of Total Deaths, and Death Rates for the 15 Leading Causes of Death in Selected Age Groups, by Race and Sex: United States, 1999*. National Center for Health Statistics, 1999.

National Institutes of Health: NIH Consensus Development Panel on the effect of corticosteroids for fetal maturation on perinatal outcomes. *JAMA* 1995;273:413.

Newman B: Neonatal imaging. *Radiol Clin North Am* 1999;37:1049.

Northway WH Jr et al: Pulmonary disease following respirator therapy of hyaline-membrane disease. *N Engl J Med* 1967;76:357.

O'Brodovich HM, Mellins RB: Bronchopulmonary dysplasia: unresolved neonatal acute lung injury. *Am Rev Respir Dis* 1986;132:694.

O'Shea et al: Randomized placebo-controlled trial of a 42-day tapering course of dexamethasone to reduce the duration of ventilator dependency in very low birth weight infants: outcome of study participants at 1-year adjusted age. *Pediatrics* 1999;104:15.

Perleman EJ et al: Pulmonary vasculature in meconium aspiration. *Hum Pathol* 1989;20:701.

Peter CS et al: Gastroesophageal reflux and apnea of prematurity: no temporal relationship. *Pediatrics* 2002;109:8.

Philips JB III: Management of the meconium-stained infant. *Neonatal Grand Rounds* 1986;3:1.

Pierce J et al: Intrapartum amnioInfusion for meconium-stained fluid: meta-analysis of prospective clinical trials. *Obstet Gynecol* 2000;95:1051.

Plavka R et al: A prospective randomized comparison of conventional mechanical ventilation and very early high frequency oscillatory ventilation in extremely premature newborns with respiratory distress syndrome. *Intensive Care Med* 1999;25:68.

Ramanathan R et al: Cardiorespiratory events recorded on home monitors: comparison of healthy infants with those at increased risk for SIDS. *JAMA* 2001;285:2199.

Ranzini AC, Chan L: Meconium and fetal-neonatal compromise. In Spitzer AR (ed): *Intensive Care of the Fetus and Neonate*. Mosby, 1996.

Rimensberger PC et al: First intention high-frequency oscillation with early lung volume optimization improves pulmonary outcome in very low birth weight infants with respiratory distress. *Pediatrics* 2000;105:1202.

Sahn SA et al: Spontaneous pneumothorax. *N Engl J Med* 2000;342:868.

Sandur S, Stoller KS: Pulmonary complications of mechanical ventilation. *Clin Chest Med* 1999; 20:223.

Schatz M et al: Increased transient tachypnea of the newborn in infants of asthmatic mothers. *Am J Dis Child* 1991;145:156.

Soll RF: *Prophylactic Natural Surfactant Extract for Preventing Morbidity and Mortality in Preterm Infants.* The Cochrane Library, 2000.

Soll RF: *Prophylactic Synthetic Surfactant for Preventing Morbidity and Mortality in Preterm Infants.* The Cochrane Library, 2000.

Soll RF: *Synthetic Surfactant for Respiratory Distress Syndrome in Preterm Infants.* The Cochrane Library, 2000.

Soll RF, Andruscavage L: The principles and practice of evidence-based neonatology. *Pediatrics* 1999;103:S215.

Soll RF, Morley CJ: *Prophylactic Versus Selective Use of Surfactant for Preventing Morbidity and Mortality in Preterm Infants.* The Cochrane Library, 2000.

Spillman T et al: Detection frequency by thin layer chromatography of phosphatidylglycerol in amniotic fluid with clinically functional pulmonary surfactant. *Clin Chem* 1988;34:1976.

Spitzer AR, Fox WW: Infant apnea. *Pediatr Clin North Am* 1986;33:561.

Stevens JC et al: Extracorporeal membrane oxygenation as treatment of severe meconium aspiration syndrome. *South Med J* 1989;82:696.

Taylor GA et al: Extracorporeal membrane oxygenation: radiographic appearance of the neonatal chest. *Am J Radiol* 1986;146:1257.

Thibeault DW: Pulmonary barotrauma: interstitial emphysema, pneumomediastinum, and pneumothorax. In Thibeault DW, Gregory GA (eds): *Neonatal Pulmonary Care.* Appleton-Century-Crofts, 1986.

Trento A et al: Extracorporeal membrane oxygenation experience at the University of Pittsburgh. *Am Thorac Surg* 1986;42:56.

Trindade O et al: Conventional vs. high-frequency jet ventilation in a piglet model of meconium aspiration: comparison of pulmonary and hemodynamic effects. *J Pediatr* 1985;107:115.

Van Marter L et al: Do clinical markers of barotrauma and oxygen toxicity explain interhospital variation in rates of chronic lung disease? *Pediatrics* 2000;105:1194.

Verder H et al: Nasal continuous positive airway pressure and early surfactant therapy for respiratory distress syndrome in newborns of less than 30 weeks' gestation. *Pediatrics* 1999;103:E24.

Watkinson M, Tiron I: Events before the diagnosis of a pneumothorax in ventilated neonates. *Arch Dis Child Fetal Neonatal Ed* 2001;85:F201.

Wilson BJ et al: A 16-year neonatal/pediatric extracorporeal membrane oxygenation transport experience. *Pediatrics* 2002;109:189.

Wiswell T et al: Delivery room management of the apparently vigorous meconium-stained neonate: results of the multicenter, International Collaborative Trial. *Pediatrics* 2000;105:1.

Wiswell TE et al: Intratracheal suctioning, systemic infection and the meconium aspiration syndrome. *Pediatrics* 1992;89:203.

Yu V et al: Pulmonary air leak in extremely low birthweight infants. *Arch Dis Child* 1986;61:239.

Yu V et al: Pulmonary interstitial emphysema in infants less than 1000g at birth. *Aust Paediatr J* 1986;22:189.

75 Renal Diseases

ACUTE RENAL FAILURE

I. **Definition.** In neonates, acute renal failure is defined as the absence of urinary output (anuria) or as urine output of <0.5 mL/kg/24 h (oliguria) with an associated increase in serum creatinine. One hundred percent of infants void by 48 h (for average times from birth to first voiding, see Table 49–1).

II. **Incidence.** In some studies, as many as 23% of neonates have some form of renal failure; prerenal factors are identified as the cause in 73%.

III. **Pathophysiology.** Normal urine output is ~1–3 mL/kg/h in newborns, and the normal newborn kidney has poor concentrating ability. Renal failure leads to problems with volume overload, hyporkalemia, acidosis, hyperphosphatemia, and hypocalcemia. Acute renal failure is traditionally divided into three categories:

A. **Prerenal failure.** Prerenal failure is due to decreased renal perfusion. Causes include dehydration (poor feeding or increased insensible losses referable to radiant warmers), perinatal asphyxia, and hypotension (septic shock, hemorrhagic shock, or cardiogenic shock resulting from congestive heart failure).

B. **Intrinsic renal failure.** If poor renal perfusion persists, acute tubular necrosis with intrinsic renal failure may result. Other causes are nephrotoxins such as aminoglycosides and methoxyflurane anesthesia, congenital anomalies (eg, renal agenesis or polycystic kidney disease), disseminated intravascular coagulation (DIC), renal vein or renal artery thrombosis, and isolated cortical necrosis.

C. **Postrenal failure.** All of the causes involve obstruction of urinary outflow. These include bilateral ureteropelvic obstruction, bilateral ureterovesical obstruction, posterior urethral valves, urethral diverticulum or stenosis, large ureterocele, neurogenic bladder, blocked urinary drainage tubes, and extrinsic tumor compression.

IV. **Risk factors.** Dehydration, sepsis, asphyxia, and administration of nephrotoxic drugs to the neonate are risk factors for acute renal failure. Maternal diabetes may increase the risk for renal vein thrombosis and subsequent renal insufficiency.

V. **Clinical presentation**

A. **Decreased or absent urine output.** Low or absent urine output is usually the presenting problem. Virtually all infants void by 48 h (see Table 49–1).

B. **Family history.** A history of urinary tract disease in other family members should be sought as well as a history of oligohydramnios, which frequently accompanies urinary outflow obstruction or severe renal dysplasia or agenesis.

C. **Physical examination.** The following abnormalities on physical examination are significant:

1. **Abdominal mass,** suggesting a distended bladder, polycystic kidneys, or hydronephrosis.

2. **Potter's facies,** associated with renal agenesis.

3. **Meningomyelocele,** associated with neurogenic bladder.

4. **Pulmonary hypoplasia,** resulting from severe oligohydramnios in utero secondary to inadequate urinary output.

5. **Urinary ascites,** which may be seen with posterior urethral valves.

6. **Prune belly** (hypoplasia of the abdominal wall musculature and cryptorchidism), associated with urinary abnormalities.

VI. Diagnosis

A. **Bladder catheterization.** Perform bladder catheterization, using a No. 5 or No. 8 French feeding tube to confirm inadequate urine output (for details of the procedure, see Chapter 18). Immediate passage of large volumes of urine suggests obstruction (eg, posterior urethral valves) or a hypotonic (neurogenic) bladder.

B. **Laboratory studies**
   1. **Serum urea nitrogen and creatinine levels**
      a. **A urea nitrogen level** >15–20 mg/dL suggests dehydration or renal insufficiency.
      b. **Creatinine level.** Normal serum creatinine values are 0.8–1.0 mg/dL at 1 day, 0.7–0.8 mg/dL at 3 days, and <0.6 mg/dL by 7 days of life. Higher values suggest renal disease except in low birth weight infants, in whom a creatinine level of <1.6 mg/dL is considered normal. (Rule of thumb: If the creatinine doubles, then 50% of the renal function has been lost.)
   2. **Urinary indices** of acute renal failure are listed in Table 75–1. Order a spot urine osmolality, a serum and spot urine sodium, and serum and urine creatinine, and calculate the fractional excretion of sodium (FeNa) and the renal failure index (RFI). These indices are of limited value if measured while the effects of diuretics such as furosemide are present.

$$\text{FeNa} = \frac{\text{Urine Na} \times \text{Plasma Cr}}{\text{Urine Cr} \times \text{Plasma Na}} \times 100$$

$$\text{RFI} = \frac{\text{Urine Na} \times \text{Serum Cr}}{\text{Urine Cr}}$$

   3. **Complete blood cell count and platelet count** may reveal thrombocytopenia, seen with sepsis or renal vein thrombosis.
   4. **Serum potassium levels** should be monitored to rule out hyperkalemia.
   5. **Urinalysis** may reveal hematuria (associated with renal vein thrombosis, tumors, or DIC; see the discussion of hematuria) or pyuria, suggesting urinary tract infection (UTI) as either the cause of renal insufficiency (sepsis) or the result of mechanical obstruction.

C. **Diagnostic fluid challenge.** If the patient does not have clinical volume overload or congestive failure, give a fluid challenge. Administer normal saline or colloid solution, 5–10 mL/kg as an intravenous bolus, and repeat once as needed. If there is no response, give furosemide, 1 mg/kg. If there is still no increase in urine output, obstruction above the level of the bladder must be ruled out by ultrasound examination. If there is no evidence of obstruction and the patient does not respond to these maneuvers, the most likely cause of anuria or oliguria is intrinsic renal failure.

D. **Radiologic studies**

TABLE 75–1. RENAL FAILURE INDICES IN THE NEONATE

	Prerenal	Renal
Urine osmolality (mOsm)	>400	<400
Urine sodium (mEq/L)	31 ± 19	63 ± 35
Urine/plasma creatinine	29 ± 16	10 ± 4
Fractional excretion of sodium	<2.5	>2.5
Renal failure index	<3.0	>3.0

1. **Abdominal ultrasonography** can delineate hydronephrosis, dilated ureters, abdominal masses, a distended bladder, or renal vein thrombosis.
2. **Intravenous urography** has limited usefulness in the neonatal period because of the poor concentrating ability of the kidney. It is of limited value in the setting of renal failure.
3. **Abdominal x-ray studies** may show spina bifida or an absent sacrum, which can cause neurogenic bladder. Displaced bowel loops suggest the presence of a space-occupying mass.
4. **Radionuclide scanning** can delineate functioning renal parenchyma (using dimercaptosuccinic acid [DMSA]) and give some indication of renal flow and function (using diethyltriamine penta-acetic acid [DTPA]). MAG-3 scanning has largely replaced these two scans, however, because it can image the parenchyma and determine function.

VII. **Management**
A. **General management**
   1. **Replace insensible fluid losses** (preterm, 50–70 mL/kg/day; term, 30 mL/kg/day) plus fluid output (urine and gastrointestinal tract).
   2. **Keep strict intake and output and frequent weight records.**
   3. **Monitor serum sodium and potassium levels** frequently, and replace losses cautiously as needed. Infants with renal failure should never be given intravenous fluids containing potassium because hyperkalemia, if it occurs, may be lethal. If hyperkalemia does occur, treat as outlined in Chapter 41.
   4. **Restrict protein** to <2 g/kg/day, and ensure adequate nonprotein caloric intake. Breast milk or formulas such as Similac PM 60/40 are frequently used for infants with renal failure.
   5. **Hyperphosphatemia and hypocalcemia frequently coexist, and phosphate binders such as aluminum hydroxide, 50–150** mg/kg/day orally, **should be used to normalize the phosphate.** Once the phosphate is normal, calcium with or without vitamin D supplements is usually needed.
   6. **For tetany or convulsions,** acute intravenous calcium replacement with 10% calcium gluconate, 40 mg/kg, or 10% calcium chloride will increase the serum calcium 1 mg/dL. Monitor ionized calcium, if available in your laboratory.
   7. **Metabolic acidosis may require chronic oral bicarbonate supplementation. Blood pressures should be monitored serially** because these infants are always at risk for chronic hypertension. Intravenous bicarbonate therapy should be given if the pH is <7.25 or the serum bicarbonate (HCO_3) is <12 mEq.

$$HCO_3 \text{ deficit} = (24 - \text{observed}) \times 0.5 \text{ body weight (kg)}$$

B. **Definitive management**
   1. **Prerenal failure** is treated by correcting the specific cause (see Acute Renal Failure, section III,A).
   2. **Postrenal failure.** Acute management involves bypassing the obstruction with a bladder catheter or by percutaneous nephrostomy drainage, depending on the level of the obstruction. Surgical correction is usually indicated at some point.
   3. **Intrinsic renal disease.** If renal disease is caused by toxins or acute tubular necrosis, renal function may recover to some extent with time.
   4. **Dialysis.** If recovery of renal function is expected or if renal transplantation is considered an option when the child is older, peritoneal dialysis is the treatment most commonly used in the neonate. On occasion, he-

modialysis, ultrafiltration, and continuous venovenous hyperfiltration may be required.

HEMATURIA

I. **Definition.** Hematuria is the presence of gross or microscopic blood in the urine. More than 3 red blood cells per high-power field (HPF) is usually considered abnormal. A red-stained diaper usually signifies hematuria but may be due to bile pigments, porphyrins, or urates.

II. **Incidence.** Hematuria is not a common problem in newborns.

III. **Pathophysiology.** Hematuria in the newborn may be caused by perinatal asphyxia, cortical or medullary necrosis, infection, trauma (birth or iatrogenic, such as bladder aspiration or catheterization), renal vein or renal artery thrombosis, hyperosmolar infusions into umbilical catheters, neoplasms (rhabdomyosarcoma or nephroblastoma), urinary tract obstruction (urolithiasis after Lasix administration) or infection, coagulopathy, and neonatal glomerulonephritis (most commonly caused by syphilis).

IV. **Risk factors** include coagulopathy, urinary tract infection, obstruction, maternal diabetes (renal vein thrombosis), indwelling urinary catheters, and traumatic delivery.

V. **Clinical presentation**
  A. **History.** A maternal history of diabetes may arouse suspicion of renal vein thrombosis. The birth history and Apgar scores may suggest perinatal asphyxia.
  B. **Physical examination** may reveal the presence of an abdominal mass (obstruction, neoplasm, or renal vein thrombosis). The presence of an umbilical or bladder catheter should be noted.

VI. **Diagnosis**
  A. **Laboratory studies**
    1. **Urinalysis.** Microscopic examination and dipstick testing will confirm the presence of blood or other causes of "red urine." **Red blood cell casts** are seen with intrinsic renal disease such as glomerulonephritis. **Bacteria or white blood cells** suggest UTI.
    2. **Urine culture.** Collection of urine by bladder aspiration or catheterization is preferred and is outlined in Chapters 17 and 18.
    3. **Serum urea nitrogen and creatinine levels** may reveal renal insufficiency.
    4. **Coagulation studies.** Prothrombin time, partial thromboplastin time, and thrombin time may provide clues to DIC or hemorrhagic disease of the newborn. Thrombocytopenia suggests renal vein thrombosis.
  B. **Radiologic studies**
    1. **Ultrasonography** will show neoplasms, renal vein thrombosis, or obstruction in the urinary tract.
    2. **Ancillary testing** such as intravenous urography, arteriography, and nuclear scans may be indicated.

VII. **Management.** Treatment is directed at the underlying cause.

URINARY TRACT INFECTION

I. **Definition.** UTI is the presence of pathogenic bacteria or fungus in the urinary tract with or without symptoms of infection. A definitive diagnosis is made by culture of any organism in a urine specimen that has been properly collected by suprapubic bladder aspiration (>10,000 col), ideally, or by gentle catheterization (>100,000 col).

II. **Incidence.** Various series report an incidence of 0.5–1.0% in term infants weighing >2500 g and higher rates (3–5%) in premature infants or infants weighing <2500 g. (*Note:* In the neonatal period, there is a greater incidence among males than females.)

III. **Pathophysiology.** When UTI is present in an infant <1 year of age, an associated urinary tract abnormality is found in ~50% of neonates. Associated anomalies that may give rise to UTI include neurogenic bladder, posterior urethral valves, vesicoureteral reflux, and ureteropelvic junction obstruction. The predominant organisms are gram-negative rods; *Escherichia coli* is the most common. In neonates, UTIs are most frequently acquired by hematogenous spread.

IV. **Risk factors** include indwelling urinary catheters, systemic sepsis with hematogenous seeding of the urinary tract, urinary tract obstruction, neurogenic bladder (myelodysplasia), and male newborns. Evidence suggests that uncircumcised males may be at higher risk for UTIs.

V. **Clinical presentation**

A. **Signs of sepsis.** The infant may have frank signs of sepsis (respiratory distress, apnea, bradycardia, hypoglycemia, or poor perfusion) or abdominal distention.

B. **Nonspecific findings.** The signs are often subtle and may include lethargy, irritability, poor feeding, vomiting, jaundice, or failure to thrive.

VI. **Diagnosis**

A. **Laboratory studies**

1. **Urine culture.** Suprapubic aspiration or bladder catheterization is mandatory for a dependable urine culture in a neonate. "Bag" urine is considered by some clinicians to be inadequate to achieve reliable culture results.

2. **Blood cultures** should be obtained before starting antibiotic therapy.

3. **Urinalysis.** Microscopic examination may show white blood cells, but the presence of bacteria is a more reliable sign of UTI in the neonate, especially when urine is collected by suprapubic aspiration.

4. **The complete blood cell count** may show leukocytosis.

5. **Serum bilirubin** may be elevated.

B. **No other studies are indicated.**

VII. **Management**

A. **Initial antibiotic treatment.** Initial antibiotic therapy usually consists of broad-spectrum intravenous antibiotics, usually ampicillin and gentamicin, or third-generation cephalosporins, until definitive urine and blood culture results are reported. (For dosages and other pharmacologic information, see Chapter 80.)

B. **Further investigations.** Further tests are necessary to rule out anatomic abnormalities in the neonate. Tests such as renal/bladder ultrasonography, contrast voiding cystourethrogram (VCUG), and renal scan are indicated; at times, an intravenous pyelogram is required for complex problems. Urologic consultation is usually recommended.

VIII. **Prognosis.** Up to one fourth of infants can have a recurrent UTI within the first year of life. Effective use of long-term suppressive antibiotics (in the presence of vesicoureteral reflux) along with any indicated corrective surgery has dramatically reduced the long-term incidence of renal scarring and renal insufficiency.

REFERENCES

Farhat W et al: The natural history of neonatal vesicoureteral reflux associated with antenatal hydronephrosis. *J Urol* 2000;164:1057.

Ginsburg CM, McCracken GH: Urinary tract infections in young infants. *Pediatrics* 1982;69:409.

Herndon CDA et al: Consensus on the prenatal management of antenatally detected urological abnormalities. *J Urol* 2000;164:1052.

Holliday MA, Bennett TM (eds): *Pediatric Nephrology,* 3rd ed. Williams & Wilkins, 1994.

Matthew OP et al: Neonatal renal failure: usefulness of diagnostic indices. *Pediatrics* 1980;65:57.

Norman ME, Asadi FK: A prospective study of acute renal failure in the newborn infant. *Pediatrics* 1979;63:475.

Stapleton FB et al: Acute renal failure in neonates: incidence, etiology and outcome. *Pediatr Nephrol* 1987;1:314.

Sweeney B et al: Reflux nephropathy in infancy: a comparison of infants presenting with and without urinary tract infection. *J Urol* 2001;166:648.

76 Retinopathy of Prematurity

I. Definitions

A. Retinopathy of prematurity (ROP) is a disorder of the developing retinal vasculature resulting from interruption of normal progression of newly forming retinal vessels. Vasoconstriction and obliteration of the advancing capillary bed are followed in succession by neovascularization extending into the vitreous, retinal edema, retinal hemorrhages, fibrosis, and traction on, and eventual detachment of, the retina. In most cases, the process is reversed before fibrosis occurs. **Advanced stages may lead to blindness.**

B. Retrolental fibroplasia. As originally described, the condition was seen only in its most advanced form, after extensive fibrosis and scarring had already occurred behind the lens. It was, therefore, termed *retrolental fibroplasia.* It is now understood that several recognizable changes occur in the developing vasculature before end-stage fibrosis occurs, making this condition a true retinopathy. Because it is found chiefly in premature infants, it is now called *retinopathy of prematurity.*

C. Cicatricial ROP. The term *cicatricial ROP* refers to fibrotic disease.

II. Incidence.
About 400–600 children per year may be blinded by ROP, representing 20% of blindness in preschool children. Of particular concern are the increasing numbers of survivors weighing <1000 g who have the highest incidence of ROP and who may account for much of the current epidemic. The US National Institutes of Health (NIH)-sponsored CRYO-ROP study, carried out in 1986–1987, showed that 65.8% of infants weighing <1251 g developed ROP of any stage. Two percent of infants weighing 1000–1250 g developed threshold stage III+ disease eligible for treatment, whereas 15.5% of infants weighing <750 g did so. **Threshold disease occurred at a median postconceptional age of 37 weeks, regardless of gestational age at birth or chronologic age.**

III. Pathophysiology

A. Historical perspective. Retrolental fibroplasia (RLF) was first described by Terry in the 1940s and was associated with the use of oxygen in newborn infants by Patz (1984). The **first epidemic,** estimated to be responsible for 30% of cases of blindness in preschool children by the end of the 1940s, occurred during a period of relatively liberal oxygen administration. After this association was recognized, oxygen use in nurseries was curtailed. Although the incidence of RLF fell, mortality rates in newborn infants increased. In the 1960s, improved oxygen monitoring techniques made possible the cautious reintroduction of oxygen into the nursery. Despite improved oxygen monitoring, however, a **second epidemic** of RLF (ROP) appeared in the late 1970s and is associated with the increased survival of very low birth weight infants.

B. Normal embryology of the eye. In the normally developing retina, there are no retinal vessels until about 16 weeks' gestation. Until then, oxygen diffuses from the underlying choroidal circulation. At 16 weeks, in response to an unknown stimulus (relative hypoxia *stimulating the release of angiogenic factors* as the retina thickens has been suggested), cells derived from mesenchyme traveling in the nerve fiber layer emanate from the optic nerve head. These cells, called *spindle cells,* are the precursors of the retinal vascular system. A fine capillary network advances through the retina to the ora serrata, or retinal edge. More mature vessels form behind this advancing network. Vascularization on the nasal side of the ora serrata is complete at about 8 months' gestation, whereas that on the temporal side is ordinarily complete at term. Once it is completely vascularized, the retinal vasculature is no longer susceptible to insults of the type that lead to ROP.

C. **Causes**
1. **There appear to be two phases in the development of ROP.**
   a. **Early vasoconstriction and obliteration of the capillary network** in response to high oxygen concentrations noted experimentally or another vascular insult.
   b. **Vasoproliferation,** which follows the period of high oxygen exposure or insult, perhaps in response to an angiogenic factor released by the hypoxic retina. Considerable evidence has been developed to support this hypothesis. Phelps and Rosenbaum (1984) studied kittens made hyperoxic and then allowed to recover in room air (21% oxygen) or 13% oxygen. Those recovering in the hypoxic environment had worse retinopathy than those recovering in room air, suggesting that retinal hypoxia may play a role. In vitro, an angiogenic factor, vascular endothelial cell growth factor (VEGF), is produced in the hypoxic retina and may play an important role in ROP.
IV. **Risk factors.** The association of ROP with oxygen alone is now not so clear. There have been many recorded instances of ROP in premature infants not exposed to elevated oxygen concentrations. Many other factors, such as extreme prematurity, maternal complications, apnea, sepsis, hyper- and hypocapnia, vitamin E deficiency, intraventricular hemorrhage, anemia, exchange transfusion, hypoxia, lactic acidosis, and bright light, have been implicated. The pathophysiology of ROP is still unclear. Experimental studies have focused chiefly on the role of oxygen, although **extreme prematurity is now known to be the most significant risk factor.**
V. **Clinical presentation.** Several methods of classification of ROP have been used. With development of the **International Classification of ROP,** there is now general agreement on the staging of active disease.

   • **Stage I:** A thin demarcation line develops between the vascularized region of the retina and the avascular zone.
   • **Stage II:** This line develops into a ridge protruding into the vitreous, in which there is histologic evidence of an arteriovenous shunt.
   • **Stage III:** Extraretinal fibrovascular proliferation occurs with the ridge. Neovascular tufts may be found just posterior to the ridge (Figure 76–1).
   • **Stage IV:** Fibrosis and scarring occur as the neovascularization extends into the vitreous. Traction occurs on the retina, resulting in retinal detachment.
   • **Plus disease** (eg, stage III+) may occur when vessels posterior to the ridge become dilated and tortuous.

VI. **Diagnosis. Ophthalmoscopic examination** by an experienced examiner usually confirms the diagnosis. A 2001 joint statement by the American Academy of Pediatrics, American Association for Pediatric Ophthalmology and Strabismus, and American Academy of Ophthalmology provided recommendations for ROP screening examinations in premature infants. It is noted that these recommendations are evolving and may change as longer-term ROP outcomes are recognized.
   A. **Infants weighing ≤1500 g or ≤28 weeks' gestation** and those weighing >1500 g with an unstable clinical course should have dilated eye examinations starting at 4–6 weeks of age or 31–33 weeks' postconceptional age. Exams should continue every 2–3 weeks until retinal maturity is reached, if no disease is present.
   B. **Infants with ROP or very immature vessels** should be examined every 1–2 weeks until vessels are mature or the risk of threshold disease has passed. Those at greatest risk should be examined every week.
VII. **Management**
   A. **Circumferential cryopexy** has been proven to be an effective treatment for progressive (stage III+) disease in an attempt to prevent further progression by destroying cells that may be releasing angiogenic factors. Results of the large, collaborative NIH-sponsored trial indicate that cryopexy carried out at

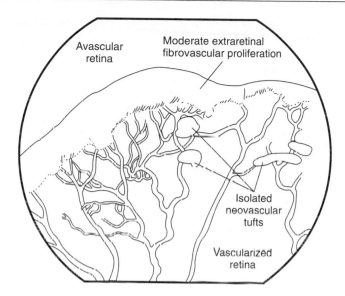

FIGURE 76–1. Schematic drawing of moderate stage III retinopathy of prematurity. Optic nerve head is shown at the bottom, and periphery of the retina is at the top. *(Reproduced, with permission, from Garner A: International classification of retinopathy of prematurity. Pediatrics 1984;74:127.)*

stage III+ can reduce the incidence of severe visual impairment by ~50% if performed within 72 h of detecting threshold disease. If both eyes are involved, cryopexy is usually performed in one eye only because there are some risks with the procedure, such as vitreal hemorrhage. If there are enough risk factors for retinal detachment, however, cryopexy may be performed in both eyes. Although myopia is a common feature of ROP, 10-year follow-up shows significant improvement in visual acuity of treated versus control eyes. It is imperative that an ophthalmologist skilled in cryopexy perform the procedure.

B. **Laser photocoagulation.** Data suggest that this technique is equally effective yet safer than cryopexy. In 1994, the Laser ROP Study Group was formed to carry out a meta-analysis of four laser-ROP trials. Treatment was based on the same criteria used in the CRYO-ROP trial. Recognizing the limitations of a meta-analysis, the study group concluded that laser therapy is at least as effective as cryotherapy for ROP, despite a small risk of cataract formation. Ten-year follow-up of a small group of patients suggests better outcomes with laser photocoagulation.

C. **Oxygen for treatment of ROP.** In an attempt to reduce angiogenic factors from the hypoxic retina and the progression of ROP from prethreshold to threshold (III+) levels, oxygen therapy was attempted in a large collaborative trial, the STOP-ROP Study. Oxygen saturations were targeted at 96–99% in the treatment group and 89–94% in the conventional group once prethreshold ROP was diagnosed. No significant difference was seen in the rate of progression to threshold disease between the two groups.

D. **Vitamin E.** The administration of pharmacologic doses of vitamin E for ROP is *controversial;* currently, there is no proof of clear benefit. Reported side effects include sepsis, necrotizing enterocolitis, and intraventricular hemorrhage. Even so, maintenance of normal serum vitamin E levels is a prudent management objective.

E. **Decreased lighting intensity.** A prospective, randomized, multicenter trial of 409 premature infants weighing <1251 g and 31 weeks' gestation concluded that a reduction in ambient light exposure does not alter the incidence of ROP (Reynolds et al, 1998).

F. **Additional experimental therapies** include inositol and D-penicillamine. Data are limited. Further work is needed.

G. **Retinal reattachment.** Stage IV disease has been treated by attempts at retinal reattachment without significant success to date. Reattachment of late retinal detachments in childhood has met with more success.

H. **Vitrectomy** has not substantially improved the outcome in cicatricial disease.

I. **Follow-up eye examinations** are advocated every 1–2 years for infants with fully regressed ROP and every 6–12 months for those with cicatricial ROP. Premature infants are at risk for myopia even in the absence of ROP and should have an eye exam by 6 months of age.

VIII. **Prognosis.** Ninety percent of cases of stage I and stage II disease regress spontaneously. Current information suggests that ~50% of cases of stage III+ disease regress spontaneously. Of those that do progress to stage III+, the incidence of severe visual impairment can be reduced by ~50% if circumferential cryopexy is carried out by a skilled ophthalmologist. Laser photocoagulation appears equally and possibly more effective than cryopexy. Sequelae of regressed disease such as myopia, strabismus, amblyopia, glaucoma, and late detachment require regular follow-up.

REFERENCES

Adamis AP et al: Inhibition of VEGF prevents ocular neovascularization in a primate. *Arch Ophthalmol* 1996;114:6671.
American Academy of Pediatrics, American Association for Pediatric Ophthalmology and Strabismus, American Academy of Ophthalmology: Joint statement: screening examination of premature infants for retinopathy of prematurity. *Pediatrics* 2001;108:809.
Cryotherapy for Retinopathy of Prematurity Cooperative Group: Multicenter trial of cryotherapy for retinopathy of prematurity: three-month outcome. *Arch Ophthalmol* 1990;108:195.
Cryotherapy for Retinopathy of Prematurity Cooperative Group: Multicenter trial of cryotherapy for retinopathy of prematurity: ophthalmological outcomes at 10 years. *Arch Ophthalmol* 2001;119:1110.
Flynn JT: Retinopathy of prematurity. *Pediatr Clin North Am* 1987;34:1847.
Garner A: International classification of retinopathy of prematurity. *Pediatrics* 1984;74:127.
Laser ROP Study Group: Laser therapy for retinopathy of prematurity. *Arch Ophthalmol* 1994;112:154.
Lucey JF, Dangman BD: A reexamination of the role of oxygen in retrolental fibroplasia. *Pediatrics* 1984;82:73.
Ng E et al: A comparison of laser photocoagulation with cryotherapy for threshold retinopathy of prematurity at 10 years: part 1. Visual function and structural outcome. *Ophthalmology* 2002;109:928.
Palmer EA et al: Incidence and early course of retinopathy of prematurity. *Ophthalmology* 1991;98:1628.
Patz A: Current concepts of the effect of oxygen on the developing retina. *Curr Eye Res* 1984;3:159.
Phelps D: Retinopathy of prematurity: clinical trials. *Neonatal Rev* 2001;2:e167.
Phelps DL: Role of vitamin E therapy in high-risk neonates. *Clin Perinatol* 1988;15:955.
Phelps DL, Rosenbaum AL: Effects of marginal hypoxemia on recovery from oxygen-induced retinopathy in the kitten model. *Pediatrics* 1984;73:1.
Reynolds JD et al: Lack of efficacy of light reduction in preventing retinopathy of prematurity. *N Engl J Med* 1998;338:1572.
Shweiki D et al: Vascular endothelial growth factor induced by hypoxia may mediate hypoxia-initiated angiogenesis. *Nature* 1992;359:843.
STOP-ROP Multicenter Study Group: Supplemental therapeutic oxygen for prethreshold retinopathy of prematurity (STOP-ROP), a randomized, controlled trial: I. Primary outcomes. *Pediatrics* 2000;105:295.

77 Disorders of Calcium and Magnesium Metabolism

OSTEOPENIA OF PREMATURITY

I. **Definition.** Osteopenia of prematurity is manifested as rickets in the preterm infant. Rickets is a chronic disorder of calcium metabolism characterized by x-ray evidence of bone demineralization and elevated serum alkaline phosphatase levels.

II. **Incidence.** The incidence of rickets in low birth weight infants is ~30%.

III. **Pathophysiology**
  A. **Chronic diseases.** Infants with chronic debilitating diseases (**notably bronchopulmonary dysplasia**) are at greatest risk for rickets. Typically, these infants require high caloric intake to sustain good weight gain. Bone demineralization can progress despite intakes of calcium, 50–60 mg/kg/day; phosphorus, 25 mg/kg/day; and vitamin D, 400 IU/day. Vitamin D metabolism is shown in Figure 77–1. These infants also have an increased incidence of rib fractures secondary to severe bone demineralization; peak occurrence is at ~2 months of age. Most infants with rickets also have received intermittent or routine doses of diuretics (especially furosemide).
  B. **Very low birth weight infants** (<1250 g). Prenatal placental insufficiency leads to low plasma phosphate concentrations in very low birth weight infants. Concomitant reduced renal tubular reabsorption of phosphate in this population exacerbates the phosphate deficiency. If untreated, 42% of these infants have been shown to develop radiologic evidence of rickets. Careful attention to appropriate calcium and phosphate supplementation prevents rickets in this group of infants.
  C. **Diuretics. Loop diuretics** (eg, furosemide and bumetanide) have a marked calciuric effect, and the increased calcium loss exacerbates calcium efflux from bones. **Thiazide diuretics** (eg, hydrochlorothiazide) tend to reduce urinary calcium losses and, therefore, can ameliorate bone demineralization.

IV. **Risk factors**
  A. Very low birth weight.
  B. Chronic diseases, especially bronchopulmonary dysplasia.
  C. Chronic stress.
  D. Malnutrition.
  E. Administration of inappropriate quantities of calcium, phosphorus, or vitamin D.
  F. Diuretics.

V. **Clinical presentation**
  A. **Poor weight gain** despite very high caloric intake is often seen in these infants.
  B. **Rib and other bone fractures** may be seen in advanced stages of rickets.
  C. **Respiratory distress** is occasionally seen.

VI. **Diagnosis**
  A. **Laboratory studies**
    1. **Alkaline phosphatase levels** are usually >280 IU/L and can be >500 IU/L.
    2. **Serum calcium levels** are usually normal.
    3. **Serum phosphorus levels** may be low (<3 mg/dL).
    4. **Vitamin D levels.** Infants with rickets typically have increased levels of 1,25-hydroxyvitamin D, which reverts to normal when the disease resolves.

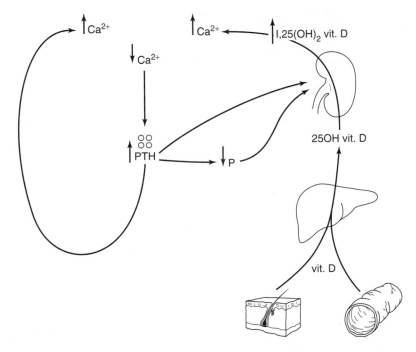

FIGURE 77-1. Vitamin D metabolism. PTH, Parathyroid hormone; P, phosphorus. *(From Tsang RC, et al: Pediatric parathyroid disorders.* Pediatr Clin North Am *1979; 26:223. Reproduced with permission from Reed Elsevier Science.)*

25-Hydroxyvitamin D levels may be depressed with active rickets, which resolves after treatment. (See Figure 77-1.)

    B. Radiologic studies. Sequential x-ray studies demonstrate gradual bone demineralization ("washed-out bones"). Some centers use the more sensitive bone mineral analyzer to monitor smaller changes in bone density, but this instrument is not widely available. X-ray films provide evidence of progressive bone demineralization. Serial films may also show lucency at the metaphyses of long bones and loss of the normal opaque line at the metaphyseal end. In advanced stages, metaphyseal fraying and cupping can be seen most markedly at the knees and wrists. Poor mineralization at the anterior aspects of the ribs ("rachitic rosary") and rib fractures may also be seen.

VII. Management and prognosis

    A. Nutrition. To sustain adequate weight gain, infants with rickets usually have an increased need for calories and for additional calcium, vitamin D, and phosphate. Use of a formula such as one of the special care formulas for premature infants or mineral supplementation in human milk (eg, Similac Special Care or Enfamil Premature), which contain 1.2–1.4 g/L of calcium and have a calcium-phosphate ratio of 2:1 with 400–800 IU of vitamin D per day, has been shown to stimulate bone mineralization and resolution of rickets. **Alkaline phosphatase levels** should be monitored every 1–2 weeks until normal levels are obtained.

    B. Calcium supplementation. Infants who are receiving nothing by mouth should be given ~45 mg/kg/day of elemental calcium intravenously with a calcium-phosphate ratio of 2–3:1 and 400–800 IU of vitamin D per day. Rarely, additional benefit can be achieved with higher doses of vitamin D. Calcitriol

(1,25-dihydroxycholecalciferol), the most potent vitamin D metabolite available, has also been used as a vitamin D supplement for rickets.

C. **Prognosis.** This condition is completely reversible with careful management. Depending on the severity of the disease, most infants should fully recover within weeks to months of detection and treatment.

HYPOCALCEMIA

I. **Definition.** In infants in intensive care nurseries, disorders of calcium metabolism frequently develop; hypocalcemia is the most common. Hypocalcemia is defined as total serum calcium concentration (tCa) levels <7 mg/dL (1.75 mmol/L) in all infants, <7.0 mg/dL (1.75 mmol/L) in preterm infants, and <8.0 mg/dL (2.00 mmol/L) in term infants. Some clinicians consider only values <6.0 mg/dL (1.50 mmol/L), in infants with no symptoms, as diagnostic of neonatal hypocalcemia. Most textbooks and reference journals indicate that serum ionized calcium (iCa) is a better value with which to evaluate hypocalcemia. The ionized fraction of calcium is considered the active component of calcium and depends on the interaction of total calcium and serum albumin level. Normal values of iCa in term infants at 24 h of age varies from 4.4 to 5.4 mg/dL (1.10–1.36 mmol/L), but some authors have suggested that iCa values >3.0 mg/dL (0.75 mmol/L) are adequate in some infants.

II. **Risk factors.** There is an increased incidence of hypocalcemia within the first 3 days of life in premature or sick neonates. The risk of hypocalcemia increases with the degree of prematurity. Some infants also are at increased risk for hypocalcemia:
A. Infants with poor enteral intake.
B. Infants of diabetic mothers.
C. Infants stressed during the perinatal period.
D. Infants receiving blood transfusions.
E. Infants with alkalosis.
F. Infants receiving diuretics.
G. Infants receiving excessive phosphate intake.
H. Infants with insufficient magnesium intake.
I. Infants with congenital hypoparathyroidism (eg, DiGeorge syndrome).

III. **Pathophysiology.** Ionized calcium is the biologically important form of calcium. The tCa levels have repeatedly been shown not to be predictive of iCa levels. Therefore, tCa levels are unreliable as criteria for true hypocalcemia. In premature infants, it has been shown that tCa levels as low as 6 mg/dL or less correspond to iCa levels >3 mg/dL.

A. **Early-onset neonatal hypocalcemia (ENH).** During the third trimester of pregnancy, the human fetus receives at least 140 mg/kg/day of elemental calcium via the umbilical cord. Most of this calcium is readily incorporated into the newly forming bones. After delivery, this massive supply of calcium is suddenly stopped, and calcium must be given enterally.

1. **A full-term infant** receiving 100–120 mL of normal formula would be receiving 50–60 mg/kg/day of calcium orally. Despite this drop in supply, full-term infants tolerate the change well and do not become hypocalcemic.

2. **Premature or sick infants** often become hypocalcemic during the first 3 days of life. Total serum calcium levels can drop to <7 mg/dL and occasionally fall below 6 mg/dL.

3. **Calcium levels** (both iCa and tCa) usually return to normal within 48–72 h regardless of whether supplemental calcium is given. It has also been shown that immunoreactive parathyroid hormone (iPTH) is often low at birth but rises to higher levels within 24–72 h after delivery. Intravenous calcium supplementation has been shown to suppress this increase in iPTH.

B. **Hypocalcemia secondary to prolonged poor enteral intake.** After 3 days of life, infants tolerating enteral feedings usually do not need calcium supplementation. Normal formula supplies adequate calcium for bone mineralization in full-term infants. Calcium-rich formula—that is, formula with an elemental calcium concentration of 1.2–1.4 g/L and a calcium-phosphate ratio of 2:1—is usually sufficient for bone growth in premature infants. However, if feedings cannot be advanced rapidly or if the infant must continue without oral feedings, parenteral calcium supplementation is needed to prevent bone demineralization. These infants often maintain normal iCa and tCa levels at the expense of bone calcium. Furthermore, magnesium deficiency secondary to malnutrition can suppress iPTH levels and thus cause hypocalcemia.

C. **Hypocalcemia secondary to maternal diabetes.** After infants of diabetic mothers are born, their serum glucose levels rapidly decline as a result of **hyperinsulinemia.** These infants also secrete higher amounts of **calcitonin,** which inhibits calcium mobilization from bone. iPTH may also be lower in these infants and may not increase as rapidly after delivery. Therefore, these infants can have a relative intolerance to phosphate and an increased risk of hypocalcemia.

D. **Hypocalcemia secondary to perinatal stress.** Stressed neonates who have suffered from perinatal sepsis, asphyxia, TORCH (*t*oxoplasmosis, *o*ther, *r*ubella, *c*ytomegalovirus, and *h*erpes simplex virus) infections, compromised placental blood flow, or meconium aspiration also have an increased risk of hypocalcemia. This is believed to be due to the effects of corticosteroids and catecholamines during stress.

E. **Hypocalcemia secondary to alkalosis.** The amount of tCa that is ionized is inversely proportionate to serum pH. Infants who are acidotic have iCa levels that are higher than expected, and alkalotic infants can likewise be clinically hypocalcemic even if their tCa level is >7 mg/dL. This is a direct pH effect.

F. **Hypocalcemia secondary to blood transfusions.** Citrate, a normal component of stored blood, forms a neutral soluble complex with calcium and thus reduces the amount of calcium that is ionized. Citrate is metabolized to bicarbonate within a few hours after administration and may induce a mild metabolic alkalosis, which will also tend to decrease the amount of iCa. The amount of citrate administered with periodic blood replacement usually does not lead to clinical hypocalcemia. However, the amount of citrate given as a result of exchange transfusion, especially repeated transfusions, is much higher and may reduce serum iCa.

G. **Hypocalcemia secondary to diuretic therapy.** Because of its action on the ascending loop of Henle and the proximal tubule, loop diuretics, especially furosemide therapy, cause hypercalciuria, which can lead to hypocalcemia, bone demineralization, or both. This effect can be most severe with chronic use of these medications.

IV. **Clinical presentation**

A. **Acute hypocalcemia.** Infants who are acutely hypocalcemic may have apnea, irritability, slight tremors of the extremities, profound tetany, or seizures. Cardiac dysfunction may occur, characterized by prolonged QT intervals and arrhythmias.

B. **Chronic hypocalcemia.** Infants who are chronically hypocalcemic may have rickets, characterized by apnea, bone demineralization, elevated alkaline phosphatase levels, and rib and long-bone fractures.

V. **Diagnosis**

A. **Laboratory studies**

1. **Total and ionized calcium.** Serum iCa levels <4.4 mg/dL (1.10 mmol/L) are diagnostic of hypocalcemia. In the absence of iCa levels, serum tCa levels <7 mg/dL (1.75 mmol/L) can be considered diagnostic of hypocalcemia.

2. **Serum magnesium levels** <1.5 mg/dL indicate hypomagnesemia, which can accompany hypocalcemia.

3. **Alkaline phosphatase levels** >225 IU/L are elevated and can be an early sign of rickets.
4. **Urinary calcium losses** can be estimated either by **random spot or 24-h urine collections.** Calcium-creatinine ratios (measured in spot urine specimens) >0.21–0.25 are indicative of hypercalciuria. Also, 24-h urinary calcium levels >4 mg/kg/24 h indicate hypercalciuria.
B. **Radiologic studies.** Bone demineralization can be grossly estimated by reviewing sequential x-ray films of ribs and long bones. Rickets can be suggested by metaphyseal lucency accompanied by metaphyseal fraying and cupping. These findings are best seen at the knees and anterior rib ends (rachitic rosary). Rib fractures can also be seen in severe cases.
C. **Other studies.** Electrocardiography may show prolonged QT intervals or arrhythmias as a result of hypocalcemia or hypomagnesemia.
VI. **Management.** Parenteral calcium therapy may be associated with significant untoward effects. These include nephrolithiasis, cardiac arrhythmias, subcutaneous calcium deposition endangering joint mobility, peripheral skin sloughs, and the possibility of metastatic calcifications in the brains of very sick neonates. **Expectant nonintervention** is, therefore, suggested for early-onset neonatal hypocalcemia, reserving treatment with parenteral calcium therapy for those cases of profound or clinical (symptomatic) hypocalcemia.
A. **ENH.** If treatment is necessary based on iCa or tCa levels or symptoms, intravenous **10% calcium gluconate** (containing 9 mg of elemental calcium/mL) should be given (for dosage, see Chapter 80). This is usually more than adequate to maintain normal ionized calcium levels. Excessive treatment can suppress iPTH levels and for this reason should be avoided. There is no real benefit to continuous-drip infusion compared with bolus administration in the treatment of ENH. When calcium gluconate is given without phosphate, most of the calcium is rapidly excreted in the urine. However, in the acute stage and during the first 3 days of life, calcium can be given every 6 h because it is impractical to give phosphate at this time.
B. **Hypocalcemia secondary to poor enteral intake.** Parenteral nutrition is usually started on days 3–4 of life, and calcium and phosphate must be started both for maintenance and to support bone growth. The intrauterine dose of 140 mg/kg/day of elemental calcium cannot be achieved by the intravenous route because of precipitation with phosphate. **An intravenous dosage of 45 mg/kg/day of elemental calcium with a calcium-phosphate ratio ranging from 1.3:1.0 to 2:1 has been shown to be optimal in promoting both calcium and phosphate retention.** Supplementation with intravenous calcium can cause hypercalciuria. If intravenous calcium is given without phosphate, most of the calcium is released in the urine and thus is not used for bone formation. Although phosphate is needed, excessive phosphate can lead to hypocalcemia. **Vitamin D supplements** of 400 IU/day should also be provided. Parenteral supplementation of calcium and phosphate may be hampered by precipitation in parenteral nutrition solutions. Factors that tend to increase the risk of precipitation include elevated pH of the solution, excessively high concentrations of calcium and phosphate, low concentrations of amino acids, high temperature, prolonged standing times, addition of calcium salts first or before final dilution, and use of the chloride salt as the source of calcium.
C. **Hypocalcemia secondary to maternal diabetes.** Because these infants are at greater risk for hypocalcemia, serum calcium levels must be closely monitored. The treatment criteria are the same as those outlined previously for ENH in section VI,A.
D. **Hypocalcemia secondary to perinatal stress.** The treatment criteria are the same as those for ENH, except when the infant is maintained alkalotic (see the following section VI,E).
E. **Hypocalcemia secondary to alkalosis.** Because alkalotic infants (eg, infants being treated for persistent pulmonary hypertension) can be clinically

hypocalcemic with tCa levels >7 mg/dL, maintenance calcium therapy should be started when blood pH levels reach 7.50.
F. Hypocalcemia secondary to blood transfusions. The amount of citrate administered with periodic blood replacement usually does not lead to clinical hypocalcemia. However, the rate of citrate given as a result of exchange transfusion is much higher and may reduce serum iCa. Hypocalcemia secondary to blood transfusion can be treated prophylactically (with calcium gluconate) or if symptoms of hypocalcemia are noted (for dosages and other pharmacologic information, see Chapter 80). Low iCa levels and clinical symptoms of hypocalcemia are rarely encountered, even when extra calcium is not given.
G. Hypocalcemia secondary to diuretic therapy. Infants receiving loop diuretics have an increased urinary loss of calcium. This loss can be demonstrated by measurement of calcium-creatinine ratios in spot urines or tCa in 24-h urine collections. If hypercalciuria exists, an attempt should be made to **substitute a thiazide diuretic (most commonly chlorothiazide) for furosemide or bumetanide.** However, if a loop diuretic is thought to be essential, a lower dose of furosemide or bumetanide in combination with a thiazide should be used. Thiazides tend to cause calcium retention and can overcome the hypercalciuric effect of the loop diuretics. These efforts will reduce the risk of nephrocalcinosis, which is directly related to the amount of calcium excreted in the urine. However, this combination can cause significant diuresis and increase urinary potassium loss. Fluids and electrolytes must, therefore, be carefully monitored if combination therapy is chosen. If >5 mEq/kg/day of potassium supplementation is required after diuretics are started, **spironolactone** therapy should also be started (for dosage, see Chapter 80). Spironolactone has little or no effect on urinary calcium loss but helps to reduce the severity of hypokalemia in infants receiving either furosemide or thiazide therapy.
VII. Prognosis. Hypocalcemia can be effectively controlled with close monitoring of calcium, phosphate, and vitamin D intake and urinary calcium losses.

HYPERCALCEMIA

I. Definition. Hypercalcemia is defined as tCa levels >11 mg/dL and iCa levels >5.4 mg/dL (1.36 mmol/L). The tCa level is not predictive of iCa levels and thus is not a reliable measure of hypercalcemia. Acidotic infants may have iCa levels >5.4 mg/dL even though tCa levels are 10 mg/dL or less.
II. Pathophysiology. Hypercalcemia may be due to parathyroid-related causes or to mechanisms unrelated to the parathyroid.
  A. Congenital primary hyperparathyroidism (rare).
  B. Congenital secondary hyperparathyroidism resulting from maternal hypoparathyroidism (rare).
  C. Subcutaneous fat necrosis (which, if extensive, may lead to hypercalcemia when large amounts of calcium are released from subcutaneous fat).
  D. Fanconi's syndrome.
  E. Benign familial hypercalcemia.
  F. Iatrogenic hypercalcemia resulting from excessive calcium supplements.
  G. Hypervitaminosis D.
  H. Hypoproteinemia.
  I. Excessive thiazide treatment.
III. Risk factors
  A. Excessive supplemental calcium.
  B. Excessive vitamin D supplement.
  C. Rare congenital hypercalcemia.

IV. Clinical presentation. Clinical symptomatology is important in establishing significant hypercalcemia. Symptoms include poor feeding with poor weight gain, depressed tone, lethargy, polyuria, and shortening of the QT interval as evidenced by electrocardiography. Seizures can also be seen in severe cases.

V. Diagnosis

A. Laboratory studies

1. **Total and ionized calcium.** Ideally, iCa levels >5.4 mg/dL (1.36 mmol/L) establish hypercalcemia. If iCa levels are not available, tCa levels >11 mg/dL can be considered abnormal. Infants who are acidotic or hypoproteinemic may have iCa levels >5.4 mg/dl even though tCa is 10 mg/dL or less. Therefore, clinical symptoms are important in establishing the diagnosis of hypercalcemia.

2. **Intakes of calcium, phosphate, and vitamin D** should be checked. The calcium-phosphate ratio should be 2:1, and vitamin D dosage should be 400–800 IU/day.

3. **Serum total protein** and the **albumin-globulin ratio** should also be obtained.

4. **Tubular resorption of phosphate** is usually reduced when hyperparathyroidism exists.

5. The **iPTH level** can be measured to establish hyperparathyroidism.

6. **Vitamin D levels.** Hypervitaminosis D can usually be determined by careful review of vitamin intake. However, if this is not clear, **25-hydroxyvitamin D** can be measured. This value is elevated if excess vitamin D has been given.

B. Radiologic studies. X-ray films are helpful in establishing the cause of hypercalcemia. Bone demineralization is typical of hyperparathyroidism, and osteosclerotic lesions are seen with hypervitaminosis D. Hypercalciuria can be very severe with excessive calcium intake or with normal calcium intake plus inadequate phosphate intake.

VI. Management

A. General. Treatment depends on the cause, but in general the calcium intake should be reduced and vitamin D supplements withheld. Some authors recommend avoidance of sunlight. After hypercalcemia has resolved, the actual calcium, phosphate, and vitamin D needs can be estimated based on normal bone mineralization without recurrence of hypercalcemia. If the infant is receiving a thiazide diuretic (which increases calcium retention in the kidneys), the drug should be discontinued.

B. Acute symptomatic hypercalcemia

1. When acute symptomatic hypercalcemia exists, **furosemide** may be effective in reducing serum calcium because of its marked hypercalciuric effect (for dosage, see Chapter 80). Fluid and electrolyte intake must be monitored closely if furosemide is used.

2. In older children and adults, calcitonin has been used for hypercalcemia associated with immobilization (patients in traction) and for acute hypercalcemic states at a dosage of 5–8 units/kg/dose intravenously or intramuscularly every 12 h. It is unlikely that calcitonin therapy would be needed in neonates.

C. Surgical intervention. Very rarely, when severe hyperparathyroidism exists, parathyroidectomy may be needed.

VII. Prognosis. Complete resolution of hypercalcemia occurs rapidly if it is treated promptly.

HYPOMAGNESEMIA

I. Definition. Hypomagnesemia is defined as a serum magnesium level <1.52 mEq/L (0.75 mmol/L).

II. Pathophysiology. Magnesium is required as a catalyst for many intracellular enzymatic reactions. Calcium homeostasis cannot be maintained if serum magnesium levels are low. The usual cause of low magnesium levels is inadequate intake after delivery.
III. Risk factors
   A. Hypocalcemia.
   B. Inadequate intake of magnesium.
IV. Clinical presentation. The most common manifestation of hypomagnesemia is hypocalcemia that fails to respond to calcium therapy.
V. Diagnosis. Serum magnesium levels should be checked in all severely stressed infants. If the level is adequate and there is normal magnesium intake, repeated checks are not necessary unless hypocalcemia occurs.
VI. Management. Acute hypomagnesemia should be treated with **magnesium sulfate** until the magnesium level is normalized or symptoms resolve. The route may be intramuscular or intravenous; however, with intravenous administration, careful electrocardiographic monitoring is indicated because of the risk for arrhythmias (for dosage, see Chapter 80). If feedings are started early, parenteral magnesium is unnecessary; however, if the infant has poor enteral intake, parenteral nutrition should include magnesium.
VII. Prognosis. This condition often goes unrecognized. However, when detected, complete resolution occurs with treatment.

HYPERMAGNESEMIA

I. Definition. Hypermagnesemia is defined as serum magnesium levels >2.3 mEq/L (1.15 mmol/L).
II. Pathophysiology. Increased serum magnesium levels depress the central nervous system and decrease skeletal muscle contractility. These effects can be reversed by increased serum iCa levels. The most common cause of hypermagnesemia in neonates is treatment of the mother with magnesium sulfate. Less commonly, it can occur with administration of a magnesium-containing antacid, especially when urine output is decreased. Hypermagnesemia can also be caused by magnesium sulfate enemas, which are absolutely contraindicated in neonates.
III. Risk factors
   A. Administration of magnesium sulfate to the mother before delivery.
   B. Administration of magnesium-containing antacids to the neonate, especially when urinary output is decreased.
IV. Clinical presentation. The symptoms of hypermagnesemia are very similar to those of hypercalcemia. These include poor feeding, lethargy, depressed tone, hyporeflexia, apnea, and decreased gastrointestinal motility with abdominal distention.
V. Diagnosis
   A. Laboratory studies. Elevated **serum magnesium levels** are diagnostic.
   B. Electrocardiography. A shortened QT interval is seen on the electrocardiogram.
VI. Management
   A. Fluids and electrolytes. If enteral feedings are not tolerated, maintenance intravenous fluids should be provided, with careful monitoring of serum electrolytes and pH.
   B. Respiratory care. In rare cases of severe apnea, intubation and mechanical ventilation are needed.
   C. Exchange transfusion can effectively reduce serum magnesium levels, but this should be reserved for extreme cases.
VII. Prognosis. Hypermagnesemia usually resolves spontaneously, provided that renal function is maintained.

REFERENCES

Bhatt DR et al: *Neonatal Drug Formulary 2002*, 5th ed.

Chan G: Growth and bone mineral status of discharged very low birth weight infants fed different formulas or human milk. *J Pediatr* 1993;123:439.

Ernst J et al: Metabolic balance studies in premature infants. *Clin Perinatol* 1995;22:177.

Faerk J et al: Diet and mineral content at term in premature infants. *Pediatr Res* 2000;47:148.

Fewtrell MS et al: Neonatal factors predicting childhood height in preterm infants: evidence for a persistent effect of early metabolic bone disease? *J Pediatr* 2000;137:668.

Koo WWK: Calcium, phosphorus, and vitamin D requirements of infants receiving parenteral nutrition. *J Perinatol* 1989;8:263.

Koo WWK, Tsang RC: Mineral requirements of low birth weight infants. *J Am Coll Nutr* 1991; 10.474.

Macmahon P et al: Association of mineral composition of neonatal intravenous feeding solutions and metabolic bone disease of prematurity. *Arch Dis Child* 1989;64:489.

Mimouni F, Tsang R: Neonatal hypocalcemia: to treat or not to treat? *J Am Coll Nutr* 1994; 13;408.

Mimouni F, Tsang RC: A pathophysiology of neonatal hypocalcemia. In Polin RA, Fox WW (eds): *Fetal and Neonatal Physiology*, vol 2. Saunders, 1992.

Moyer-Mileur LJ et al: Daily physical activity program increases bone mineralization and growth in preterm very low birth weight infants. *Pediatrics* 2000;106:1088.

Pohlandt F: Prevention of postnatal bone demineralization in very low birth weight infants by individually monitored supplementation with calcium and phosphorus. *Pediatr Res* 1994; 35:125.

Schanler RJ, Rifka M: Calcium, phosphorus and magnesium needs for the low birth weight infant. *Acta Paediatr* 1994;405:111.

Schanler RJ et al: Parenteral nutrient needs of very low birth weight infants. *J Pediatr* 1994; 125:961.

Shankaran S et al: Mineral excretion following furosemide compared with bumetanide therapy in premature infants. *Pediatr Nephrol* 1995;9:159.

Vileisis RA: Furosemide effect on mineral status of parenterally nourished neonates with chronic lung disease. *Pediatrics* 1990;85:316.

78 Surgical Diseases of the Newborn

ALIMENTARY TRACT OBSTRUCTION

VASCULAR RING

I. **Definition.** *Vascular ring* denotes a variety of anomalies of the aortic arch and its branches that create a "ring" of vessels around the trachea and esophagus.

II. **Pathophysiology.** Partial obstruction of the trachea or the esophagus, or both, may result from extrinsic compression by the encircling ring of vessels.

III. **Clinical presentation.** Dysphagia or stridor (respiratory insufficiency), or both, are the modes of presentation.

IV. **Diagnosis** is by barium swallow, which identifies extrinsic compression of the esophagus in the region of the aortic arch.

V. **Management** consists of surgical division of a portion of the constricting ring of vessels. The specific surgical plan must be tailored to the particular type of aortic arch anomaly present.

ESOPHAGEAL ATRESIA

I. **Definition.** The esophagus ends blindly ~10–12 cm from the nares. In 85% of cases, the distal esophagus communicates with the posterior trachea (distal tracheoesophageal fistula [TEF]).

II. **Pathophysiology.** Prime morbidity is pulmonary. Complete esophageal obstruction results in inability of the infant to handle his or her own secretions, producing "excess salivation" and aspiration of pharyngeal contents. More important, the direct communication between the stomach and the tracheobronchial tree via the distal TEF allows the crying newborn to greatly distend the stomach with air; embarrassment of diaphragmatic excursion promotes basilar atelectasis and subsequent pneumonia. Additionally, the distal TEF permits reflux of gastric secretion directly into the tracheobronchial tree, causing chemical pneumonitis, which may be complicated by bacterial pneumonia.

III. **Clinical presentation.** The pregnancy may have been complicated by polyhydramnios. After delivery, the infant typically is unable to swallow saliva, which drains from the corners of the mouth and requires frequent suctioning. Attempts at feeding will result in prompt regurgitation, coughing, choking, and cyanosis.

IV. **Diagnosis is established by attempting to pass a nasogastric tube and meeting resistance at 10–12 cm from the nares followed by chest x-ray film for confirmation.** Chest x-ray film will show the tube to end or coil in the region of the thoracic inlet. The x-ray film should also be examined for possible skeletal anomalies, pulmonary infiltrates, cardiac size and shape, and abdominal bowel gas patterns. The absence of gas in the gastrointestinal (GI) tract implies esophageal atresia without TEF (10% of cases), surgical management of which will probably differ from that of the more common esophageal atresia with TEF. Careful contrast x-ray study of the proximal esophageal pouch can also be performed to delineate the precise length of the proximal pouch and to rule out the rare proximal TEF.

V. **Management**

    A. **Preoperative treatment** should focus on protecting the lungs by evacuating the proximal esophageal pouch with an indwelling Repogle tube or frequent suctioning and by placing the baby in a relatively upright (45°) position to lessen the likelihood of reflux of gastric contents up the distal esophagus into the trachea. **Broad-spectrum antibiotics** should be administered.

B. Surgical therapy. The steps and timing of surgical therapy must be individualized. Some surgeons perform preliminary gastrostomy to decompress the stomach and provide additional protection against reflux. Ligation of the TEF and esophageal anastomosis are the essential steps in total surgical correction.

DUODENAL OBSTRUCTION

I. **Definition.** Obstruction of the lumen of the duodenum may be either complete or partial, pre- or postampullary, and caused by either intrinsic or extrinsic problems.
II. **Pathophysiology**
  A. **Duodenal atresia** results in complete obstruction of the lumen of the duodenum, whereas symptoms of partial obstruction result from a stenotic lesion.
  B. **Annular pancreas** is a congenital anomaly of pancreatic development, which results in an encircling "napkin ring" of pancreatic tissue about the descending duodenum. It can result in either complete or, more commonly, partial duodenal obstruction.
  C. **Malrotation** may cause complete or partial duodenal obstruction in one of two ways. In uncomplicated malrotation, peritoneal attachments (Ladd's bands) may compress the duodenum, resulting in total or, more commonly, partial obstruction. Midgut volvulus may complicate nonrotation and nonfixation of the intestine. The entire midgut may twist on the pedicle of its blood supply, the superior mesenteric artery, resulting in duodenal obstruction and eventual nonviability of the midgut.
III. **Clinical presentation**
  A. **General.** Infants with duodenal obstruction typically experience vomiting (often bilious). Abdominal distention is not usually a prominent feature. Polyhydramnios may be evident.
  B. **Duodenal atresia.** The presence of Down syndrome, esophageal atresia, or imperforate anus suggests duodenal atresia.
  C. **Midgut volvulus** typically presents with symptoms of duodenal obstruction (bilious vomiting) and evidence of intestinal ischemia (mucoid bloody stools), usually in an infant who for days or weeks has eaten and stooled normally.
IV. **Differential diagnosis** includes duodenal atresia (stenosis), annular pancreas, and malrotation with or without the complication of midgut volvulus.
V. **Diagnosis.** The exact cause of the obstruction may not be known until a laparotomy is performed.
  A. **Abdominal x-ray study.** In complete duodenal obstruction, the pathognomonic x-ray finding is a **"double bubble."** Two large gas collections, one in the stomach and the other in the first portion of duodenum, are the only lucencies in the GI tract.
  B. **Radiologic contrast studies**
    1. **Partial obstructions** will probably require an upper GI series to identify the site of difficulty.
    2. **Malrotation.** It is important to eliminate malrotation as a possibility because its complication, midgut volvulus, is a true surgical emergency. This is best done by an upper GI series, identifying a transverse portion of the duodenum leading to a fixed ligament of Treitz, or by barium enema, localizing the cecum to its normal, right lower quadrant position.
VI. **Management**
  A. **Duodenal atresia or annular pancreas.** In cases of atresia or annular pancreas, gastric suction will control vomiting and allow "elective" surgical correction.
  B. **Malrotation mandates immediate surgical intervention** because the viability of the intestine from the duodenum to the transverse colon may be at risk from midgut volvulus.

PROXIMAL INTESTINAL OBSTRUCTION

I. Definition. Proximal intestinal obstruction is obstruction of the jejunum.

II. Pathophysiology. Jejunal obstruction typically results from atresia of that segment of the bowel, usually caused by a vascular accident in utero.

III. Clinical presentation. Infants with jejunal obstruction usually have bilious vomiting associated with minimal abdominal distention, because few loops of intestine are involved in the obstructive process.

IV. Diagnosis. A plain **abdominal x-ray study** reveals only a few dilated small bowel loops with no gas distally.

V. Management. Surgical correction is required.

DISTAL INTESTINAL OBSTRUCTION

I. Definition. The term *distal intestinal obstruction* denotes partial or complete obstruction of the distal portion of the GI tract. It may be either small bowel (ileum) or large bowel obstruction. The list of causes includes the following:
  A. Ileal atresia.
  B. Meconium ileus
    1. **Uncomplicated (simple) obstruction of the terminal ileum** by pellets of inspissated meconium.
    2. **Complicated meconium ileus,** implying compromise of bowel viability either prenatally or postnatally.
  C. Colonic atresia.
  D. Meconium plug–hypoplastic left colon syndrome.
  E. Hirschsprung's disease (congenital aganglionic megacolon).

II. Clinical presentation. Infants with obstructing lesions in the distal intestine have similar signs and symptoms. They typically have distended abdomens, fail to pass meconium, and vomit bilious material.

III. Diagnosis
  A. Abdominal x-ray studies show multiple dilated loops of intestine; the site of obstruction (distal small bowel vs colon) cannot be determined on plain x-ray films.
  B. Contrast radiologic studies. The preferred diagnostic test is contrast enema. It may identify colonic atresia, outline microcolon (which may signify complete distal small bowel obstruction), or suggest a transition zone (which may signify Hirschsprung's disease). The procedure can identify and treat meconium plug–hypoplastic left colon syndrome. If the test is normal, ileal atresia, meconium ileus, and Hirschsprung's disease are possibilities.
  C. Sweat test. A sweat test may be needed to document cystic fibrosis in cases of meconium ileus (unlikely to be helpful in the first few weeks of life).
  D. Mucosal rectal biopsy for histologic detection of ganglion cells is the safest and most widely available screening test for Hirschsprung's disease. However, laparotomy is often necessary to determine the exact nature of the problem in infants with normal results of barium enema.

IV. Management
  A. Nonoperative management is "curative" in cases of meconium plug and hypoplastic left colon.
    1. **Passage of time and colonic stimulation by digital examination and rectal enemas** promote return of effective peristalsis.
    2. **In infants who achieve apparently normal bowel function,** one must rule out Hirschsprung's disease by mucosal rectal biopsy; a small percentage of patients with meconium plug will prove to have aganglionosis.
    3. **Interestingly, uncomplicated meconium ileus, if identified, can often be treated by nonoperative means.** Repeated enemas with Hypaque or acetylcysteine (Mucomyst) may disimpact the inspissated meconium in the terminal ileum and relieve the obstruction.
  B. Surgical therapy. Surgical intervention is required for atresia of the ileum or colon, for complicated meconium ileus, and when the diagnosis is in doubt.

Hirschsprung's disease is usually treated in the neonatal period by colostomy through ganglionic bowel. Some surgeons are performing "one-stage" pull-through procedures, without preliminary colostomy.

IMPERFORATE ANUS

I. **Definition.** Imperforate anus is the lack of an anal opening of proper location or size. There are two types: high and low.
   A. **High imperforate anus.** The rectum ends above the puborectalis sling, the main muscle responsible for maintaining fecal continence. There is never an associated fistula to the perineum. In males, there may be a rectourinary fistula, and in females, a rectovaginal fistula.
   B. **Low imperforate anus.** The rectum has traversed the puborectalis sling in the correct position. Variants include anal stenosis, imperforate anus with perineal fistula, and imperforate anus without fistula.
II. **Diagnosis** is by inspection and calibration of any perineal opening. All patients with imperforate anus should have x-ray studies of the lumbosacral spine and urinary tract because there is a high incidence of dysmorphism in these areas.
III. **Management.** Surgical therapy in the neonate consists of colostomy for high anomalies and perineal anoplasty or dilation of fistula for low lesions. If the level is not known, colostomy is preferable to blind exploration of the perineum. If colostomy is done, a contrast x-ray study of the distal limb should be performed to ascertain the level at which the rectum ends and to determine the presence or absence of an associated fistula.

CAUSES OF RESPIRATORY DISTRESS

CHOANAL ATRESIA

I. **Definition.** Choanal atresia is a congenital blockage of the posterior nares caused by persistence of a bony septum (90%) or a soft tissue membrane (10%).
II. **Pathophysiology.** Unilateral or bilateral obstruction at the posterior nares may be secondary to soft tissue or bone. Choanal atresia, which is complete and bilateral, is one of the causes of respiratory distress immediately after delivery. The effects of upper airway obstruction are compounded because neonates are obligate nose-breathers and will not "think" to breathe through the mouth.
III. **Clinical presentation.** Respiratory distress resulting from partial or total upper airway obstruction is the mode of presentation.
IV. **Diagnosis** is based on an **inability to pass a catheter into the nasopharynx via either side of the nose.**
V. **Management.** Simply making the infant cry and thereby breathe through the mouth will temporarily improve breathing. Insertion of an oral airway will maintain the ability to breathe until the atresia is surgically corrected.

PIERRE ROBIN SYNDROME

I. **Definition.** This anomaly consists of mandibular hypoplasia in association with cleft palate.
II. **Pathophysiology.** Airway obstruction is produced by posterior displacement of the tongue associated with the small size of the mandible.
III. **Clinical presentation.** Severity of symptoms varies, but most infants manifest a high degree of partial upper airway obstruction.
IV. **Management**
   A. **Infants with mild involvement** can be cared for in the prone position and fed through a special Breck nipple. Adjustment to the airway compromise will occur over days or weeks.

B. More severe cases require nasopharyngeal tubes or surgical procedures to hold the tongue in an anterior position. Tracheostomy is generally a last resort.

VASCULAR RING

Airway compromise is rarely severe and usually presents as stridor.

LARYNGOTRACHEAL ESOPHAGEAL CLEFT

I. **Definition.** Laryngotracheal esophageal cleft is a rare congenital anomaly in which there is incomplete separation of the larynx (and sometimes the trachea) from the esophagus, resulting in a common channel of esophagus and airway. This communication may be short or may extend almost the entire length of the trachea.

II. **Pathophysiology.** The persistent communication between the larynx (and occasionally a significant portion of the trachea) and the esophagus results in recurring symptoms of aspiration and respiratory distress with feeding.

III. **Clinical presentation.** Respiratory distress during feeding is the presenting symptom.

IV. **Diagnosis.** Contrast swallow may suggest the anomaly, but endoscopy is essential in firmly establishing the diagnosis and delineating the extent of the defect.

V. **Management.** Laryngotracheal esophageal cleft is treated by surgical correction, which is difficult and often unsuccessful.

H-TYPE TRACHEOESOPHAGEAL FISTULA

I. **Definition.** This anomaly is the third most common type of TEF, making up 5% of cases. Esophageal continuity is intact, but there is a fistulous communication between the posterior trachea and the anterior esophagus.

II. **Pathophysiology.** If the fistula is small, as is usually the case, "silent" aspiration occurs during feedings with resulting pneumonitis. If the fistula is unusually large, coughing and choking may accompany each feeding.

III. **Clinical presentation.** Symptoms, as noted previously, depend on the size of the fistula.

IV. **Diagnosis.** Barium swallow is the initial diagnostic study and may identify the fistula. The most accurate procedure, however, is bronchoscopy (perhaps combined with esophagoscopy); this should allow discovery and perhaps cannulation of the fistula.

V. **Management.** Surgical correction is required. The approach (via the neck or chest) is determined by location of the fistula.

INTRINSIC ABNORMALITIES OF THE AIRWAY

I. **Definition.** Abnormalities of, or within, the airway that cause partial obstruction fall into this category. Examples include laryngomalacia, paralyzed vocal cord, subglottic web, and hemangioma.

II. **Pathophysiology.** These lesions result in partial obstruction of the airway and cause stridor and respiratory distress of varying severity.

III. **Clinical presentation.** See section II: Pathophysiology.

IV. **Diagnosis.** The diagnosis is established by endoscopy of the airway.

V. **Management** is individualized. Some problems, such as laryngomalacia, will be outgrown if the child can be supported through the period of acute symptoms. Other lesions, such as subglottic webs, may be amenable to endoscopic resection or laser therapy.

CONGENITAL LOBAR EMPHYSEMA

I. **Definition.** *Lobar emphysema* is a term used to denote hyperexpansion of the air spaces of a segment or lobe of the lung.

II. Pathophysiology. Inspired air is trapped in an enclosed space. As the cyst of entrapped air enlarges, the normal lung is increasingly compressed. Cystic problems are more common in the upper lobes.

III. Clinical presentation. Small cysts may cause few or no symptoms and are readily seen on x-ray film. Giant cysts may cause significant respiratory distress, with mediastinal shift and compromise of the contralateral lung.

IV. Diagnosis. Usually, the cysts are easily seen on plain chest x-ray films. However, the radiologic findings may be confused with those of tension pneumothorax.

V. Management. Therapeutic options include observation for small asymptomatic cysts, repositioning of the endotracheal tube to selectively ventilate the uninvolved lung for 6–12 h, bronchoscopy for endobronchial lavage, and operative resection of the cyst with or without the segment or lobe from which it arises.

CYSTIC ADENOMATOID MALFORMATION

I. Definition. The term *cystic adenomatoid malformation* encompasses a spectrum of congenital pulmonary malformation involving varying degrees of adenomatosis and cyst formation.

II. Pathophysiology. Severity of symptoms is related to the amount of lung involved and particularly to the degree to which the normal ipsilateral and contralateral lung is compressed.

III. Clinical presentation. Signs of respiratory insufficiency such as tachypnea and cyanosis are modes of presentation.

IV. Diagnosis. The characteristic pattern on chest x-ray film is multiple discrete air bubbles, occasionally with air-fluid levels, involving a region of the lung. The radiographic appearance can mimic that of congenital diaphragmatic hernia (CDH).

V. Management. Treatment is surgical resection of the involved lung, allowing reexpansion of compressed normal pulmonary tissue.

CONGENITAL DIAPHRAGMATIC HERNIA

I. Definition. A patent pleuroperitoneal canal through the foramen of Bochdalek is the essential defect in CDH.

II. Pathophysiology

  A. Prenatal. The abnormal communication between the peritoneal and pleural cavities allows herniation of intestine into the pleural space as the developing GI tract returns from its extracoelomic phase at 10–12 weeks' gestation. Depending on the degree of pulmonary compression by herniated intestine, there may be marked diminution of bronchial branching, limited multiplication of alveoli, and persistence of muscular hypertrophy in pulmonary arterioles. These anatomic abnormalities are most notable on the side of the CDH (usually the left); they are also present to some degree in the contralateral lung.

  B. Postnatal. After delivery, the anatomic anomaly may contribute to the development of either or both of the following pathologic conditions:

  1. Pulmonary parenchymal insufficiency. Infants with CDH have an abnormally small functional lung mass. Some have so few conducting air passages and developed alveoli—a condition known as *pulmonary parenchymal insufficiency*—that survival is unlikely.

  2. Pulmonary hypertension. Infants with CDH are predisposed anatomically to pulmonary hypertension of the newborn (PHN), also known as persistent fetal circulation (PFC). In this condition, blood is shunted around the lungs through the foramen ovale and patent ductus arteriosus. Shunting promotes acidosis and hypoxia, both of which are potent stimuli to additional pulmonary vasoconstriction. Thus, a vicious cycle of clinical deterioration is established.

III. Clinical presentation. Most infants with CDH exhibit significant respiratory distress within the first few hours of life.

IV. Diagnosis. Prenatal diagnosis can reliably be made by ultrasonography. Delivery should occur in a neonatal center with extracorporeal membrane oxygenation (ECMO) capability. Afflicted infants tend to have scaphoid abdomens because there is a paucity of the GI tract located in the abdomen. Auscultation reveals diminished breath sounds on the affected side. Diagnosis is established by a chest x-ray film that reveals a bowel gas pattern in one hemithorax, with shift of mediastinal structures to the other side and compromise of the contralateral lung.

V. Management

A. **Indwelling arterial catheter.** Blood gas levels should be monitored by an indwelling arterial catheter.

B. **Supportive care.** Appropriate respiratory and metabolic support should be provided. CDH lungs are surfactant deficient, and replacement therapy appears to be helpful. Avoidance of aggressive conventional hyperventilation, permissive hypercapnia, seems to improve survival and decrease complications.

C. **Nasogastric intubation** should be performed to lessen gaseous distention of the stomach and intestine. For the same reason, any positive-pressure ventilation must be delivered by endotracheal tube, never by mask.

D. **Surgical correction** is by reduction of intrathoracic intestine and closure of the diaphragmatic defect. Surgical intervention is obviously an essential element of treatment, but it is not the key to survival. Formerly, surgery was performed on an urgent or emergent basis. Current thinking favors a delayed approach, allowing the newborn to stabilize a hyperreactive pulmonary vascular bed and to improve pulmonary compliance. If indicated, ECMO can be instituted and repair performed while on support 1 or 2 days after decannulation.

E. **ECMO** is used in the treatment of neonates with severe respiratory failure. Exposure of venous blood to the extracorporeal circuit allows correction of Po_2 and Pco_2 abnormalities as well as recovery of the lungs from the trauma associated with positive-pressure ventilation (see Chapter 11).

VI. Prognosis. Mortality rates for infants with CDH are still in the range of 50%. This high rate has prompted a search for other modes of treatment in addition to the expensive, labor-intensive modality ECMO.

A. **Fetal surgery** has been performed successfully on a limited basis, with the idea that in utero intervention will lessen the risk for development of pulmonary hypoplasia, which may be incompatible with life after delivery. Formal operative correction of CDH in the fetus has been abandoned, but several centers currently perform in utero tracheal occlusion in selected patients. This appears to result in increased lung fluid and to promote pulmonary growth.

B. **Medications.** Another major area of research is the attempt to develop a pharmacologic agent to selectively decrease pulmonary vascular resistance. Such an agent would help solve the problem of PHN (PFC).

ABDOMINAL MASSES

RENAL MASSES

In most clinical series, the majority of abdominal masses in neonates are renal in origin. They may be unilateral or bilateral, solid or cystic. After physical examination, evaluation begins with ultrasonography, which is simple and safe to perform. Ultrasonography should define the solid or cystic nature of the mass, determine the presence or absence of normal kidneys, and yield information on other intra-abdominal abnormalities. In selected instances, more involved procedures such as renal scan, computed tomography (CT) scan, retrograde pyelography, venography, and arteriography may be needed to define the problem and plan appropriate therapy.

I. **Multicystic kidney** is a form of renal dysplasia and the most common renal cystic disease of the newborn. Fortunately, it is usually unilateral. Ultrasonography can define the nature of the disorder, and CT/nuclear renal scans are useful in assessing the remainder of the urinary system. Nephrectomy is appropriate treatment.

II. Hydronephrosis. Urinary obstruction, depending on its location, can cause unilateral or bilateral flank and abdominal masses. Treatment is by correction of the obstructing lesion or decompression proximal to it. A kidney rendered nonfunctional by back pressure is usually best removed. Obstructive uropathy may be one category of lesion suitable for in utero intervention. Surgery on the developing fetus to decompress the obstructed urinary system may improve the postnatal status and increase survival.

III. Infantile polycystic kidney disease. Inherited in an autosomal recessive fashion, this entity involves both kidneys and carries a grim prognosis.

IV. Renal vein thrombosis. The typical presentation is one or more flank masses and hematuria, usually within the first 3 days of life. Risk factors are maternal diabetes and dehydration. In general, conservative nonoperative management is recommended.

V. Wilms' tumor. See p 580.

OVARIAN MASSES

Simple ovarian cyst has been called the most frequently palpated abdominal mass in the female neonate. It presents as a relatively mobile, smooth-walled abdominal mass. It is not associated with cancer, and excision with preservation of any ovarian tissue is curative.

HEPATIC MASSES

The liver can be enlarged, often to grotesque proportions, by a variety of problems. When physical examination, ultrasonography, and other x-ray studies suggest hepatic origin, CT or angiography should be performed. These studies may be diagnostic and will aid in surgical planning. Lesions include the following:

I. Hepatic cysts.

II. Solid, benign tumors.

III. Vascular tumors

    A. Hemangiomas of the liver may cause heart failure, thrombocytopenia, and anemia. Therapeutic options include digitalis, corticosteroid administration, embolization, hepatic artery ligation, and liver resection.

    B. Hemangioendothelioma.

IV. Malignant tumors. Hepatoblastoma is by far the most common liver cancer in the neonate. Serum alpha-fetoprotein may be elevated. Although surgical resection remains the key to achieving cure, new chemotherapeutic protocols (cisplatin [Platinol] and doxorubicin [Adriamycin]) may significantly improve the formerly dismal prognosis for infants with this tumor.

GASTROINTESTINAL MASSES

Palpable abdominal masses that arise from the GI tract are unusual and tend to be cystic, smooth walled, and mobile (depending on the size). Causes include intestinal duplication and mesenteric cyst.

RETROPERITONEAL TUMORS

NEUROBLASTOMA

I. Definition. Neuroblastoma is a primitive malignant neoplasm that arises from neural crest tissue. It is probably the most common congenital tumor and is usually located in the adrenal gland.

II. Clinical presentation. This tumor typically presents as a firm, fixed, irregular mass extending obliquely from the costal margin, occasionally across the midline and into the lower abdomen.

III. Diagnosis

   A. Laboratory studies. A 24-h urine collection should be analyzed for vanillylmandelic acid and other metabolites.

   B. Radiologic studies. A plain abdominal x-ray film may reveal calcification within the tumor. Intravenous pyelogram (IVP) and CT scan typically show extrinsic compression and inferolateral displacement of the kidney. Search for possible metastatic deposits involves bone marrow aspiration and biopsy, bone scan, chest x-ray study, and chest CT scan.

IV. Management. Planned therapy should take into account the well-recognized but poorly understood fact that neuroblastoma is notably less aggressive in the young infant than in the older child.

WILMS' TUMOR (NEPHROBLASTOMA)

I. Definition. Wilms' tumor is an embryonal renal neoplasm in which blastemic, stromal, and epithelial cell types are present. Renal involvement is usually unilateral but may be bilateral (5% of cases).

II. Clinical presentation. A palpable abdominal mass extending from beneath the costal margin is the usual mode of presentation.

III. Risk factors include aniridia, hemihypertrophy, certain genitourinary anomalies, and a family history of nephroblastoma.

IV. Diagnosis

   A. Laboratory studies. There is no tumor marker for Wilms' tumor.

   B. Radiologic studies. Ultrasonography is generally followed by CT scan, which reveals intrinsic distortion of the caliceal system of the involved kidney. The possibility of tumor thrombus in the renal vein and inferior vena cava should be evaluated by ultrasonography and venography, if necessary.

V. Management

   A. Unilateral renal involvement. Nephrectomy is the first step in treatment. Surgical staging determines the administration of radiotherapy and chemotherapy; both are very effective.

   B. Bilateral renal involvement. Treatment of bilateral Wilms' tumor is highly individualized.

TERATOMA

I. Definition. Teratoma is a neoplasm containing elements derived from all three germ cell layers: endoderm, mesoderm, and ectoderm. Teratomas in the neonate are primarily sacrococcygeal in location and are believed to represent a type of abortive caudal twinning.

II. Clinical presentation. This tumor is usually grossly evident as a large external mass in the sacrococcygeal area. Occasionally, however, it may be presacral and retroperitoneal in location and may present as an abdominal mass.

III. Diagnosis. See section II: Clinical Presentation. Digital rectal examination of the presacral space is important.

IV. Management. Because the incidence of malignancy in these tumors increases with age, prompt surgical excision is required.

ABDOMINAL WALL DEFECTS

GASTROSCHISIS

I. Definition. Gastroschisis is a centrally located, full-thickness abdominal wall defect with two distinctive anatomic features.

   A. The extruded intestine never has a protective sac covering it.

B. **The umbilical cord is an intact structure** at the level of the abdominal skin, just to the left of the defect. Typically, the opening in the abdominal wall is 2–4 cm in diameter, and the solid organs (the liver and spleen) reside in the peritoneal cavity.

II. **Pathophysiology.** Exposure of unprotected intestine to irritating amniotic fluid in utero results in its edematous, indurated, foreshortened appearance. Because of these intestinal abnormalities, development of appropriate peristalsis and effective absorption is significantly delayed, usually by several weeks. Fortunately, associated congenital anomalies are rare in patients with gastroschisis.

III. **Clinical presentation.** See sections I, Definition, and II, Pathophysiology.

IV. **Diagnosis.** The key differential diagnosis is ruptured omphalocele, although the diagnosis is readily apparent in most cases. Increasingly, prenatal ultrasonography identifies gastroschisis.

V. **Management**
   A. **General considerations.** All agree that infants with gastroschisis should be delivered at a neonatal center equipped and staffed to provide definitive care. Less certain is the recommended mode of delivery. Some experts argue that abdominal wall defect is an indication for cesarean section. However, other investigators note that, in the absence of other factors, vaginal delivery does not increase the mortality, morbidity, or length of hospital stay for newborns with gastroschisis.
   B. **Specific measures**
      1. **Temperature regulation.** Immediate attention should be directed toward maintenance of normal body temperature. The tremendous intestinal surface area exposed to the environment puts these infants at great risk for hypothermia.
      2. **Protective covering.** It is best not to keep replacing moist, saline-soaked gauze over the exposed intestine because doing so promotes evaporative heat loss. It is better to apply a dry (or moist) protective dressing and then wrap the abdomen in layers of cellophane. A warm, controlled environment should be provided.
      3. **Nasogastric decompression** is helpful.
      4. **Broad-spectrum antibiotic coverage** is appropriate, given the unavoidable contamination.
      5. **Total parenteral nutrition.** A protracted ileus is to be expected, and appropriate intravenous nutritional support must be provided.
      6. **Surgical correction.** As soon as the infant's condition permits, operative correction should be undertaken. Complete reduction of herniated intestine, with primary closure of the abdominal wall, or placement of unreduced intestine in a protective prosthetic silo, with subsequent staged reduction over 7–14 days, is usually performed.

OMPHALOCELE

I. **Definition.** An omphalocele is a herniation of abdominal contents into the base of the umbilical cord. The gross appearance of omphalocele differs from that of gastroschisis in two important respects.
   A. **A protective membrane encloses the malpositioned abdominal contents** (unless rupture has occurred, eg, during the birth process).
   B. **Elements of the umbilical cord course individually over the sac and come together at its apex to form a normal-appearing umbilical cord.**

II. **Associated anomalies.** Significant associated congenital anomalies occur in ~25–40% of infants with omphalocele. Problems include chromosomal abnormalities, CDH, and a variety of cardiac defects.

III. **Clinical presentation.** There are different sizes of omphaloceles. The smaller ones typically contain only intestine; large or giant omphaloceles contain liver and spleen as well as the GI tract. The peritoneal cavity in infants with large or giant

omphaloceles is very small because growth has proceeded without the solid organs in proper position.
IV. Diagnosis. The anomaly is usually apparent. Ruptured omphalocele may be confused with gastroschisis; both defects are characterized by exposed intestine, but infants with omphalocele do not possess an intact umbilical cord at the level of the abdominal wall to the left of the defect. Careful studies to identify associated congenital anomalies should be performed.
V. Management. Reduction, even in stages over a lengthy period, may be very difficult to achieve. Therapeutically, infants with omphalocele fall into two main groups.
   A. Ruptured sac. Infants with ruptured sacs resemble those with gastroschisis. The unprotected intestine should be cared for as described for gastroschisis (see Abdominal Wall Defects, Gastroschisis, section V,B,2, p 581), and the problem should be corrected surgically on an emergent basis.
   B. Intact sac. Intact omphalocele is a less urgent surgical problem. The protective membrane conserves heat and in most cases allows effective peristalsis. This sac should be carefully protected. Some surgeons favor daily dressing changes with gauze pads impregnated with povidone-iodine until the sac toughens and desiccates. The timing of surgery is influenced by a number of factors, including the dimensions of the defect, size of the infant, and presence of other anomalies. Nonoperative staged reduction using compressive dressings has been described.

EXSTROPHY OF THE BLADDER

I. Definition. Exstrophy of the bladder is a congenital malformation of the lower anterior abdominal wall. In this defect, the internal surface of the posterior wall of the urinary bladder extrudes through the abdominal wall defect. The problem occurs in varying degrees of severity, ranging from epispadias to complete extroversion of the bladder, with exposure of the ureteral orifices.
II. Clinical presentation. The lower abdominal wall defect is obvious; exposed bladder mucosa is markedly edematous and friable.
III. Diagnosis. Diagnosis is by inspection. Radiologic evaluation of the proximal urinary tract is advisable.
IV. Management
   A. Protective covering. The bladder should be carefully protected with Vaseline gauze or cellophane wrap. Attention should also be paid to protection of the surrounding skin.
   B. Surgical repair. In most centers, primary closure of the bladder is attempted within the first 48–72 h of life, while the sacroiliac joints are still pliable and the pelvis can be "molded" to allow better approximation of the pubic rami.

CLOACAL EXSTROPHY

I. Definition. Cloacal exstrophy is a rare but devastating complex of anomalies, including imperforate anus, exstrophy of the bladder, omphalocele, and vesicointestinal fistula, frequently with prolapse of bowel through the fistula onto the bladder mucosa.
II. Clinical presentation. See section I: Definition.
III. Diagnosis. Diagnosis is by inspection. Evaluation of the genitourinary system and GI tract is appropriate.
IV. Management
   A. Protective covering. Exposed mucosa, both bladder and intestine, should be protected with Vaseline gauze or cellophane wrap. Ointments should be applied to the surrounding skin to prevent maceration.
   B. Surgical care. Prompt surgery to separate the fecal and urinary streams is imperative.

MISCELLANEOUS SURGICAL CONDITIONS

NECROTIZING ENTEROCOLITIS

In most centers, necrotizing enterocolitis (NEC) is the most common indication for operation in neonates (see also Chapter 71). Abdominal exploration is usually reserved for infants with full-thickness necrosis of the intestine, usually manifested by pneumoperitoneum (best identified by serial left lateral decubitus x-ray films). Other, less common indications for surgery include cellulitis and induration of the abdominal wall and an unchanging abdominal mass. Delayed stricture formation, which is most common on the left side of the colon, complicates NEC in 15–25% of cases.

HYPOSPADIAS

I. **Definition.** Hypospadias is a developmental anomaly in which the external opening of the urethra is present on the underside of the penis or on the perineum rather than in its normal position at the end of the penile shaft.
II. **Clinical presentation.** There are different anatomic classifications, depending on the location of the meatal opening and the degree of chordee (curvature of the penis). There is a high incidence of associated cryptorchidism in these patients. Severe cases of hypospadias may be confused with ambiguous genitalia.
III. **Diagnosis.** The anomaly is readily apparent (see sections I, Definition, and II, Clinical Presentation). Radiologic evaluation of the urinary system is appropriate to screen for other anomalies.
IV. **Management.** Surgical correction usually should not be attempted in the newborn. Because foreskin tissue may be needed for later surgical correction, **circumcision must be avoided in infants with hypospadias.**

INGUINAL HERNIA AND HYDROCELE

I. **Definition.** Persistence of a patent processus vaginalis (related to testicular descent) is responsible for inguinal hernia and hydrocele in the neonate.
   A. **Inguinal hernia.** The opening of the patent processus at the internal ring is large enough to allow a loop of intestine to extrude from the abdominal cavity with an increase in intra-abdominal pressure.
   B. **Hydrocele.** The patent processus is too narrow to permit egress of intestine; peritoneal fluid drips down along the course of the narrow patent processus and accumulates in the scrotum.
II. **Diagnosis**
   A. **Inguinal hernias** tend to present as lumps or bulges that come and go at the pubic tubercle. Less commonly, they descend into the scrotum.
   B. **Hydroceles** typically are scrotal in location, transilluminate, and are not reducible.
III. **Management**
   A. **Inguinal hernia** carries a 5–15% risk of incarceration during the first year of life. Accordingly, they are usually surgically repaired when the infant's general medical condition permits.
   B. **Hydrocele** frequently resolves without specific treatment because the obliteration of the narrow patent processus continues after birth. Persistence of hydrocele beyond 6–12 months is an indication for surgical repair.

UMBILICAL HERNIA

I. **Definition.** This hernia is a skin-covered fascial defect at the umbilicus that allows protrusion of intra-abdominal content.
II. **Diagnosis.** Transmission of intra-abdominal pressure via fascial defect at the umbilicus establishes the diagnosis.

III. Management. In infancy, surgical intervention for an umbilical hernia is seldom warranted. Complications such as incarceration and skin breakdown are exceedingly rare. The natural history is one of gradual closure of the umbilical fascial defect, often leading to complete resolution of the problem.

UNDESCENDED TESTICLES (CRYPTORCHIDISM)

Undescended testicles occur in ~33% of premature and 3% of term male infants. Many undescended testes will descend in the first few months after birth. Unless there is an associated inguinal hernia, surgical correction is usually not performed until the infant is between 1 and 2 years of age, although some surgeons favor earlier correction.

POSTERIOR URETHRAL VALVES

I. Definition. Posterior urethral valves are abnormal valves in the urethra at the verumontanum. They represent the most common cause of congenital obstructive uropathy in males.

II. Pathophysiology. The high degree of bladder outlet obstruction caused by posterior urethral valves results in proximal dilatation. The urinary bladder enlarges, the ureters become dilated and tortuous, and back pressure in the collecting systems compromises developing renal parenchyma.

III. Clinical presentation

   A. Prenatal ultrasonography currently identifies many infants with posterior urethral valves.

   B. After birth, neonates with this anomaly have bilateral flank masses, a distended bladder, and poor urinary stream (with dribbling).

IV. Diagnosis. Voiding cystourethrography documents the abnormal valves.

V. Management. The goal of therapy is preservation of renal function and avoidance of renal failure.

   A. Renal function and the infant's general status should be evaluated.

   B. Stabilization, rehydration, correction of electrolyte abnormalities, and treatment of urinary tract infection should be accompanied by transurethral drainage of the bladder, using a No. 5 French infant feeding tube.

   C. Surgical therapy

   1. **Ablation of valves** is the initial operative procedure favored by most pediatric urologists.

   2. **Urinary diversion** may be indicated.

REFERENCES

Albanese CT (ed): Abdominal masses in the newborn. *Semin Pediatr Surg* 2000;9:107.

Bianchi A: One stage neonatal reconstruction without stoma for Hirschsprung's disease. *Semin Pediatr Surg* 1998;7:170.

Chwals WJ et al: Surgery-associated complications in necrotizing enterocolitis: a multiinstitutional study. *J Pediatr Surg* 2001;36:1722.

Dimmitt RA et al: Venoarterial versus venovenous extracorporeal membrane oxygenation in congenital diaphragmatic hernia: the extracorporeal life support organization registry, 1990–1999. *J Pediatr Surg* 2001;36:1199.

Greenholz SK: Congenital diaphragmatic hernia: an overview. *Semin Pediatr Surg* 1996;5:216.

Langer JC: Gastroschisis and omphalocele. *Semin Pediatr Surg* 1996;5:124.

Moss RL et al: A meta-analysis of peritoneal drainage versus laparotomy for perforated necrotizing enterocolitis. *J Pediatr Surg* 2001;36:1210.

Nuchtern JG, Harberg FJ: Congenital lung cysts. *Semin Pediatr Surg* 1994;3:233.

O'Neill JA et al (eds): *Pediatric Surgery*, 5th ed. Mosby-Year Book, 1998.

Pena A: Imperforate anus and other hindgut malformations. *Semin Pediatr Surg* 1997;6:165.

Wong JT et al: Congenital diaphragmatic hernia: survival treated with very delayed surgery, spontaneous respiration and no chest tube. *J Pediatr Surg* 1995;30:406.

79 Thyroid Disorders

Disorders of thyroid function in infants often present a diagnostic dilemma. Signs of thyroid dysfunction are rarely present at birth, and initial signs and symptoms are often subtle or misleading. A good understanding of the unique thyroid physiology and the assessment of thyroid function in neonates is necessary in order to recognize, diagnose, and treat thyroid disorders.

GENERAL CONSIDERATIONS

I. **Fetal and neonatal thyroid function**
   A. **Embryogenesis** begins during the third week of gestation and continues through 10–12 weeks' gestation. At that time, thyroid-stimulating hormone (TSH) can be detected. Thyroid activity remains low until midgestation and then increases slowly until term.
   B. **Thyroid hormones** undergo rapid and dramatic changes in the immediate postnatal period.
      1. **An acute release of TSH occurs within minutes after birth.** Peak values of 60–80 µU/mL are seen at 30–90 min. Levels decrease to <5 µU/mL by 3–5 days.
      2. **Stimulated by the TSH surge,** thyroxine (T_4), free T_4 (FT_4), and triiodothyronine (T_3) rapidly increase, reaching peak levels by 24 h. Levels decrease slowly over the first few weeks of life.
   C. **Thyroid function in the premature infant.** Identical changes in TSH, T_4, and T_3 are seen in premature infants; however, absolute values are lower. TSH levels return to normal by 3–5 days of life regardless of gestational age.
II. **Physiologic action of thyroid hormones.** Thyroid hormones have profound effects on growth and neurologic development. They also influence O_2 consumption, thermogenesis, and the metabolic rate of many processes.
III. **Biochemical steps to thyroid hormone synthesis.** Thyroid hormone production includes the stages of iodide transport, thyroglobulin synthesis, organization of iodide, monoiodotyrosine and diiodotyrosine coupling, thyroglobulin endocytosis, proteolysis, and deiodination.
IV. **Assessment of thyroid function.** Thyroid tests are intended to measure the level of thyroid activity and to identify the cause of thyroid dysfunction.
   A. **T_4 concentration** is the most important parameter in the evaluation of thyroid function. More than 99% of T_4 is bound to thyroid hormone–binding proteins. Therefore, changes in these proteins may affect T_4 levels. Serum levels for term newborn infants range between 7.3 and 22.9 mcg/dL.
   B. **Free T_4** reflects the availability of thyroid hormone to the tissues. Serum levels vary widely by gestational age: newborn term infants, 2.0–5.3 ng/dL; preterm infants of 31–36 weeks' gestation, 1.3–4.7 ng/dL; and infants of 25–30 weeks' gestation, 0.6–3.3 ng/dL.
   C. **TSH measurement** is one of the most valuable tests in evaluating thyroid disorders, particularly primary hyperthyroidism. Serum levels over all gestational ages of 25–42 weeks range from 2.5 to 18.0 µU/mL.
   D. **T_3 concentration** is particularly useful in the diagnosis and treatment of hyperthyroidism. Serum levels of T_3 are very low in the fetus and cord blood samples (20–75 ng/dL). Shortly after birth, levels exceed 100 ng/dL, up to 260 ng/dL. In hyperthyroid states, levels may exceed 400 ng/dL. In sick preterm infants, a very low T_3 (hypothyroid range) may signal the euthyroid sick syndrome, also known as the nonthyroidal illness syndrome.

E. **Thyroid-binding globulin (TBG)** can be measured directly by radioimmunoassay. T_3 resin uptake provides an indirect measurement of TBG and is now considered an outdated test, unless it is factored with the T_4 level to give an FT_4 index, using the infant's T_4 level and T_3 uptake against a normal control T_3 uptake. TBG may be decreased in preterm infants, in those with malnutrition, and in those with chronic illness. It is increased by estrogens and heroin. Drugs such as Dilantin (phenytoin), diazepam, heparin, and furosemide compete with T_4 for TBG binding sites, resulting in falsely low T_4 levels.

F. **The thyrotropin-releasing hormone (TRH) stimulation test** can assess pituitary and thyroid responsiveness. It is used to differentiate between secondary and tertiary hypothyroidism.

G. **Thyroid imaging**
  1. **Thyroid scanning** with iodine 123 or technetium Tc 99m pertechnetate is used to identify functional thyroid tissue. Iodine 123 is the preferable isotope for children.
  2. **Ultrasonography** is useful in evaluating anatomy but is not a reliable alternative to a scan.

CONGENITAL HYPOTHYROIDISM

I. **Definition.** Congenital hypothyroidism is defined as a significant decrease in, or the absence of, thyroid function present at birth.

II. **Incidence.** The overall incidence is 1 in 3500 to 1 in 4500 births. Sporadic cases account for 85% of patients diagnosed; 15% are hereditary. It is more prevalent among females than males by a ratio of 2:1. It is more common in Hispanic and Asian infants (1 in 3000 births) and less common in blacks (1 in 32,000 births). The incidence is significantly increased in Down syndrome (1 in 140).

III. **Etiologic classification**
  A. **Primary hypothyroidism**
    1. Developmental defects such as ectopic thyroid (most common), thyroid hypoplasia, or agenesis.
    2. Inborn errors of thyroid hormone synthesis.
    3. Maternal exposure to radioiodine, propylthiouracil, or methimazole during pregnancy.
    4. Iodine deficiency (endemic cretinism).
  B. **Secondary hypothyroidism:** TSH deficiency.
  C. **Tertiary hypothyroidism:** TRH deficiency.
  D. **Hypopituitary hypothyroidism:** associated with other hormonal deficiencies.

IV. **Molecular pathogenesis.** Autosomal recessive inheritance of mutations of thyroid peroxidase, thyroglobulin, NIS (sodium iodide symporter) and pendrin genes, all encoding for sodium iodide transporters, have been identified in patients with congenital hypothyroidism. The autosomal recessively inherited thyroid-stimulating receptor gene has been identified in patients with congenital hypothyroidism and thyroid hypoplasia, as have autosomal dominant mutations of the *PAX-8* gene and genes coding for other transcription factors in thyroid dysgenesis.

V. **Clinical presentation.** Symptoms are usually absent at birth; however, subtle signs may be detected during the first few weeks of life.
  A. **Early manifestations.** Signs at birth include prolonged gestation, large size for gestational age, large fontanelles, and respiratory distress syndrome. Manifestations that may be seen by 2 weeks include hypotonia, lethargy, hypothermia, prolonged jaundice, and feeding difficulty.
  B. **Late manifestation.** Classic features usually appear after 6 weeks and include puffy eyelids, coarse hair, large tongue, myxedema, and hoarse cry.

Late manifestations in borderline hypothyroidism detected in screening programs can present as significant hearing impairment with speech delays.

VI. Diagnosis

A. Screening. Newborn screening for congenital hypothyroidism is mandatory in most states.

1. **Method.** Most programs use a twofold process with the filter paper spot technique. A T_4 measurement is followed by a measurement of TSH in specimens with low T_4 values (T_4 in the 10th percentile).

2. **Timing.** The ideal time for screening is between days 2 and 6 of life. Infants discharged before 48 h should be screened before discharge; however, this increases the number of false-positive results because of the TSH surge that occurs at birth. A repeat test at 2 to 6 weeks identifies about 10% of cases.

3. **Results.** A low T_4 level (<7 mcg/dL) and TSH concentrations >40 μU/mL are indicative of congenital hypothyroidism. Borderline TSH levels (20–40 μU/mL) should be repeated.

B. Diagnostic studies

1. **Serum** for confirmatory measurements of T_4 and TSH concentrations should be tested. If an abnormality of TBG is suspected, FT_4 and TBG concentrations should also be evaluated.

2. **Thyroid scan** remains the most accurate diagnostic modality to determine the cause of congenital hypothyroidism.

VII. Management

A. Consultation with a pediatric endocrinologist is recommended.

B. Treatment. Sodium L-thyroxine is the drug of choice because of its uniform potency and reliable absorption. The average starting dose is 10–15 mcg/kg/ day. Usually, term infants receive a 50-μg tablet daily; preterm infants, 25 mcg daily. The goal of therapy is to maintain T_4 concentration in the upper normal range (10–16 mcg/dL) and TSH <10 μU/mL.

C. Follow-up. Frequent T_4 and TSH measurements are required to ensure optimal treatment. Recommended follow-up is as follows:

1. **At 2 and 4 weeks** after initiation of therapy.

2. **Every 1–2 months** for the first year.

3. **Two weeks** after changing dosage.

VIII. Prognosis. Prognosis is dependent on prudent initiation of therapy and subsequent management in an effort to mitigate the deficits in neurocognitive areas.

NEONATAL THYROTOXICOSIS

I. Definition. Neonatal thyrotoxicosis is defined as a hypermetabolic state resulting from excessive thyroid hormone activity in the newborn.

II. Causes

1. This disorder usually results from transplacental passage of thyroid-stimulating immunoglobulin from a mother with Graves' disease.

2. Congenital non-autoimmune hyperthyroidism has been identified, resulting from activating mutations in the thyrotropin receptor as well as stimulatory G protein.

III. Incidence. This is a rare disorder occurring in only ~1 of 70 thyrotoxic pregnancies (autoimmune disease). (The incidence of maternal thyrotoxicosis in pregnancy is 1–2 per 1000 pregnancies.)

IV. Clinical presentation. Fetal tachycardia in the third trimester may be the first manifestation. Signs are usually apparent within hours after birth unless the mother was taking antithyroid medications, in which case the presentation may be delayed 2–10 days. Thyrotoxic signs include irritability, tachycardia, flushing, tremor, poor weight gain, thrombocytopenia, and arrhythmias. A goiter is usually present and may be large enough to cause tracheal compression.

V. Diagnosis
  A. History and physical examination. A maternal history of Graves' disease and the presence of a goiter are most consistent with thyrotoxicosis.
  B. Laboratory studies. Diagnosis is confirmed by demonstrating increased levels of T_4, FT_4, and T_3 with suppressed levels of TSH.
VI. Management. Although the disorder is usually self-limited, therapy depends on the severity of the symptoms.
  A. Mild. Close observation is required. Therapy is not necessary.
  B. Moderate. Administer one of the following antithyroid medications:
    1. Lugol's solution (iodine), 1 drop every 8 h.
    2. Propylthiouracil, 5–10 mg/kg/day in 3 divided doses.
    3. Methimazole, 0.5–1 mg/kg/day in 3 divided doses.
  C. Severe. In addition to the medications just listed, during extreme conditions, prednisone, 2 mg/kg/day; propranolol, 1–2 mg/kg/day in 2–4 divided doses; and digitalis (in preventing cardiovascular collapse) may be used.
  D. Non-autoimmune hyperthyroidism requires thyroid gland ablation or near-total thyroidectomy.
VII. Prognosis. The disorder is usually self-limited and disappears spontaneously within 2–4 months. Mortality in affected infants is ~15% if the disorder is not recognized and treated properly.

TRANSIENT DISORDERS OF THYROID FUNCTION IN THE NEWBORN

I. Euthyroid sick syndrome
  A. Definition. Transient alteration in thyroid function associated with severe nonthyroidal illness.
  B. Incidence. The syndrome is frequently seen in premature infants because of their increased susceptibility to neonatal morbidity. Preterm infants with respiratory distress syndrome have been the most frequently reported patients with this disorder.
  C. Diagnosis. A low T_3 level is usually present, associated with low or normal T_4 and normal TSH. Infants are euthyroid (normal TSH).
  D. Treatment. Treatment has not been shown to be beneficial. Abnormal thyroid functions return to normal as the sick infant improves.
II. Transient hypothyroxinemia
  A. Incidence. All preterm infants have some degree of hypothyroxinemia (>50% have T_4 levels <6.5 mcg/dL).
  B. Pathophysiology. The condition is presumed to be related to immaturity of the hypothalamic-pituitary axis.
  C. Diagnosis is low T_4 and FT_4 with normal TSH and normal response to the TRH stimulation test.
  D. Treatment. No treatment is required. This disorder corrects spontaneously with progressive maturation, usually in 4–8 weeks. Attempts to supplement preterm infants born before 30 weeks' gestation with thyroxine to improve neurologic outcome have been unsuccessful.

REFERENCES

Adams L et al: Reference ranges for newer thyroid function tests in pre-mature infants. *J Pediatr* 1995;126:122.
American Academy of Pediatrics, Section on Endocrinology and Committee on Genetics, American Thyroid Association, Committee on Public Health: Newborn screening for congenital hypothyroidism: recommended guidelines. *Pediatrics* 1993;9:1203.
Biswas S et al: Thyroid function in very preterm infants. *Pediatrics* 2002;2:222.
Fisher DA: Thyroid function in premature infants. The hypothyroxinemia of prematurity. *Clin Perinatol* 1998;25:999.

Hunter MK et al: Follow-up of newborns with low thyroxine and nonelevated thyroid-stimulating hormone-screening concentrations: results of the 20-year experience in the Northwest Regional Newborn Screening Program. *J Pediatr* 1998;132:70.

Krude H et al: Molecular pathogenesis of neonatal hypothyroidism. *Horm Res* 2000;53(suppl 1):12.

LaFranchi S: Congenital hypothyroidism: etiologies, diagnosis, and management *Thyroid* 1999; 9:735.

Osborn DA: Thyroid hormone for preventing of neurodevelopmental impairment in preterm infants. *Cochrane Database Syst Rev* 2001;4:CD001070.

Polk DH, Fisher DA: Fetal and neonatal thyroid physiology. In Polin RA, Fox WW (eds): *Fetal and Neonatal Physiology*, 2nd ed, vol 2. Saunders, 1998.

Rose SR: Metabolic and endocrine disorders. In Fanaroff AA, Martin RJ (eds): *Neonatal-Perinatal Medicine—Diseases of the Fetus and Infant*, 7th ed. Mosby-Year Book, 2002.

Rovet J et al: Long-term sequelae of hearing impairment in congenital hypothyroidism. *J Pediatr* 1996;128:776.

Skuza K et al: Prediction of neonatal hyperthyroidism in infants born to mothers with Graves' disease. *J Pediatr* 1996;128:264.

Zimmerman D: Fetal and neonatal Hyperthyroidism. *Thyroid* 1999;9:727.

80 Commonly Used Medications

Acetaminophen (APAP) (Liquiprin, Tempra, Tylenol)
INDICATIONS AND USE: Analgesic-antipyretic.
ACTIONS: Mechanism of analgesic effect is unclear. Reduction of fever is produced by direct action on the hypothalamic heat-regulating center.
SUPPLIED: Suppositories, elixir, liquid, drops (preferred).
ROUTE: PO, PR.
DOSAGE: 5–10 mg/kg/dose q4–6h as needed.
ADVERSE EFFECTS: Hepatic necrosis with overdosage, rash, fever, and blood dyscrasias (neutropenia, pancytopenia, leukopenia, and thrombocytopenia). May be hepatotoxic with chronic use.

Acetazolamide (Diamox)
INDICATIONS AND USE: For use as a mild diuretic or as an anticonvulsant in refractory neonatal seizures. To decrease cerebrospinal fluid (CSF) production in posthemorrhagic hydrocephalus; also used in the treatment of renal tubular acidosis.
ACTIONS: Carbonic anhydrase inhibitor. Appears to retard abnormal discharge from central nervous system (CNS) neurons. Beneficial effects may be related to direct inhibition of carbonic anhydrase or may be due to the acidosis produced. Also produces urinary alkalosis, useful in the treatment of renal tubular acidosis.
SUPPLIED: Injection, tablets. (Suspension can be compounded by the pharmacist.)
ROUTE: IV, PO.
DOSAGE:

- Diuretic: 5 mg/kg/dose qd–qod.
- Anticonvulsant: 8–30 mg/kg/day PO divided q6–8h.
- To alkalinize urine: 5 mg/kg/dose 2–3 times over 24 h.
- To decrease CSF production: 50–100 mg/kg/day divided q6–8h.

ELIMINATION: Unchanged in urine. Half-life is 4–10 h.
ADVERSE EFFECTS: Gastrointestinal (GI) irritation, anorexia, transient hypokalemia, drowsiness, and paresthesias.
COMMENTS: Limited clinical experience in neonates. Used as an adjunct to other medications in refractory seizures. Tolerance to diuretic effect with long-term use.

Acyclovir (Zovirax)
CLASSIFICATION: Antiviral agent.
ACTION AND SPECTRUM: Indicated in herpes simplex and varicella-zoster viral infections. Virostatic activated in virally infected cells, inhibits viral DNA polymerase, and is a viral chain terminator. Good activity against herpes simplex (types 1 and 2) and varicella-zoster viruses. Poor activity against Epstein-Barr virus and cytomegalovirus. CSF concentrations are 50% of those of plasma.
SUPPLIED: Injection, topical, suspension.
ROUTE: Topical, IV, PO.
DOSAGE:

- Topical: Apply sufficient amount to cover the lesion q3h.
- IV: 30–40 mg/kg/day divided q8h for 10–14 days (dilute to a final concentration of 7 mg/mL and infuse over 60 min).
- PO (varicella): 20 mg/kg/dose q6h initiated at the first sign of disease. Continue for 5 days.

ADVERSE EFFECTS: Transient elevation of serum creatinine, thrombocytosis, jitters, rash, and hives.

COMMENTS: Drug of choice for documented or suspected herpes encephalitis (suggest 40 mg/kg/day IV in divided doses for 14 days).

Adenosine (Adenocard)

INDICATIONS AND USE: Conversion to sinus rhythm of paroxysmal supraventricular tachycardia.

ACTIONS: A purine nucleoside naturally occurring in all human cells. Slows conduction time through the atrioventricular (AV) node and interrupts reentry pathways through the AV node to restore normal sinus rhythm. Its electrophysiologic effects are mediated by depression of calcium slow-channel conduction, an increase in potassium conductance, and possibly indirect antiadrenergic effects.

SUPPLIED: Injection, 6 mg/2 mL.

ROUTE: IV.

DOSAGE: 0.1–0.2 mg/kg by rapid IV push over 1–2 s.

ADVERSE EFFECTS: Do not use in second- or third-degree AV block. May produce a short-duration first-, second-, or third-degree heart block; hypotension; brief dyspnea; and facial flushing. Half-life is <10 s; duration is 20–30 s. Carbamazepine increases the degree of heart block caused by adenosine. Methylxanthines (eg, caffeine and theophylline) are competitive antagonists; **larger adenosine doses may be required.**

Albumin, Human (Various)

INDICATIONS AND USE: Plasma volume expander. Treatment of hypoproteinemia.

ACTIONS: Maintains plasma colloid oncotic pressure. IV administration causes a shift of fluid from the interstitial spaces into the circulation. Serves as a carrier for many substances, such as bilirubin. Limited nutritional value.

SUPPLIED: Injection, 50 mg/mL (5%), 250 mg/mL (25%) (contains 130–160 mEq of sodium per liter).

ROUTE: IV.

DOSAGE: 0.5–1 g/kg IV (or 10–20 mL/kg of 5% IV bolus) repeated as necessary. Maximum: 6 g/kg/day.

ADVERSE EFFECTS: Infrequent. Rapid infusion may cause vascular overload and precipitation of congestive heart failure. Hypersensitivity reactions may include chills, fever, nausea, and urticaria.

COMMENTS: More purified than plasma protein fraction and thus less likely to cause hypotension.

Albuterol (Proventil, Ventolin)

INDICATIONS AND USE: Manage bronchospasm in reversible airway obstruction, increase maximal expiratory flow in infants with respiratory distress syndrome (RDS), and improve lung mechanics in ventilator-dependent infants and those with bronchopulmonary dysplasia (BPD).

ACTIONS: Primarily β_2-adrenergic stimulation (bronchodilation and vasodilation) with minor β_1 stimulation (increased myocardial contractility and conduction). Duration of action is ~3–8 h.

SUPPLIED: 0.083% (0.83 mg/mL), 3-mL unit-dose; 0.5% (5 mg/mL), 20-mL bottle.

ROUTE: Nebulization.

DOSAGE:

- 0.5%: 0.04 mL/kg/dose (= 0.2 mg/kg/dose).
- 0.083%: 0.2 mL/kg/dose (= 0.2 mg/kg/dose).
  Dilute in 2 mL of normal saline and give q4–6h.

ADVERSE EFFECTS: Tachycardia, tremors, CNS stimulation, hypokalemia, and hypertension.

COMMENTS: Titrate the dose to the heart rate and clinical effect.

Alprostadil (Prostaglandin E₁) (Prostin VR)

INDICATIONS AND USE: Any state in which blood flow must be maintained through the ductus arteriosus to sustain either pulmonary or systemic circulation until corrective or palliative surgery can be performed. Examples are pulmonary atresia, pulmonary stenosis, tricuspid atresia, transposition of the great arteries, aortic arch interruption, coarctation of the aorta, and severe tetralogy of Fallot (TOF).

ACTIONS: Vasodilator and platelet aggregation inhibitor. Smooth muscle of the ductus arteriosus is especially sensitive to its effects, responding to the drug with marked dilatation. Decreased response after 96 h of infusion. Maximal improvement in Pao_2, usually within 30 min in cyanotic infants, 1.5–3 h in acyanotic infants.
SUPPLIED: Injection.
ROUTE: IV.
DOSAGE: 0.05 mcg/kg/min. Decrease to the lowest rate that will maintain response.
ADVERSE EFFECTS: Cutaneous vasodilation, seizure-like activity, jitteriness, temperature elevation, hypocalcemia, apnea, thrombocytopenia, and hypotension. May cause apnea. Have an intubation kit at the bedside if the patient is not already intubated.
COMMENTS: Use cautiously in infants with bleeding tendencies.

Alteplase, Recombinant (Activase, t-PA)

INDICATIONS AND USE: Used to restore patency of occluded central venous catheters and for lysis of large-vessel thrombus (systemic use).
ACTIONS: Alteplase is a thrombolytic. Enhances conversion of plasminogen to plasmin, which then cleaves fibrin, fibrinogen, factor V, and factor VIII, resulting in clot breakdown.
SUPPLIED: Injection: 50 mg (= 29 million units/vial) lyophilized powder with 50-mL diluent (sterile water for injection).
ROUTE: IV.
DOSAGE:

- Lysis of large vessel thrombus (systemic use): Dose is *controversial,* ranging from 0.1 to 1 mg/kg/h for hours to days. (For a discussion of doses that have been used, see Zenk et al: Alteplase. In *Neonatal Medications and Nutrition,* 3rd ed. NICU Ink Santa Rosa, 2003.)
- Occluded central venous catheter: ≤2.5 kg: 0.25 mg diluted in normal saline (NS) to volume required to fill line. 2.5–10 kg: 0.5 mg diluted in NS to volume required to fill line.

Instill into lumen of catheter slowly and carefully so as not to inject the drug into the systemic circulation. Dwell time is 2–4 h. Concentration: 0.5–1 mg/mL in dextrose or saline. Check for catheter malposition with x-ray film before alteplase administration. (See Choi et al: The use of alteplase to restore patency of central venous lines in pediatric patients: a cohort study. *J Pediatr* 2001;139:152.)
ADVERSE EFFECTS:

- Large-vessel thrombus (systemic use): Not recommended with preexisting intraventricular hemorrhage or cerebral ischemic changes. Correct hypertension before use. May cause bleeding from puncture sites or internally. Severe bleeding complications may occur. Monitoring methods are *controversial;* the following have been used by various investigators: Frequent reassessment of thromboses usually by ultrasonography; daily cranial sonography; after fibrin/fibrinogen degradation products and/or D-dimers; after fibrinogen with a lower limit of usually 100 mg/dL, but >150 mg/dL in one study (*J Pediatr* 1998;133:133).
- Occluded central venous catheter: Bleeding may occur if excessive tissue plasminogen activator (t-PA) is inadvertently injected into the systemic circulation. Excessive pressure on instillation may force the clot into the systemic circulation.

COMMENTS: Increases risk of bleeding in infants concurrently on heparin, warfarin (Coumadin), or indomethacin.

Amikacin Sulfate (Amikin)

CLASSIFICATION: Aminoglycoside.
ACTION AND SPECTRUM: Primarily bactericidal against gram-negative organisms by inhibiting protein synthesis. Active against gram-negative bacteria, including most *Pseudomonas* and *Serratia* spp. No activity against anaerobic organisms.
SUPPLIED: Injection.
ROUTE: IM, IV (infuse over 30 min).

DOSAGE: Dosage should be monitored and adjusted by use of pharmacokinetics. Initial empiric dosing based on body weight.

- <1.2 kg and 0–4 weeks' postnatal age: 7.5 mg/kg/dose q18–24h.
- 1.2–2 kg:
  0–7 days: 7.5 mg/kg/dose q12–18h.
  >7 days: 7.5 mg/kg/dose q8–12h.
- >2 kg:
  0–7 days: 10 mg/kg/dose q12h.
  >7 days: 10 mg/kg/dose q8h.

ELIMINATION: Renal (glomerular filtration); half-life is 4–8 h; volume of distribution is 0.6 L/kg.

COMMENTS: Lowest overall resistance of all the aminoglycosides and thus should be reserved for infections with organisms resistant to other aminoglycosides Adjust the dosage according to serum peak and trough levels. Draw serum levels at about the fourth maintenance dose (draw a serum trough sample 30 min to just before the dose and a serum peak sample 30 min after infusion is complete). Therapeutic peak level is 25–35 mcg/mL, and trough level is 10 mcg/mL. Nephrotoxicity is associated with serum trough concentrations >10 mcg/mL; ototoxicity, with serum peak concentrations >35–40 mg/mL (more cochlear damage than vestibular).

Amphotericin B (Fungizone), amphotericin B, liposomal (AmBisome)

CLASSIFICATION: Antifungal agent.

ACTION AND SPECTRUM: Acts by binding to sterols and disrupting the fungal cell membranes. Broad spectrum of activity against *Candida* spp and other fungi.

SUPPLIED: Injection.

ROUTE: IV.

DOSAGE:

- Initially: Test dose of 0.25 mg/kg IV over 4 h. Use 0.1 mg/mL concentration in 5% dextrose in water (D_5W). Incompatible with NaCl.
- Increment: Increase the daily dosage by 0.25 mg/kg/day qd–qod as tolerated to a maximum daily or alternate-day dosage of 0.75–1.5 mg/kg. A total dosage of 30–35 mg/kg should be given over 6 weeks or longer, although a lower dose may suffice. In general, infusions should be given over 2–6 h, although infusion over 1–2 h may be used if tolerated.
- Intrathecal or intraventricular: Reconstitute with sterile water at 0.25 mg/mL; dilute with CSF and reinfuse. Usual dose: 0.25–0.5 mg.
- Liposomal amphotericin B: 5 mg/kg IV infused over 1–2 h. Consider using liposomal amphotericin B in infants on parenteral nutrition (PN) who have limited IV access and/or are nutritionally depleted, because it can be infused in a shorter period of time with fewer adverse effects than conventional amphotericin B, thus minimizing the time the PN is interrupted.

ELIMINATION AND METABOLISM: Slow renal excretion.

ADVERSE EFFECTS: Few adverse effects in neonates as opposed to adults. May cause fever, chills, vomiting, thrombophlebitis at injection sites, renal tubular acidosis, renal failure, hypomagnesemia, hypokalemia, bone marrow suppression with reversible decline in hematocrit, hypotension, hypertension, wheezing, and hypoxemia. Fewer adverse effects with liposomal amphotericin B.

COMMENTS: Irritation at the infusion site may be reduced by addition of heparin (1 unit/mL). Protect the solution from light. Monitor serum potassium, magnesium, urea nitrogen, creatinine, alkaline phosphatase, and aspartate transaminase (AST [serum glutamic oxaloacetic transaminase, or SGOT]) qd–qod until the dosage is stabilized, then every week. Monitor complete blood cell count (CBC) every week. Discontinue if blood urea nitrogen (BUN) is >40 mg/dL, serum creatinine is >3 mg/dL, or liver function tests are abnormal.

Ampicillin (Polycillin, Others)

CLASSIFICATION: Semisynthetic penicillinase-sensitive penicillin.

ACTION AND SPECTRUM: The penicillins are bactericidal and act by inhibiting the late stages of cell wall synthesis. As effective as penicillin G in pneumococcal, streptococcal, and meningococcal infections and also is active against many strains of *Salmonella* spp, *Shigella* spp, *Proteus mirabilis, Escherichia coli,* and *Listeria* spp, and most strains of *Haemophilus influenzae*. Inactivated by staphylococcal and *H. influenzae* β-lactamases.

SUPPLIED: Powder to make pediatric drops, oral suspension, and injection.

ROUTE: PO, IM, IV.

DOSAGE:

- Meningitis:
  Age 0–7 days: 100–200 mg/kg/day IV or IM divided q12h.
  Age >7 days: 200–300 mg/kg/day IV or IM divided q6–8h; maximum: 400 mg/kg/day.
- Other indications:
  Age 0–7 days: 100 mg/kg/day PO, IV, or IM divided q12h.
  Age >7 days: 100 mg/kg/day PO, IV, or IM divided q6–8h.

ELIMINATION AND METABOLISM: 90% excreted unchanged in urine. Half-life in neonates is 2 h.

ADVERSE EFFECTS: Hypersensitivity, rubella-like rash, abdominal discomfort, nausea, vomiting, diarrhea, and eosinophilia. Very large doses may cause CNS excitation or convulsions.

COMMENTS: The penicillin of choice in combination with an aminoglycoside in the prophylaxis and treatment of infections with group B streptococci, group D streptococci (enterococci), and *Listeria monocytogenes*. Contains 3 mEq of sodium per gram.

Ampicillin Sodium/Sulbactam Sodium (Unasyn)

CLASSIFICATION: Combination β-lactamase inhibitor and β-lactam agent.

ACTION AND SPECTRUM: The bactericidal spectrum of ampicillin is extended by the addition of sulbactam, a β-lactamase inhibitor, to include β-lactamase-producing strains of *Staphylococcus aureus, Staphylococcus epidermidis,* enterococci, *Haemophilus influenzae, Branhamella catarrhalis,* and *Klebsiella* spp, including *K. pneumoniae*. Also has good activity against *Bacteroides fragilis*, making it a suitable choice for single-drug treatment of intra-abdominal and pelvic infections caused by susceptible organisms.

SUPPLIED: Injection.

ROUTE: IV, IM.

- Meningitis:
  Age 0–7 days: 100–200 mg/kg/day IV q12h.
  Age >7 days: 200–300 mg/kg/day IV or IM q6–8h.
- Other indications:
  Age 0–7 days: 100 mg/kg/day IV or IM q12h.
  Age >7 days: 100 mg/kg/day IV or IM q6–8h.

ELIMINATION: See Ampicillin, above.

ADVERSE EFFECTS: See Ampicillin, above.

COMMENTS: See Ampicillin, above.

Arginine HCl (R-Gene 10)

INDICATIONS AND USE: Treatment of alkalosis, growth hormone reserve test, and treatment of certain neonatal-onset urea cycle disorders.

ACTIONS: Corrects severe metabolic alkalosis resulting from the chloride content of arginine. Arginine stimulates pituitary release of growth hormone.

SUPPLIED: Injection: 10% = 100 mg/mL (contains 0.475 mEq chloride)

ROUTE: IV, PO.

DOSAGE:

- Metabolic alkalosis: IV, PO

$$\text{MEq Cl} / \text{kg} = 0.2 \text{ L} / \text{kg} \times (103 - \text{serum Cl}) \text{ (mEq} / \text{L)}$$

or

$$0.3 \, L/kg \times \text{Base Excess (mEq/L)}$$

or

$$0.5 \, L/kg \times (\text{serum HCO}_3 - 24) \, (\text{mEq/L})$$

Give ½ to ½ of the calculated dose, then reevaluate. IV: May use undiluted or dilute with saline or dextrose. Infuse over at least 30 min or over 24 h in maintenance IV. Maximum: 1 g/kg/h (= 10 mL/kg/h of 10% solution). PO: May use the injectable form, diluted.
Growth hormone reserve test: IV
500 mg/kg (= 5 mL/kg of the 10% solution) infused IV over 30 min. (Use only IV, not PO administration for this test.)
Urea cycle disorders: Consult specialists in metabolic disorders and specialized references if a urea cycle disorder is suspected (see Urea Cycle Disorders Conference Group: Consensus statement from a conference for the management of patients with urea cycle disorders. *J Pediatr* 2001;138:S1.)
ADVERSE EFFECTS: Not a first-line treatment for metabolic acidosis; try sodium, potassium, or ammonium chlorides first. May be toxic in infants with arginase deficiency. Do not use in patients sensitive to arginine HCl or in those with hepatic or renal failure. May cause: hyperchloremic metabolic acidosis, elevated gastrin, glucagon and growth hormone; flushing and GI upset with rapid IV administration; hyperglycemia, hypoglycemia, hyperkalemia; tissue necrosis on extravasation, vein irritation; allergic reactions; elevated BUN and creatinine.
COMMENTS: Monitor IV site, blood glucose, chloride, and blood pressure.

Atropine Sulfate (Various)
INDICATIONS AND USE: Sinus bradycardia, cardiopulmonary resuscitation (CPR), and reversal of neuromuscular blockade. Used preoperatively to inhibit salivation and reduce excessive secretions of the respiratory tract.
ACTIONS: A competitive antagonist of acetylcholine at smooth muscle, cardiac muscle, and various glandular cells, leading to increased heart rate, reduced GI motility and tone, urinary retention, cycloplegia, and decreased salivation and sweating.
SUPPLIED: Injection, ophthalmic ointment, ophthalmic solution.
ROUTE: IV, IM, SC, PO, intratracheal.
DOSAGE:

- Bradycardia in infants and children: 0.02–0.03 mg/kg/dose q5min prn. Maximum: 1 mg.
- Preanesthetic: 0.03 mg/kg/dose.

ADVERSE EFFECTS: Xerostomia, blurred vision, mydriasis, tachycardia, palpitations, constipation, urinary retention, ataxia, tremor, and hyperthermia. Toxic effects are especially likely in children receiving low doses.
COMMENTS: Contraindicated in thyrotoxicosis, tachycardia secondary to cardiac insufficiency, and obstructive GI disease. In low doses, may cause paradoxic bradycardia secondary to its central actions.

AZT: See Zidovudine.

Aztreonam (Azactam)
CLASSIFICATION: Monobactam antibiotic.
ACTION AND SPECTRUM: Antibacterial activity resulting from inhibition of mucopeptide synthesis in the cell wall. Bactericidal against most Enterobacteriaceae and *Pseudomonas aeruginosa* but little or no activity against gram-positive aerobic or anaerobic bacteria.
SUPPLIED: Injection.
ROUTE: IV.

DOSAGE:

* Premature infants: 50 mg/kg/dose q12h.
* Term infants: 50 mg/kg/dose q8h.

ELIMINATION: Renal (glomerular filtration and secretion). Half-life is ~6–10 h. Volume of distribution is 0.26–0.36 L/kg.

ADVERSE EFFECTS: Diarrhea, nausea, vomiting, rash irritation at the infusion site, increased prothrombin time, and transient eosinophilia.

COMMENTS: Used primarily for *Pseudomonas* infections.

Beractant (Survanta): See also Surfactant

INDICATIONS AND USE: Prevention and treatment of respiratory distress syndrome of preterm infants.

ACTIONS: A natural bovine lung extract containing phospholipids, neutral lipids, fatty acids, and surfactant-associated proteins to which dipalmitoylphosphatidylcholine (DPPC), palmitic acid, and tripalmitin are added to mimic the surface tension–lowering properties of natural lung surfactant. Surfactant lowers surface tension on alveolar surfaces during respiration and stabilizes the alveoli against collapse.

SUPPLIED: Suspension in single-use vials containing 25 mg of phospholipids per milliliter, 8 mL. Refrigerate.

ROUTE: Intratracheal using a No. 5 French end-hole catheter.

DOSAGE: 4 mL/kg (100 mg of phospholipids per kilogram) birth weight. Give in 4 increments, repositioning the infant with each dose. Inject each ¼ dose gently into the catheter over 2–3 s. Ventilate the infant after each ¼ dose for at least 30 s or until stable. Four doses of 4 mL/kg can be given in the first 48 h of life, no more frequently than q6h. Wean ventilator settings rapidly after administration.

ADVERSE EFFECTS: Most adverse effects are associated while administering the beractant to the infant: transient bradycardia and oxygen desaturation.

LESS FREQUENT ADVERSE EFFECTS: Endotracheal tube (ET) reflux, pallor, vasoconstriction, hypotension, ET blockage, hypertension, hypocarbia, hypercarbia, and apnea. In two studies, the rate of intracranial hemorrhage was significantly higher in infants who received beractant than in controls. When all study results were pooled, however, there was no difference in intracranial hemorrhage rates.

Bumetanide (Bumex)

INDICATIONS AND USE: Management of edema associated with congenital heart disease, congestive heart failure, and hepatic or renal disease.

ACTIONS: Inhibition of the active chloride and, possibly, sodium transport systems of the loop of Henle. Urinary excretion of sodium, chloride, potassium, hydrogen, calcium, magnesium, ammonium, phosphate, and bicarbonate increases with bumetanide-induced diuresis. Renal blood flow increases substantially as a result of renovascular dilation.

SUPPLIED: Injection, 0.25 mg/mL; tablets.

ROUTE: PO, IV, IM.

DOSAGE: 0.015 mg/kg/dose up to 0.1 mg/kg/day.

ADVERSE EFFECTS: Hypokalemia, hypochloremia, hyponatremia, metabolic alkalosis, and hypotension.

COMMENTS: Patients refractory to furosemide may respond to bumetanide for diuretic therapy. Although patients may respond differently, bumetanide is ~40 times more potent on a milligram-per-milligram basis than furosemide.

Caffeine Citrate

INDICATIONS AND USE: Apnea of prematurity.

ACTIONS: Similar to those of other methylxanthine drugs (eg, theobromine and theophylline). Caffeine appears to be more active on and less toxic to the CNS and the respiratory system. Proposed mechanisms of action include increased production of cyclic adenosine monophosphate (cAMP) and alterations of intracellular calcium concentrations. Stimulates the CNS and exerts a positive inotropic effect on the myocardium. Stimulates voluntary skeletal muscle and gastric acid secretion. Increases renal blood flow and glomerular filtration rate. Stimulates glycogenolysis and lipolysis.

SUPPLIED: Injection: 20 mg/mL as caffeine citrate (10 mg/mL as caffeine base). Oral: 20 mg/mL as caffeine citrate (10 mg/mL as caffeine base).
ROUTE: IV (not IM), PO.
DOSAGE:

- Loading dose: 20 mg of caffeine citrate (10-mg caffeine base) IV or PO.
- Maintenance dose (caffeine base): 2.5–5.0 mg/kg/day as a single daily dose.

ADVERSE EFFECTS: Nausea, vomiting, gastric irritation, agitation, tachycardia, and diuresis. Symptoms of overdosage include arrhythmias and tonic-clonic seizures.
COMMENTS: Contraindicated in hypersensitivity to the drug. Therapeutic levels are 5–25 mcg/mL, severe toxicity is associated with levels >50 mcg/mL. Initial half-life in neonates is 90–100 h, decreasing to 6 h at ~60 weeks' postconceptual age. Serum levels should be monitored.

Calcium Chloride (Various)

INDICATIONS AND USE: Symptomatic hypocalcemia such as neonatal tetany. Last-resort agent in cardiac arrest when other agents have failed to improve myocardial contraction. Overdose of calcium channel blocker.
ACTIONS: Calcium is essential for the functional integrity of the nervous, muscular, skeletal, and cardiac systems and for clotting function.
SUPPLIED: Injection, 100 mg/mL (10%, 10 mL), contains 27 mg (1.35 mEq) of elemental calcium and 1.35 mEq of chloride per milliliter.
ROUTE: IV, PO.
DOSAGE:

- Cardiac arrest (as a last resort): 20–30 mg/kg/dose (10% solution) IV q10min prn.
- Maintenance in Infants: 70 mg/kg/day IV divided q8h, or as infusion.

ADVERSE EFFECTS: Arrhythmias (eg, bradycardia) and deterioration of cardiovascular function. Extravasation may cause skin sloughing. May potentiate digoxin-related arrhythmias.
COMMENTS: Contraindicated in ventricular fibrillation or hypercalcemia. Use with caution in digitalized patients. Chloride salt is preferred to the gluconate form (see Calcium Gluconate) during cardiac arrest because the calcium in the chloride is already ionized and the gluconate requires metabolism to release the calcium ion. Precipitates when mixed with sodium bicarbonate.

Calcium Gluconate (Various)

INDICATIONS AND USE: Treatment of asymptomatic hypocalcemia, prevention of hypocalcemia in susceptible neonates, and prevention of hypocalcemia during exchange transfusion.
ACTIONS: See Calcium Chloride. Calcium gluconate must be metabolized to release calcium ion.
SUPPLIED: Injection 10% = 100 mg/mL (9 mg [0.45 mEq] of elemental calcium per milliliter).
DOSAGE:

- Maintenance IV: 200–700 mg/kg/day divided q6h, or as infusion; maximum rate: 200 mg/kg over 10 min.
- Maintenance PO: 200–800 mg/kg/day divided q6h mixed in feedings.
- Exchange transfusion: 0.45 mEq (1 mL 10%)/dL of citrated blood.

ADVERSE EFFECTS: See Calcium Chloride. Oral form may cause constipation.

Captopril (Capoten)

INDICATIONS AND USE: Congestive heart failure and hypertension.
ACTIONS: Competitive inhibitor of angiotensin-converting enzyme. Causes fall in angiotensin II and aldosterone levels, decrease in systemic vascular resistance, and augmentation of cardiac output.
SUPPLIED: Tablets. (Tablets can be dissolved in water and administered PO within 30 min, or an oral liquid can be compounded by the pharmacist.)
ROUTE: PO.

DOSAGE:

- Neonates: Initial: 0.05 mg/kg/dose, then 0.1–0.4 mg/kg/dose 1–4 times daily.
- Infants: 0.05 mg/kg/dose, then 0.5–6 mg/kg/day divided q6–24h.

ADVERSE EFFECTS: Hypotension, rash, fever, eosinophilia, neutropenia, and GI disturbances. A low initial dose is used because some infants have experienced a dramatic drop in blood pressure.
COMMENTS: Use with caution in patients with low renal perfusion pressure. Reduce the dose with renal impairment and in sodium- and water-depleted patients.

Carbamazepine (Tegretol)
INDICATIONS AND USE: Anticonvulsant. Prophylaxis against partial (especially complex partial), primary generalized tonic-clonic seizures and mixed seizures, including the above. Not effective for absence (petit mal) seizures.
ACTIONS: Acts by reducing polysynaptic responses and blocking the posttetanic potentiation.
PHARMACOKINETICS: Absorbed slowly from the GI tract. Protein binding is 76%. Metabolized in the liver to active epoxide by cytochrome P450 3A4. Induces liver enzymes and increases its own metabolism. Eliminated 72% in urine and 28% in feces. Half-life in neonates is 8–28 h. Therapeutic range is 4–12 mcg/mL.
INTERACTIONS: Erythromycin, isoniazid, and cimetidine may inhibit hepatic metabolism of carbamazepine, resulting in increased carbamazepine serum concentrations. Concurrent phenobarbital may lower carbamazepine serum levels. Carbamazepine may induce metabolism of warfarin, phenytoin, theophylline, benzodiazepines, and corticosteroids. Thyroid function tests may show decreased values with carbamazepine.
SUPPLIED: Suspension, 20 mg/mL. Shake well.
ROUTE: PO. No parenteral form available.
DOSAGE: 5 mg/kg/day PO initially. May increase weekly to 10 mg/kg/day, then to a maximum of 20 mg/kg/day if needed. Administer the daily dose in 3–4 divided doses. Administer with feedings.
ADVERSE EFFECTS GI: Nausea and vomiting. *Hematologic:* Leukopenia, thrombocytopenia, aplastic anemia, and agranulocytosis. *Cardiovascular:* Congestive heart failure, heart block, and cardiovascular collapse. *CNS:* Dystonia, drowsiness, and behavioral changes. *Ophthalmic:* Eyes: scattered punctate cortical lens opacities. *Endocrine/metabolic:* Syndrome of inappropriate antidiuretic hormone (SIADH). *Hepatic:* Hepatitis and cholestasis. *Dermatologic:* Rash and Stevens-Johnson syndrome. *Genitourinary:* Urine retention, azotemia, oliguria, and anuria. Monitor CBC, liver function, and urinalysis; perform periodic eye exam. Do not discontinue abruptly because seizures may result in epileptic patients.
COMMENTS: Avoid switching between Tegretol and generic carbamazepine if possible because changes in carbamazepine serum concentration and seizure activity may result; monitor serum concentrations.

Cefazolin Sodium (Ancef, Kefzol)
CLASSIFICATION: First-generation cephalosporin.
ACTION AND SPECTRUM: A broad-spectrum semisynthetic β-lactam antibiotic bactericidal by virtue of its inhibition of cell wall synthesis. Good activity against gram-positive cocci (except enterococci), including penicillinase-producing staphylococci. Gram-negative coverage includes *Escherichia coli*, most *Klebsiella* spp, many strains of *Haemophilus influenzae*, and indole-positive *Proteus* spp. Organism resistance is primarily due to elaboration of β-lactamases, which inactivate the antibiotic through hydrolysis.
SUPPLIED: Injection.
ROUTE: IM, IV (infuse over 20–30 min).
DOSAGE:

- Newborn and premature infants:
  - <2000 g: 40 mg/kg/day divided q12h.
  - >2000 g and >7 days: 60 mg/kg/day divided q12h.
- Age 1 month and older: 25–100 mg/kg/day divided q6–8h.

ELIMINATION AND METABOLISM: 100% excreted unchanged in urine. Half-life is 1.5–4 h.
ADVERSE EFFECTS: Infrequent except for allergic reactions, including fever, rash, and urticaria. May cause leukopenia, thrombocytopenia, and a positive Coombs' test reaction. Excessive dosage (especially in renal impairment) may result in CNS irritation with seizure activity.
COMMENTS: Use with caution in patients with a history of severe allergic reactions to penicillins. Dosage reduction is required in moderate to severe renal failure. Contains 2 mEq of sodium/g.

Cefotaxime Sodium (Claforan)

CLASSIFICATION: Third-generation cephalosporin.
ACTION AND SPECTRUM: Mechanism of action is identical to that of other β-lactam antibiotics and is bactericidal. Active chiefly against gram-negative organisms (except *Pseudomonas* spp), including *Escherichia coli*, *Enterobacter* spp, *Klebsiella* spp, *Haemophilus influenzae* (including ampicillin-resistant strains), *Proteus mirabilis*, and indole-positive *Proteus* spp, *Serratia marcescens*, *Neisseria gonorrhoeae*, and *Neisseria meningitidis*. Generally poor activity against gram-positive aerobic organisms.
SUPPLIED: Injection.
ROUTE: IM, IV (infuse over 30 min).
DOSAGE:

- Meningitis: 200 mg/kg/day divided q6h.
- Other indications:
  <7 days old: 100 mg/kg/day divided q12h.
  >7 days old: 150 mg/kg/day divided q8h.

ELIMINATION AND METABOLISM: Excreted principally unchanged in the urine. Half-life in neonates is 1–4 h.
ADVERSE EFFECTS: Hypersensitivity reactions, thrombophlebitis, serum sickness–like reaction with prolonged administration, diarrhea, and, rarely, blood dyscrasias, hepatic dysfunction, or renal damage.
COMMENTS: Should be reserved for suspected or documented gram-negative meningitis or sepsis. When used as empiric therapy, combine with ampicillin or aqueous penicillin G to provide gram-positive coverage (ie, group B streptococci, pneumococci, and *Listeria monocytogenes*). High degree of stability to β-lactamases. Third-generation cephalosporins have been proven to induce the emergence of multi-drug-resistant bacteria when used excessively and without proper clinical indications. Contains 2.2 mEq of sodium/g.

Cefoxitin (Mefoxin)

INDICATIONS AND USE: Treatment of infections from gram-negative enteric organisms, ampicillin-resistant *Haemophilus influenzae*, and anaerobic bacteria, including *Bacteroides fragilis* spp.
ACTIONS: A second-generation cephalosporin. A β-lactam antibiotic bactericidal by inhibiting cell wall synthesis.
SUPPLIED: Powder for injection, 1-, 2-, and 10-g vials.
ROUTE: IV, IM.
DOSAGE:

- <2 kg and >7 days old: 90 mg/kg/day divided q8h.
- ≥3 months old: 80–160 mg/kg/day divided q4–6h.

ADVERSE EFFECTS: Usually well tolerated. May cause rash, thrombophlebitis, a positive direct Coombs' test, eosinophilia, and increase in liver enzymes.

Ceftazidime (Fortaz, Tazidime)

CLASSIFICATION: Third-generation cephalosporin.
ACTION AND SPECTRUM: A broad-spectrum gram-negative semisynthetic β-lactam antibiotic bactericidal by virtue of its inhibition of cell wall synthesis. Has poor gram-positive activity compared with first-generation cephalosporins but good activity against gram-negative aerobic bacteria, including *Neisseria meningitidis*, *Haemophilus influenzae*, and most of the Enterobacteriaceae. Has excellent activity

against *Pseudomonas aeruginosa* (the best of all third-generation cephalosporins). Little activity against *Listeria monocytogenes* and enterococci.

SUPPLIED: IV.

ROUTE: IM, IV (infuse over 20–30 min).

DOSAGE:

- <2000 g and <7 days old: 30 mg/kg/dose IV q12h.
- >2000 g and <7 days old: 30 mg/kg/dose IV q8h.
- >2000 g and >7 days old: 30 mg/kg/dose IV q8h.

ELIMINATION: Renal (glomerular filtration), 100% excreted unchanged. Half-life is 2.2–4.7 h.

ADVERSE EFFECTS: Infrequent except for allergic reactions, including fever, rash, and urticaria. May cause transient leukopenia, neutropenia, and thrombocytopenia; a direct positive Coombs' test; and transient elevation in the liver function test.

COMMENTS: Penetrates well into CSF; concentrations approximate 25–50% of serum concentrations. In combination with ampicillin (for *Listeria* spp), can be used to treat suspected gram-negative meningitis in the neonate. Also an alternative to aminoglycosides for *P. aeruginosa* therapy, particularly in patients with renal failure.

Ceftriaxone Sodium (Rocephin)

CLASSIFICATION: Third-generation cephalosporin.

ACTION AND SPECTRUM: Mechanism of action is identical to that of other β-lactam antibiotics. High degree of stability to β-lactamases and good activity against both gram-negative and gram-positive organisms except *Pseudomonas* spp, enterococci, methicillin-resistant staphylococci, and *Listeria monocytogenes*. Has longest serum half-life of all currently available cephalosporins.

SUPPLIED: Injection.

ROUTE: IM, IV (infuse over 30 min).

DOSAGE:

- Meningitis: 100 mg/kg/day divided q12h.
- Other indications: 50 mg/kg/day divided q12–24h.

ELIMINATION AND METABOLISM: Both biliary and renal excretion. Half-life is 5.2–8.4 h.

ADVERSE EFFECTS: Mild diarrhea and eosinophilia are most common. May also cause neutropenia, rash, thrombophlebitis, and bacterial (GI) or fungal overgrowth. Rare reports of increased prothrombin times. Increases free and erythrocyte-bound bilirubin in premature infants with hyperbilirubinemia; use with caution in infants with hyperbilirubinemia.

COMMENTS: Many clinical studies support once-a-day dosing. Do not use as the sole drug in infections caused by staphylococci or pseudomonas. Combine with ampicillin for initial empiric therapy of meningitis (ceftriaxone has poor activity against *Listeria* spp). Generally no dosage reduction is required in renal or hepatic dysfunction. Contains 2.4 mEq of sodium/g.

Cefuroxime Sodium (Kefurox, Zinacef)

CLASSIFICATION: Second-generation cephalosporin.

ACTION AND SPECTRUM: Mechanism of action identical to that of other β-lactam antibiotics. Active against both gram-positive and gram-negative organisms, including streptococci (except enterococci), both penicillinase-producing and non-penicillinase-producing staphylococci (not including methicillin-resistant staphylococci), *Escherichia coli*, *Haemophilus influenzae* (including ampicillin-resistant strains), *Klebsiella* spp, *Neisseria gonorrhoeae*, *Neisseria meningitidis*, *Proteus mirabilis*, *Salmonella* spp, *Shigella* spp, and *Enterobacter* spp.

SUPPLIED: Injection.

ROUTE: IM, IV (IV preferred; infuse over 30 min).

DOSAGE: 100 mg/kg/day divided q12h.

ELIMINATION AND METABOLISM: Primarily excreted unchanged in the urine. Half-life is 5–8 h in infants <4 days old and 1.6–3.8 h in infants >8 days of age.

ADVERSE EFFECTS: Generally free of adverse effects but may cause hypersensitivity reactions, thrombophlebitis, elevated serum transaminases, mildly elevated BUN, diarrhea, and, rarely, blood dyscrasias (transient neutropenia, leukopenia, and thrombocytopenia).

COMMENTS: The only first- or second-generation cephalosporin that crosses the blood-brain barrier. Provides no activity against *Listeria* spp, so ampicillin should be added in initial empiric therapy. Has added gram-negative coverage over first-generation cephalosporins while retaining very good gram-positive coverage. Decrease the dosage in renal failure. Contains 2.4 mEq of sodium/g. Limited experience in neonates.

Cephalothin Sodium (Keflin)

CLASSIFICATION: First-generation cephalosporin.

ACTION AND SPECTRUM: Mechanism of action identical to that of other β-lactam antibiotics. Active against both gram-positive and gram-negative organisms, including streptococci (except enterococci), both penicillinase-producing and non-penicillinase-producing staphylococci (but not methicillin-resistant staphylococci), *Escherichia coli, Proteus mirabilis, Klebsiella* spp, *Haemophilus influenzae, Salmonella* spp, and *Shigella* spp.

SUPPLIED: Injection.

ROUTE: IV (Infuse over 30 min).

DOSAGE:

- <2000 g and 0–7 days old: 40 mg/kg/day divided q12h.
- <2000 g and >7 days old: 60 mg/kg/day divided q8h.
- >2000 g and 0–7 days old: 60 mg/kg/day divided q8h.
- >2000 g and >7 days old: 80 mg/kg/day divided q6h.

ELIMINATION AND METABOLISM: 75% excreted unchanged in the urine.

ADVERSE EFFECTS: Hypersensitivity reactions, thrombophlebitis, serum sickness–like reaction with prolonged use, diarrhea, neutropenia, leukopenia, and transient elevation of AST (SGOT). May falsely elevate serum creatinine.

COMMENTS: Generally better activity against gram-positive organisms than second- or third-generation drugs. Dosage adjustment required in renal failure. Contains 2.8 mEq of sodium/g.

Chloral Hydrate (Aquachloral Supprettes, Noctec)

INDICATIONS AND USE: Sedation.

ACTIONS: CNS depressant. Mechanism of action not completely understood. Usual doses produce mild CNS depression and quiet, deep sleep; higher doses can result in general anesthesia with concurrent respiratory depression.

SUPPLIED: Syrup, suppositories.

ROUTE: PO, PR.

DOSAGE: 20–40 mg/kg/dose PO or rectally q6–8h prn. Sedation before electroencephalography and other procedures: 30–75 mg/kg/dose once PO, PR. Usually, 50 mg/kg/dose once, with orders to repeat with 25 mg/kg/dose once if needed. Use the lowest effective dose.

ADVERSE EFFECTS: GI irritation resulting in nausea, vomiting, and diarrhea; paradoxic excitation; and respiratory depression, particularly if administered with opiates and barbiturates. Direct hyperbilirubinemia with chronic use. Overdose can be lethal.

COMMENTS: Contraindicated with marked renal or hepatic impairment.

Chloramphenicol (Chloromycetin)

CLASSIFICATION: Antibiotic.

ACTION AND SPECTRUM: A broad-spectrum agent. Interferes with or inhibits protein synthesis. Bactericidal for *Haemophilus influenzae* and *Neisseria meningitidis;* bacteriostatic for *Escherichia coli, Klebsiella* spp, *Serratia* spp, *Enterobacter* spp, *Salmonella* spp, *Shigella* spp, *Neisseria gonorrhoeae,* staphylococci, *Streptococcus pneumoniae,* and groups A, B, C, nonenterococcal D, and G streptococci. Drug of choice for *Salmonella typhi* infection.

SUPPLIED: Injection, oral suspension, ophthalmic solution.

ROUTE: PO, IM, IV (infuse over 5–15 min).

DOSAGE:

- <2000 g and 0–7 days old: 25 mg/kg/day q24h.
- <2000 g and >7 days old: 25 mg/kg/day q24h.
- >2000 g and 0–7 days old: 25 mg/kg/day q24h.
- >2000 g and >7 days old: 50 mg/kg/day divided q12h.
- Ophthalmic solution: 1 drop in each eye q6–12h.

ELIMINATION AND METABOLISM: Metabolized by the liver. Half-life is 9–27 h.

ADVERSE EFFECTS: Idiosyncratic reactions result in aplastic anemia (irreversible and rare), reversible bone marrow suppression (dose-related), allergy (rash and fever), diarrhea, vomiting, stomatitis, glossitis, *Candida* superinfection, and "gray baby" syndrome (early signs are hyperammonemia and unexplained metabolic acidosis; other signs are abdominal distention, hypotonia, gray skin color, and cardiorespiratory collapse).

COMMENTS: Avoid use where possible. Must monitor serum levels. Desired peak is 10–25 mcg/mL; levels >50 mcg/mL are strongly associated with "gray baby" syndrome. Monitor CBC with differential, platelet count, and reticulocyte count every 3 days.

Chlorothiazide (Diuril)
INDICATIONS AND USE: Fluid overload, pulmonary edema, and hypertension.

ACTIONS: The thiazide diuretics enhance the excretion of NaCl and water by interfacing with transport of sodium ions across the renal tubular epithelium in the cortical nephron. Potassium, bicarbonate, magnesium, phosphate, and iodide excretion are also enhanced, whereas calcium excretion is decreased. Duration of action of chlorothiazide and hydrochlorothiazide is 6–12 h; onset of action is within 2 h, and peak action is at 3–6 h.

SUPPLIED: Suspension; injection, 500 mg (as sodium) per 20-mL vial.

ROUTE: PO, IV.

DOSAGE: 10–30 mg/kg/day divided q12h.

ADVERSE EFFECTS: Hypokalemia, hypochloremic alkalosis, prerenal azotemia, hyperuricemia, hyperglycemia, hypermagnesemia, volume depletion, and dilutional hyponatremia may occur in situations of excessive fluid intake.

COMMENTS: Do not use in patients with anuria or hepatic dysfunction.

Cholestyramine Resin (Questran)
CLASSIFICATION: Resin-binding agent.

INDICATIONS AND USE: For use as a resin-binding agent in patients with chronic diarrhea and short-gut syndrome to decrease fecal output.

ACTION: Cholestyramine resin releases chloride ion and absorbs bile acid in the intestine, forming a nonabsorbable complex preventing enterohepatic recirculation of bile salts.

SUPPLIED: Powder.

ROUTE: PO.

DOSAGE: 1–2 g/dose bid–qid.

ELIMINATION: Not absorbed; excreted in the feces.

ADVERSE EFFECTS: Constipation. High doses can cause hyperchloremic acidosis and increase urinary calcium excretion.

COMMENTS: May bind concurrent oral medications.

Cimetidine (Tagamet)
INDICATIONS AND USE: Duodenal and gastric ulcers and hypersecretory conditions (eg, Zollinger-Ellison syndrome).

ACTIONS: A histamine (H_2) receptor antagonist; competitively inhibits the action of histamine on the parietal cells, decreasing gastric acid.

SUPPLIED: Oral liquid, injection.

ROUTE: IV, PO.

DOSAGE:

- Neonates: 5–10 mg/kg/day IV or PO divided q8–12h.
- Infants: 20 mg/kg/day IV or PO divided q6h.

ADVERSE EFFECTS: CNS toxicity such as alterations in consciousness, antiandrogenic effects, cholestatic jaundice, and increased serum concentrations of hepatic-metabolized drugs. Reduce the theophylline dose 50% if used concurrently.
COMMENTS: Limited use in neonates. May add daily dose to the PN regimen and infuse over 24 h to avoid the need for q6–8h administration.

Clindamycin (Cleocin)

ACTION AND SPECTRUM: Bactericidal activity by inhibiting protein synthesis. Active against both aerobic and anaerobic streptococci (except enterococci), most staphylococci (except methicillin-resistant strains), Bacteroides spp (except Bacteroides melaninogenicus), Fusobacterium varium, Actinomyces israelii, Clostridium perfringens, and Clostridium tetani. Chiefly used against the above anaerobes. Not effective against gram-negative organisms or many clostridial species.
SUPPLIED: Injection, oral solution.
ROUTE: PO, IM, IV (infuse over 10–20 min).
DOSAGE:

- <1200 g: 10 mg/kg/day divided q12h.
- <2000 g and 0–7 days old: 10 mg/kg/day divided q12h.
- <2000 g and >7 days old: 15 mg/kg/day divided q8h.
- >2000 g and 0–7 days old: 15 mg/kg/day divided q8h.
- >2000 g and >7 days old: 20 mg/kg/day divided q6h.

ELIMINATION AND METABOLISM: Primarily hepatic metabolism.
ADVERSE EFFECTS: Sterile abscess formation at the IM injection site. Vomiting and diarrhea occur frequently. Pseudomembranous colitis resulting from suppression of normal flora and overgrowth of Clostridium difficile is uncommon but potentially fatal (treated with oral vancomycin or metronidazole). Rash, glossitis, and pruritus occur occasionally. Serum sickness, anaphylaxis, hematologic (granulocytopenia and thrombocytopenia), and hepatic abnormalities occur rarely.
COMMENTS: Does not cross the blood-brain barrier; therefore, do not use to treat meningitis.

Clonidine (Catapres)

INDICATIONS AND USE: Management of hypertension (not commonly used in infants), neonatal abstinence syndrome, and iatrogenic narcotic dependency and for growth hormone testing. Although preliminary data show that clonidine produces a dramatic reduction in the severity of neonatal withdrawal symptoms, more experience is needed before clonidine is routinely used to treat opioid withdrawal in infants. Use with caution and monitor infant for hypotension.
ACTIONS: Stimulates CNS α_2-adrenergic receptors, results in decreased peripheral vascular resistance, systolic and diastolic blood pressure, and heart rate. Reduces circulating plasma renin levels. Single doses of the drug produce pronounced increase in growth hormone concentration in normal, but not in growth hormone–deficient, children.
SUPPLIED: Tablet: 0.1 mg, 0.2 mg. An oral liquid is not commercially available; however, a suspension can be prepared by the pharmacist.
ROUTE: PO. May administer with feedings or water to decrease GI upset.
DOSAGE: Use the lowest effective dose. Reduce dose in renal dysfunction.

- Hypertension:
  PO: 5–10 mcg/kg/day divided q8–12 h. May increase dose gradually, if needed, allowing 5–7 days between dose adjustments. Maximum: 20 mcg/kg/day divided every 6 h.
- Opioid withdrawal:
  2 mcg/kg/day divided q6h. Maximum: 4 mcg/kg/day PO divided q6h. Weaning: Wean gradually over 1–2 weeks. Adjust the dose to avoid hypotension and oversedation; individualize dose per patient tolerance.
  Growth hormone provocation test: 0.1–0.15 mg/m^2 PO as a single dose. Levels for growth hormone are usually drawn in blood samples 30, 60, and 90 min after PO clonidine. Monitor for drowsiness, pallor, and hypotension.

ADVERSE EFFECTS: Hypotension, bradycardia; severe rebound hypertension with abrupt discontinuation (or missing of several consecutive doses) discontinue gradually over 27 days; drowsiness, weakness, anxiety, hypothermia; dry mouth, GI upset; urine retention, decrease in plasma renin activity in hyperreninemic patients; rash; thrombocytopenia (rare); transient weight gain resulting from sodium and water retention. Infants and children may be especially sensitive to the effects of clonidine; use with caution. Retinal degeneration has been observed in laboratory animals; consider periodic eye exams.

OVERDOSE: CNS depression, apnea, bradycardia, arrhythmia, profound hypotension, transient hypertension, hyporeflexia, hypothermia, miosis, irritability, and dry mouth.

COMMENTS: Observe for excessive CNS and/or respiratory depression. Monitor blood pressure, heart rate, and rhythm. Ensure that the drug is not abruptly discontinued.

Cosyntropin (Cortrosyn)

INDICATIONS AND USE: Aid in the diagnosis of adrenocortical insufficiency.

ACTIONS: Stimulates the adrenal cortex to secrete cortisol (hydrocortisone) and other substances.

DOSAGE: 0.015 mg/kg (1 dose only).

SUPPLIED: Injection, 0.25 mg/vial; dilution: 0.25 mg/mL.

ROUTE: IM, IV (infuse initial dilution over 2 min).

COMMENTS: For rapid diagnostic screening of adrenocortical insufficiency, plasma cortisol concentrations should be measured before and 60 min after administration of cosyntropin; 0.25 mg = 25 USP units of corticotropin.

Curare: See Tubocurarine

Dexamethasone (Decadron, Others)

INDICATIONS: Resistant neonatal hypoglycemia and airway edema. Used in weaning infants with BPD from the ventilator.

ACTIONS: Used primarily as an anti-inflammatory or immunosuppressive agent. Because of its minimal mineralocorticoid activity, not indicated for replacement therapy in adrenocortical insufficiency. A long-acting, potent glucocorticoid lacking sodium-retaining activity with low to moderate doses. Increases urinary calcium excretion.

SUPPLIED: Injection; solution; inhalation (aerosol), 200 mcg/spray.

ROUTE: IV, IM, PO, inhalation.

DOSAGE:

- BPD (dosage not well established): A suggested regimen is: 0.05–0.1 mg/kg/dose q12h for 2–3 days. Maximum: 7 days.
- Lower dexamethasone doses and shorter durations of therapy are now more commonly used than high-dose (initial dose ≥0.5 mg/kg/day), long-duration regimens because of adverse effects such as hyperglycemia, hypertension, growth suppression, and concerns for neurodevelopmental compromise. Steroid trials in patients with BPD are not routine. When using steroids, use the lowest dose for the shortest period of time.
- Neonatal hypoglycemia (dosage not well established): 0.25 mg/kg/dose repeated q12h prn.
- Airway edema: 0.25 mg/kg/dose q12h generally beginning 24 h before planned extubation and continued for 2–4 doses afterward.

ADVERSE EFFECTS: With long-term use, increased susceptibility to infection, osteoporosis, growth retardation, hyperglycemia, fluid and electrolyte disturbances, cataracts, myopathy, GI perforation, hypertension, and acute adrenal insufficiency.

Diazepam (Valium)

INDICATIONS: Status epilepticus, convulsions refractory to other combined anticonvulsant agents, and hyperglycinemia.

ACTIONS: Exact action is unknown; appears to act at the CNS to produce sedative, hypnotic, skeletal muscle relaxant, and anticonvulsant effects.

DOSAGE:

- Status epilepticus: 0.1–0.3 mg/kg/dose IV q15–30min to a maximum total dose of 2–5 mg.
- Continuous refractory convulsions: 0.1–0.3 mg/kg/dose IV bolus followed by 0.3 mg/kg/h as continuous IV (dilute in saline to 0.1 mg/mL).

- Hyperglycinemia: 1.5–3 mg/kg/day PO divided q6–8h (in combination with sodium benzoate, 125–200 mg/kg/day PO divided q6–8h).
- Drug withdrawal: 0.1–0.3 mg/kg/dose PO or slowly IV given every 6–8 hours, as needed. Maximum: 1 mg/kg/dose. See Chapter 67.

ADVERSE EFFECTS: May cause drowsiness, ataxia, rash, vasodilation, respiratory arrest, and hypotension.

COMMENTS: Observe for and be prepared to manage respiratory arrest.

Diazoxide (Hyperstat IV, Proglycem)

INDICATIONS AND USE: Hypertension and persistent neonatal hypoglycemia.

ACTIONS: Nondiuretic thiazide with antihypertensive and hyperglycemic effects. Reduces total peripheral vascular resistance by direct relaxation of arteriolar smooth muscle. Inhibits pancreatic insulin release.

SUPPLIED: Oral suspension, 50 mg/mL; injection, 300 mg/20 mL.

ROUTE: IV, PO.

DOSAGE:

- IV: 3–5 mg/kg/dose; repeat in 20 min if no effect.
- PO: 8–15 mg/kg/day in 2–3 divided doses q8–12h.

ADVERSE EFFECTS: When given for short periods, adverse effects are rare. May cause bilirubin displacement from albumin, hypotension, hyperglycemia, hyperuricemia, rash, fever, leukopenia, thrombocytopenia, and ketosis.

Digoxin (Lanoxin)

INDICATIONS AND USE: Congestive heart failure, atrial fibrillation or flutter, and paroxysmal AV nodal tachycardia.

ACTIONS: Exerts a positive inotropic effect on the myocardium. Antiarrhythmic actions are due to an increase in the AV nodal refractory period produced by increased vagal activity and by a sympatholytic effect.

SUPPLIED: Pediatric injection, 100 mcg/mL; elixir, 50 mcg/mL.

ROUTE: IV, PO, IM.

DOSAGE: TDD (total digitalizing dose) to be divided ½, ¼, and ¼ q8h. *Note:* Oral doses (elixir) are ~20% higher than IV doses listed below.

- Premature infants (up to 2.5 kg)—TDD: 10–20 mcg/kg IV; maintenance: 2.5 mcg/ kg/dose q12h IV.
- Term infants—TDD: 30 mcg/kg IV; maintenance: 4 mcg/kg/dose q12h IV.
- Infants 1–12 months—TDD: 35 mcg/kg IV; maintenance: 4–5 mcg/kg/dose q12h IV.
- Reduce dose in renal dysfunction.

Therapeutic levels: 0.5–2.0 ng/mL, up to 3 ng/mL. Considerable overlap exists between toxic and therapeutic serum levels.

ADVERSE EFFECTS: Persistent vomiting is usually the most common sign of digoxin toxicity in infants. Other adverse effects are anorexia, nausea, dysrhythmias (paroxysmal ventricular contractions, blocks, tachycardia, and other), and delirium. Toxicity is markedly enhanced by hypokalemia.

Management of toxicity: Give Fab fraction of specific digoxin antibody (digoxin immune Fab [ovine] [**Digibind**]) IV in equimolar amounts (ie, 60 mg of Fab/1 mg of digoxin). Give KCl if hypokalemic.

COMMENTS: Contraindicated in second- and third-degree block, idiopathic hypertrophic subaortic stenosis, and atrial flutter or fibrillation with slow ventricular rates.

Dobutamine Hydrochloride (Dobutrex)

INDICATIONS AND USE: To increase cardiac output during states of depressed contractility, such as septic shock, organic heart disease, or cardiac surgical procedures.

ACTIONS: A direct β_1-agonist; actions on β_2- and α-adrenergic receptors are much less marked than those of dopamine. Unlike dopamine, dobutamine does not cause release of endogenous norepinephrine, nor does it have any effect on dopaminergic receptors.

SUPPLIED: Injection, 250 mg/20 mL.

ROUTE: IV.

DOSAGE: 2–10 mcg/kg/min by continuous infusion. Maximum: 40 mcg/kg/min.
ADVERSE EFFECTS: Generally dose related. Chiefly ectopic heart beats, increased heart rate, and blood pressure elevations.
COMMENTS: Contraindicated in idiopathic subaortic stenosis and atrial fibrillation.

Dopamine Hydrochloride (Dopastat, Intropin)

INDICATIONS AND USE: To increase tissue perfusion after adequate fluid volume replacement in septic states, improve cardiac output and stroke volume with severe congestive heart failure refractory to digoxin and diuretics, and increase cardiac output, blood pressure, and urine flow in patients in shock.
ACTIONS: Actions are dose-dependent. Low doses act directly on dopaminergic receptors to produce renal and mesenteric vasodilation; in moderate doses, β_1-adrenergic effects become prominent, resulting in a positive inotropic effect on the myocardium; high doses stimulate α-adrenergic receptors, producing increased peripheral resistance and renal vasoconstriction.
SUPPLIED: Injection, 40, 80, and 160 mg/mL.
ROUTE: IV by continuous infusion.
DOSAGE: *Note:* Dose–effect relationship is speculative in neonates.

- Low dose: 0.5–5 mcg/kg/min causes increased renal perfusion.
- Moderate dose: 5–10 mcg/kg/min causes increased cardiac output.
- High dose: 10–40 mcg/kg/min causes systemic vasoconstriction.

Suggested drip administration:

mg of dopamine / 100 mL of solution =

$$\frac{6 \times \text{infant's weight (kg)} \times \text{desired dose (mcg/kg/min)}}{\text{rate (mL/h)}}$$

ADVERSE EFFECTS: Dopamine may cause ectopic heartbeats, tachycardia, hypotension, hypertension, and excessive diuresis. Gangrene of the extremities has occurred with high doses over prolonged periods. Extravasation may cause tissue necrosis and sloughing of surrounding tissues; if this occurs, inject phentolamine, 0.1–0.2 mg/kg diluted to 1 mL of saline, throughout the affected area.
COMMENTS: Administration of phenytoin IV to patients receiving dopamine may result in severe hypotension and bradycardia; therefore, use with extreme caution.

Doxapram Hydrochloride (Dopram)

INDICATIONS AND USE: Apnea of prematurity resistant to methylxanthine therapy.
ACTIONS: Analeptic agent with potent respiratory and CNS stimulant properties.
SUPPLIED: Injection, 20 mg/mL.
ROUTE: IV.
DOSAGE: 0.5–1.5 mg/kg/h (maximum: 2.5 mg/kg/h) by continuous IV infusion; decrease the infusion rate when control of apnea is achieved.
Therapeutic range: <5 mcg/mL. At a dose of 1.5 mg/kg/h, the mean serum concentration reported was 3.2 mcg/mL (assay not available in most centers).
ADVERSE EFFECTS: Increases in blood pressure, heart rate, cardiac output, and skeletal muscle hyperactivity may occur. Abdominal distention, increased gastric residuals, vomiting, jitteriness, hyperglycemia, glycosuria, and seizures have been reported in neonates.
COMMENTS: Efficacy of doxapram in premature neonates with severe idiopathic apnea resistant to theophylline has been documented. Use cautiously because of its side effects. Should not be given during the first few days of life, when hypertensive episodes may be associated with an increased risk of intraventricular hemorrhage. Has a narrow therapeutic range, and its use warrants serum drug level monitoring. Contraindicated in cardiovascular and seizure disorders. Benzyl alcohol is contained in the formulation, which may accumulate to toxic levels after prolonged use.

Enalapril (PO)/Enalaprilat (IV) (Vasotec)

INDICATIONS AND USE: Manage hypertension and heart failure.

ACTIONS: Inhibits conversion of angiotensin I to angiotensin II and the breakdown of bradykinin, causing vasodilation.
SUPPLIED: Injection: 1.25 mg/mL. PO: Immediately before administration, dissolve 2.5 mg (½ of a 5-mg tablet) in 25 mL of sterile water (= 100 mcg/mL). Draw up the appropriate dose using a calibrated oral syringe. Discard the unused portion.
ROUTE: IV, PO.
DOSAGE:

- IV: 5–10 mcg/kg/dose q8–24h.
- PO: 100 mcg/kg/dose as a single daily dose. May increase gradually over 2 weeks as needed to a maximum of 500 mcg/kg/day PO. Reduce the dose in renal dysfunction.
- Use a low initial dose to avoid a profound drop in blood pressure, especially in patients on diuretics who are hyponatremic or hypovolemic. Monitor blood pressure hourly for the first 12 h.

ADVERSE EFFECTS: Hypotension, hyperkalemia, decreased renal function, oliguria, cough, decreased hemoglobin and hematocrit, and, rarely, bone marrow depression, neutropenia, and thrombocytopenia.
COMMENTS: Note that the IV dose is much smaller than the PO dose. Use caution to adjust the dose when changing routes of administration.

Epinephrine (Various)
INDICATIONS AND USE: Bradycardia, cardiac arrest, cardiogenic shock, anaphylactic reactions, and bronchospasm.
ACTIONS: Acts directly on both α- and β-adrenergic receptors, β₂ effects predominate at lower doses. Exerts both positive chronotropic and inotropic effects on the heart and relaxes bronchial smooth muscle. The α-adrenergic stimulation produces an increase in systolic blood pressure and constriction of renal blood vessels.
SUPPLIED: Injection, 0.1 mg/mL (1:10,000) and 1 mg/mL (1:1000).
ROUTE: IV, ET.
DOSAGE: 1:10,000 used IV.

- IV bolus: 0.1–0.3 mL/kg/dose q5min prn.
- IV infusion: Start with 0.1 mcg/kg/min. Maximum: 1.5 mcg/kg/min (titrate).
- Intratracheal: 0.1–0.3 mL/kg/dose diluted 1:1 with NS.

ADVERSE EFFECTS: Hypertension, tachycardia, nausea, pallor, tremor, cardiac arrhythmias, increased myocardial oxygen consumption, and decreased renal and splanchnic blood flow.

Erythromycin (Ilosone, Others)
CLASSIFICATION: Macrolide antibiotic.
ACTION AND SPECTRUM: Acts by suppression of protein synthesis. Action may be bactericidal or bacteriostatic at normal therapeutic concentrations. Spectrum of activity is broad and includes the streptococci (except enterococci), Staphylococcus aureus, Clostridium spp, Corynebacterium diphtheriae, Listeria monocytogenes, Haemophilus influenzae, Bordetella pertussis, Brucella spp, Campylobacter fetus, Branhamella catarrhalis, Neisseria gonorrhoeae, Legionella micdadei, Legionella pneumophila, Rickettsia spp, Mycoplasma pneumoniae, Chlamydia trachomatis, Treponema pallidum, and some Bacteroides spp. Ophthalmic form is routinely instilled into the eyes of newborn infants as prophylaxis against ophthalmia neonatorum.
SUPPLIED: Oral suspension, oral drops, erythromycin base (Ilotycin Ophthalmic) ointment, injection.
ROUTE: PO, IV over 60 min, ophthalmic.
DOSAGE:

- <1200 g: 20 mg/kg/day divided q12h.
- 0–7 days old: 20 mg/kg/day divided q12h.
- >7 days old: 30 mg/kg/day divided q8h.
- Ophthalmic as prophylaxis: Instill 0.5–1 cm in each eye once.
- Ophthalmic for acute infection: Instill 0.5–1 cm in each eye q6h.

ELIMINATION AND METABOLISM: Hepatic metabolism, excreted via the bile and kidneys. Half-life is 1.5–3 h (prolonged in renal failure).

ADVERSE EFFECTS: Stomatitis, epigastric distress, and oral or perianal candidiasis. Transient cholestatic hepatitis and allergic reactions occur rarely. May cause increased serum levels of theophylline, digoxin, and carbamazepine. Infantile hypertrophic pyloric stenosis (IHPS) may occur in neonates given postexposure prophylaxis with erythromycin PO after possible exposure to pertussis. Cardiac toxicity requiring CPR may occur with IV erythromycin; reduce risk of arrhythmias by slowly infusing over 1 h.

COMMENTS: Parenteral forms are painful and irritative; dilute to 5 mg/mL and infuse over 60 min. Do not use IM. Lactobionate formulation contains 180 mg of benzyl alcohol/g erythromycin.

Erythropoietin/Epoetin Alfa (Epogen, Procrit)
Synomyms: EPO, rEpo

INDICATIONS AND USE: Treatment of anemia of prematurity.

ACTIONS: A reticulocyte response may occur within 72–96 h after initiation of EPO therapy, but a change in hematocrit may not occur for 5–7 days depending on the volume of ongoing phlebotomy losses.

SUPPLIED: Injection: 2000, 3000, 4000 units/mL (and others).

ROUTE: SC, IV.

DOSAGE: Various dose regimens have been used ranging from 500 to 1400 units/kg/week, given in divided doses per week or as a single dose each week.

EPO is usually administered with iron; however, some clinicians are concerned about the use of iron in the first 2 weeks of life because of its oxidation potential and because the long-term effects of giving iron in the first 2 weeks of life are not known. Iron supplementation is given PO as ferrous sulfate drops if tolerated or IV as iron dextran.

ADVERSE EFFECTS: EPO should be used in conjunction with restrictive transfusion guidelines and minimizing of phlebotomy losses. EPO is not a substitute for emergency blood transfusion. Do not use in patients with uncontrolled hypertension. May cause hypertension, edema, fever, rash, possible seizures, transient early thrombocytosis and late neutropenia, polycythemia, and local skin reaction at injection site.

Ethacrynic Acid (Edecrin)
INDICATIONS AND USE: When prompt diuresis is needed in patients refractory to other diuretics. Other diuretics should be tried first because ethacrynic acid is more toxic.

ACTIONS: Loop diuretic. Inhibits reabsorption of sodium and chloride in the proximal and distal tubules and the loop of Henle. Inhibits sodium reabsorption to a greater degree than other diuretics. Does not appear to have a direct effect on the pulmonary vasculature, as furosemide does.

SUPPLIED: Injection, 50 mg in 50-mL vials for reconstitution; tablet, 25 mg (scored). (No oral liquid is available.)

ROUTE: PO, IV.

DOSAGE: 0.5–1 mg/kg/dose qd in preterm infants; q12h in full-term neonates; or more frequently, if needed, in older infants. Maximum: 2 mg/kg IV or 6 mg/kg PO.

ADVERSE EFFECTS: Inject the IV dose slowly over several minutes. May cause dehydration, electrolyte depletion, diarrhea, GI upset, GI bleeding, hearing loss, rash, local irritation and pain, hematuria, and, rarely, hypoglycemia and neutropenia.

Fentanyl (Sublimaze)
INDICATIONS AND USE: Analgesia, anesthesia, and sedation.

ACTIONS: A synthetic opiate agonist. Acts similarly to morphine and meperidine but without the cardiovascular effects of those drugs and with shorter respiratory depressant effects.

SUPPLIED: Injection, 50 mcg/mL.

ROUTE: IV.

DOSAGE:

• Analgesia: 1–2 mcg/kg/dose q2–4h prn or by continuous infusion at 0.1–3 mcg/kg/h.

- Anesthesia: Major surgery, 25–50 mcg/kg/dose; minor surgery, 2–10 mcg/kg/dose.
- Sedation: 2 mcg/kg/dose q2–4h prn or by continuous infusion of 0.5–1 mcg/kg/h (titrate).

ADVERSE EFFECTS: Bradycardia, muscular rigidity with reduced pulmonary compliance or apnea, bronchoconstriction, and laryngospasm.
COMMENTS: Limited experience in neonates; 0.1 mg of fentanyl = 10 mg of morphine or 75 mg of meperidine. Concurrent ventilatory assistance is suggested with its use. Tachyphylaxis occurs after several days of therapy. Adheres to extracorporeal membrane oxygenation (ECMO) filter membranes; may have to adjust the dose.

Ferrous Sulfate (20% Elemental Iron) (Various)
INDICATIONS AND USE: Treatment and prevention of iron deficiency anemia.
ACTIONS: Iron is needed for the production of heme proteins. The use of iron-fortified formulas during the first year of life will usually prevent iron deficiency anemia in both the preterm and term infants. Iron-fortified formulas can be fed safely to preterm infants. Of the ferrous salts available (sulfate, fumarate, and gluconate), sulfate is preferred.
SUPPLIED: Drops (proferred), 75 mg/0.6 ml (15 mg of elemental iron); elixir, 220 mg/5 mL (44 mg of elemental iron); syrup, 90 mg/5 mL (18 mg of elemental iron).
ROUTE: PO.
DOSAGE: Recommendations of the American Academy of Pediatrics; dosages are for elemental iron

- Term infants: 1 mg/kg/day starting no later than 2 months of age.
- Preterm infants: 2 mg/kg/day starting no later than 2 months of age.
- Iron deficiency anemia: 6 mg/kg/day in 4 divided doses.
- Iron supplementation with erythropoietin. 6 mg/kg/day.

ADVERSE EFFECTS: GI irritation (vomiting, diarrhea, constipation, and darkened stool color).
COMMENTS: Caution parents to guard against iron poisoning from accidental ingestion. Antidote is chelation with deferoxamine; consult specialized references and regional Poison Control Center for further information.

Fluconazole (Diflucan)
INDICATIONS AND USE: Antifungal agent for systemic candidiasis and meningitis. Advantages over amphotericin B are once-a-day dosing, good distribution characteristics with similar CSF and serum levels, oral as well as IV administration, and fewer adverse effects. Check the sensitivity of the organism.
ACTIONS: Inhibits fungal cytochrome P450 and sterol C-14 α-demethylation, resulting in a fungistatic effect.
SUPPLIED: PO, 10-mg/mL and 40-mg/mL suspensions; injection, 2 mg/mL.
ROUTE: PO, IV.
DOSAGE: 6 mg/kg/day as a single daily dose. Infuse IV over 1–2 h. Reduce the dose in renal dysfunction.
ADVERSE EFFECTS: Usually well tolerated. Vomiting, diarrhea, rash, and elevations in liver function tests.
COMMENTS: Monitor liver function tests. Use caution in preexisting renal dysfunction. Cimetidine and rifampin decrease fluconazole levels. Hydrochlorothiazide increases fluconazole levels. Fluconazole increases phenytoin and zidovudine levels and increases the prothrombin time for patients on warfarin.

Flucytosine (Ancobon)
CLASSIFICATION: Antifungal agent.
ACTION AND SPECTRUM: Penetrates fungal cells, where it acts as an antimetabolite, ultimately interfering with protein synthesis. It is active in vivo against some strains of *Cryptococcus* and *Candida*. May be synergistic with amphotericin B.

SUPPLIED: Capsules. (The pharmacist can compound an oral liquid.)
ROUTE: PO.
DOSAGE:

- 50–100 mg/kg/day divided q6h. Renal impairment: 12.5–25 mg/kg/day divided as follows:
  q12h for a creatinine clearance of 20–40 mL/min.
  q24h for a creatinine clearance of 10–20 mL/min.
  q24–48h for a creatinine clearance of <10 mL/min.

Serum concentrations: 24–120 mcg/mL.
PHARMACOKINETICS: Volume of distribution, 0.68 L/kg; half-life, 3–5 h; renal elimination.
ADVERSE EFFECTS: Vomiting, diarrhea, rash, anemia, leukopenia, thrombocytopenia, elevated liver function tests, increased BUN and creatinine, and CNS disturbances.

Fludrocortisone (Florinef)
INDICATIONS AND USE: Fludrocortisone is a mineralocorticoid used for partial replacement therapy for adrenocortical insufficiency and treatment of salt-losing forms of congenital adrenogenital syndrome. Usually used with concurrent hydrocortisone and sodium chloride.
ACTIONS: Acts on the distal tubule to increase loss of potassium and hydrogen ion and increases reabsorption of sodium with subsequent water retention. Fludrocortisone has some glucocorticoid activity.
SUPPLIED: Scored tablet: 0.1 mg/tablet (= 100 mcg/tablet).
ROUTE: PO.
DOSAGE: 0.05–0.2 mg/day (= 50–200 mcg/day) as a single daily dose. (*Note:* Doses are the same regardless of patient weight or age. Newborns are quite insensitive to the drug and may require larger doses than adults.) May administer with feedings.
ADVERSE EFFECTS: Hypertension, congestive heart failure, GI upset, hypokalemia, growth suppression, hyperglycemia, salt and water retention, edema, suppression of endogenous steroid production, osteoporosis, muscle weakness resulting from excessive potassium loss. Rarely causes anaphylaxis and rash. Monitor serum electrolytes (particularly sodium and potassium).
COMMENTS: Fludrocortisone 0.1 mg has a sodium retention activity equal to deoxycorticosterone acetate (DOCA) 1 mg.

Furosemide (Lasix)
INDICATIONS AND USE: Fluid overload, pulmonary edema, congestive heart failure, and hypertension.
ACTIONS: Inhibits active chloride transport in the ascending limb of the loop of Henle. Furosemide-induced diuresis results in enhanced excretion of NaCl, potassium, calcium, magnesium, bicarbonate, ammonium, hydrogen, and possibly phosphate. IV administration increases venous capacitance independently of its diuretic effect, resulting in rapid improvement of pulmonary edema.
SUPPLIED: Oral solution, 10 mg/mL; injection, 10 mg/mL.
ROUTE: PO, IV, IM.
DOSAGE:

- PO: 1–2 mg/kg/dose q12h as initial dose and increase slowly if needed, because more may be required as a result of highly variable bioavailability.
- IV or IM: 1 mg/kg/dose q12–24h slowly. If there is no increase in urine output, double the above doses and repeat.

ADVERSE EFFECTS: Hypokalemia, hypocalcemia, and hyponatremia. With prolonged use, nephrocalcinosis and hypochloremic metabolic alkalosis.

Gentamicin Sulfate (Garamycin, Others)
CLASSIFICATION: Aminoglycoside.
ACTION AND SPECTRUM: Bactericidal activity by inhibition of bacterial protein synthesis. Active chiefly against gram-negative aerobic bacteria, including most *Pseudomonas, Proteus,* and *Serratia* spp. Some activity against coagulase-positive staphylococci but ineffective against anaerobes and streptococci. Provides some synergistic effect against group D streptococci (enterococci) when used in combination with a penicillin.

SUPPLIED: Injection, intrathecal injection, ophthalmic solution.

ROUTE: IM, IV (infuse over 30 min).

DOSAGE: Base the initial dose on body weight, then monitor levels and adjust using pharmacokinetics.

- IV (preferred), IM:
  <7 days' postnatal age:
  <1 kg and <28 weeks' gestational age: 2.5 mg/kg/dose q24h.
  <1.5 kg and <34 weeks' gestational age: 2.5 mg/kg/dose q18h.
  >1.5 kg and >34 weeks' gestational age: 2.5 mg/kg/dose q12h.
  >7 days' postnatal age:
  <1.2 kg: 2.5 mg/kg/dose q18–24h.
  >1.2 kg: 2.5 mg/kg/dose q8h.

- *Note:* Once-a-day dosing using 4-mg/kg IV has been reported in a few studies in term infants and for infants >34 weeks' gestation with normal renal function.
- Intrathecal or intraventricular: 1–2 mg qd.
- Ophthalmic solution: Instill 1 drop into each eye q4–12h.

ELIMINATION AND METABOLISM: Renal excretion by glomerular filtration. Half-life is 4–8 h initially.

ADVERSE EFFECTS: Irreversible vestibular injury, proteinuria, uremia, oliguria, and macular rash.

COMMENTS: Desired serum peak is 4–10 mcg/mL (sample obtained 30 min after infusion has been completed), and desired serum trough is <2 mcg/mL (sample obtained 30 min before next dose). In general, a set of peak and trough levels should be obtained at about the fourth maintenance dose. Monitor serum creatinine. Excessive serum peak levels are associated with ototoxicity; excessive trough levels, with nephrotoxicity. The aminoglycosides should not be used alone against gram-positive pathogens.

Glucagon

INDICATIONS AND USE: Hypoglycemia as seen in infants of diabetic mothers (IDMs); hypoglycemia resulting from other causes unresponsive to routine treatment. Bowel spasm during barium enema.

ACTIONS: Glucagon, a hormone produced by the alpha cells of the pancreas, causes increased breakdown of glycogen to form glucose and inhibition of glycogen synthetase. Blood glucose elevation occurs. Produces relaxation of the smooth muscle in the GI tract when the drug is administered parenterally.

SUPPLIED: Injection, 1-mg (1-unit) vials.

ROUTE: SC, IM, IV.

DOSAGE: 0.025–0.3 mg/kg/dose; may repeat in 20 min prn. In IDMs: 0.3 mg/kg/ dose. Maximum: 1 mg.

ADVERSE EFFECTS: Hypersensitivity, nausea, and vomiting.

COMMENTS: Incompatible with electrolyte-containing solutions; compatible with dextrose solutions. *Caution:* Do not delay initiation of glucose infusion while observing for glucagon effect.

Heparin Sodium (Various)

INDICATIONS AND USE: Primary role is as an anticoagulant. Used to diagnose and treat disseminated intravascular coagulation and to maintain patency of arterial or venous catheters.

ACTIONS: In combination with antithrombin III (heparin cofactor), heparin inactivates coagulation factors IX, X, XI, and XII and thrombin, inhibiting the conversion of fibrinogen to fibrin.

SUPPLIED: Injection, 10, 100, 1000, and 5000 units/mL.

ROUTE: SC, IV.

DOSAGE:

- Loading dose: 50 units/kg as IV bolus.
- Maintenance DOSAGE: 10–20 units/kg/h as continuous infusion.
- To maintain catheter patency: 0.5–1 unit/mL of fluid.

- Antidote: Protamine sulfate, 1 mg for each 100 units of heparin given in the preceding 3–4 h up to a maximum dose of 50 mg.

Hepatitis B Immune Globulin (H-BIG, Others)
INDICATIONS AND USE: Prophylaxis of hepatitis B exposure.
ACTIONS: Passive immunization agent. Immune serum provides protection against the hepatitis B virus by directly providing specific antibody to hepatitis B surface antigen (HBsAg). The immunity is transient, usually lasting ~30 days.
SUPPLIED: Injection, 1-, 4-, and 5-mL vials.
ROUTE: IM only.
DOSAGE: 0.5 mL administered within 12 h after delivery. (Repeat at 3 months and 6 months if the vaccine was not given.)
ADVERSE EFFECTS: Swelling, warmth, erythema, and soreness at the injection site. Rarely, rash, fever, and urticaria.
COMMENTS: Do not use in patients with immunoglobulin (Ig) A deficiency, thrombocytopenia, or coagulopathy. Do not administer IV.

Hepatitis B Vaccine (Heptavax-B, Recombivax HB, Engerix B)
INDICATIONS AND USE: Prophylaxis for hepatitis B.
ACTIONS: Induces protective antibody formation to hepatitis B virus (anti-HBs).
SUPPLIED: Injection: Recombivax HB, 10 mcg/mL; Engerix B, 20 mcg/mL and 10 mcg/ 0.5 mL.
ROUTE: IM only.
DOSAGE: 0.5 mL IM (= Recombivax HB, 5 mcg; Engerix B, 10 mcg).
ADVERSE EFFECTS: Swelling, warmth, erythema, soreness at the injection site, and, rarely, vomiting, rash, and low-grade fever.
COMMENTS: Do not give IV or intradermally. Administer in the anterolateral thigh.

Hyaluronidase (Wydase)
INDICATIONS AND USE: Treatment of extravasation injuries.
ACTIONS: An enzyme that temporarily breaks down hyaluronic acid (tissue "cement") and thereby allows the infiltrated drug or solution to be absorbed over a larger surface area. This speeds absorption and reduces tissue contact time with the irritant substance.
SUPPLIED: Injection, 150 units/mL as a lyophilized powder or a stabilized solution. The solution must be refrigerated.
ROUTE: SC.
DOSAGE: Dilute to 15 units/mL in normal saline. Before it is removed, inject 0.2 mL into the needle that was used to infuse the IV, and four 0.2-mL injections into the leading edge of the extravasation. Elevate the extremity. Do not apply heat. May repeat if necessary.
ADVERSE EFFECTS: Usually well tolerated. Urticaria (rare). Administer hyaluronidase within 1 h of the extravasation, if possible.

Hydralazine Hydrochloride (Apresoline Hydrochloride)
INDICATIONS AND USE: For hypertension and as an afterload reducing agent to treat congestive heart failure.
ACTIONS: Direct-acting vasodilator that reduces peripheral resistance and blood pressure and relaxes venous capacitance vessels. Reflex increases in heart rate, cardiac output, and stroke volume are probably produced in response to the decrease in peripheral vascular resistance.
SUPPLIED: Injection, 20 mg/mL; tablets, 10 mg (oral liquid can be compounded by the pharmacist).
ROUTE: IM, IV, PO.
DOSAGE:

- IM or IV: 0.1–0.5 mg/kg/dose q6h (maximum: 2 mg/kg/dose).
- PO: 0.5–7.0 mg/kg/day divided q6–8h.

ADVERSE EFFECTS: Most frequent are headache, palpitations, and tachycardia; most serious is a reversible lupus-like syndrome. Tachyphylaxis often occurs on chronic therapy.

COMMENTS: Contraindicated in mitral valve rheumatic heart disease.

Hydrochlorothiazide (Various)

INDICATIONS AND USE: Hypertension and pulmonary edema.
ACTIONS: See Chlorothiazide.
SUPPLIED: Solution, 50 mg/5 mL and 100 mg/mL.
ROUTE: PO.
DOSAGE: Up to 1–3 mg/kg/day divided q12h.
ADVERSE EFFECTS AND COMMENTS: See Chlorothiazide.

Hydrocortisone (Various)

INDICATIONS AND USE: Acute adrenal insufficiency, congenital adrenal hyperplasia, and shock.
ACTIONS: A steroid possessing glucocorticoid activity with some mineralocorticoid effects; most effects probably result from modification of enzyme activity, thus affecting almost all body systems. Promotes protein catabolism, gluconeogenesis, renal excretion of calcium, capillary wall permeability and stability, and red blood cell production; suppresses immune and inflammatory responses.
SUPPLIED: Injection (acetate, sodium phosphate, and sodium succinate), oral suspension (cypionate), topical ointment and cream (acetate).
ROUTE: PO, IV, IM, topical.
DOSAGE:

- Acute adrenal insufficiency. 1–2 mg/kg/dose IV bolus; then 25–150 mg q24h divided q6h.
- Congenital adrenal hyperplasia: Initial dose, 0.5–0.7 mg/kg/day divided ¼ in the morning, ¼ at noon, and ½ at night; maintenance dose, 0.3–0.4 mg/kg/day divided as above.
- Topical (0.5%): Apply to the area 3 times daily.

ADVERSE EFFECTS AND COMMENTS: See Dexamethasone. Application to large body surface areas may produce absorption with systemic effects. Avoid facial application.

Immune Globulin, Intravenous (IVIG) (Gamimune N, Sandoglobulin, Gammagard)

INDICATIONS AND USE: Immunodeficiency syndromes and suspected sepsis (controversial). Sandoglobulin is also indicated for treatment of idiopathic thrombocytopenic purpura.
ACTIONS: Establishes immediate (passive) IgG antibody serum levels.
SUPPLIED: Injection, 50 mg/mL (Gamimune N, 10 and 50 mL) or powder for injection (Sandoglobulin, 1 g/vial).
ROUTE: IV only.
DOSAGE:

- Suspected sepsis: IV IgG 400–500 mg/kg/dose for 1–2 doses; repeat weekly.
- Immunodeficiency syndrome:
    Sandoglobulin: 200 mg/kg (initial rate: 0.08–0.1 mL/kg/min) once per month. If the desired clinical response or level of IgG is insufficient, then increase the dose to 300 mg/kg or repeat the dose more frequently.
    Gamimune N: 100 mg/kg or 2 mL/kg (at an initial flow rate of 0.01–0.02 mL/kg/min for 30 min, may dilute in D_5W) once per month. If no adverse effects are observed, then increase the rate to 0.02–0.04 mL/kg/min. If the desired clinical response is not achieved or the level of IgG is insufficient, increase the dose to 200 mg/kg (4 mL/kg) or repeat the dose more frequently than once per month.
    Gammagard: 100 mg/kg once per month (initial rate of 0.5 mL/kg/h). If the desired clinical response is not achieved or the level of IgG is insufficient, increase the dose to 200–400 mg/kg to maintain a serum IgG level >500 mg/dL.
- Idiopathic thrombocytopenia purpura:
    Sandoglobulin: 400 mg/kg/day for 5 consecutive days. (See above administration rate for immunodeficiency syndrome.)

ADVERSE EFFECTS: Hypotension and anaphylaxis. If either occurs, the rate of infusion should be decreased or stopped until resolved, then resumed at a slower rate as tolerated. Preparations contain antibodies to group B streptococcus and *Escherichia coli.* Substantial variation among lots and manufacturers.

Indomethacin (Indocin IV)
INDICATIONS AND USE: Pharmacologic closure of patent ductus arteriosus (PDA).
ACTIONS: Nonsteroidal anti-inflammatory drug (NSAID) with analgesic and antipyretic properties. Action is principally by inhibition of prostaglandin synthesis, thus inhibiting cyclooxygenase, an enzyme that catalyzes the formation of prostaglandin precursors (endoperoxides) from arachidonic acid. Decreases cerebral blood flow.
SUPPLIED: Powder for injection, 1-mg vials.
ROUTE: IV.
DOSAGE: PDA closure: IV at 12- to 24-h intervals. Indocin should be given q12h unless the patient has decreased urinary output.

- Initial dose: 0.2 mg/kg.
- Second dose:
  <48 h: 0.1 mg/kg.
  2–7 days: 0.2 mg/kg.
  >8 days: 0.25 mg/kg.
- Third dose:
  <48 h: 0.1 mg/kg.
  2–7 days: 0.2 mg/kg.
  >8 days: 0.25 mg/kg.
- Prevention of intraventricular hemorrhage: 0.1 mg/kg IV at 6 and 12 h postnatal and q24h for 2 more doses.

ADVERSE EFFECTS: May cause decreased platelet aggregation, transient oliguria (decreased glomerular filtration rate), increased serum creatinine, and increased serum concentrations of renally eliminated drugs such as gentamicin, hyponatremia, hyperkalemia, and hypoglycemia. Displaces bilirubin from albumin binding sites but is not considered clinically significant.
COMMENTS: Contraindicated in necrotizing enterocolitis (NEC) or when the stool Hematest >3+, BUN >30 mg/dL, serum creatinine >1.8 mg/dL, or urine output <0.6 mL/kg/h for the preceding 8 h; in thrombocytopenia (<60,000/mm^3); with active bleeding; or if there has been intraventricular bleeding within the preceding 7 days (*controversial*).

Insulin, Regular (Various)
INDICATIONS AND USE: Hyperglycemia, hyperkalemia, and increasing caloric intake in infants with glucose intolerance on PN.
ACTIONS: Hormone derived from the beta cells of the pancreas and the principal hormone required for glucose utilization. In skeletal and cardiac muscle and adipose tissue, insulin facilitates transport of glucose into these cells. Stimulates lipogenesis and protein synthesis and inhibits lipolysis and release of free fatty acids from adipose cells. Promotes intracellular shift of potassium and magnesium.
SUPPLIED: Injection, 100 units/mL; Humulin R (human insulin that is prepared using recombinant DNA technology).
Note: Should be diluted by the pharmacy to 1 unit/mL in diluent provided by the manufacturer to improve accuracy in measurement and avoid overdose.
ROUTE: IV, SC.
DOSAGE:

- Hyperglycemia: Loading dose, 0.1 unit/kg/dose infused IV over 15–20 min; maintenance dose, 0.02–0.1 unit/kg/h by continuous IV infusion (titrate with hourly determinations of blood glucose until stable, then q4h) (dilute insulin as above).
- Hyperkalemia: Give calcium gluconate, 50 mg/kg/dose IV, and sodium bicarbonate IV, 1 mEq/kg/dose IV, first; then give dextrose, 600–800 mg/kg/dose, and insulin, 0.2 unit/kg/dose IV (3–4:1 glucose-insulin ratio).

• Increase caloric intake for infants on PN: 0.02–0.1 unit/kg/h IV as continuous infusion. Monitor serum glucose every hour until stable, then q4h.

ADVERSE EFFECTS: Hypoglycemia (may cause coma and severe CNS injury), hyperglycemic rebound (Somogyi effect), urticaria, and anaphylaxis.

COMMENTS: Human insulin (preferred) is less antigenic than pork-derived insulin, which is less antigenic than beef-derived insulin. Insulin adsorbs to plastic surfaces of IV systems. In concentrations of 10 units/L, ~50% of the insulin binds to the tubing. At greater concentrations, ~5 units/L binds to the IV tubing. Adjust the dose as needed.

Ipratropium Bromide (Atrovent)
INDICATIONS AND USE: Bronchodilator.
ACTIONS: Anticholinergic drug that acts by antagonizing acetylcholine at the parasympathetic sites, thereby inhibiting parasympathetic bronchoconstriction.
SUPPLIED: Solution for nebulization, 500 mcg/2.5 mL.
ROUTE: Nebulization.
DOSAGE: Nebulization: 250 mcg given q8h. Dilute to 3 mL with NS or concurrent albuterol.
ADVERSE EFFECTS: Rebound airway hyperresponsiveness after discontinuation. Nervousness, dizziness, nausea, blurred vision, dry mouth, exacerbation of symptoms, airway irritation, cough, palpitations, rash, and urinary difficulty. Use with caution in narrow-angle glaucoma or bladder neck obstruction.
COMMENTS: Compatible when admixed with albuterol if given within 1 h.

Iron Dextran (INFeD, DexFerrum)
INDICATIONS AND USE: Used to treat iron deficiency anemia, as an iron supplement for infants on epoetin, and for infants on long-term PN. Oral iron is much safer than the parenteral form; the parenteral form is usually reserved for patients who cannot take oral iron.
ACTIONS: Iron is a component in the formation of hemoglobin, and adequate amounts are necessary for erythropoiesis and oxygen transport capacity of blood.
SUPPLIED: Injection: 50 mg Fe/mL
ROUTE: IV, IM
DOSAGE:

• Iron deficiency anemia: Total deficit or required dose in mg of iron can be calculated with this formula:

$$\text{Dose Fe (mg/kg)} = (12 \text{ g/dL} - \text{Hgb [g/dL]}) \times 4.5$$

Divide this total dose into daily increments (or less frequently), usually not more than 25 mg Fe/day for infants weighing <5 kg and 50 mg Fe/day for infants 5–10 kg.
Iron dextran has been admixed in the PN solution 1 mg/kg/day (or 3–5 mg/kg as a single weekly dose). The drug has also been infused by Y-site injection into the PN catheter (institutional experience).
ADVERSE EFFECTS: Iron accumulation in patients with serious liver dysfunction; anaphylaxis, fever, and arthralgia.

• IV: Pain and redness at IV site, rash, shivering; hypotension and flushing with rapid infusion.
• IM: Possible sarcomas (controversial), pain and redness or sores at injection site; infection associated with large IM doses in infants. Staining at IM site can be minimized by using Z-track technique by displacing the skin laterally before injection and using a separate needle to withdraw the drug from the vial.

Isoniazid (INH, Laniazid, Nydrazid)
CLASSIFICATION: Antituberculous agent.
ACTION AND SPECTRUM: Bactericidal effect on growing tubercle bacilli by interfering with lipid and protein synthesis. Spectrum includes *Mycobacterium* spp (eg, *M. tuberculosis, M. kansasii,* and *M. avium*).

SUPPLIED: Injection, 100 mg/mL; syrup, 50 mg/5 mL.

ROUTE: PO, IM.

DOSAGE:

- Primary tuberculosis: 10–15 mg/kg/day divided q12–24h with rifampin for 9–12 months.
- Skin test conversion: 10–15 mg/kg/day PO q24h for 9 months.

ADVERSE EFFECTS: Peripheral neuropathy, seizures, encephalopathy, blood dyscrasias, and allergy.

Isoproterenol (Isuprel, Others)

INDICATIONS AND USE: Shock, cardiac arrest, Adams-Stokes syndrome, ventricular arrhythmias resulting from AV block, and bronchospasm.

ACTIONS: Acts on both β_1- and β_2-adrenergic receptors with minimal or no effect on alpha receptors in therapeutic doses. Relaxes bronchial smooth muscle, cardiac stimulation (inotropic and chronotropic), and peripheral vasodilation (reduces cardiac afterload).

SUPPLIED: Injection (1:5000), 0.2 mg/mL; solution for nebulization, aerosol (various strengths).

ROUTE: IV, inhalation.

DOSAGE:

- IV: 0.05–0.5 mcg/kg/min (titrate).
- Inhalation/nebulization: 0.1 mL to a maximum of 0.5 mL/dose. Dilute to 2 mL with normal saline, given q4h prn.

ADVERSE EFFECTS: Tremor, vomiting, hypertension, tachycardia, and cardiac arrhythmias.

COMMENTS: Contraindicated in hypertension, degenerative heart disease, hyperthyroidism, tachycardia caused by digoxin toxicity, and preexisting cardiac arrhythmias. Increases cardiac oxygen consumption disproportional to the increase in cardiac oxygen output. Not considered an inotropic agent of choice.

Kanamycin Sulfate (Kantrex)

CLASSIFICATION: Aminoglycoside.

ACTION AND SPECTRUM: Mechanism of action is identical to that of gentamicin sulfate. Active primarily against gram-negative aerobic bacteria, including *Escherichia coli; Klebsiella, Enterobacter, Serratia,* and *Proteus* spp; and some *Pseudomonas* spp. Some activity against staphylococci and mycobacteria. Not active against other gram-positive organisms or anaerobes.

SUPPLIED: Injection.

ROUTE: IV (infuse over 30 min), IM.

DOSAGE: Base the initial dose on body weight, then monitor levels and adjust using pharmacokinetics.

- <1.2 kg, 0–4 weeks old: 7.5 mg/kg/dose q18–24h.
- 1.2–2 kg:
  0–7 days old: 7.5 mg/kg/dose q12–18h.
  >7 days old: 7.5 mg/kg/dose q8–12h.
- >2 kg:
  0–7 days old: 10 mg/kg/dose q12h.
  >7 days old: 10 mg/kg/dose q8h.

ELIMINATION AND METABOLISM: Primarily renally excreted by glomerular filtration. Half-life is 4–8 h.

ADVERSE EFFECTS: See Gentamicin Sulfate.

COMMENTS: See Gentamicin Sulfate. Desired serum peak is 25–35 mcg/mL (sample obtained 30 min after infusion is complete), and serum trough is <10 mcg/mL (sample obtained 30 min to just before next dose). In general, a set of serum peak and trough levels should be obtained at about the fourth maintenance dose. Monitor serum creatinine every 3–4 days. Excessive serum peak levels are associated with ototoxicity; excessive trough levels, with nephrotoxicity.

Ketamine Hydrochloride (Ketalar)

INDICATIONS AND USE: Ketamine is a rapid-acting general anesthetic agent for short diagnostic and minor surgical procedures that do not require skeletal muscle relaxation.

ACTIONS: Dissociates the cortex from the limbic system. Induces coma, analgesia, and amnesia. The patient appears to be awake but is immobile and unresponsive to pain. Increases cerebral blood flow and cerebral oxygen consumption; improves pulmonary compliance and relieves bronchospasm.

PHARMACOKINETICS: Onset and duration: Unconsciousness:

- IV: 30 s, lasts 5–10 min.
- IM: 3–4 min, lasts 12–25 min.
- Analgesia lasts 30–40 min.
- Amnesia lasts for 1–2 h. Concurrent narcotics or barbiturates prolong recovery time.
- SUPPLIED: Injection, 10, 50, and 100 mg/mL.

ROUTE: IV, IM, PO.

DOSAGE:

- IV: 0.5–1 mg/kg/dose.
- IM: 3–7 mg/kg/dose.
- PO: 6 mg/kg/dose.
- Dilute before administration. Repeat doses are ½ of initial doses. Reduce the dose in hepatic dysfunction.

Avoid use of ketamine in patients in whom increased intracranial pressure, cerebral blood flow, CSF pressure, cerebral metabolism, or significant elevation in blood pressure may present a risk. *Cardiovascular:* Elevated blood pressure (frequent), tachycardia, arrhythmia, hypotension, bradycardia, increased cerebral blood flow, and decreased cardiac output may occur. *Respiratory:* Respiratory stimulation, transient and minimal respiratory depression, and apnea after rapid IV administration of high doses; laryngospasm; and hypersalivation. Gag and cough reflexes are generally preserved. *Ophthalmic:* Nystagmus, increased intraocular pressure. *CNS:* Emergence reactions (psychic disturbances such as hallucinations and delirium lasting up to 24 h). Minimize by reducing verbal, tactile, and visual simulation in the recovery period. These occur less commonly in pediatric patients than in adults. Severe reactions can be treated with a benzodiazepine. Increased muscle tone that may resemble seizures and extensor spasm with opisthotonos may occur in infants receiving high, repeated doses. *Dermatologic:* Rash as well as pain and redness at the IM injection site.

COMMENTS: Pretreatment with a benzodiazepine 15 min before ketamine may reduce side effects such as psychic, circulatory, increased intracranial pressure and cerebral blood flow; tachycardia; and jerky movements. Monitor heart rate, respiratory rate, blood pressure, and pulse oximetry. Observe for CNS side effects during the recovery period. Have equipment for resuscitation available.

Ketoconazole (Nizoral)

CLASSIFICATION: Antifungal agent.

ACTION AND SPECTRUM: A broad-spectrum antifungal agent that acts by disrupting cell membranes. Fungicidal against *Blastomyces dermatitidis, Candida* spp, *Coccidioides immitis, Histoplasma capsulatum, Paracoccidioides brasiliensis,* and *Phialophora* spp. Development of resistance is rare.

SUPPLIED: Tablet, 200 mg. Oral suspension may be prepared by the pharmacist.

ROUTE: PO.

DOSAGE: 2.5–5 mg/kg/day q24h.

ELIMINATION AND METABOLISM: Hepatic metabolism.

ADVERSE EFFECTS: Gastric distress is the most common side effect. Hepatic damage is rare.

COMMENTS: Penetration into CSF is poor, so do not use in the treatment of fungal meningitis. Minimum period of treatment for candidiasis is 1–2 weeks, but duration should be based on clinical response. Monitor liver function tests. Limited experience in neonates.

Labetalol Hydrochloride (Normodyne)

INDICATIONS AND USE: Treatment of hypertension. IV form is used to control severe hypertension.

ACTIONS: Causes a dose-related decrease in blood pressure through α-, β_1-, and β_2-blocking actions without causing significant reflex tachycardia or a decrease in heart rate. Reduces elevated renins.

PHARMACOKINETICS: Peak effect PO is 1–4 h after the dose; peak effect IV is 5–15 min. Metabolized in the liver by glucuronidation. Oral labetalol has a bioavailability of only 25% because of extensive first-pass effect. Oral absorption is improved by taking with food. Concomitant oral cimetidine may increase the bioavailability of oral labetalol.

SUPPLIED: Injection, 5 mg/mL multidose vials. No oral liquid is commercially available. Labetalol oral liquid, 40 mg/mL, can be compounded by the pharmacist from tablets and a sweetened vehicle (see *Am J Health Syst Pharm* 1996;53:2304).

ROUTE: PO, IV, continuous IV infusion.

DOSAGE: Limited experience in neonates; carefully monitor blood pressure, heart rate, and electrocardiogram, and adjust the dose accordingly. Use the lowest effective dose.

- PO: 3–4 mg/kg/day PO in 2 divided doses.
- IV: 0.2–0.5 mg/kg/dose over 2–3 min.
- Continuous IV infusion: 0.2–1 mg/kg/h (1 mg/mL dilution).

ADVERSE EFFECTS: Orthostatic hypotension, bronchospasm, nasal congestion, edema, congestive heart failure, bradycardia, myopathy, and rash. Intensifies AV block. Reversible hepatic dysfunction (rare). Do not discontinue chronic labetalol abruptly; rather, discontinue gradually over 1–2 weeks. Do not use in patients with asthma, overt cardiac failure, heart block, cardiogenic shock, or severe bradycardia. May cause a paradoxic increase in blood pressure in patients with pheochromocytoma. Use with caution in hepatic dysfunction. Incompatible with sodium bicarbonate.

COMMENTS: Use caution in converting from the PO to IV route of administration because a much smaller dose is required IV than PO.

Levothyroxine Sodium (T₄) (Synthroid)

INDICATIONS AND USE: Treatment of congenital hypothyroidism.

ACTIONS: Thyroid hormones increase the metabolic rate of body tissues, noted by increases in oxygen consumption; respiratory rate; body temperature; cardiac output; heart rate; blood volume; rates of fat, protein, and carbohydrate metabolism; enzyme system activity; growth; and maturation. Thyroid hormones are very important in CNS development. Deficiency in infants results in growth retardation and failure of brain growth and development.

SUPPLIED: Injection, 200 mcg per vial as a lyophilized powder; scored tablets, 0.025, 0.05, 0.075, 0.088, 0.1, 0.112, 0.125, 0.15, and 0.175 mg. Tablets may be crushed and mixed with water or a small amount of infant formula and administered immediately after mixing. Discard the unused portion.

ROUTE: IV, IM, PO.

DOSAGE: *Note:* The parenteral dose should be approximately ½ the previously established oral dose.

- 0–6 months: 25–50 mcg/day PO (8–10 mcg/kg/day).
- 6–12 months: 50–75 mcg/day PO (6–8 mcg/kg/day).
- Alternatively, 8–10 mcg/kg/day PO has been recommended for infants from birth to 1 year.

ADVERSE EFFECTS: Adverse effects are usually due to excessive dose. If the following occur, discontinue and reinstitute at a lower dose: tachycardia, cardiac arrhythmias, tremors, diarrhea, weight loss, and fever.

Lidocaine (Xylocaine, Others)

INDICATIONS AND USE: IV lidocaine is used almost exclusively for the short-term control of ventricular arrhythmias (premature beats, tachycardia, and fibrillation) or for prophylactic treatment of such arrhythmias. Skin infiltration as a local anesthetic.

ACTIONS: Type I antiarrhythmic agent, with most activity related to blockade of the fast sodium channels in Purkinje fibers. Also a CNS depressant with sedative, analgesic, and anticonvulsant properties.

SUPPLIED: IV forms: Injection (premixed) in D_5W, 2 mg/mL (500 mL), 4 mg/mL (250 mL), and 8 mg/mL (250 mL); injection (for IV bolus), 10 mg/mL (5 mL); injection (for IV admixture [must be diluted]), 40 mg/mL (25 mL). Solution, 0.5% and 1%, for local anesthesia.

ROUTE: IV, SC, or intratracheal.

DOSAGE: 1 mg/kg/dose as IV bolus q5min to a maximum total dose of 5 mg/kg, followed by IV infusion of 10–50 mcg/kg/min.

Therapeutic levels: 1–5 mcg/mL. Toxicity associated with levels >5 mcg/mL.

ADVERSE EFFECTS: Adverse effects generally involve the CNS: drowsiness, dizziness, tremulousness, and paresthesias. Muscle twitching, seizures, coma, respiratory depression, and respiratory arrest may also occur.

COMMENTS: Primarily metabolized by the liver; dosage adjustment is necessary in liver failure. Contraindicated in sinoatrial or AV nodal block.

Lidocaine/Prilocaine Cream (EMLA)

INDICATIONS AND USE: Produces local analgesia of intact skin for minor procedures such as insertion of intravenous catheters, venipuncture, and lumbar puncture in infants ≥37 weeks gestational age.

ACTIONS: EMLA (eutectic mixture of local anesthetics) contains two local anesthetics: lidocaine and prilocaine. Local anesthetics inhibit conduction of nerve impulses from sensory nerves by changing the cell membrane's permeability to ions.

SUPPLIED: Cream: lidocaine 2.5% with prilocaine 2.5% with Tegaderm dressings.

ROUTE: Topical

DOSAGE: Maximum EMLA dose, application area and application time

- 0–3 months or <5 kg: Maximum:1 g over 10 cm² for 1 h.
- 3–12 months and >5 kg: Maximum: 2 g over 20 cm² for 4 h.
- 1–6 years and >10 kg: Maximum: 10 g over 100 cm² for 4 h.
- Reduce amount in infants with impaired hepatic and/or renal function.
- Do not rub into skin. Cover with occlusive dressing such as Tegaderm.

ADVERSE EFFECTS: Not for use on mucous membranes or ophthalmic use. May cause methemoglobinemia. Not for use in infants <37 weeks' gestational age or infants <12 months old receiving concurrent methemoglobin-inducing agents (sulfonamides, acetaminophen, nitroprusside, nitric oxide, phenobarbital and others).

Lorazepam (Ativan)

INDICATIONS AND USE: Treatment of status epilepticus resistant to conventional anticonvulsant therapy (ie, phenobarbital or phenytoin).

ACTIONS: A benzodiazepine. Facilitates γ-aminobutyric acid (GABA), which mediates transmission and mimics the actions of glycine at its receptor sites. Penetrates the blood-brain barrier more slowly than diazepam; however, the duration of action of lorazepam in the control of seizure activity in children studied was at least 3 h in 83% of cases and 24 h or longer in nearly 59% of cases. Median onset of seizure control is 10 min.

SUPPLIED: Oral solution, 2 mg/mL; injection, 2 mg/mL.

ROUTE: PO, IM, IV.

DOSAGE: Status epilepticus:

- Initial DOSAGE: 0.05 mg/kg/dose IV. If no response after 15 min, repeat the initial dose. May dilute with an equal volume of sterile water, NS, or D_5W. Infuse the dose over 2–3 min.
- Sedation, anxiety: 0.05-0.1 mg/kg/dose IV q4–8h prn.

ADVERSE EFFECTS: May cause respiratory depression, apnea, hypotension, bradycardia, cardiac arrest, and seizure-like activity. Paradoxic CNS stimulation may occur, usually early in therapy; the drug should be discontinued if this effect occurs. Overdose may be reversed using flumazenil (Romazicon), 5–10 mcg/kg/dose IV.

Magnesium Sulfate (Various)

INDICATIONS AND USE: Hypomagnesemia and refractory hypocalcemia.

ACTIONS: May depress CNS and peripheral neuromuscular transmission by decreasing acetylcholine release. Acts on cardiac muscle to slow sinoatrial nodal impulse formation and prolong conduction time.

SUPPLIED: Injection, oral.

ROUTE: IM, IV, PO.

DOSAGE: Hypomagnesemia or refractory hypocalcemia:

- Initial DOSAGE: 0.2 mEq/kg/dose IV or IM q6h until the serum magnesium level is normal or symptoms resolve, or 0.8–1.6 mEq/kg/dose PO 4 times daily.
- Maintenance DOSAGE: 0.25–0.5 mEq/kg/24 h IV (add to infusion or give IV).

ADVERSE EFFECTS: Hypotension, flushing, depression of reflexes, depressed cardiac function, and CNS and respiratory depression.

COMMENTS: Contraindicated in renal failure. Monitor serum magnesium, calcium, and phosphate levels. Infuse IV magnesium sulfate over several hours.

Meperidine Hydrochloride (Demerol)

INDICATIONS AND USE: Preoperative medication and for relief of moderate to severe pain.

ACTIONS: Stimulates opiate receptors in the CNS. Meperidine produces respiratory depression proportionate to the drug dose. Duration of respiratory depression can extend several hours beyond the plasma half-life.

SUPPLIED: Injection, 25 mg/mL; syrup, 50 mg/mL.

ROUTE: PO, IM, IV, SC.

DOSAGE: 0.5–1.5 mg/kg/dose. Maximum: 2 mg/kg/dose IM, IV, and SC, and 4 mg/kg/dose PO.

ADVERSE EFFECTS: Normeperidine (active metabolite) has excitant effects that may precipitate tremors, myoclonus, or seizures. Other side effects include respiratory and circulatory depression, nausea, vomiting, constipation, and sedation.

COMMENTS: Effects can be reversed by naloxone, 0.1 mg/kg IV.

Methadone Hydrochloride

INDICATIONS AND USE: Long-acting narcotic analgesic used for severe pain and neonatal abstinence syndrome.

ACTIONS: CNS opiate receptor agonist resulting in analgesia and sedation.

SUPPLIED: Injection, 10 mg/mL; oral liquid, 1, 2, and 10 mg/mL.

ROUTE: IV, IM, PO, SC.

DOSAGE: 0.05–0.2 mg/kg/dose given q12–24h. The daily dose can be divided q8h.

ADVERSE EFFECTS: Respiratory depression, bronchospasm, constipation, hypotension, bradycardia, CNS depression, sedation, increased intracranial pressure, urinary tract spasm, urine retention, biliary tract spasm, and dependence with prolonged use. *Caution:* Methadone may accumulate; reassess for the need to adjust the dose downward after 3–5 days to avoid overdose. Smaller doses or less frequent administration may be required in renal and hepatic dysfunction.

COMMENTS: Taper by 10–20% weekly, based on the infant's symptoms of withdrawal. Tapering is difficult with methadone because of its long duration of action; consider morphine instead. Treat overdose with naloxone.

Methicillin Sodium (Staphcillin)

CLASSIFICATION: Penicillinase-resistant penicillin.

ACTION AND SPECTRUM: Mechanism of action identical to that of other β-lactam antibiotics. Active chiefly against penicillinase-positive and penicillinase-negative staphylococci. Less effective than penicillin G against other gram-positive cocci. No activity against enterococci.

SUPPLIED: Injection.

ROUTE: IM, IV (infuse over 20 min).
DOSAGE:

- Meningitis:
  <2000 g and 0–7 days old: 100 mg/kg/day divided q12h.
  <2000 g and >7 days old: 150 mg/kg/day divided q8h.
  >2000 g and 0–7 days old: 150 mg/kg/day divided q8h.
  >2000 g and >7 days old: 200 mg/kg/day divided q6h.
- Other indications:
  <2000 g and 0–7 days old: 50 mg/kg/day divided q12h.
  <2000 g and >7 days old: 75 mg/kg/day divided q8h.
  >2000 g and 0–7 days old: 75 mg/kg/day divided q8h.
  >2000 g and >7 days old: 100 mg/kg/day divided q6h.

ELIMINATION AND METABOLISM: Renal. Half-life is variable (60–120 min or longer).
ADVERSE EFFECTS: Nephrotoxicity (interstitial nephritis) occurs more often with methicillin than with other penicillins. May cause hypersensitivity reactions, anemia, leukopenia, thrombocytopenia, phlebitis at the infusion site, and hemorrhagic cystitis (in poorly hydrated patients).
COMMENTS: In cases of methicillin resistance, vancomycin becomes the antistaphylococcal drug of choice. Dosage adjustment is necessary in renal impairment. Monitor serum urea nitrogen and creatinine. Contains 2.9 mEq of sodium/g.

Methyldopa (Aldomet)
INDICATIONS AND USE: Hypertension.
ACTIONS: Mechanism of action is not fully understood. Metabolized to α-methylnorepinephrine in the CNS, where it lowers arterial pressure by stimulation of central α-adrenergic receptors. Reduction of plasma renin may also play a role in its antihypertensive effect.
SUPPLIED: Injection, suspension.
ROUTE: IV, PO.
DOSAGE: 5–40 mg/kg/day divided q6–8h.
ADVERSE EFFECTS: Most common adverse effect is drowsiness, which occurs within the first 48–72 h and may cause marked depression, orthostatic hypotension, sodium retention, edema, a positive direct Coombs' test reaction in 10–20% of patients (reversible), and drug fever. Causes fluid and sodium retention and should be given with a diuretic.
COMMENTS: Preferred route of administration is oral, but absorption from the GI tract is unpredictable (10–15%). Contraindicated with active hepatic disease.

Metoclopramide Hydrochloride (Reglan, Others)
INDICATIONS AND USE: Used in a variety of GI disorders. In neonates and infants, the drug has been used investigationally for feeding intolerance and gastroesophageal reflux.
ACTIONS: Dopamine antagonist acting on the CNS and on other organs. GI smooth muscle stimulant. Increases the resting tone of the esophageal sphincter. In neonates, metoclopramide resulted in a significant decrease in gastric aspirate, increased weight gain, shortened GI transit time, and increased food intake.
SUPPLIED: Syrup, injection.
ROUTE: IM, IV, PO.
DOSAGE: 0.1–0.2 mg/kg/dose given q6h 20 min before feedings.
ADVERSE EFFECTS: CNS effects include restlessness, drowsiness, and fatigue. Extrapyramidal reactions may occur but usually subside 24 h after discontinuance of the drug, and most patients will respond rapidly to diphenhydramine.
COMMENTS: Contraindicated with bowel obstruction and seizure disorders.

Metronidazole (Flagyl)
CLASSIFICATION: Bactericidal antibiotic.
ACTION AND SPECTRUM: The mechanism of action is not established. Good activity against anaerobic protozoa, including *Trichomonas vaginalis, Entamoeba histolytica, Giardia lamblia,* and *Balantidium coli.* Good activity also against gram-positive bacte-

ria (*Clostridium, Peptococcus, Peptostreptococcus,* and *Veillonella* spp) and anaerobic gram-negative bacteria (*Bacteroides* and *Fusobacterium* spp). Nonsporulating gram-positive bacilli are often resistant (eg, *Propionibacterium* and *Actinomyces* spp), and the drug has minimal activity against aerobic and facultative anaerobic bacteria.

SUPPLIED: Tablets (suspension can be compounded by pharmacist), injection.

ROUTE: PO, IV (infuse commercial dilution over 1 h).

DOSAGE:

- <2000 g: 15 mg/kg/day divided q12h.
- >2000 g and 0–7 days old: 15 mg/kg/day divided q12h.
- >2000 g and >7 days old: 30 mg/kg/day divided q12h.

ELIMINATION AND METABOLISM: Hepatic metabolism with final excretion via the urine and feces. Large volume of distribution (penetrates into all body tissues and fluids).

ADVERSE EFFECTS: Occasional vomiting, diarrhea, insomnia, weakness, rash, phlebitis at the injection site, and, rarely, leukopenia. Mutagenicity and carcinogenicity may occur, but this has not been established in humans.

COMMENTS: Some texts recommend an initial loading dose of 15 mg/kg, with the first maintenance dose either 48 h later (for premature infants <2000 g) or 24 h later (for the infant >2000 g at birth). Effectively penetrates into the CSF and, therefore, is indicated for meningitis resulting from susceptible anaerobic pathogens.

Note: Some centers use empiric coverage with ampicillin and gentamicin for NEC. Use of metronidazole in NEC remains *controversial.*

Mezlocillin Sodium (Mezlin)

CLASSIFICATION: Semisynthetic extended-spectrum penicillin.

ACTION AND SPECTRUM: Mechanism of action identical to that of other β-lactam antibiotics. Effective principally against gram-negative organisms, including *Haemophilus influenzae, Klebsiella pneumoniae, Proteus mirabilis, Escherichia coli, Pseudomonas aeruginosa,* and some *Serratia* spp. Active also against many anaerobes, including *Peptococcus, Peptostreptococcus,* and *Bacteroides* spp (eg, *Bacteroides fragilis*).

SUPPLIED: Injection.

ROUTE: IM, IV (infuse over 30 min).

DOSAGE:

- 0–7 days: 150 mg/kg/day divided q12h.
- >7 days: 225 mg/kg/day divided q8h.

ELIMINATION AND METABOLISM: Excreted primarily unchanged with urine; <10% hepatically metabolized.

ADVERSE EFFECTS: See Penicillin G (Aqueous), Parenteral.

COMMENTS: Does not cause platelet dysfunction. Avoid IM use if possible. Adjust the dosage in renal impairment. Contains 1.85 mEq of sodium/g.

Note: Limited experience in neonates.

Midazolam Hydrochloride (Versed)

INDICATIONS AND USE: Antianxiety agent. May be used for infants on assisted ventilation who are agitated and need sedation or as a sedative before procedures.

ACTIONS: Short-acting benzodiazepine.

SUPPLIED: Injection, 1 and 5 mg/mL. Contains 1% benzyl alcohol.

ROUTE: IV, IM, IV continuous infusion.

DOSAGE:

- Intermittent: 0.05–0.2 mg/kg/dose IV q2–4h prn.
- Continuous infusion:
    Loading dose: 0.2 mg/kg IV.
    Infusion: 0.4–0.6 mcg/kg/min.
    Maximum: 6 mcg/kg/min.

ADVERSE EFFECTS: Respiratory depression and arrest with excessive doses or rapid IV infusions. May cause hypotension. Infuse IV slowly. Use caution, particularly if fentanyl is being used concurrently.

Morphine Sulfate (Various)

INDICATIONS AND USE: Analgesia, preoperative sedation, supplement to anesthesia, and acute pulmonary edema.

ACTIONS: CNS opiate receptor agonist resulting in analgesia, drowsiness, and alterations in mood and pain perception. Vasodilatory (especially in coronary vessels).

SUPPLIED: Injection, oral solution.

ROUTE: IM, IV, SC.

DOSAGE: 0.05–0.2 mg/kg/dose q2–4h or continuous administration of 0.01–0.04 mg/kg/h.

ADVERSE EFFECTS: Dose-dependent side effects include miosis, respiratory depression, drowsiness, bradycardia, and hypotension. Constipation, sedation, GI upset, urine retention, histamine release, and sweating may occur. Causes physiologic dependence; taper the dose gradually after long-term use to avoid withdrawal.

Mupirocin (Bactroban)

INDICATIONS AND USE: Topical treatment of impetigo resulting from *Staphylococcus aureus* (including methicillin-resistant and β-lactamase-producing strains), β-hemolytic *Streptococcus* spp, and *Streptococcus pyogenes*. Used for minor bacterial skin infections resulting from susceptible organisms.

ACTIONS: A topical antibacterial ointment. Inhibits protein and RNA synthesis by binding to bacterial isoleucyl-tRNA synthetase.

SUPPLIED: Topical ointment 2%, 15 g.

ROUTE: Topical.

DOSAGE: Apply sparingly 3 times a day. Reevaluate in 3–5 days if no response.

ADVERSE EFFECTS: Burning, rash, erythema, and pruritus.

COMMENTS: Use with caution in burn patients and patients with impaired renal function. Avoid contact with eyes; not for ophthalmic use. When applied to extensive open wounds or burns, the possibility of absorption of the polyethylene glycol vehicle, resulting in serious renal toxicity, should be considered.

Nafcillin Sodium (Unipen)

CLASSIFICATION: Semisynthetic penicillinase-resistant penicillin.

ACTION AND SPECTRUM: Mechanism of action identical to that of other β-lactam antibiotics. Spectrum identical to that of methicillin (ie, primarily antistaphylococcal).

SUPPLIED: Injection.

ROUTE: IV (infuse over 30 min), IM (avoid–very irritating).

DOSAGE:

- <2000 g and 0–7 days old: 50 mg/kg/day divided q12h.
- <2000 g and >7 days old: 75 mg/kg/day divided q8h.
- >2000 g and 0–7 days old: 50 mg/kg/day divided q8h.
- >2000 g and >7 days old: 75 mg/kg/day divided q6h.

ELIMINATION AND METABOLISM: Hepatic metabolism; concentrated in bile.

ADVERSE EFFECTS: Thrombophlebitis, hypersensitivity, and leukopenia. Severe tissue injury after IV extravasation.

COMMENTS: Avoid IM use. Contains 2.9 mEq of sodium/g.

Naloxone Hydrochloride (Narcan)

INDICATIONS AND USE: Narcotic reversal and investigationally for the treatment of septic shock.

ACTIONS: A pure opiate antagonist with little or no agonistic activity. It has minimal or no pharmacologic effect, even in high doses, in patients who have not received opiates. Onset of action is within 1–2 min after IV injection and 2–5 min after SC or IM injection. Duration of action is generally 45 min to 4 h.

SUPPLIED: Injection, 0.4 and 1.0 mg/mL.

ROUTE: IV, IM, SC, intratracheal.

DOSAGE: 0.1 mg/kg. May repeat in 5 min.

COMMENTS: Avoid in infants of narcotic-addicted mothers because naloxone may precipitate acute withdrawal syndrome. Infants must be monitored for reappearance of respiratory depression and the need for repeated doses.

Neomycin Sulfate (Mycifradin, Others)

CLASSIFICATION: Aminoglycoside.

ACTION AND SPECTRUM: Mechanism of action identical to that of gentamicin sulfate. Indicated in the treatment of diarrhea resulting from enteropathogenic *Escherichia coli* and as preoperative prophylaxis before intestinal surgery.

SUPPLIED: Oral solution, 125 mg/5 mL.

ROUTE: PO.

DOSAGE: 50–100 mg/kg/day divided q4–6h.

ELIMINATION AND METABOLISM: Renal excretion if systemic absorption occurs; otherwise, fecally excreted.

ADVERSE EFFECTS: Sensitization with allergic reaction.

COMMENTS: Poorly absorbed from the GI tract, but significant levels can occur, especially in impaired renal function. Inactive against anaerobic organisms.

Neostigmine Methylsulfate (Prostigmin)

INDICATIONS AND USE: Improvement of muscle strength in the treatment of myasthenia gravis. Reversal of nondepolarizing neuromuscular blocking agents (eg, tubocurarine and pancuronium) and occasionally for postoperative distention and urinary retention).

ACTIONS: Neostigmine inhibits hydrolysis of acetylcholine and thus produces generalized cholinergic responses.

SUPPLIED: Injection, 0.25, 0.5, and 1 mg/mL.

ROUTE: IM, IV, SC, PO.

DOSAGE:

- Myasthenia gravis:
- Diagnosis: 0.04 mg/kg/dose IM once or 0.02 mg/kg/dose IV once.
- Treatment: 0.01–0.04 mg/kg/dose IM, IV, or SC q2–3h prn.
- Reversal of nondepolarizing neuromuscular blocking agents:
- Infants: 0.025–0.1 mg/kg/dose. (Use with atropine: Dose: 0.01–0.04 mg/kg or 0.4 mg of atropine for each 1 mg of neostigmine.)

ADVERSE EFFECTS: Cholinergic crisis, which may include bronchospasm, increased bronchial secretions, vomiting, diarrhea, bradycardia, respiratory depression, seizures, and coma.

COMMENTS: Antidote is atropine, 0.01–0.04 mg/kg/dose. Reversal of the blocking agent should not be attempted for at least 30 min after a dose of pancuronium or tubocurarine.

Netilmicin Sulfate (Netromycin)

CLASSIFICATION: Aminoglycoside.

ACTION AND SPECTRUM: See Gentamicin Sulfate.

SUPPLIED: Injection.

ROUTE: IM, IV (infuse over 30 min).

DOSAGE: Monitor and adjust by pharmacokinetics. Initial empiric dosing is based on body weight.

- <1.2 kg: 2.5 mg/kg/dose q18–24h.
- <2 kg and 0–7 days: 2.5 mg/kg/dose q12–18h.
- <2 kg and >7 days: 2.5 mg/kg/dose q8–12h.
- >2 kg and 0–7 days: 2.5 mg/kg/dose q12h.
- >2 kg and >7 days: 2.5 mg/kg/dose q8h.

ELIMINATION AND METABOLISM: Renal excretion. Half-life is 4–8 h.

ADVERSE EFFECTS: Ototoxicity is associated with serum peak concentrations >12 mcg/mL; nephrotoxicity is associated with serum trough concentrations >4 mcg/mL.

COMMENTS: Therapeutic range is 6–10 mcg/mL (sample obtained 30 min after the infusion is completed); serum trough concentrations are <3 mcg/mL (sample obtained 30 min to just before the next dose). Obtain an initial set of serum peak and trough levels at about the fourth maintenance dose. Monitor serum creatinine every 3–4 days. For other comments, see Gentamicin Sulfate. Limited experience in neonates.

Nitric Oxide (INOmax for Inhalation; NO, inhaled nitric oxide [iNO]

INDICATIONS AND USE: iNO is indicated for the treatment of term and near-term (≥34 weeks) neonates with hypoxic respiratory failure associated with clinical or echocardiographic evidence of persistent pulmonary hypertension of the newborn (PPHN).

ACTIONS: iNO is a selective pulmonary vasodilator without significant effects on the systemic circulation. Excess iNO is quickly bound to and inactivated, producing methemoglobin. The half-life of iNO is <5 s. Exogenous iNO causes vasodilation by acting on the receptors in the muscle wall of blood vessels. Guanylyl cyclase activation leads to production of cyclic guanosine monophosphate and subsequent smooth muscle relaxation—the same mechanism as endogenous NO.

SUPPLIED: Portable aluminum cylinders containing NO gas in 800 and 100 ppm concentration in nitrogen.

ROUTE: Given as a gas by inhalation.

DOSAGE: Term infants and those >34 weeks' gestation: Begin with 20 ppm. Reduce dose to lowest possible level. Maximum: Per manufacturer, doses above 20 ppm are usually not used because of the increased risk of methemoglobinemia and elevated NO_2.

Maintain treatment up to 14 days or until the underlying oxygen desaturation has resolved and the infant is ready to be weaned from iNO.

ADVERSE EFFECTS: Do not use in neonates dependent on right-to-left shunting of blood. Direct pulmonary injury from excess levels of NO_2 and ambient air contamination may occur. May cause methemoglobinemia and elevated NO_2. Risk of adverse effects increases when iNO is given at doses >20 ppm. Conflicting data have been published on whether or not iNO inhibits platelet aggregation and prolongs bleeding time. Monitor methemoglobin levels, iNO, NO_2, and O_2 levels. iNO therapy should be directed by physicians qualified by education and experience in its use and offered only at centers that are qualified to provide multisystem support, generally including on-site ECMO capability or with a collaborating ECMO center. Consult the manufacturer's product literature and specialized references for complete information on the use of iNO. (See American Academy of Pediatrics, Committee on Fetus and Newborn: Use of inhaled nitric oxide. *Pediatrics* 2000;106:344.)

Nitroprusside Sodium (Nipride, Nitropress)

INDICATIONS AND USE: Severe hypertension and hypertension crisis, congestive heart failure, and congenital heart lesions that have resulted in pulmonary hypertension with increased pulmonary vascular resistance.

ACTIONS: Direct-acting vasodilator (arterial and venous) that reduces peripheral vascular resistance (afterload). Venous return is reduced (preload). Acts within seconds to lower blood pressure; when discontinued, the effect dissipates within minutes. Rapidly metabolized to thiocyanate, which is eliminated by the kidneys.

SUPPLIED: Injection.

ROUTE: Continuous IV infusion.

DOSAGE: 0.5–8 mcg/kg/min (titrate to the desired response) by IV infusion.

ADVERSE EFFECTS: Generally related to too-rapid reduction in blood pressure. Thiocyanate may accumulate, especially in patients receiving high doses or those who have impaired renal function. Cyanide toxicity can develop abruptly if large doses are administered rapidly. Cyanide causes early persistent acidosis. Thiocyanate toxicity appears at plasma levels of ~5–10 mg/dL; levels of 20 mg/dL have been associated with death. Thiocyanate levels should be monitored in any patient receiving 5 mcg/kg/min or more of nitroprusside, especially those with renal impairment. Toxicity is treated with 20% sodium thiosulfate (10 mg/kg/min for 15 min).

COMMENTS: Contraindicated with increased intracranial pressure, hypertension secondary to arteriovenous shunts, or coarctation of the aorta. Reconstitute contents of a 50-mg vial in 2–3 mL of D_5W, then further dilute in D_5W for infusion. Protect from light.

Norepinephrine Bitartrate (Levarterenol Bitartrate) (Levophed)

INDICATIONS AND USE: Vasoconstriction and cardiac stimulation as adjunctive therapy to correct shock after fluid volume replacement. Prolongation of local anesthetics by decreasing vascular absorption.

ACTIONS: Direct effect on α-adrenergic receptors and β-adrenergic receptors of the heart (β_1) but not those of the bronchi or peripheral blood vessels (β_2). Norepinephrine has less effect on β_1 receptors than does epinephrine or isoproterenol.

SUPPLIED: Injection.

ROUTE: IV infusion.

DOSAGE: 0.02–0.1 mcg/kg/min initially, titrated to attain desired perfusion.

ADVERSE EFFECTS: Respiratory distress, arrhythmias, bradycardia or tachycardia, hypertension, and vomiting.

COMMENTS: In case of extravasation, use phentolamine, 0.1–0.2 mg/kg SC, infiltrated into the area of extravasation within 12 h.

Nystatin (Mycostatin, Nilstat)

ACTION AND SPECTRUM: Fungistatic and fungicidal in vitro against a wide variety of yeasts and yeast-like fungi. Acts by disrupting cell membranes. Neonatal indications include oral candidiasis (thrush), *Candida* diaper rash, and benign mucocutaneous candidiasis.

SUPPLIED: Oral suspension, 100,000 units/mL; topical cream; powder; ointment.

ROUTE: PO, topical.

DOSAGE:

- Oral thrush: 0.5–1 mL to each side of the mouth qid after feedings for 7–10 days.
- Diaper rash: Topical cream applied tid–qid for 7–10 days.

ELIMINATION AND METABOLISM: Poorly absorbed. Most is passed unchanged in the stool.

ADVERSE EFFECTS: Side effects are uncommon but may cause diarrhea.

Octreotide (Sandostatin)

INDICATIONS AND USE: Short-term management of persistent hyperinsulinemic hypoglycemia of nesidioblastosis. A few patients have been treated for as long as 5 years. Has also been used to treat hypersecretory diarrhea and fistulas in infants. Significant reductions in stool or ileal output were achieved with this drug.

ACTIONS: A long-acting analog of somatostatin that suppresses pancreatic insulin release. Inhibits serotonin, glucagon, and growth hormone release. Reduces splanchnic blood flow and both exocrine and hormonal GI secretions. Duration of action is 6–12 h.

SUPPLIED: Injection, 0.05, 0.1, 0.2, 0.5, and 1 mg/mL. Refrigerate.

ROUTE: Continuous IV infusion, SC. Continuous SC infusion using a portable pump has been used in two infants with nesidioblastosis.

DOSAGE:

- Hypoglycemia: Starting dose is 2–10 mcg/kg/day divided q6–8h, up to 40 mcg/kg/day divided q4–8h. Adjust the dose to maintain symptomatic control. Continuous SC infusion: 2–10 mcg/kg/day.
- Diarrhea: 1–10 mcg/kg/dose given q12h. Adjust the dose to maintain symptomatic control.
- Postoperative chylothorax (limited experience): 10 mcg/kg/day SC in 3 divided doses. Increase dose stepwise by 5–10 mcg/kg/day q72–96h to 40 mcg/kg/day. Consider weaning after 3 days of insignificant chyle output (<10 mL/day). (See Cheung Y et al: *J Pediatr* 2001;139:157.)

ADVERSE EFFECTS: Possible growth retardation during long-term treatment; gallbladder microlithiasis reported in adolescents; flushing, hypertension, insomnia, fever, chills, seizures, Bell's palsy, hair loss, bruising, rash, hypoglycemia, hyperglycemia, galactorrhea, hypothyroidism, diarrhea, abdominal distention, constipation, hepatitis, jaundice, local injection site pain, thrombophlebitis, muscle weakness, increased creatine kinase, muscle spasm, tremor, oliguria, shortness of breath, and rhinorrhea.

COMMENTS: Tachyphylaxis may occur.

Oxacillin Sodium (Bactocill, Prostaphlin)

CLASSIFICATION: Semisynthetic penicillinase-resistant penicillin.

ACTION AND SPECTRUM: Mechanism of action is identical to that of other β-lactam antibiotics. Spectrum of activity is identical to that of nafcillin sodium and methicillin sodium.

SUPPLIED: Injection.

ROUTE: IM, IV (infuse over 30 min).

DOSAGE:

- <2000 g and 0–7 days old: 50 mg/kg/day divided q12h.
- <2000 g and >7 days old: 100 mg/kg/day divided q8h.
- >2000 g and 0–7 days old: 75 mg/kg/day divided q8h.
- >2000 g and >7 days old: 150 mg/kg/day divided q6h.

ELIMINATION AND METABOLISM: Metabolized chiefly in the liver and excreted in bile. Renal excretion is substantial but requires no adjustment in renal failure.

ADVERSE EFFECTS: Hypersensitivity reactions (rash), thrombophlebitis, mild leukopenia, and elevation in AST (SGOT).

COMMENTS: Avoid IM injection. Contains 2.8 mEq of sodium/g.

Pancuronium Bromide (Pavulon)

INDICATIONS AND USE: To increase pulmonary compliance in an uncooperative neonate during mechanical ventilation. To produce skeletal muscle relaxation during surgery.

ACTIONS: Nondepolarizing neuromuscular blocking agent that produces skeletal muscle paralysis mainly by causing a decreased response to acetylcholine at the myoneural junction. Pancuronium may cause an increase in heart rate. The onset of action is generally 30–60 s, with a duration of action of ~40–60 min, but it may be much longer in neonates.

SUPPLIED: Injection, 1 mg/mL.

ROUTE: IV.

DOSAGE:

- Initial DOSAGE: 0.03 mg/kg IV; repeat prn.
- Maintenance DOSAGE: 0.03–0.09 mg/kg IV q1–4h prn to maintain paralysis.

ADVERSE EFFECTS: Tachycardia may occur.

COMMENTS: Neonates are particularly sensitive to its actions; prolonged paralysis may be noted. Ventilation must be supported during neuromuscular blockade. Many centers place a sign over the patient's bedside to alert all medical personnel that the infant is paralyzed. Neostigmine methylsulfate and atropine sulfate are used for reversal (for dosage, see pages 624 and 595 respectively).

Papaverine Hydrochloride (Various)

INDICATIONS AND USE: Peripheral arterial spasms.

ACTIONS: Directly relaxes vascular smooth muscle and results in vasodilation.

SUPPLIED: Injection, tablets.

ROUTE: PO, IM, IV (infuse over 1–2 min).

DOSAGE: 6 mg/kg/24 h in 4 divided doses.

COMMENTS: IV infusion should be performed under a physician's supervision because arrhythmias and fatal apnea may result from rapid injection.

Note: Limited experience in neonates.

Paraldehyde (Paral)

INDICATIONS AND USE: Status epilepticus resistant to conventional therapy (ie, phenobarbital, phenytoin, diazepam, and lorazepam).

ACTIONS: A rapid-acting hypnotic agent effective against all types of seizures when administered in large doses. Precise mechanism of action is unknown.

SUPPLIED: Oral solution, rectal liquid.

ROUTE: PO, PR.

DOSAGE: 0.3 mL/kg/dose q4–6h if needed. For rectal use, dilute in an equal volume of olive or mineral oil. For oral use, dilute in infant formula.

ADVERSE EFFECTS: Side effects severely limit use. May cause pulmonary edema and hemorrhage, severe coughing, irritation to GI mucosa, and thrombophlebitis. Overdose may cause cardiac and respiratory depression. Rectal administration may cause proctitis.

COMMENTS: Routine use in infants is discouraged. Contraindicated in pulmonary or hepatic disease.

Note: Dissolves plastic and reacts with rubber stoppers in bottles and syringes. Do not use plastic equipment for administration. For rectal administration, use glass syringes. Discard a container opened >24 h, discolored solution, or solution smelling of acetic acid (vinegar) because it may be toxic.

Penicillin G (Aqueous), Parenteral

ACTION AND SPECTRUM: Mechanism of action is identical to that of other β-lactam antibiotics. Effective mainly against streptococci, some community-acquired staphylococci (except methicillin-resistant and penicillinase-producing strains), *Neisseria gonorrhoeae*, *Neisseria meningitidis*, *Bacillus anthracis*, *Clostridium tetani*, *Clostridium perfringens*, *Bacteroides* (oropharyngeal strains), *Leptospira* spp, and *Treponema pallidum*.

SUPPLIED: Injection, as the potassium or sodium salt.

ROUTE: IM, IV (infuse over 30 min).

DOSAGE:

- Meningitis:
    <2000 g and 0–7 days old: 100,000 units/kg/day divided q12h.
    <2000 g and >7 days old: 150,000 units/kg/day divided q8h.
    >2000 g and 0–7 days old: 150,000 units/kg/day divided q8h.
    >2000 g and >7 days old: 200,000 units/kg/day divided q6h.
- Other indications:
    <2000 g and 0–7 days old: 50,000 units/kg/day divided q12h.
    <2000 g and >7 days old: 75,000 units/kg/day divided q8h.
    >2000 g and 0–7 days old: 50,000 units/kg/day divided q8h.
    >2000 g and >7 days old: 100,000 units/kg/day divided q6h.

ELIMINATION AND METABOLISM: Renal.

ADVERSE EFFECTS: Allergic reactions, rash, fever, change in bowel flora, *Candida* superinfection, diarrhea, and hemolytic anemia. Very large doses may cause seizures. Rapid IV push of potassium penicillin G may cause cardiac arrhythmias and arrest because of the potassium component. Infuse slowly over 30 min.

COMMENTS: 1600 units = 1 mg. Some strains of group B streptococci are penicillinase producers, thus requiring the addition of an aminoglycoside antibiotic for synergistic bactericidal effect. Good activity against anaerobes. Drug of choice for tetanus neonatorum. Contains 1.7 mEq of sodium or potassium per million units.

Penicillin G Benzathine (Bicillin L-A, Permapen)

ACTION AND SPECTRUM: See Penicillin G (Aqueous), Parenteral. A drug of choice in the treatment of asymptomatic congenital syphilis.

SUPPLIED: Injection.

ROUTE: IM only. (Viscosity requires ≥23-gauge needle.)

DOSAGE: 50,000 units/kg once.

ELIMINATION AND METABOLISM: Renally excreted over a prolonged interval owing to slow absorption from the injection site.

ADVERSE EFFECTS AND COMMENTS: See Penicillin G (Aqueous), Parenteral. 1211 units = 1 mg. Not often used.

Penicillin G Procaine (Wycillin)

ACTION AND SPECTRUM: See Penicillin G (Aqueous), Parenteral. A drug of choice in the treatment of symptomatic or asymptomatic congenital syphilis.

SUPPLIED: Injection.

ROUTE: IM only. (Viscosity requires ≥23-gauge needle.)

DOSAGE: 50,000 units/kg/dose q24h.

ELIMINATION AND METABOLISM: See Penicillin G (Aqueous), Parenteral.

ADVERSE EFFECTS: See Penicillin G (Aqueous), Parenteral. May also cause sterile abscess formation at the injection site. Contains 120 mg of procaine per 300,000 units, which may cause allergic reactions, myocardial depression, or systemic vasodilation. There is cause for much greater concern about these effects in the neonate than in older patients.

COMMENTS: 1000 units = 1 mg. Not often used.

Pentobarbital Sodium (Nembutal)

INDICATIONS AND USE: Sedative/hypnotic. Used for agitation, for pre-procedure sedation, or as an anticonvulsant.

ACTIONS: Short-acting barbiturate.

SUPPLIED: Injection, 50 mg/mL; elixir, 18.2 mg/5 mL (18% alcohol), suppositories. (Suppositories should be used for the older, larger infant only because 30 mg is the smallest size available, and it is recommended that they not be divided.)

ROUTE: PO, PR, IM, IV.

DOSAGE:

- Sedative: 2–6 mg/kg/day divided tid. Maximum: 100 mg/day.
- Hypnotic and anticonvulsant: 3–5 mg/kg/dose. Maximum: 100 mg/dose.

ADVERSE EFFECTS: Inject the IV dose slowly in fractional doses. Observe the IV site closely during administration because this drug may cause extravasation injury. Tolerance and physical dependence may occur with continued use. May cause somnolence, apnea, bradycardia, rash, pain on IM injection, thrombophlebitis, osteomalacia from prolonged use (rare), and excitability. May increase reaction to painful stimuli. Rapid IV administration may cause hypotension and apnea.

PGE₁: See Alprostadil

Phenobarbital (Various)

INDICATIONS AND USE: Tonic-clonic and partial seizures, neonatal withdrawal syndrome, and neonatal jaundice.

ACTIONS: Anticonvulsant that limits the spread of seizure activity and increases the threshold for electrical stimulation of the motor cortex. In neonates, the initial half-life is 100–120 h or longer, gradually declining to 60–70 h at ~3–4 weeks of age. Reduction in serum bilirubin levels is attributed to increased levels of glucuronyl transferase and intracellular Y-binding protein. More effective in reducing bilirubin levels in full-term infants than in premature infants and must be administered at least 2–3 days before detectable reductions can be observed. Effective in controlling symptoms of neonatal withdrawal syndrome, with the exception of vomiting and diarrhea.

SUPPLIED: Oral elixir, tablets, injection.

ROUTE: IV, IM, PO.

DOSAGE:

- Seizures:
  Loading dose: 20–30 mg/kg IV or IM over 15–30 min. May give in 2 divided doses.
  Maintenance dose: 2.5–4 mg/kg/day as a single dose or divided q12h. For neonates <30 weeks' gestational age, start 1–3 mg/kg/day.
  Hyperbilirubinemia: Dose is not clearly established. Generally, 4–5 mg/kg/day.
  Neonatal withdrawal syndrome: 5–10 mg/kg/day in 4 divided doses. Monitor serum phenobarbital concentrations and withdrawal score.

ADVERSE EFFECTS: Sedation, lethargy, paradoxic excitement, GI distress, ataxia, and rash.

COMMENTS: Contraindicated in porphyria. Monitor serum levels, and adjust the dosage to maintain between 15 and 40 mcg/mL for anticonvulsant activity.

Phentolamine (Regitine)

INDICATIONS AND USE: Treatment of extravasation from IV dopamine or norepinephrine bitartrate (levarterenol bitartrate [Levophed]). Helps prevent dermal necrosis and sloughing.

ACTIONS: Phentolamine is an α-adrenergic blocking drug that works to reverse the severe vasoconstriction from extravasation of vasopressors such as dopamine.
SUPPLIED: Injection, 5 mg/mL.
ROUTE: SC.
DOSAGE: 0.1–0.2 mg/kg diluted to 1 mL of saline injected into the area of extravasation within 12 h.
ADVERSE EFFECTS: Hypotension, tachycardia, cardiac arrhythmias, flushing, and GI upset.

Phenytoin (Dilantin)

INDICATIONS AND USE: Seizures unresponsive to phenobarbital.
ACTIONS: Raises seizure threshold of the motor cortex to electrical or chemical stimuli. Precise mechanism of anticonvulsant activity has not been determined. Bilirubin displaces phenytoin from albumin binding sites, increasing the percentage of unbound drug; this may complicate the interpretation of serum levels. Follows zero-order pharmacokinetics, in which small dosage adjustments may result in large changes in serum drug concentrations. Neonates and other infants absorb phenytoin poorly from the GI tract. Use in the long-term management of seizures in neonates is questionable because of the difficulty in appropriate dosing.
SUPPLIED: Oral suspension, injection.
ROUTE: PO, IV.
DOSAGE:

- IV: 15–20 mg/kg as a loading dose at a rate not >0.5 mg/kg/min, followed by a maintenance dose of 5–8 mg/kg/day divided q12–24h.
- PO: Highly variable, from 5–8 mg/kg/day to 8 mg/kg/dose q12h.

Fosphenytoin IV, IM (not available PO): 75 mg is equivalent to phenytoin 50 mg. The dose of fosphenytoin is expressed as phenytoin equivalents (PE): 1 mg phenytoin = fosphenytoin 1 mg PE. For example, "an initial maintenance dose of 4–6 mg PE/kg/day is suggested." Order fosphenytoin in PE as in this example to avoid error. Fosphenytoin has been associated with fewer adverse effects in general than phenytoin (adults). Experience in neonates is very limited.
ADVERSE EFFECTS: Few reports of toxicity in neonates, probably because of the difficulty of physically assessing the common toxic manifestations. In adults and children, adverse effects include nystagmus, ataxia, lethargy, slurred speech, diplopia, headache, hirsutism, behavioral changes, and gum hyperplasia. Hypotension occurs with rapid IV administration.
COMMENTS: Therapeutic levels are between 10 and 20 mcg/mL (may be lower in preterm infants). Multiple drug interactions.

Phosphorus (Various)

INDICATIONS AND USE: Treatment of hypophosphatemia, provision of maintenance phosphorus in PN solutions, and treatment of nutritional rickets of prematurity.
ACTIONS: Phosphorus is an intracellular ion required for formation of energy-transfer enzymes such as ADP and ATP. Phosphorus is also needed for bone metabolism and mineralization.
SUPPLIED: Injection, sodium phosphates, 3 mmol of elemental phosphorus/mL and 4 mEq of sodium/mL; potassium phosphates, 3 mmol of elemental phosphorus/mL and 4.4 mEq of potassium/mL.
ROUTE: IV, PO.
DOSAGE:

- Severe hypophosphatemia: 0.15–0.3 mmol/kg/dose (= 5–9 mg of elemental phosphorus/kg/dose). Infuse slowly over several hours or dilute in daily 24-h maintenance IV solution (preferred).
- Maintenance: 0.5–2 mmol/kg/day (= 16–63 mg of elemental phosphorus/kg/day). For oral use, may use parenteral form and give PO in divided doses, diluted in infant's feedings.

ADVERSE EFFECTS: Hyperphosphatemia, hypocalcemia, and hypotension. GI discomfort may occur with oral administration. Rapid IV bolus of potassium phosphates can cause cardiac arrhythmias.

Piperacillin Sodium (Pipracil)

CLASSIFICATION: Semisynthetic extended-spectrum penicillin.
ACTION AND SPECTRUM: See Mezlocillin Sodium. Good in vivo activity against *Pseudomonas aeruginosa*.
SUPPLIED: Injection.
ROUTE: IM, IV (infuse over 30 min).
DOSAGE:

- <2000 g and 0–7 days old: 150 mg/kg/day divided q12h.
- <2000 g and >7 days old: 225 mg/kg/day divided q8h.
- >2000 g and 0–7 days old: 225 mg/kg/day divided q8h.
- >2000 g and >7 days old: 300 mg/kg/day divided q6h.

ELIMINATION AND METABOLISM: Excreted unchanged in the urine.
ADVERSE EFFECTS: See Mezlocillin Sodium. Hypokalemia and leukopenia are less pronounced.
COMMENTS: Avoid IM use where possible. Should be reserved for cases resistant to ticarcillin disodium. Contains 1.85 mEq (42.5 mg) of sodium/g.

Pneumococcal 7-Valent Conjugate Vaccine (Diphtheria CRM$_{197}$) Protein PVC (Prevnar)

INDICATIONS AND USE: PCV is recommended for active immunization of infants and toddlers against *Streptococcus pneumoniae* invasive disease caused by the 7 capsular serotypes in the vaccine for all children 2–23 months of age. It is also recommended for certain children 24–59 months of age. *S. pneumoniae* causes invasive infections such as bacteremia and meningitis, pneumonia, otitis media, and sinusitis.
ACTIONS: The vaccine is a sterile solution of saccharides of the capsular antigens of *S. pneumoniae* serotypes 4, 6B, 9V, 14, 18C, 19F, and 23F conjugated to diphtheria CRM$_{197}$ protein. CRM$_{197}$ protein is a nontoxic variant of diphtheria toxin. These 7 serotypes cause about 80% of invasive pneumococcal disease in children <6 years of age in the US.
SUPPLIED: Injection: 0.5-mL vials. Refrigerate.
ROUTE: IM.
DOSAGE: 0.5 mL/dose as a single dose IM at 2, 4, 6, and 12–15 months of age. Shake well before administration.
The schedule usually begins at 2 months of age, but as young as 6 weeks of age is acceptable. *Three* doses of 0.5 mL each are given at about 2-month intervals, followed by a fourth dose of 0.5 mL at 12 months to 15 months of age. Give the fourth dose 2 or more months after the third dose.
ADVERSE EFFECTS: May cause decreased appetite, drowsiness, irritability, fever, and injection site local tenderness, redness, and edema. This vaccine is not a treatment of active infection. Do not give if patient is hypersensitive to any component of the vaccine. Immune response in preterm infants has not been studied. Use of this vaccine does not replace the use of the 23-valent pneumococcal polysaccharide vaccine in children ≥24 months old with sickle cell disease, chronic illness, asplenia, HIV, or immunocompromise. May be given simultaneously with other immunizing agents as part of the routine immunization schedule.

Potassium Chloride (KCl) (Various)

INDICATIONS AND USE: To correct hypokalemia and as maintenance potassium provision. Also corrects hypochloremia.
ACTIONS: Potassium is essential for maintaining intracellular tonicity; transmission of nerve impulses; contraction of cardiac, skeletal, and smooth muscle; and maintenance of normal renal function.
SUPPLIED: Injection, 2 mEq/mL; oral liquid, 10, 15, 20, 30, and 40 mEq/15 mL.
ROUTE: IV, PO.

DOSAGE: Maintenance: 2–3 mEq/kg/day diluted in 24-h maintenance IV solution. Higher doses are often required in infants receiving diuretics. Titrate the dose with the previous day's requirements and daily serum potassium determination. Maximum rate: Infants on a cardiac monitor: 0.5 mEq/kg/h; infants not on a cardiac monitor: 0.3 mEq/kg/h. Dilute bolus doses in 6–8 h of IV solution if possible. For oral use, the injectable form of the drug may be given in divided doses PO and diluted in the infant's formula.

ADVERSE EFFECTS: Avoid rapid IV injection. Excessive dose or rate may cause cardiac arrhythmias (peaked T waves, widened QRS, flattened P waves, bradycardia, and heart block), respiratory paralysis, and hypotension with rapid infusion. Potassium accumulates with renal dysfunction. Causes severe vein irritation; do not give undiluted in a peripheral vein. Dilute to 0.08 mEq/mL if possible.

Prazosin Hydrochloride (Minipress)

INDICATIONS AND USE: Hypertension and congestive heart failure. Experimental in infants and should be used only when traditional therapy has failed.

ACTIONS: Postsynaptic α-adrenergic blocking agent that reduces peripheral vascular resistance and blood pressure.

SUPPLIED: Capsules, 1 mg.

ROUTE: PO.

DOSAGE:

- Test: 5–10 mcg/kg PO.
- Maintenance: Up to 25 mcg/kg/dose q6h.

ADVERSE EFFECTS: Dizziness, weakness, fatigue, palpitations, headache, and nausea. The most severe adverse effect in adults is the "first-dose phenomenon," in which severe orthostatic hypotension occurs.

Prednisone (Liquid Pred, Prednisone Intensol Concentrate)

INDICATIONS AND USE: Resistant neonatal hypoglycemia, airway edema, and weaning of infants with BPD from the ventilator. Used chiefly as an anti-inflammatory or immunosuppressive agent. Not indicated for adrenocortical insufficiency because of minimal mineralocorticoid activity.

actions: An intermediate-acting glucocorticoid. Prednisone has four times the anti-inflammatory potency of hydrocortisone, and half the mineralocorticoid potency.

SUPPLIED: Tablets, 1, 2.5, 5, and 10 mg (scored); oral solution, 5 mg/5 mL (5% alcohol) and 5 mg/mL (30% alcohol).

ROUTE: PO.

DOSAGE: 0.1–2 mg/kg/day qd or divided q12h.

ADVERSE EFFECTS: Cataracts, leukocytosis, peptic ulcer, nephrocalcinosis, myopathy, osteoporosis, diabetes, growth failure, hyperlipidemia, hypocalcemia, hypokalemic alkalosis, sodium retention and hypertension, and increased susceptibility to infection. Withdraw the dose gradually after prolonged therapy to prevent acute adrenal insufficiency.

Procainamide Hydrochloride (Various)

INDICATIONS AND USE: As prophylaxis to maintain normal sinus rhythm in paroxysmal atrial tachycardia, atrial fibrillation, premature atrial and ventricular contractions, and ventricular tachycardia.

ACTIONS: Class I antiarrhythmic agent similar to quinidine sulfate. Partially metabolized by the liver to the active metabolite N-acetylprocainamide (NAPA).

SUPPLIED: Capsules, tablets, injection.

ROUTE: PO, IM, IV.

DOSAGE:

- IV (monitor the electrocardiogram and blood pressure): 1.5–2 mg/kg (dilute to 10 mg/mL) over 10–30 min. Repeat as needed to a maximum dose of 10–15 mg/kg, then continuous infusion of 20–60 mcg/kg/min.
- PO: 5–15 mg/kg q4–6h.

THERAPEUTIC LEVELS:

- Procainamide, 3–10 mcg/mL: Toxicity associated with levels >12 mcg/mL.
- NAPA, 10–20 mcg/mL: Toxicity associated with levels >30 mcg/mL.

ADVERSE EFFECTS: Serious toxic effects if given rapidly IV, including asystole, myocardial depression, ventricular fibrillation, hypotension, and reversible lupus-like syndrome. May cause nausea, vomiting, diarrhea, anorexia, skin rash, tachycardia, agranulocytosis, and hepatic toxicity.

COMMENTS: Contraindicated in second- or third-degree heart block, bundle branch block, digitalis intoxication, and allergy to procaine. Do not use in atrial fibrillation or flutter until the ventricular rate is adequately controlled to avoid a possible paradoxic increase in ventricular rate. Quinidine sulfate (see p 634) is generally used for long-term therapy because it has less associated toxicity. Phenylephrine should be available to treat severe hypotension caused by IV procainamide. QRS or QT prolongation >35% of baseline is an indication to withhold further doses of procainamide.

Propranolol (Inderal, Others)

INDICATIONS AND USE: Hypertension, supraventricular tachycardia, premature ventricular contractions, tachycardia, and tetralogy spells.

ACTIONS: Nonselective β-adrenergic blocking agent. Inhibits adrenergic stimuli by competitively blocking β-adrenergic receptors within the myocardium and bronchial and vascular smooth muscle. Decreases heart rate, myocardial contractility, and cardiac output.

SUPPLIED: Oral liquid, injection.

ROUTE: PO, IV.

DOSAGE:

- Arrhythmias:
  IV: 0.025–0.15 mg/kg/dose to a maximum of 1 mg/dose as slow push.
  PO: 0.5–2 mg/kg/day divided q6–8h. May increase to 1 mg/kg/dose q6h or more as tolerated.
- Hypertension:
  0.5–2 mg/kg/day PO divided q6–12h. May increase as tolerated.
- Tetralogy spells:
  0.15–0.25 mg/kg/dose slow IV. May repeat q15min prn or 1–2 mg/kg/dose PO q6h prn.

ADVERSE EFFECTS: Generally dose-related hypotension, nausea, vomiting, bronchospasm, heart block, depression, hypoglycemia, and depressed myocardial contractility.

COMMENTS: Contraindicated in obstructive pulmonary disease, asthma, heart failure, shock, second- or third-degree heart block, and hypoglycemia. Use with caution in renal or hepatic failure.

Prostaglandin E₁: See Alprostadil

Protamine Sulfate (Various)

INDICATIONS AND USE: Reversal of heparin and heparin overdose.

ACTIONS: Combines with heparin, forming a stable salt complex. Devoid of anticoagulant activity. Effect on heparin is almost immediate and persists for ~2 h.

SUPPLIED: Injection.

ROUTE: IV.

DOSAGE: For every 100 units of heparin estimated to remain in the patient, give 1 mg by slow infusion over 3–5 min or not >5 mg/min. Maximum: 50 mg.

ADVERSE EFFECTS: May cause a fall in blood pressure, bradycardia, dyspnea, and anaphylaxis. Excessive administration beyond that needed to reverse a heparin effect may have an anticoagulant effect.

Pyridoxine (Vitamin B₆) (Various)

INDICATIONS AND USE: For treatment of pyridoxine-dependent seizures and to prevent or treat vitamin B₆ deficiency.

ACTIONS: Vitamin B_6 is essential in the synthesis of GABA, an inhibitory neurotransmitter in the CNS; GABA increases the seizure threshold. Vitamin B_6 is also required for heme synthesis and amino acid, carbohydrate, and lipid metabolism.
SUPPLIED: Tablets, injection.
ROUTE: PO, IM, IV.
DOSAGE: For vitamin B_6-dependent seizures, give 100 mg IV as a single test dose, followed by a 30-min observation period. If a definite response is seen, begin maintenance of 50–100 mg PO daily.

Pyrimethamine (Daraprim)

ACTION AND SPECTRUM: Folic acid antagonist selective for plasmodial dihydrofolate reductase. Activity highly selective for plasmodia (cidal) and *Toxoplasma gondii*.
SUPPLIED: Tablets.
ROUTE: PO.
DOSAGE: For toxoplasmosis, give 1 mg/kg/day divided q12h for 4 weeks. Combine with sulfadiazine.
ELIMINATION AND METABOLISM: Hepatic metabolism.
ADVERSE EFFECTS: Anorexia, vomiting, megaloblastic anemia, leukopenia, thrombocytopenia, pancytopenia, atrophic glossitis, rash, seizures, and shock.
COMMENTS: Give folinic acid (leucovorin), 1 mg PO daily or 3 mg twice weekly, if leukopenia or thrombocytopenia occurs. Administer with feedings if vomiting persists. Give sulfadiazine alone in empiric therapy of toxoplasmosis until the diagnosis is ruled out. Reduce the dosage in hepatic dysfunction.

Quinidine (Various)

INDICATIONS AND USE: Restoration of normal sinus rhythm in atrial flutter or fibrillation once the ventricular rate is controlled by digoxin. Prevention of atrial and ventricular arrhythmias.
ACTIONS: Group I antiarrhythmic agent with cardiac effects similar to those of procainamide hydrochloride. Direct depressant effect on myocardial contractility, conduction velocity, and excitability. Causes increases in PR, QRS, and QT intervals.
SUPPLIED: Tablets (as sulfate, gluconate, or polygalacturonate), injection (as gluconate).
ROUTE: PO, IM (IV not recommended).
DOSAGE: 5–15 mg/kg q6h PO or 2–4 mg/kg q2–4h IM. Total daily dose: 10–30 mg/kg. Therapeutic levels: 3–7 mcg/mL.
ADVERSE EFFECTS: Severe hypotension with IV use. Adverse reactions in ~30% of patients include nausea, vomiting, diarrhea, blood dyscrasias, and drug fever. Overdose may cause cinchonism or respiratory depression.
COMMENTS: Contraindicated with AV nodal block.

Ranitidine (Zantac)

INDICATIONS AND USE: Duodenal and gastric ulcers, gastroesophageal reflux, and hypersecretory conditions (eg, Zollinger-Ellison syndrome).
ACTIONS: Histamine (H_2) receptor antagonist; competitively inhibits the action of histamine on the parietal cells, decreasing gastric acid.
SUPPLIED: Injection, oral liquid.
ROUTE: PO, IV.
DOSAGE: 1–2 mg/kg/day divided q8h IV; 3–4 mg/kg/day divided q12h PO. Maximum: 6 mg/kg/day. Continuous IV infusion: 1.5 mg/kg/day. Reduce the dose in renal dysfunction.
ADVERSE EFFECTS: Constipation, diarrhea, sedation, and, rarely, tachycardia.
Note: Does not interact with other drugs. Injection contains 0.5% phenol. No short-term toxicity is noted. May add the daily dose to the total PN regimen and infuse over 24 h to avoid the need for separate q8h dosing.

Respiratory Syncytial Virus Immune Globulin (RSV-IGIV) (RespiGam)

INDICATIONS AND USE: Prevention of serious lower respiratory tract infection from RSV. Consider prophylactic use of RSV-IGIV in patients <2 years old who have BPD and are receiving oxygen therapy or have received oxygen in the past 6 months and infants with a gestational age of ≤32 weeks, even if there is no BPD. RSV-IGIV should not be given to infants with cyanotic congenital heart disease because of safety concerns. Immunization with measles-containing vaccines should be delayed for 9 months after the last dose of RSV-IGIV, but no changes need to be made in all other routinely given vaccines. (See American Academy of Pediatrics: Respiratory syncytial virus immune globulin intravenous: indications for use. *Pediatrics* 1997;99:645.) RSV-IGIV may be substituted for IGIV during the RSV season for severely immunocompromised infants and children who receive IGIV monthly.

ACTIONS: Passive immunization to RSV. RSV-IGIV contains IgG, which contains antibody to neutralize RSV pooled from adult human plasma having high titers of neutralizing antibody against RSV. Reduces the number of RSV hospitalizations. Reduces the frequency and severity of RSV infections by 40–60%.

PHARMACOKINETICS: Mean half-life is 22–28 days.

SUPPLIED: Injection, 2500 mg/50-mL vial (= 50 mg/mL). Refrigerate.

ROUTE: IV.

DOSAGE: 750 mg/kg (= 15 mL/kg) once per month during flu season (November–April). Infuse at 1.5 mL/kg/h for the first 15 min, then at 3 mL/kg/h for the next 15 min, then increase the rate to 6 mL/kg/h until the end of the infusion.

Monitor vital signs frequently during administration for increases in heart rate, respiratory rate, retractions, and rales; observe for fluid overload or allergic reaction during infusion. Furosemide should be available for management of fluid overload. If severe allergic reaction occurs, discontinue infusion and consider epinephrine.

ADVERSE EFFECTS: Many adverse effects relate to the rate of infusion. Respiratory distress, tachycardia, fever, allergic reactions, rash, gastroenteritis, local site inflammation, and fluid overload in fluid-sensitive patients. Aseptic meningitis syndrome may occur (rare). Do not use in patients who previously had severe reactions to human Ig preparations or in those with IgA deficiency or allergy to any component in the product.

Rifampin (Rifadin, Rimactane)

ACTION AND SPECTRUM: A broad-spectrum antibiotic that exerts its bacteriostatic action by inhibiting DNA-dependent RNA polymerase activity. Effective against mycobacteria, *Neisseria* spp, and gram-positive cocci (eg, staphylococci). Resistance develops rapidly, so the drug should always be used in combination with other agents for synergistic effect.

SUPPLIED: Capsules (oral liquid can be compounded from the capsules by the pharmacist in 10 mg/mL concentration), injection.

ROUTE: PO, IV.

DOSAGE: 10–20 mg/kg/day divided q12h.

ELIMINATION AND METABOLISM: Hepatic. Half-life is ~3 h.

ADVERSE EFFECTS: GI irritation (anorexia, vomiting, and diarrhea), hypersensitivity (rash, pruritus, and eosinophilia), drowsiness, ataxia, blood dyscrasias (leukopenia, thrombocytopenia, and hemolytic anemia), hepatitis (rare), and elevation of serum urea nitrogen and uric acid levels. Causes pink to red discoloration of urine.

COMMENTS: Crosses into CSF. When used, should always be in combination with other agents to provide synergistic effect (eg, vancomycin hydrochloride plus gentamicin sulfate, with or without rifampin, for infection with vancomycin-resistant or tolerant staphylococci).

Note: A potent enzyme inducer of hepatic metabolism. Patients receiving phenytoin, phenobarbital, or theophylline may have a substantial decrease in the serum concentration of these drugs after starting rifampin. Careful monitoring of serum drug concentrations is necessary.

Sodium Bicarbonate (Various)

INDICATIONS AND USE: Metabolic acidosis. Treatment of certain intoxications (eg, salicylates and phenothiazines) and renal tubular acidosis. Adjunctive treatment of hyperkalemia.

ACTIONS: Alkalinizing agent that dissociates to provide bicarbonate ion.

SUPPLIED: Injection.

ROUTE: PO, IV.

DOSAGE:

- Cardiac arrest (no longer recommended for routine use):
  Initial dose: 1–2 mEq/kg IV slowly over 2 min.

Subsequent doses: Number of milliequivalents = 0.3 × weight (kg) × base deficit.

- Renal tubular acidosis:
  Distal: 2–3 mEq/kg/day.
  Proximal: 5–10 mEq/kg/day as the initial dose; adjust prn for maintenance.

ADVERSE EFFECTS: Rapid correction of metabolic acidosis with sodium bicarbonate can lead to intraventricular hemorrhage, hyperosmolality, metabolic alkalosis, hypernatremia, and hypokalemia.

COMMENTS: Use with close monitoring of arterial blood pH.

Sodium Polystyrene Sulfonate (Kayexalate)

INDICATIONS AND USE: Treatment of hyperkalemia.

ACTIONS: Cation exchange resin that releases sodium in exchange for other cations such as potassium. Each gram of resin exchanges 1 mEq of sodium for each milliequivalent of potassium removed. Other cations, such as calcium, magnesium, and iron, are also bound.

SUPPLIED: Powder for suspension, suspension (in 33% sorbitol) (1.25 g/5 mL, containing 4.1 mEq of sodium ion/g).

ROUTE: PO, PR (prepare in ~25% sorbitol solution).

DOSAGE: 1 g of resin will exchange 1 mEq of potassium. Usual dose: 1 g/kg/dose PO q6h or q2–6h PR.

ADVERSE EFFECTS: Large doses may cause fecal impaction. Hypokalemia, hypocalcemia, hypomagnesemia, and sodium retention may occur.

Spironolactone (Aldactone)

INDICATIONS AND USE: Primarily used in conjunction with a thiazide diuretic in the treatment of hypertension, congestive heart failure, and edema when prolonged diuresis is desirable.

ACTIONS: Mild diuretic with potassium-sparing effects. Competitive antagonist of aldosterone.

SUPPLIED: Tablets, 25 mg. (A 4-mg/mL suspension can be compounded by the pharmacist.)

ROUTE: PO.

DOSAGE: 1–3 mg/kg/day divided q12h.

ADVERSE EFFECTS: Hyperkalemia, dehydration, hyponatremia, and gynecomastia (usually reversible).

COMMENTS: Contraindicated in hyperkalemia, anuria, and rapidly deteriorating renal function. Monitor potassium closely when giving potassium supplements. More expensive but more effective than potassium supplements. Peak effect after 2–3 days.

Streptokinase (Kabikinase, Streptase)

INDICATIONS AND USE: Deep venous thrombosis and femoral artery thrombosis after cardiac catheterization.

ACTIONS: Thrombolytic enzyme that converts plasminogen to the enzyme plasmin (fibrinolysin). Plasmin degrades fibrin, fibrinogen, and other plasma procoagulant proteins.

SUPPLIED: Powder for injection.

ROUTE: IV.

DOSAGE:

- Loading dose: 1500–2000 units/kg infused over 30–60 min.
- Maintenance dose: 1000 units/kg/h as continuous infusion for 24–72 h. Titrate the dose to maintain the thrombin time at 2–5 times the normal control value.

ADVERSE EFFECTS: May cause severe spontaneous bleeding, hypersensitivity and anaphylactic reactions, fever (common), and chills.

COMMENTS: Before starting therapy, obtain a baseline thrombin time, activated partial thromboplastin time, prothrombin time, hematocrit, and platelet count; repeat all tests q12h. It is desired to maintain the thrombin time at 2–5 times normal and the prothrombin time and activated partial thromboplastin time as 1.5–2 times normal. Prepare final infusion solution to a concentration of 1000 units/mL in D₅W. At the end of streptokinase therapy, begin IV heparin. Antidote: Aminocaproic acid (loading dose

200 mg/kg IV or PO stat, followed by a maintenance dose of 100 mg/kg/dose IV or PO q6h for up to 10 days after the procedure). *Note:* Limited experience in neonates.

Sulfacetamide Sodium (Isopto Cetamide, Sodium Sulamyd, Others)
ACTION AND SPECTRUM: For mechanism, see Sulfadiazine. Indicated in acute conjunctivitis. Spectrum includes *Staphylococcus aureus*, *Streptococcus pneumoniae*, *Haemophilus influenzae*, and *Moraxella* spp.
SUPPLIED: Ophthalmic solution (10%), ophthalmic ointment.
ROUTE: Topical.
DOSAGE: Instill 1–2 drops into each eye q2h initially, then increase the time interval as the condition responds, or ointment in each eye q1–6h for 7 10 days.
COMMENTS: For adverse effects, see Sulfadiazine. May cause local irritation. Ophthalmic solution is preferred over the neomycin-containing ophthalmic preparation because of decreased incidence of local irritation and allergic response.

Sulfadiazine (Various)
ACTION AND SPECTRUM: Acts via competitive antagonism of *p*-aminobenzoic acid, an essential factor in folic acid synthesis. Spectrum of action includes both gram-positive and gram-negative organisms. In neonatology, used chiefly against *Toxoplasma gondii* in combination with pyrimethamine.
SUPPLIED: Tablets.
ROUTE: PO.
DOSAGE: For toxoplasmosis, give 120 mg/kg/day divided q6h for 4 weeks. Combine with pyrimethamine.
ELIMINATION AND METABOLISM: Rapid renal excretion.
ADVERSE EFFECTS: Hypersensitivity (fever, rash, hepatitis, vasculitis, and lupus-like syndrome), neutropenia, agranulocytosis, thrombocytopenia, aplastic anemia, Stevens-Johnson syndrome, and crystalluria (keep urine alkaline and output high). Kernicterus may occur.
COMMENTS: Avoid use in neonates, except for treatment of congenital toxoplasmosis. See comments under Pyrimethamine regarding folinic acid use.

Surfactant (Exosurf Neonatal)
INDICATIONS AND USE: Surfactant therapy is indicated for the prophylactic treatment of infants with a birth weight <1350 g who are at risk of any type of RDS or for infants with a birth weight >1350 g with coexisting, proven pulmonary immaturity or compromise. Exosurf Neonatal is also indicated for neonates with established surfactant deficiency syndrome.
ACTIONS: Surfactant acts to decrease the work of breathing, increase lung compliance, and increase alveolar expansion and stability by decreasing surface tension, preventing atelectasis at end expiration. As a result, surfactant directly acts to reverse surfactant deficiency syndrome; prevent or reduce the development of pulmonary interstitial edema, which may progress to other forms of RDS; and reduce oxygen positive-pressure mechanical ventilation requirements. The pharmacologic activity of commercial surfactant results from the combined action of three synthetic components: dipalmitoylphosphatidylcholine (DPPC), cetyl alcohol, and tyloxapol. DPPC, the major component of natural surfactant, rapidly and efficiently acts to dramatically decrease alveolar surface tension. Cetyl alcohol facilitates the dispersion and adsorption of DPPC onto the air-liquid interface of the alveoli. Cetyl alcohol modulates this physiologically essential function without the increased risk or immunogenicity of infectious potential associated with foreign protein substances. Tyloxapol provides the product with a hydrophilic agent that allows for reconstitution of the lyophilized powder. Tyloxapol also plays a minor role in distribution of the active components into the smaller airways.
SUPPLIED: Exosurf Neonatal is supplied in a kit containing a 10-mL vial containing DPPC, 108 mg; cetyl alcohol, 12 mg; tyloxapol, 8 mg; and NaCl, 46.75 mg (tonicity agent). Also supplied as a 10-mL vial of sterile water for injection, and ET adapters of varying sizes. Before reconstitution, the drug requires no special storage requirements. Once reconstituted using exactly 8 mL of sterile water, the milky white suspension is stable for up to 12 h either at room temperature or under refrigeration.

ROUTE: Surfactant can only be administered endotracheally using a special ET tube adapter supplied with the drug kit, without the interruption of mechanical ventilation and after radiographic confirmation of the location of the ET tip in the trachea unless impractical because of time restraints.

DOSAGE AND ADMINISTRATION: Before administration of surfactant, the infant should be well suctioned, and suctioning should be withheld for 2 h after the dose unless clinically necessary. Prophylactic surfactant is administered as a single 5-mL/kg dose as soon as RDS is clinically confirmed after birth. Second and third doses may be subsequently administered if necessary while the infant remains mechanically ventilated and under respiratory distress. Rescue treatment for infants who acutely develop RDS is administered as two 5-mL/kg doses; the first dose is given at the time of diagnosis and the second administered 12–24 h later.

Administration of the dose requires intubation and should be done in ½ doses, with the first half given over 1–2 min using the appropriately sized ET adapter with the infant positioned at the midline position. The adapter fits into the ventilator line and has a Luer-Lok syringe port, through which the drug is administered while maintaining the closed system of the respirator. The infant's head and torso are then rotated 45° to the right and held in that position for 30 s. The infant is then returned to midline, and the remaining drug is administered in the same manner, with the head and torso rotated to the left for 30 s. Wean ventilator pressures rapidly after administration.

ADVERSE EFFECTS: Significant adverse effects associated with Exosurf Neonatal during clinical use to this point include increased incidence of pulmonary hemorrhage, apnea, and methylxanthine dosage requirements. Other adverse effects associated with the use of the drug involve increased risk of PDA, thrombocytopenia, and acute changes in respiratory status, the latter of which may be a direct result of the pharmacologic activity of the drug and require rapid adjustment of mechanical ventilatory parameters.

COMMENTS: Administration of surfactant requires close and continuous monitoring during and 30 min after administration of the dose to ensure maximum safety, efficacy, and benefit. This should include blood gas monitoring, rapid weaning of mechanical ventilatory parameters, and monitoring of changes in clinical signs and symptoms consistent with changes in oxygenation and pulmonary function.

Survanta: See Beractant

Theophylline (Various)

INDICATIONS AND USE: Apnea of prematurity. There is evidence that theophylline can improve lung compliance and aid in weaning infants from respiratory support in diseases such as BPD.

ACTIONS: A methylxanthine. Probably acts by virtue of adenosine antagonism. Neonates have the unique ability to convert theophylline to caffeine in a ratio of 1:0.3, respectively, and caffeine may approach 50% of theophylline serum levels. Thus, it is impossible to distinguish the pharmacodynamic effects of theophylline from those of caffeine in the neonate. Theophylline produces excitation throughout all levels of the CNS; produces modest decreases in peripheral vascular resistance; increases cardiac output; relaxes pulmonary airway smooth muscle, with a resultant increase in vital capacity; decreases diaphragmatic fatigue; and may cause marked increases in cerebrovascular resistance, resulting in decreased cerebral blood flow. In premature infants at risk for ventricular hemorrhage, the latter effect may be deleterious.

SUPPLIED: Oral solution, injection.

ROUTE: IV, PO.

DOSAGE:

- Apnea of prematurity: 5–6 mg/kg PO or IV (infused over 15–30 min) as a loading dose, followed by a maintenance dose of 2 mg/kg q12h starting 12 h after the loading dose.
- Ventilator weaning: 6.5 mg/kg PO or IV as a loading dose, followed by a maintenance dose of 3–4 mg/kg q12h.

ADVERSE EFFECTS: Side effects and toxicity include hyperglycemia, diuresis, dehydration, feeding intolerance, tachycardia and other arrhythmias, hyperreflexia, jitteriness, and seizures.

COMMENTS: Levels for apnea are 6–11 mcg/mL. Toxicity is associated with levels >15–20 mcg/mL. Monitor serum levels on day 4 of therapy: peak level 1 h after an IV dose is completed or 2 h after an oral dose, and trough level 30 min before the next dose. Levels of caffeine and theophylline should ideally be monitored any time toxicity is suspected or when apnea spells appear to be increasing in frequency.

Ticarcillin Disodium (Ticar)

CLASSIFICATION: Semisynthetic extended-spectrum penicillin.
ACTION AND SPECTRUM: See Mezlocillin Sodium.
SUPPLIED: Injection.
ROUTE: IM, IV (infuse over 30 min).
DOSAGE:

- <2000 g and 0–7 days old: 150 mg/kg/day divided q12h.
- <2000 g and >7 days old: 225 mg/kg/day divided q8h.
- >2000 g and 0–7 days old: 225 mg/kg/day divided q8h.
- >2000 g and >7 days old: 300 mg/kg/day divided q6h.

ELIMINATION AND METABOLISM: Renally excreted.
ADVERSE EFFECTS: See Mezlocillin Sodium. Hypokalemia is pronounced.
COMMENTS: Drug of first choice when considering an extended-spectrum penicillin. Avoid IM use if possible. Contains 5.2 mEq of sodium/g.

Ticarcillin Disodium and Clavulanate Potassium (Timentin)

CLASSIFICATION: Combination antibiotic of ticarcillin (a carboxypenicillin) and clavulanic acid (a β-lactamase inhibitor).
Spectrum: Good antipseudomonal activity similar to that of ticarcillin except for additional coverage of lactamase-producing species, particularly gram-positive cocci (eg, Staphylococcus aureus, Streptococcus pneumoniae, and group B streptococcus). Good coverage against gram-negative organisms, including Escherichia coli, Klebsiella spp, and Proteus spp. Also demonstrated activity against anaerobes such as Clostridium spp and Peptostreptococcus spp.
SUPPLIED: Injection.
ROUTE: IV.
DOSAGE:

- <2000 g and 0–7 days old: 150 mg/kg/day divided q12h.
- <2000 g and >7 days old: 225 mg/kg/day divided q8h.
- >2000 g and 0–7 days old: 225 mg/kg/day divided q8h.
- >2000 g and >7 days old: 300 mg/kg/day divided q6h.

ELIMINATION: Ticarcillin, renal (tubular secretion); clavulanic acid, hepatic and renal.
ADVERSE EFFECTS: See Ticarcillin Disodium.

Tobramycin Sulfate (Nebcin)

CLASSIFICATION: Aminoglycoside.
ACTION AND SPECTRUM: Mechanism of action and spectrum identical to those of gentamicin sulfate.
SUPPLIED: Injection, ophthalmic drops, ophthalmic ointment.
ROUTE: IM, IV (infuse over 30 min), topical (ophthalmic).
DOSAGE:

- IM or IV: Monitor and adjust by pharmacokinetics. Initial empiric dosing based on body weight.
  <1.2 kg: 2.5 mg/kg/dose q18–24h.
  <2 kg and 0–7 days old: 2.5 mg/kg/dose q12–18h.
  <2 kg and >7 days old: 2.5 mg/kg/dose q8–12h.
  >2 kg and 0–7 days: 2.5 mg/kg/dose q12h.
  >2 kg and >7 days old: 2.5 mg/kg/dose q8h.
- Ophthalmic: Instill 1–2 drops into each eye 2–6 times a day or more often prn, or apply a small amount of ointment into each eye q3–4h.

ELIMINATION AND METABOLISM: Renal.
ADVERSE EFFECTS: See Gentamicin Sulfate.

COMMENTS: Reserve for cases resistant to gentamicin sulfate. Obtain serum peak and trough concentrations at about the fourth maintenance dose. Desired serum peak concentration is 4–10 mcg/mL (sample obtained 30 min after the infusion is complete); desired serum trough concentration is <2 mcg/mL (sample obtained 30 min to just before the next dose).

Tolazoline Hydrochloride (Priscoline)

INDICATIONS AND USE: Hypoxia caused by persistent pulmonary hypertension.
ACTIONS: α-Adrenergic blocking agent with histaminergic properties. Results in pulmonary and systemic vasodilator effects. Histaminic effects stimulate gastric secretion and peripheral vasodilation and increase salivary, lacrimal, respiratory tract, and pancreatic secretions. Response is marked by cutaneous flushing followed by increased Pao_2.
SUPPLIED: Injection.
ROUTE: IV.
DOSAGE: 1–2 mg/kg IV as the initial dose (infused over 5–10 min), followed by a continuous infusion of 0.3–0.6 mg/kg/h. Some infants respond rapidly; others may require 30 min or more.
ADVERSE EFFECTS: Tachycardia, nausea, vomiting, diarrhea, GI bleeding, increased GI secretions, increased pilomotor activity, sweating, thrombocytopenia, agranulocytosis, and hypotension.
COMMENTS: Contraindicated in renal failure, hypotension shock, and intraventricular hemorrhage. Dopamine and dobutamine are often used to support systemic pressure in neonates with persistent pulmonary hypertension; both drugs may have adverse effects on peripheral vascular resistance, especially at higher dosages. For severe hypotension, use ephedrine (0.2 mg/kg/dose) to increase peripheral vascular resistance or dopamine (<10 mcg/kg/min) to improve cardiac output. Epinephrine administered with tolazoline may cause a paradoxic reduction in blood pressure followed by an exaggerated rebound blood pressure elevation.

Tromethamine (THAM)

INDICATIONS AND USE: Metabolic acidosis when sodium bicarbonate is contraindicated because of elevated serum sodium (eg, metabolic acidosis in persistent fetal circulation treated with multiple doses of sodium bicarbonate).
ACTIONS: Alkalinizing agent that acts as a proton (hydrogen ion) acceptor; combines with hydrogen ions and their associated anions of acids (lactic, pyruvic, carbonic, and other metabolic acids). The resulting salts are then renally excreted.
SUPPLIED: Injection, 0.3-mol solution (36 mg/mL).
ROUTE: IV.
DOSAGE:

- Loading dose: 3–5 mL/kg of undiluted solution infused over 1 h, or dose = weight (kg) × 1.1 × base deficit (mEq/L).
- Maintenance dose: 3 mL/kg/h (undiluted solution) as continuous infusion. Titrate the dose to the desired response via frequent blood gas monitoring.

ADVERSE EFFECTS: Respiratory depression, thrombophlebitis, venospasm, alkalosis, transient hypocalcemia or hypoglycemia, and hyperkalemia. Extravasation may cause sloughing of the skin.
COMMENTS: Contraindicated in anuria, uremia, and chronic respiratory acidosis. Do not administer for periods >24 h. Hyperkalemia is a problem, especially with decreased renal function.

Tubocurarine (Curare)

INDICATIONS AND USE: To improve oxygenation in the uncooperative neonate during mechanical ventilation. To provide muscle relaxation during general anesthesia.
ACTIONS: Nondepolarizing (competitive) neuromuscular blocking agent. Rapid IV administration may cause hypotension, bradycardia, and possibly circulatory collapse. Atropine is an effective prophylactic agent. Onset of paralysis is generally 1–2 min after IV administration. Duration of paralysis depends on the number of doses and the total dosage delivered and may persist for 20–90 min.

SUPPLIED: Injection, 3 mg/mL.
ROUTE: IV, IM (only if IV access is not available).
DOSAGE: Infuse undiluted over 1 min or more to minimize cardiovascular effects.

- Initial dose: 0.25–0.5 mg/kg IV.
- Maintenance dose: 0.15 mg/kg/dose IV prn.

ADVERSE EFFECTS: Hypotension, bradycardia, possibly circulatory collapse, and allergic reactions.
COMMENTS: For reversal, give neostigmine, with atropine, IV. For dose, see pages 595 and 624.

Vancomycin Hydrochloride (Vancocin, Others)

ACTION AND SPECTRUM: Bactericidal action by interference with bacterial cell wall synthesis. Active against most gram-positive cocci and bacilli, including streptococci, staphylococci (including methicillin-resistant staphylococci), clostridia (including *Clostridium difficile*), *Corynebacterium* spp, and *Listeria monocytogenes*. Bacteriostatic against enterococci. No cross-resistance with other antibiotics has been reported. The drug of choice against methicillin-resistant staphylococci and *C. difficile*.
SUPPLIED: Injection, oral solution.
ROUTE: IV, PO.
DOSAGE:

- IV: Monitor and adjust by pharmacokinetics. Initial empiric dosing based on body weight.
  <1.2 kg and 0–4 weeks' postnatal age: 15 mg/kg/dose q24h.
  1.2–2 kg and 0–7 days: 15 mg/kg/dose q12–18h.
  1.2–2 kg and >7 days: 15 mg/kg/dose q8–12h.
  >2 kg and 0–7 days: 15 mg/kg/dose q12h.
  >2 kg and >7 days: 15 mg/kg/dose q8h.
- PO: To treat pseudomembranous colitis resulting from *C. difficile* or staphylococcal enterocolitis, give 20–40 mg/kg/day divided q6h for 5–7 days.

ELIMINATION AND METABOLISM: Renally excreted. Half-life is 7–9 h.
ADVERSE EFFECTS: Allergy (rash and fever), ototoxicity (with serum peak levels >40 mcg/mL), and thrombophlebitis at the site of injection. A too-rapid infusion may cause rash, chills, and fever ("red-man" syndrome) mimicking anaphylactic reaction. Rapid infusion may cause apnea and bradycardia without other signs of "red-man" syndrome. Infuse dose over at least 60 min.
COMMENTS: Therapeutic range: 20–40 mcg/mL (sample drawn 60 min after the infusion is complete) and serum trough levels of 5–10 mcg/mL (sample drawn 30 min to just before the next dose). In general, draw serum peak and trough levels at about the fourth maintenance dose. Monitor serum creatinine. If staphylococci exhibit tolerance to the drug, combine it with an aminoglycoside, with or without rifampin. Oral doses are poorly absorbed. Powder for injection, diluted and flavored, is the most economic means of oral dosing.

Varicella-Zoster Immune Globulin (VZIG)

INDICATIONS AND USE: For protection of infants of mothers with varicella-zoster infections (chickenpox) within 5 days before or 48 h after delivery, of postnatally exposed preterm infants <1000 g or <28 weeks' gestation regardless of maternal history, and of postnatally exposed premature infants whose maternal history is negative for varicella.
ACTIONS: Passive immunity through infusion of IgG antibody. Protection lasts 1 month or longer. VZIG does not reduce the incidence but acts to decrease the risk of complications.
SUPPLIED: Injection, 125 units/1.25-mL vial.
ROUTE: IM only.
DOSAGE: 0–10 kg: 125 units IM as a single dose injected at one site.
ADVERSE EFFECTS: Pain, erythema, swelling, rash at the site of injection, and, rarely, anaphylaxis.

COMMENTS: Best results are achieved if VZIG is given within 96 h after exposure. It is obtained through the American Red Cross Blood Services. *Note:* Do not give IV.

Vecuronium Bromide (Norcuron)

INDICATIONS AND USE: Skeletal muscle relaxation and paralysis in infants requiring mechanical ventilation.

ACTIONS: Nondepolarizing muscle relaxant that competitively antagonizes autonomic cholinergic receptors. Onset of action is 1–2 min with a duration that varies with dose and age.

SUPPLIED: Powder for injection.

ROUTE: IV.

DOSAGE: 0.03–0.15 mg/kg IV push q1–2h to maintain paralysis.

ADVERSE EFFECTS: May cause hypoxemia.

COMMENTS: Causes less tachycardia than pancuronium bromide. When used with narcotics, decreases in heart rate and blood pressure have been observed.

Vidarabine (Vira-A)

ACTION AND SPECTRUM: Antiviral agent for treatment of herpes encephalitis. Inhibits viral DNA formation. Good activity against herpes simplex type 1, poor activity against adenoviruses or RNA viruses. Activity against varicella-zoster virus is unconfirmed.

SUPPLIED: Injection (monohydrate), 200 mg/mL, equivalent to 187.4 mg of vidarabine; ophthalmic ointment, 3%.

ROUTE: Ophthalmic, IV (dilute to 1 mg/2.2 mL and infuse over 12–24 h).

DOSAGE:

Ophthalmic: Instill a small amount into each eye q3h.

- IV:
    <1 month: 15–30 mg/kg/day as an 18- to 24-h infusion.
    >1 month: 10–15 mg/kg/day as a 12-h or longer infusion.

ADVERSE EFFECTS: Rash and pain at the injection site. Decreased reticulocyte count, white blood cell count, and platelet count. Elevated total bilirubin and AST (SGOT).

COMMENTS: Rarely used. Volume necessary for IV infusion may cause fluid overload. Acyclovir is the usual agent of choice. Must filter the final solution (use a 0.45-μmol filter).

Vitamin D$_2$ (Ergocalciferol, Calciferol) (Drisdol)

INDICATIONS AND USE: To prevent or treat rickets and to manage hypocalcemia resulting from vitamin D deficiency.

ACTIONS: Regulation of plasma calcium and phosphate, supporting normal mineralization of bone.

SUPPLIED: Oral solution, 8000 units/mL; injection, 500,000 units/mL for IM use only.

ROUTE: PO, IM.

DOSAGE: 400–800 units/day.

COMMENTS: Excessive doses may lead to hypervitaminosis D, manifested by hypercalcemia and its associated complications.

Vitamin E (DL-α-Tocopherol Acetate) (Aquasol E)

INDICATIONS AND USE: Investigational for treatment or prevention of anemia of prematurity, retinopathy of prematurity, BPD, and intraventricular hemorrhage.

ACTIONS: A potent free radical scavenger. An antioxidant to prevent destruction of unsaturated fatty acids and cell membranes by uncontrolled free radicals. At birth, tissue stores of α-tocopherol (active form) are low.

SUPPLIED: Drops, 50 units/mL.

ROUTE: PO.

DOSAGE:

- Requirements: Recommendations currently followed in infant formulas are:
    Full-term infants: 0.3 unit/100 kcal or 0.7 unit/g of linoleic acid.
    Premature infants: 1 unit/g of linoleic acid.
- Anemia of prematurity: Prevention or treatment requires only adequate nutritional intake of vitamin E.
- Alternative:

Prophylaxis: 25–50 units/day PO until 2–3 months of age.
Treatment: 50–200 units/day PO for 2 weeks.

COMMENTS: Physiologic serum levels for premature infants are 1–3 mg/dL. Serum levels should be monitored when pharmacologic doses of vitamin E are administered. Liquid preparation is very hyperosmolar (3000 mOsm/L) and should be diluted. (1 mg of DL-α-tocopherol acetate = 1 unit).

Vitamin K$_1$ (Phytonadione) (AquaMEPHYTON, Mephyton)

INDICATIONS AND USE: Prevention and treatment of hemorrhagic disease of the newborn and vitamin K deficiency.

ACTIONS: Required for the synthesis of blood coagulation factors II, VII, IX, and X. Because vitamin K$_1$ may require 3 h or more to stop active bleeding, fresh-frozen plasma, 10 mL/kg, may be necessary when bleeding is severe. The drug has no antagonistic effects against heparin.

SUPPLIED: Tablets, injection.

ROUTE: PO, IM, IV, SC. (For IV use, dilute in D$_5$W and infuse over 30 min or longer.)

DOSAGE:

- Neonatal hemorrhagic disease:
  Prevention: 1 mg IM at birth; if the infant is <1500 g, give 0.5 mg IM at birth.
  Treatment: 1 mg as a single dose.
- Deficiency state: 1 mg/dose PO, IM, or slowly IV.

ORAL ANTICOAGULANT OVERDOSE: 1–2 mg/dose IV q4–8h prn. (Monitor the serial prothrombin time and partial thromboplastin time for response.)

ADVERSE EFFECTS: Relatively nontoxic. Hemolytic anemia and kernicterus have been reported in neonates given menadiol sodium diphosphate (vitamin K$_3$ [Synkayvite]); however, vitamin K$_1$ has not been associated with toxic symptoms or hypersensitivity. No association between exposure to vitamin K at birth and an increased risk of any childhood cancer or of all childhood cancers combined were found using data from the Collaborative Perinatal Project, although a slightly increased risk could not be ruled out.

Zidovudine (AZT) (Retrovir)

INDICATIONS AND USE: Management of patients with HIV infection. Prevention of maternal-fetal HIV transmission.

ACTIONS: Virostatic. Inhibits HIV viral polymerases and DNA replication.

SUPPLIED: Syrup, 10 mg/mL; injection, 10 mg/mL.

ROUTE: IV, PO.

DOSAGE:

- 0–2 weeks old: 2 mg/kg/dose PO q6h.
- 2–4 weeks old: 3 mg/kg/dose PO q6h.
- >4 weeks old: 90–180 mg/m^2/dose PO q6h; 0.5–1.8 mg/kg/h IV continuous infusion; 100–120 mg/m^2/dose q6h over 1 h with a maximum concentration of 4 mg/mL in D$_5$W.
- Reduce the dose by 30% in children with zidovudine toxicity with hemoglobin <8 g/dL.
- Give the PO dose 30 min before or 1 h after feedings with water.

ADVERSE EFFECTS: The most frequent are granulocytopenia and severe anemia. Others include thrombocytopenia, leukopenia, diarrhea, fever, seizures, insomnia, and cholestatic hepatitis.

COMMENTS: Use with caution in patients with impaired hepatic function, bone marrow compromise, or folic acid or vitamin B$_{12}$ deficiency.

INTERACTIONS: Concurrent acetaminophen, probenecid, cimetidine, indomethacin, morphine, and benzodiazepines may increase toxicity as a result of decreased glucuronidation or reduced renal excretion of zidovudine. Concomitant acyclovir may cause neurotoxicity; ganciclovir may cause severe hematologic toxicity as a result of synergistic myelosuppression. Ribavirin and zidovudine are antagonistic and should not be used concurrently.

81 Effects of Drugs and Substances on Lactation and Breast-Feeding

The drugs and substances listed below are those for which reliable data on their effect during lactation have been compiled. This listing is undoubtedly incomplete because it is impossible to list every possible medication. Clinical judgment about the possible effects of maternal drug intake while nursing must always be exercised.

Drug or Substance	Compatibility With Breast-Feeding, Effect on Lactation, and Adverse Effects on Infant
Acetaminophen	Generally compatible with breast-feeding.
Acyclovir	Generally compatible with breast-feeding.
Albuterol	Generally compatible with breast-feeding. Monitor for agitation and spitting up. Use inhaled form to decrease maternal absorption.
Alcohol	Generally compatible with breast-feeding with moderate use. Passes freely into breast milk. Monitor for drowsiness, diaphoresis, weakness, and failure to thrive. Intake of 1 g/kg/day may decrease maternal milk ejection reflex.
Allopurinol	Generally compatible with breast-feeding.
Alprazolam	Avoid during lactation
Amantadine	Contraindicated. Causes release of levodopa in central nervous system (CNS).
Amikacin	Generally compatible with breast-feeding. Low concentrations in breast milk because of poor oral absorption.
Aminoglycosides	Generally compatible with breast-feeding. All antibiotics are excreted in breast milk in limited amounts. Apparently safe; not absorbed in newborn gastrointestinal tract. Monitor for diarrhea.
Aminophylline	Generally compatible with breast-feeding. Monitor for irritability.
Amiodarone	Breast-feeding not recommended because of iodine contained in each dose and possible accumulation of amiodarone in the infant. Possible hypothyroidism.
Amitriptyline	Milk-plasma ratio of 1.0. Use in breast-feeding may be of concern.
Amoxapine	Active metabolites in milk. Use in breast-feeding may be of concern.
Amoxicillin	Generally compatible with breast-feeding. Monitor for diarrhea.
Amphetamines	Avoid. Monitor for irritability and poor sleeping pattern.
Ampicillin	Generally compatible with breast-feeding. Monitor for diarrhea.
Aspartame	Generally compatible with breast-feeding. Use cautiously in carrier of phenylketonuria.
Aspirin	Use with caution. Monitor for spitting up or bleeding. May affect platelet function. Increased risk with high doses used for rheumatoid arthritis (3–5 g/day). Metabolic acidosis may occur.
Atenolol	Use with caution. Monitor for signs of β-blockade such as bradycardia.
Atropine	Generally compatible with breast-feeding. No adverse effects reported.
Aztreonam	Generally compatible with breast-feeding.
Baclofen	Generally compatible with breast-feeding.
Bethanechol	Generally compatible with breast-feeding. May cause abdominal pain and diarrhea.
Bismuth subsalicylate	Use with caution because of potential for adverse effects from salicylates.
Bromides	Breast-feeding not recommended because of possible drowsiness and rash.
Bromocriptine	Contraindicated. Suppresses lactation.
Brompheniramine	Generally compatible with breast-feeding. Monitor for agitation, poor sleeping pattern, and feeding problems.
Bupropion	Avoid in breast-feeding. Effects not known. Excreted in milk.
Butorphanol	Generally compatible with breast-feeding.
Caffeine	Generally compatible with breast-feeding. Monitor for irritability and poor sleeping pattern. No effect with moderate intake (2–3 cups/day).
Calcitonin	May inhibit lactation.
Captopril	Generally compatible with breast-feeding.
Carbamazepine	Generally compatible with breast-feeding. Risk of bone marrow suppression if taken chronically.

Drug or Substance	Compatibility With Breast-Feeding, Effect on Lactation, and Adverse Effects on Infant
Carbimazole	Generally compatible with breast-feeding. Monitor for goiter.
Cascara sagrada	Generally compatible with breast-feeding. Monitor for diarrhea.
Cefaclor	Generally compatible with breast-feeding. Monitor for diarrhea.
Cefadroxil	Generally compatible with breast-feeding. Monitor for diarrhea.
Cefamandole	Generally compatible with breast-feeding. Monitor for diarrhea.
Cefazolin	Generally compatible with breast-feeding. Monitor for diarrhea.
Cefonicid	Generally compatible with breast-feeding. Monitor for diarrhea.
Cefoperazone	Generally compatible with breast-feeding. Monitor for diarrhea.
Ceforanide	Generally compatible with breast-feeding. Monitor for diarrhea.
Cefotaxime	Generally compatible with breast-feeding. Monitor for diarrhea.
Cefotetan	Generally compatible with breast-feeding. Monitor for diarrhea.
Cefoxitin	Generally compatible with breast-feeding. Monitor for diarrhea.
Cefprozil	Generally compatible with breast-feeding. Monitor for diarrhea.
Ceftazidime	Generally compatible with breast-feeding. Monitor for diarrhea.
Ceftizoxime	Generally compatible with breast-feeding. Monitor for diarrhea.
Ceftriaxone	Generally compatible with breast-feeding. Monitor for diarrhea.
Cefuroxime	Generally compatible with breast-feeding. Monitor for diarrhea.
Cephalexin	Generally compatible with breast-feeding. Monitor for diarrhea.
Cephalosporins	Generally compatible with breast-feeding. All antibiotics excreted in breast milk in limited amounts. Monitor for rash; sensitization possible.
Cephalothin	Generally compatible with breast-feeding. Monitor for diarrhea.
Cephapirin	Generally compatible with breast-feeding. Monitor for diarrhea.
Cephradine	Generally compatible with breast-feeding. Monitor for diarrhea.
Chloral hydrate	Generally compatible with breast-feeding. Monitor for sedation and rash.
Chloramphenicol	Discontinue during breast-feeding. Risk of bone marrow toxicity. Wait 24 h after last dose before breast-feeding.
Chloroquine	Generally compatible with breast-feeding. Insufficient amounts excreted in breast milk to provide adequate protection against malaria.
Chlorothiazide	Generally compatible with breast-feeding but may suppress lactation, especially in first month of lactation. Adverse effects have not been reported, but infant's electrolytes and platelets should be monitored.
Chlorpheniramine	Generally compatible with breast-feeding. Monitor for agitation, poor sleeping pattern, and feeding problems.
Chlorpromazine	Effects unknown. Use with caution. Monitor for sedation. Galactorrhea in adults.
Chlorpropamide	Contraindicated. Excreted in breast milk and may cause hypoglycemia.
Chlortetracycline	Generally compatible with breast-feeding. Monitor for diarrhea.
Chocolate	Generally compatible with breast-feeding. Irritability or increased bowel activity if mother consumes excessive amounts (>16 oz/day).
Cimetidine	Use with caution. May suppress gastric acidity in infant, inhibit drug metabolism, and cause CNS stimulation.
Ciprofloxacin	Avoid. Wait 48 h after last dose before breast-feeding.
Clemastine	Use with caution. Drowsiness and CNS effects may occur.
Clindamycin	Discontinue during breast-feeding. Risk of gastrointestinal bleeding. Wait 24 h after last dose before breast-feeding.
Clofazimine	Avoid if possible. Increased skin pigmentation may occur.
Clonazepam	Generally compatible with breast-feeding. Monitor for respiratory and CNS depression.
Clonidine	Contraindicated. Excreted in breast milk.
Cloxacillin	Generally compatible with breast-feeding. Monitor for diarrhea.
Cocaine	Contraindicated. Causes cocaine intoxication in infant from maternal intranasal use (hypertension, tachycardia, mydriasis, and apnea) and from topical use on mother's nipples (apnea and seizures).
Codeine	Generally compatible with breast-feeding. Monitor for sedation. Milk ejection reflex (letdown) may be inhibited.
Contraceptives, oral	May cause poor weight gain and breast enlargement in infants. May decrease milk production. Use with caution. Monitor infant's weight gain.
Coumadin (warfarin, dicumarol)	Generally compatible with breast-feeding.
Cyclophosphamide	Contraindicated. Possible immune suppression. Unknown effect on growth or association with carcinogenesis. May cause neutropenia.
Cyclosporine	Possible immune suppression; unknown effect on growth or association with carcinogenesis.

Drug or Substance	Compatibility With Breast-Feeding, Effect on Lactation, and Adverse Effects on Infant
Cyproheptadine	Generally compatible with breast-feeding. Monitor for agitation, poor sleeping pattern, and feeding problems.
Desipramine	Effects on infant unknown but may be of concern.
Dextroamphetamine	Contraindicated. May cause infant stimulation.
Diazepam	Contraindicated. May cause infant sedation. May accumulate in breast-fed infants.
Diazoxide	Contraindicated. May cause hyperglycemia.
Dicumarol	See Coumadin.
Digoxin	Generally compatible with breast-feeding. Monitor for spitting up, diarrhea, and heart rate changes.
Diphenhydramine	Generally compatible with breast-feeding. Monitor for agitation, poor sleeping pattern, and feeding problems.
Dipyridamole	Generally compatible with breast-feeding.
Disopyramide	Generally compatible with breast-feeding.
Doxepin	Avoid. Excreted into milk. Serious, potentially lethal adverse effects reported in one infant.
Doxorubicin	Contraindicated. Concentrated in milk. May cause immune suppression and other adverse effects.
Doxycycline	Generally compatible with breast-feeding. Monitor for diarrhea.
Enalapril	Generally compatible with breast-feeding.
Enoxaparin	Generally compatible with breast-feeding.
Ephedrine	Generally compatible with breast-feeding. Monitor for agitation.
Ergotamine	Contraindicated. Causes vomiting, diarrhea, and convulsions. May hinder lactation.
Erythromycin	Generally compatible with breast-feeding. Monitor for diarrhea.
Ethambutol	Generally compatible with breast-feeding.
Ethanol	See Alcohol.
Ethosuximide	Generally compatible with breast-feeding. Rare occurrence of bone marrow suppression and gastrointestinal upset. Excreted freely into breast milk. Use lowest effective dose and monitor blood levels in mother and infant.
Famotidine	Generally compatible with breast-feeding.
Fava beans	Generally compatible with breast-feeding. Hemolysis in patients with glucose-6-phosphate dehydrogenase (G6PD) deficiency.
Fenoprofen	Excreted in breast milk in small quantities.
Flecainide	Generally compatible with breast-feeding.
Fluconazole	Generally compatible with breast-feeding.
Fluoride	No reports of adverse effects.
Fluoxetine	Avoid. Colic, irritability, sleep disorders, and poor weight gain may occur.
Folic acid	Generally compatible with breast-feeding.
Furosemide	Generally compatible with breast-feeding.
Gallium 67	Discontinue during breast-feeding. Radioactivity can remain in breast milk for 2 weeks.
Gentamicin	Generally compatible with breast-feeding. Monitor for diarrhea and bloody stools.
Gold salts	Contraindicated. May cause rash and inflammation of kidney and liver.
Guanethidine	Generally compatible with breast-feeding.
Haloperidol	Use may be of concern. Effects on infant unknown. Possible decline in developmental score.
Halothane	Generally compatible with breast-feeding.
Heparin	Generally compatible with breast-feeding.
Heroin	Contraindicated. Monitor for depression and withdrawal.
Hydralazine	Generally compatible with breast-feeding.
Hydrochlorothiazide	Generally compatible with breast-feeding. See Chlorothiazide.
Hydromorphone	Generally compatible with breast-feeding. Monitor for sedation. Milk ejection reflex (letdown) may be inhibited.
Ibuprofen	Generally compatible with breast-feeding.
Imipramine	Use may be of concern. Effects on infant unknown.
Indomethacin	Generally compatible with breast-feeding. One case of seizure in infant.
Insulin	Generally compatible with breast-feeding.
Interferon alfa	Generally compatible with breast-feeding.
Iodine	Generally compatible with breast-feeding. May cause goiter.
Iodine-125	Contraindicated. Risk of thyroid cancer. Radioactivity present in milk for 12 days.
Iodine-131	Contraindicated. Radioactivity in milk for 2–14 days.
Isoniazid	Generally compatible with breast-feeding. Monitor for rash, diarrhea, and constipation. Substantial excretion into milk.

Drug or Substance	Compatibility With Breast-Feeding, Effect on Lactation, and Adverse Effects on Infant
Isoproterenol	Generally compatible with breast-feeding. Monitor for agitation and spitting up. Use aerosol form to decrease maternal absorption.
Isotretinoin	Contraindicated.
Kanamycin	Generally compatible with breast-feeding. Low concentrations in breast milk because of poor oral absorption. Monitor for diarrhea.
Labetalol	Generally compatible with breast-feeding. Monitor for hypotension and bradycardia.
Lamotrigine	May be of concern. Consider monitoring infant's serum lamotrigine concentration.
Levodopa	Contraindicated. Inhibitory effect on prolactin release.
Levothyroxine (T$_4$)	Generally compatible with breast-feeding. Probably does not interfere with neonatal thyroid screening.
Lidocaine	Generally compatible with breast-feeding.
Liothyronine (T$_3$)	Generally compatible with breast-feeding. Probably does not interfere with neonatal thyroid screening.
Lithium	Contraindicated during breast-feeding. Milk levels average 40% of maternal serum concentration. Monitor infant for cyanosis, hypotonia, bradycardia, and other lithium toxicities.
Loperamide	Generally compatible with breast-feeding.
Loratadine	Generally compatible with breast-feeding.
Lorazepam	Generally compatible with breast-feeding. Monitor for sedation, especially if exposure is prolonged.
Lovastatin	Avoid. Potential for adverse effect in infant.
Magnesium sulfate	Generally compatible with breast-feeding.
Marijuana	Avoid. Long-term effects of exposure unknown.
Meperidine	Generally compatible with breast-feeding. Monitor for sedation. Milk ejection reflex (letdown) may be inhibited.
Meprobamate	Generally compatible with breast-feeding but excreted in milk in high amounts. Monitor for sedation.
Metaproterenol	Generally compatible with breast-feeding. Monitor for agitation and spitting up. Use aerosol form to decrease maternal absorption.
Methadone	Generally compatible with breast-feeding when mother is receiving ≤20 mg/day. Monitor for sedation, depression, and withdrawal on cessation of methadone treatment.
Methimazole	Usually compatible with breast-feeding. Potential for interfering with thyroid function.
Methotrexate	Contraindicated. Possible immune suppression. Effects on growth and association with carcinogenesis unknown.
Methyldopa	Generally compatible with breast-feeding. Risk of hemolysis and increased liver enzymes.
Methyprylon	Generally compatible with breast-feeding. Monitor for drowsiness.
Metoclopramide	Generally compatible with breast-feeding with maternal dose of ≤45 mg/day. Increases milk production.
Metoprolol	Generally compatible with breast-feeding. Monitor for bradycardia and hypotension.
Metronidazole	Discontinue during breast-feeding. Do not nurse until 12–24 h after discontinuing to allow excretion of drug.
Mexiletine	Generally compatible with breast-feeding.
Midazolam	Effects on nursing infant may be of concern.
Minoxidil	Generally compatible with breast-feeding. Monitor for hypotension.
Misoprostol	Contraindicated. Could cause significant diarrhea in infant.
Monosodium glutamate	Generally compatible with breast-feeding.
Morphine	Generally compatible with breast-feeding. Monitor for sedation. Milk ejection reflex (letdown) may be inhibited.
Moxalactam	Usually compatible with breast feeding.
Nadolol	Generally compatible with breast-feeding. Monitor for bradycardia and hypotension.
Naproxen	Generally compatible with breast-feeding. Adverse effects unknown.
Nicotine	May be of concern. Excessive amounts may cause diarrhea, vomiting, tachycardia, irritability, decreased milk production, and decreased weight gain.
Nifedipine	Generally compatible with breast-feeding.
Nitrofurantoin	Generally compatible with breast-feeding. Excreted in milk in small amounts. Monitor infants with G6PD deficiency for hemolytic anemia.

Drug or Substance	Compatibility With Breast-Feeding, Effect on Lactation, and Adverse Effects on Infant
Nizatidine	Generally compatible with breast-feeding.
Nystatin	Generally compatible with breast-feeding.
Oral contraceptives	Contraindicated. Can cause poor weight gain, breast enlargement, and proliferation of vaginal epithelium in infants.
Oxacillin	Generally compatible with breast-feeding. Monitor for diarrhea.
Oxazepam	Generally compatible with breast-feeding. Monitor for sedation and depression.
Oxprenolol	Generally compatible with breast-feeding. Monitor for hypotension and bradycardia.
Oxycodone (Percodan, Percocet)	Generally compatible with breast-feeding. Monitor for drowsiness.
Paroxetine	Effect on nursing infant is unknown but may be of concern.
Penicillins	Generally compatible with breast-feeding. All antibiotics are excreted in breast milk in limited amounts. Monitor for rash, diarrhea, and spitting up.
Pentoxifylline	Avoid. Excreted in milk.
Phencyclidine	Contraindicated. Excreted in high amounts in breast milk.
Phenobarbital	Use with caution. Monitor for sucking problems, sedation, rashes, and withdrawal.
Phenylbutazone	Generally compatible with breast-feeding.
Phenylpropanolamine	Generally compatible with breast-feeding. Monitor for agitation.
Phenytoin	Generally compatible with breast-feeding. Monitor for methemoglobinuria (rare). Keep maternal phenytoin in therapeutic range.
Phytonadione	Generally compatible with breast-feeding. Breast-fed infants should receive prophylactic vitamin K at birth because content in breast milk is low and hemorrhagic disease may occur.
Pindolol	Generally compatible with breast-feeding. Monitor for hypotension and bradycardia.
Piperacillin	Generally compatible with breast-feeding. Monitor for diarrhea.
Potassium iodide	Contraindicated. Goiter and allergic reactions may be seen.
Prednisone	Generally compatible with breast-feeding. Safety of long-term therapy has not been established. If maternal dose is more than 2 times physiologic, avoid breast-feeding.
Primidone	Use with caution. Monitor for sucking problems, sedation, rashes, and withdrawal.
Procainamide	Avoid. Excreted in and accumulates in milk.
Prochlorperazine	Generally compatible with breast-feeding. Monitor for sedation.
Propoxyphene	Generally compatible with breast-feeding. Monitor for withdrawal after long-term high-dose maternal use.
Propranolol	Generally compatible with breast-feeding. Monitor for hypotension and bradycardia.
Propylthiouracil	Generally compatible with breast-feeding. Monitor thyroid function of infant periodically.
Pseudoephedrine	Generally compatible with breast-feeding. Monitor for agitation.
Psychotropic drugs	May be of concern. Long half-life. Long-term neurodevelopmental effects cannot be determined.
Pyridoxine	Generally compatible with breast-feeding.
Pyrimethamine	Generally compatible with breast-feeding.
Quinidine	Generally compatible with breast-feeding. Monitor for rash, anemia, and arrhythmias. Risk of optic neuritis with chronic use.
Radiopharmaceuticals (generally)	Discontinue during breast-feeding. Consult nuclear medicine physician for selection of radionuclide with shortest excretion time.
Ranitidine	Generally compatible with breast-feeding. May increase infant's gastric pH.
Reserpine	Generally compatible with breast-feeding. Monitor for infantile galactorrhea.
Riboflavin	Generally compatible with breast-feeding.
Rifampin	Generally compatible with breast-feeding.
Saccharin	Generally compatible with breast-feeding.
Secobarbital	Generally compatible with breast-feeding.
Senna	Generally compatible with breast-feeding.
Sertraline	Effect on nursing infant is unknown but may be of concern. Concentrated in human milk.
Silicone breast implants	The AAP does not classify as contraindicated but more information is needed.
Sotalol	Avoid. Milk levels 3–5 times maternal serum levels. Could cause bradycardia and hypotension.

Drug or Substance	Compatibility With Breast-Feeding, Effect on Lactation, and Adverse Effects on Infant
Sucralfate	Generally compatible with breast-feeding.
Sulfamethoxazole, sulfisoxazole	Avoid in ill, stressed, or preterm infants and with hyperbilirubinemia or G6PD deficiency.
Sumatriptan	Generally compatible with breast-feeding.
Technetium 99m	Contraindicated. Radioactivity present in breast milk for 15 h to 3 days.
Terbutaline	Generally compatible with breast-feeding. Monitor for agitation and spitting up. Use inhaled form to decrease maternal absorption if available.
Tetracyclines	Generally compatible with breast-feeding. Monitor for diarrhea.
Theophylline	Generally compatible with breast-feeding. Monitor for irritability.
Thiamine	Generally compatible with breast-feeding.
Ticarcillin	Generally compatible with breast-feeding. Monitor for diarrhea.
Timolol	Generally compatible with breast-feeding. Monitor for hypotension and bradycardia.
Tobramycin	Generally compatible with breast-feeding. Poor oral absorption. Monitor for diarrhea.
Tolbutamide	Generally compatible with breast-feeding. Monitor for jaundice.
Trazodone	Avoid. Excreted in milk. Effects unknown but may be of concern.
Trimethoprim	Generally compatible with breast-feeding.
Valproic acid	Generally compatible with breast-feeding per AAP but carries risk of fatal hepatotoxicity.
Vegetarian diet	Generally compatible with breast-feeding. Monitor for vitamin B_{12} deficiency (failure to thrive, psychomotor retardation, and megaloblastic anemia).
Vitamin B_{12}	Generally compatible with breast-feeding.
Vitamin D	Generally compatible with breast-feeding. Monitor for increased calcium levels.
Vitamin K	Generally compatible with breast-feeding. Breast-fed infants should receive prophylactic vitamin K at birth because content in breast milk is low and hemorrhagic disease may occur.
Warfarin	Generally compatible with breast-feeding.

REFERENCES

American Academy of Pediatrics: The transfer of drugs and other chemicals into human milk. *Pediatrics* 2001;108:776.

Briggs GG et al: *Drugs in Pregnancy and Lactation*, 6th ed. Lippincott Williams & Wilkins, 2002.

Manufacturer's product information for specific medication listed.

82 Effects of Drugs and Substances Taken During Pregnancy

The drugs listed below include a fetal risk category to indicate a systemically absorbed drug's potential for causing birth defects or neonatal disorders. Regardless of the designated risk category or presumed safety, no drug or substance should be used during pregnancy unless it is clearly needed. Please refer to the manufacturer's product literature or references listed at the end of this chapter for further information.

US FOOD AND DRUG ADMINISTRATION (FDA) FETAL RISK CATEGORIES

CATEGORY A

Adequate studies in pregnant women have not demonstrated a risk to the fetus in the first trimester of pregnancy; there is no evidence of risk in the last two trimesters.

CATEGORY B

Animal studies have not demonstrated a risk to the fetus, but there are no adequate studies in pregnant women.
or
Animal studies have shown an adverse effect, but adequate studies in pregnant women have not demonstrated a risk to the fetus during the first trimester of pregnancy and there is no evidence of risk in the last two trimesters.

CATEGORY C

Animal studies have shown an adverse effect on the fetus, but there are no adequate studies in humans. The benefits from the use of the drug in pregnant women may be acceptable despite its potential risks.
or
There are no animal reproduction studies and no adequate studies in humans.

CATEGORY D

There is evidence of human fetal risk, but the potential benefits from the use of the drug in pregnant women may be acceptable despite its potential risks.

CATEGORY X

Studies in animals or humans or adverse reaction reports, or both, have demonstrated fetal abnormalities. The risk of use in pregnant women clearly outweighs any possible benefit.

Drug or Substance	FDA Fetal Risk Category, Adverse Effects, and Clinical Comments
Acebutolol	Category B. May cause bradycardia and hypotension in infant exposed near term. Carefully monitor blood pressure and heart rate.
Acetaminophen	Category B. Safe for short-term use in therapeutic doses. If medication is required to treat fever or pain, use acetaminophen rather than aspirin.
Acetazolamide	Category C. Not associated with major or minor malformations.

Drug or Substance	FDA Fetal Risk Category, Adverse Effects, and Clinical Comments
Acetohexamide	Category D. Pregnant diabetics should be managed with insulin, not oral hypoglycemics. Causes symptomatic hypoglycemia resulting from hyperinsulinemia in newborn. Monitor infant's serum glucose for 5 days after birth.
Acetophenazine	Category C. No reports of fetal risk available.
Acetylcholine	Category C. No reports of fetal risk available. Significant transplacental passage not expected.
Acyclovir	Category C. Report of 2 infants exposed in utero who exhibited no toxicity. Fetal risk minimal, but insufficient data exist to establish safety.
Adenosine	Category C. No adverse effects in fetus and newborn reported. High intravenous doses could potentially produce fetal toxicity.
Albumin	Category C. No known problems associated with use in pregnancy.
Albuterol	Category C. Used to prevent premature labor, as is terbutaline and ritodrine. May cause fetal tachycardia (>160 beats/min) and hypoglycemia in newborn. Decreases incidence of neonatal respiratory distress syndrome.
Alcohol	Category D or X if used excessively. Causes multiple congenital anomalies. Causes fetal alcohol syndrome (prenatal and postnatal growth deficiency, facial dysmorphogenesis, CNS abnormalities, and impairment in mental and motor function), spontaneous abortion, renal anomalies, alcohol withdrawal syndrome, and other abnormalities.
Alfentanil	Category C. No adverse effects reported. Could cause respiratory depression, reversible with naloxone.
Allopurinol	Category C. No adverse reports in humans.
Alprazolam	Category D. Freely crosses placenta. Neonatal withdrawal may occur.
Alteplase (t-PA)	Category C. May be used if mother's condition warrants.
Amantadine	Category C. Teratogenic in animals in high doses. In 1 reported case, exposure in first trimester may have caused a single ventricle with pulmonary atresia.
Ambenonium	Category C. No reports of fetal risk available. Intravenous anticholinesterases could potentially induce premature labor.
Amikacin	Category C. No reports of adverse effects on fetus. Testing for ototoxicity recommended because other aminoglycosides (eg, kanamycin and streptomycin) have been associated with eighth cranial nerve damage.
Amiloride	Category B. Hypospadias reported in 1 infant.
Aminocaproic acid	Category C. No fetal toxicity occurred in 1 patient given aminocaproic acid in second trimester.
Aminoglutethimide	Category D. Possible virilization when given throughout pregnancy.
Aminophylline	Category C. At birth, transient tachycardia, irritability, and vomiting may occur, especially if mother's serum concentrations above therapeutic range. No congenital defects reported.
Aminopterin	Category X. Several reports have described fetal malformations when used unsuccessfully to induce abortion in first trimester.
p-Aminosalicylic acid (PAS)	Category C. In 1 study, congenital defects were found in 5 infants; other studies have reported no fetal risk.
Amiodarone	Category D. Transient bradycardia and IUGR may occur. Also, because this drug contains iodine, there is potential concern regarding fetal thyroid gland. Test thyroid function of newborn. Use with caution, if at all, during pregnancy.
Amitriptyline	Category C. Malformations, neonatal withdrawal, and urinary retention in neonate are potential problems. Most evidence indicates amitriptyline is relatively safe in pregnancy and may be preferred over other antidepressants during gestation.
Ammonium chloride	Category B. Three possible malformations (inguinal hernia if taken during first trimester, cataracts, and benign tumors) reported. Acidoses may occur in mother and fetus when taken near term.
Amobarbital	Category D. Increased incidence of congenital defects reported. May cause withdrawal syndrome.
Amoxapine	Category C. Three major birth defects (type unknown) reported from first-trimester exposure.
Amoxicillin	Category B. No evidence of fetal or neonatal risk.
Amphetamines	Category C. With amphetamine abuse, increased incidence of preterm labor, placental abruption, fetal distress, postpartum hemorrhage, IUGR, feeding difficulty, drowsiness, and lassitude that may last several months.
Amphotericin B	Category B. No adverse effects on fetus reported.
Ampicillin	Category B. Probably not teratogenic.
Amyl nitrite	Category C. Insufficient data to draw conclusions regarding safety during pregnancy.

Drug or Substance	FDA Fetal Risk Category, Adverse Effects, and Clinical Comments
Anileridine	Category B. Potential risk of withdrawal syndrome and respiratory depression from maternal use of this narcotic analgesic.
Antacids	Category C. No teratogenic effects reported. Avoid chronic use of high doses.
Aspartame	Category B. Not a risk to fetus.
Aspirin	Category C. May cause increased risk of hemorrhage, closure of ductus arteriosus, and prolonged labor. First-trimester use does not increase risk of congenital heart defects. Risk is greatest in last 3 months of pregnancy. High doses may cause increased perinatal mortality and IUGR. If medication required to treat fever or pain, use acetaminophen rather than aspirin.
Atenolol	Category D. May cause bradycardia and hypotension in infant exposed near term. Carefully monitor blood pressure and heart rate. May cause IUGR.
Atracurium	Category C. No adverse effects reported.
Atropine	Category C. No association with malformations reported in 1 large survey. In another survey, possible association with limb reduction in 2 infants.
Aurothioglucose	Category C. No reports of fetal risk available; however, experience with use during pregnancy limited.
Azatadine	Category B. Not associated with birth defects.
Azathioprine	Category D. Most investigators have found azathioprine to be relatively safe. In a few cases, however, abnormalities reported, including leukopenia and thrombocytopenia, immunosuppression, transient chromosomal aberrations, and congenital defects. Interferes with effectiveness of intrauterine contraceptive device.
Azithromycin	Category B. Macrolide antibiotics are not considered major human teratogens. More study needed.
Aztreonam	Category B. No reports of adverse effects located.
Bacampicillin	Category B. No reports of fetal risk available.
Bacitracin	Category C. Not associated with birth defects.
Baclofen	Category C. No reports of adverse effects located. Limited data.
BCG (bacille Calmette-Guérin) vaccine	Category C. Animal studies not done. If possible, avoid use in pregnancy. Live, attenuated vaccine.
Belladonna	Category C. Associated with fetal malformations of varying severity in general and with minor malformations when used in first trimester.
Benazepril	Category D (Category C in first trimester). Discontinue as soon as pregnancy detected. ACE inhibitors have caused fetal death and malformations.
Benzocaine	Category C. No adverse effects reported.
Benzoyl peroxide	Category C. No adverse effects reported.
Benzthiazide	Category D. Thiazide-related diuretics may cause increased risk of congenital defects if taken during first trimester. May also cause hypoglycemia, thrombocytopenia, hyponatremia, hypokalemia, and death. May inhibit labor. Use during pregnancy only if required for patients with heart disease. Carefully monitor infant's electrolytes, platelet count, and serum glucose after birth.
Benztropine	Category C. May cause decreased intestinal motility in infant.
Beta-carotene	Category C. No reports of fetal risk available.
Betamethasone	Category C. Stimulates fetal lung maturation, thus reducing incidence and severity of respiratory distress syndrome. No reports of congenital defects associated with human use of corticosteroids in pregnancy.
Bethanechol	Category C. No reports of fetal risk available, but data limited.
Biperiden	Category C. No reports of fetal risk available.
Bisacodyl	Category C. Bulk-forming (methylcellulose) or surfactant (docusate) laxatives preferred for use in pregnancy over this stimulant laxative.
Bismuth subsalicylate (Pepto-Bismol)	Category C. Contains salicylates. See Aspirin.
Bleomycin	Category D. If possible, avoid during pregnancy. Two normal infants born to mothers receiving bleomycin and other antineoplastic agents in second and third trimesters.
Bretylium	Category C. No reports of fetal risk available; however, may cause maternal hypotension, with potential risk to fetus from reduced uterine blood flow and hypoxia.
Bromides	Category D. Possible association with polydactyly, GI malformations, clubfoot, and congenital dislocation of hip. May cause neonatal bromism (poor sucking, diminished Moro's reflex, and hypotonia). Monitor serum bromide concentrations in newborn.
Bromocriptine	Category C. Does not pose significant risk to fetus.

Drug or Substance	FDA Fetal Risk Category, Adverse Effects, and Clinical Comments
Brompheniramine	Category C. Increased risk of fetal malformations if taken during first trimester. Increased risk of retrolental fibroplasia in premature infant exposed to antihistamines during last 2 weeks in utero.
Buclizine	Category C. Possible increased risk of fetal malformations. Increased risk of retrolental fibroplasia in premature infant exposed to antihistamines during last 2 weeks in utero.
Budesonide	Category C. Not a major teratogenic risk.
Busulfan	Category D. Use during pregnancy associated with fetal malformations and low birth weight.
Butalbital	Category C. No association with fetal malformations reported. However, withdrawal syndrome may occur; observe infant for 48 h after birth.
Butorphanol	Category B. No association with fetal malformations reported; however, respiratory depression and withdrawal syndrome may occur.
Caffeine	Category B. Moderate consumption of caffeine probably does not pose risk to fetus; even so, prudent to avoid or limit consumption. Consumption of 6–8 cups of coffee/day may be associated with decreased fertility, spontaneous abortion, and low birth weight.
Calcifediol	Category A for RDA amounts; category D for therapeutic and higher doses. Vitamin D analog. High doses of vitamin D teratogenic in animals but not in humans. Because vitamin D raises calcium levels, it may be associated with supravalvular aortic stenosis syndrome, which is often associated with hypercalcemia of infancy.
Calcitonin	Category B. No reports of fetal risk available.
Calcitriol	Category C; category D for doses higher than RDA. High doses of vitamin D teratogenic in animals but not in humans. Because vitamin D raises calcium levels, may be associated with supravalvular aortic stenosis syndrome, which is often associated with hypercalcemia of infancy.
Camphor	Category C. No reports of fetal risk with topical application available. May cause fetal death and respiratory failure with maternal ingestion.
Captopril	Category D; category C in first trimester. Discontinue as soon as pregnancy detected. ACE inhibitors have caused malformations and fetal death.
Carbachol	Category C. No reports of fetal risk available.
Carbamazepine	Category D. May cause craniofacial defects, fingernail hypoplasia, and developmental delay (similar to fetal hydantoin syndrome). May cause spina bifida.
Carbarsone	Category D. Contains arsenic, which has been associated with CNS lesions. If possible, avoid during pregnancy.
Carbenicillin	Category B. Has been used in a large number of pregnancies; no malformations associated with use.
Carbimazole	Category D. May cause aplasia cutis (scalp defects). For treatment of hyperthyroidism during pregnancy, use propylthiouracil rather than carbimazole or methimazole.
Carbinoxamine	Category C. No reports of fetal risk available, but data limited.
Carphenazine	Category C. No reports of fetal risk available, but data limited.
Casanthranol	Category C. No reports of fetal anomalies reported in 109 infants exposed to this drug during pregnancy.
Cascara sagrada	Category C. Higher than expected risk for benign tumors in 1 study, but confirmation needed.
Castor oil	Category C. May cause premature labor.
Cefaclor	Category B. Increased risk of congenital defects, but other factors may be involved.
Cefadroxil	Category B. No association with congenital defects.
Cefamandole	Category B. Data limited, but no abnormalities noted in 1 infant exposed in first trimester.
Cefazolin	Category B. No reports of fetal risk available.
Cefonicid	Category B. No reports of fetal risk available.
Cefoperazone	Category B. No adverse newborn effects noted.
Ceforanide	Category B. No reports of fetal risk available.
Cefotaxime	Category B. No reports of fetal risk available.
Cefotetan	Category B. Not teratogenic or fetotoxic in animals. Cephalosporins are usually considered safe during pregnancy.
Cefoxitin	Category B. No adverse newborn effects noted when administered to mother at term.

Drug or Substance	FDA Fetal Risk Category, Adverse Effects, and Clinical Comments
Ceftazidime	Category B. Not teratogenic in animals. No data on human pregnancy outcome available.
Ceftizoxime	Category B. No adverse newborn effects noted when administered to mother at term.
Ceftriaxone	Category B. No adverse newborn effects noted when administered to mother at term.
Cefuroxime	Category B. No adverse newborn effects noted.
Cephalexin	Category B. Increased risk of congenital defects, but other factors may be involved.
Cephalothin	Category B. No adverse newborn effects noted.
Cephapirin	Category B. No data available.
Cephradine	Category B. Increased risk of congenital defects, but other factors may be involved.
Chloral hydrate	Category C. No adverse effects reported.
Chlorambucil	Category D. Reports of unilateral agenesis of kidney and ureter and cardiovascular anomalies. May cause low birth weight.
Chloramphenicol	Category C. No congenital defects reported. Avoid at term because of risk for gray syndrome (cardiovascular collapse).
Chlordiazepoxide	Category D. Some studies found increased risk of fetal malformations; however, others have not confirmed this. When given at term, neonatal depression with hypotonia persisting for up to 1 week reported. Neonatal withdrawal syndrome may occur.
Chlorhexidine	Category B. No reports of adverse effects in the newborn have been reported.
Chloroquine	Category C. Generally considered safe, but there may be a small increased risk of birth defects.
Chlorothiazide	Category D. Thiazide-related diuretics may cause increased risk of congenital defects if taken during first trimester. May also cause hypoglycemia, thrombocytopenia, hyponatremia, hypokalemia, and death. May inhibit labor. Use in pregnancy only if required for patients with heart disease. Monitor infant's electrolytes, platelet count, and serum glucose carefully after birth.
Chlorpheniramine	Category B. Possible association with fetal malformations reported, but statistical significance unknown. Increased risk of retrolental fibroplasia in premature infant exposed to antihistamines during last 2 weeks in utero.
Chlorpromazine	Category C. Probably safe and effective for treatment of vomiting and nausea of pregnancy when used occasionally at low doses. Avoid administration at term because it may cause hypotension. May cause extrapyramidal syndrome (tremors and increased muscle tone) in infant when administered near term.
Chlorpropamide	Category C. Pregnant diabetics should be managed with insulin, not oral hypoglycemics. Causes symptomatic hypoglycemia as a result of hyperinsulinemia in newborn. Monitor infant's serum glucose for 5 days after birth.
Chlortetracycline	Category D. Tetracyclines should be avoided during pregnancy because they may cause adverse effects, including yellow staining of teeth, inhibition of bone growth, maternal liver toxicity, and congenital defects.
Chlorthalidone	Category D. Thiazide-related diuretics may cause increased risk of congenital defects if taken during first trimester. May also cause hypoglycemia, thrombocytopenia, hyponatremia, hypokalemia, and death. May inhibit labor. Use in pregnancy only if required for patients with heart disease. Carefully monitor infant's electrolytes, platelet count, and serum glucose after birth.
Cholecalciferol	Category A for RDA amounts; category D for higher doses. Vitamin D analog. High doses of vitamin D teratogenic in animals but not in humans. Because vitamin D raises calcium level, it may be associated with supravalvular aortic stenosis syndrome, which is often associated with hypercalcemia of infancy.
Cholera vaccine	Category C. Inactivated bacterial vaccine. Indications for vaccine not altered by pregnancy, but should be given only in unusual outbreak situations.
Cholestyramine	Category B. Not systemically absorbed but may bind fat-soluble vitamins in GI tract and cause vitamin deficiency in fetus, although this effect not reported.
Ciclopirox	Category B. No adverse effects reported.
Cimetidine	Category B. One report of transient liver impairment in newborn not confirmed by other investigators. Has antiandrogenic effects; feminization observed in some animals and in nonpregnant humans. More data needed.
Ciprofloxacin	Category C. No congenital defects reported. Use a safer alternative in pregnancy because of arthropathy in immature animals.

Drug or Substance	FDA Fetal Risk Category, Adverse Effects, and Clinical Comments
Cisapride	Category C. Does not appear to be a major human teratogen.
Cisplatin	Category D. Data limited. A few case reports document normal infants after use of cisplatin during pregnancy.
Citrate and citric acid (Shohl solution, Bicitra, Polycitra)	Category C. Avoid sodium citrate in toxemic patients (contains 1 mEq/mL sodium).
Clemastine	Category B. Possible association with limb reduction defects, but other factors may have been involved. Increased risk of retrolental fibroplasia in premature infant exposed to antihistamines during last 2 weeks in utero.
Clindamycin	Category B. No adverse effects reported.
Clofazimine	Category C. May cause temporary skin pigmentation.
Clofibrate	Category C. No adverse effects reported; however, data limited. Avoid administration near term, especially in preterm infant, because of limited capacity for glucuronidation of this compound.
Clomiphene	Category X. May cause neural tube defects and other fetal malformations. Start each new course after pregnancy excluded.
Clomipramine	Category D. Infant lethargy, hypotonia, cyanosis, jitteriness, irregular respirations, respiratory acidosis, hypothermia, seizures, and withdrawal may occur.
Clonazepam	Category C. May cause apnea.
Clonidine	Category C. Data limited; however, no adverse effects reported.
Clorazepate	Category D. Multiple anomalies with first-trimester exposure in one case. Congenital malformations associated with in utero exposure to other benzodiazepines.
Clotrimazole	Category B. No adverse effects reported.
Cloxacillin	Category B. No adverse effects reported.
Coal tar	Category C. No adverse effects reported.
Cocaine	Category C; category X for nonmedicinal use. May cause withdrawal syndrome, multisystem abnormalities as a result of vasoconstrictive properties of the drug, including urogenital anomalies, prematurity, spontaneous abortions, fetal growth retardation, neurobehavioral deficits, electroencephalogram abnormalities, cerebral infarctions, cardiorespiratory pattern abnormalities, and abruptio placentae.
Codeine	Category C. May cause malformations, respiratory depression, and withdrawal syndrome.
Colchicine	Category D. Use by father before conception possibly associated with atypical Down syndrome. No malformations reported from maternal consumption. Teratogenicity occurs in animals. Use with caution. Limited data.
Colestipol	Category B. Not systemically absorbed but may bind fat-soluble vitamins in GI tract and cause vitamin deficiency in fetus, although this effect not reported.
Colistimethate	Category C. No adverse effects reported.
Contraceptives, oral	Category X. May affect development of sexual organs and may cause hyperbilirubinemia in newborn.
Corticotropin	Category C. No adverse effects reported.
Cortisone	Category C (D if used in first trimester). No association with congenital malformations found in 1 large study; however, other studies reported abnormalities, including cataracts, cyclopia, intraventricular septal defect, gastroschisis, and other abnormalities.
Coumadin	See warfarin.
Cromolyn	Category B. Generally considered safe for use in pregnancy.
Crotamiton	Category C. No adverse effects reported. One of the preferred drugs for treatment of scabies in pregnant women.
Cyclacillin	Category B. Has been used in a large number of pregnancies and has not been associated with malformations.
Cyclamate	Category C. No adverse effects reported.
Cyclizine	Category B. Teratogenic in animals but not in humans. Increased risk of retrolental fibroplasia in premature infant exposed to antihistamines during last 2 weeks in utero.
Cyclophosphamide	Category D. May cause fetal malformations from first-trimester exposure, possible pancytopenia, and low birth weight. Use by father before conception may cause malformations in infant.
Cycloserine	Category C. No adverse fetal effects reported. Use with caution. Limited data.
Cyclosporine	Category C. Not a human teratogen, based on limited data.

Drug or Substance	FDA Fetal Risk Category, Adverse Effects, and Clinical Comments
Cyproheptadine	Category B. No adverse effects reported.
Cytarabine	Category D. May cause chromosomal abnormalities and congenital anomalies with maternal or paternal use before conception and low birth weight; however, normal infants have been delivered.
Dacarbazine	Category C. No data available.
Dactinomycin	Category C. Stillbirth and low birth weight may occur; however, normal infants have been delivered.
Dalteparin	Category B. Probably no more fetal or newborn risk than from standard, unfractionated heparin.
Danazol	Category X. May cause virilization with ambiguous genitalia of female infants.
Danthron	Category C. One study reported higher than expected risk of benign tumors, but confirmation needed.
Dantrolene	Category C. No fetal or newborn adverse effects reported when used in a limited number of patients shortly before delivery.
Dapsone	Category C. Does not present a major risk to fetus or newborn.
Daunorubicin	Category D. Successful pregnancies with normal infants reported; however, abnormalities such as low birth weight, anemia, hypoglycemia, intrauterine death, and myocardial necrosis may occur. Paternal use may result in congenital defects in infant.
Deferoxamine	Category C. No abnormalities reported. May cause low iron levels in infant, requiring iron supplementation.
Demeclocycline	Category D. Tetracyclines should be avoided during pregnancy because they may cause adverse effects, including yellow staining of teeth, inhibition of bone growth, maternal liver toxicity, and congenital defects.
Desipramine	Category C. Withdrawal syndrome reported.
Desmopressin	Category B. No adverse effects reported.
Dexamethasone	Category C (D if used in first trimester). No known congenital defects reported. Given in premature labor to stimulate fetal lung maturation.
Dextroamphetamine	Category C. May cause congenital defects such as cardiac abnormalities, biliary atresia, and eye defects; may cause withdrawal syndrome.
Dextromethorphan	Category C. Not a major teratogen.
Diatrizoate	Category D. Monitor thyroid function because this drug may suppress fetal thyroid gland when administered by intra-amniotic injection.
Diazepam	Category D. May cause hypotonia, lethargy, sucking difficulties, and withdrawal syndrome. May also cause craniofacial abnormalities, sullen and expressionless face, low Apgar scores, apneic spells, delayed motor development, and hypotonia.
Diazoxide	Category C. May cause transient fetal bradycardia and hyperglycemia.
Diclofenac	Category B (D if used in third trimester). May close ductus arteriosus in utero, cause PPHN, inhibition of labor, and spontaneous abortion.
Dicloxacillin	Category B. No adverse effects reported.
Dicumarol	Category D. Coumadin (warfarin) derivative. Significant risk of congenital defects. May cause fetal warfarin syndrome (hypoplastic, flattened nasal bridge; stippled epiphyses; and possibly other features, such as low birth weight, eye defects, developmental retardation, congenital heart disease, and death). May also cause hemorrhage. If anticoagulation required during pregnancy, heparin given at lowest effective dose is probably safer choice.
Didanosine	Category B. CDC recommends that antiretrovirals be continued during pregnancy with the possible exception of the first trimester).
Dienestrol	Category X. Contraindicated during pregnancy. May lead to high estrogen concentrations in blood, leading to fetal malformations.
Diethylstilbestrol	Category X. May result in complications of reproductive system, including carcinoma of cervix and vagina. Hirsutism and irregular menses may result, but this is *controversial*. Genitourinary abnormalities, including neoplasms, may also occur in male offspring.
Digitalis, digoxin, and digitoxin	Category C. No congenital defects reported. Neonatal death has resulted from maternal overdose of digitoxin.
Dihydrotachysterol	Category A for RDA amounts; category D for therapeutic and higher doses. Vitamin D analog. High doses of vitamin D teratogenic in animals but not in humans. Because vitamin D raises calcium levels, it may be associated with supravalvular aortic stenosis syndrome, which is often associated with hypercalcemia of infancy.

Drug or Substance	FDA Fetal Risk Category, Adverse Effects, and Clinical Comments
Diltiazem	Category C. Compared with controls, no increase in the risk of major congenital malformations was found in 78 women exposed to calcium channel blockers in the first trimester.
Dimenhydrinate	Category B. Has not been associated with major or minor fetal malformations. May have oxytocic effect. Increased risk of retrolental fibroplasia in premature infant exposed to antihistamines during last 2 weeks in utero.
Diphenhydramine	Category B. May cause cleft palate, withdrawal. Probably safe for use in pregnancy. Increased risk of retrolental fibroplasia in premature infant exposed to antihistamines during last 2 weeks in utero. Diphonhydramine taken concurrently with temazepam has resulted in stillbirth; avoid this combination.
Diphenoxylate (combined with atropine, Lomotil)	Category C. No abnormalities reported.
Diphtheria and tetanus toxoids	Category C. No data available on safety of diphtheria toxoid; therefore, manufacturer does not recommend use of combination product in pregnancy.
Dipyridamole	Category C. No abnormalities reported.
Disopyramide	Category C. No abnormalities reported.
Disulfiram	Category C. Not a major teratogen. Of course, alcohol should not be consumed while on this drug.
Dobutamine	Category B. No adverse effects reported, but data limited.
Docusate	Category C. No fetal malformations reported. Possible hypomagnesemia with use throughout pregnancy.
Dopamine	Category C. No adverse effects reported.
Doxepin	Category C. Possible decrease in GI motility if given at term.
Doxorubicin	Category D. Normal pregnancies have occurred in mothers treated with this drug; however, fetal malformations have also been reported.
Doxycycline	Category D. Tetracyclines should be avoided during pregnancy because they may cause adverse effects, including yellow staining of teeth, inhibition of bone growth, maternal liver toxicity, and congenital defects.
Doxylamine	Category B. Probably not associated with malformations.
Droperidol	Category C. No adverse effects reported.
Echinacea	Category C. Safety in pregnancy needs to be established.
Echothiophate	Category C. No information available, but transplacental passage not likely because of chemical structure.
Edrophonium	Category C. No adverse effects reported. May cause premature labor.
Enalapril	Category D (category C in first trimester). Discontinue as soon as pregnancy detected. ACE inhibitors have caused malformations and fetal death.
Encainide	Category B. Not teratogenic, but experience limited.
Enoxaparin	Category B. Because of relatively high molecular weight, not expected to cross placenta to fetus.
Ephedrine	Category C. Minor fetal malformations may be associated with use during first trimester. May cause fetal tachycardia.
Epinephrine	Category C. May cause fetal malformations with first-trimester use and inguinal hernia with use any time during pregnancy. May cause decreased uterine blood flow.
Epoetin alfa	Category C. No major risk to fetus, but experience limited.
Epoprostenol	Category B. Not teratogenic in animals, but human data are limited. Transplacental passage of this drug is unlikely. Benefits of this drug in treating maternal pulmonary hypertension appear to outweigh potential risks to fetus.
Ergocalciferol	Category A for RDA amounts; category D for therapeutic and higher doses. Vitamin D analog. High doses of vitamin D teratogenic in animals but not in humans. Because vitamin D raises calcium levels, it may be associated with supravalvular aortic stenosis syndrome, which is often associated with hypercalcemia of infancy.
Ergotamine derivatives	Category X. May cause intrauterine fetal death from drug-induced increase in uterine motility and placental vasoconstriction. The combination of ergotamine, caffeine, and propranolol potentiates vasoconstriction.
Erythromycin	Category B. No abnormalities reported.
Esmolol	Category C. May decrease uterine blood flow, resulting in fetal hypoxia. Bradycardia, hypoglycemia, poor feeding, and hypotonia may occur.
Estradiol	Category X. Estrogenic hormones contraindicated during pregnancy. In utero exposure may cause developmental changes in psychosexual performance of boys, less heterosexual experience, and fewer masculine interests.

Drug or Substance	FDA Fetal Risk Category, Adverse Effects, and Clinical Comments
Estrogens (conjugated)	Category X. Estrogenic hormones contraindicated during pregnancy. May cause fetal malformations.
Ethacrynic acid	Category D. May decrease placental perfusion and may cause ototoxicity. Not recommended for use in pregnancy.
Ethambutol	Category B. No abnormalities reported.
Ethinylestradiol	Category X. Estrogenic hormones contraindicated during pregnancy. In utero exposure may cause developmental changes in psychosexual performance of boys, less heterosexual experience, and fewer masculine interests.
Ethiodized oil	Category D. May cause neonatal hypothyroidism.
Ethionamide	Category C. May cause Down syndrome (2 cases). Some reports documented no association with birth defects.
Ethisterone	Category D. Possible association with congenital anomalies.
Ethosuximide	Category C. May cause congenital anomalies and spontaneous hemorrhage in neonate.
Ethynodiol	Category D. May cause modified development of sexual organs and hyperbilirubinemia of the newborn.
Famotidine	Category B. No adverse effects reported, but data limited.
Felodipine	Category C. Compared with controls, no increase in the risk of major congenital malformations was found in 78 women exposed to calcium channel blockers in the first trimester.
Fenoprofen	Category B; category D if used near term. No congenital malformations reported. May cause constriction of ductus arteriosus in utero, PPHN, and inhibition of labor.
Fenoterol	Category B. No malformations reported. Inhibits uterine activity at term.
Fentanyl	Category C; category D with prolonged high doses. No malformations reported. May cause respiratory depression and withdrawal syndrome.
Ferrous sulfate	Category B. No adverse effects reported.
Flecainide	Category C. No congenital defects reported. May cause hyperbilirubinemia. Several publications report successful use of flecainide for treatment of fetal tachycardia.
Fluconazole	Category C. Continuous first trimester doses of 400 mg/day or more may be teratogenic.
Flucytosine	Category C. No defects reported, although its metabolite (fluorouracil) may produce fetal malformations.
Fludrocortisone (Florinef)	Category C. Observe infant for signs of adrenocortical insufficiency, and treat if required.
Fluoride	Category C. Crosses placenta. No information available on fetal effects.
Fluorouracil	Category D. May cause fetal malformations (first-trimester use), cyanosis and jerking extremities (third-trimester use), and low birth weight (used any time during pregnancy).
Fluoxetine	Category C. Not associated with increased risk of major congenital defects. More studies are needed of the potential effects on the developing CNS to exclude the possibility of permanent changes. Weigh maternal benefits against fetal risks before use.
Fluphenazine	Category C. Extrapyramidal effects; possible congenital malformations in 1 infant.
Flurazepam	Category X. Active metabolite crosses placenta. Drowsiness if given preceding delivery. No congenital anomalies reported; however, other agents in this class may cause fetal abnormalities.
Folic acid	Category A. Folate deficiency may result in congenital anomalies.
Foscarnet	Category C. Observe for fetal renal toxicity by monitoring amniotic fluid volume.
Fosinopril	Category D. Discontinue as soon as pregnancy detected. ACE inhibitors have caused malformations and fetal death.
Furazolidone	Category C. No congenital defects reported. Could cause hemolytic anemia in G6PD-deficient infant if given at term.
Furosemide	Category C. No congenital defects reported. Generally not indicated in pregnancy except in patients with cardiovascular disorders.
Gabapentin	Category C. Limited data. No pattern of malformations reported.
Ganciclovir	Category C. Toxic effects in animals. Potential for fetal toxicity. Reserve use for life-threatening disease or in immunocompromised patients with major CMV infections such as retinitis.
Gentamicin	Category C. No congenital defects reported. Potentiation of magnesium sulfate-induced neuromuscular weakness. Monitor infant for ototoxicity because this has occurred with other aminoglycosides (eg, kanamycin and streptomycin).
Ginkgo biloba	Category C. Controversial. Limited data. Avoid.

Drug or Substance	FDA Fetal Risk Category, Adverse Effects, and Clinical Comments
Glyburide, glipizide	Category C. May cause neonatal hypoglycemia. Insulin is drug of choice for treating diabetes during pregnancy.
Glycopyrrolate	Category B. Minor fetal malformations may occur but are unlikely.
Gold sodium thiomalate	Category C. Probably no risk to fetus, but experience limited.
Griseofulvin	Category C. Teratogenic in animals, but no data available for humans.
Guaifenesin	Category C. May cause inguinal hernias with first-trimester use.
Haloperidol	Category C. Limb reductions in 2 reports, but other studies have not confirmed this.
Heparin	Category C. No reports of congenital defects reported. Heparin preferred over oral anticoagulants during pregnancy.
Hepatitis B immune globulin (HBIG)	Category B. No adverse effects reported.
Hepatitis B vaccine	Category C. No adverse effects reported.
Heroin	Category B; category D with prolonged high-dose use. May cause congenital malformations, jaundice, RDS, low Apgar scores, withdrawal, low birth weight, and increased perinatal mortality.
Hexachlorophene	Category C. Increased risk of anomalies with excessive first-trimester use.
Hexamethonium	Category C. No congenital abnormalities reported.
Homatropine	Category C. Possible association with minor malformations.
Hyaluronidase	Category C. No adverse effects reported.
Hydralazine	Category C. No congenital abnormalities reported.
Hydrochlorothiazide	Category D. See Chlorothiazide.
Hydrocodone	Category B; category D with prolonged high-dose use. No malformations reported; however, respiratory depression or withdrawal syndrome may occur.
Hydromorphone	Category B; category D with prolonged high-dose use. No malformations reported; however, respiratory depression or withdrawal syndrome may occur.
Hydroxychloroquine	Category C. Probably not a significant risk to fetus, especially at lower doses. CDC states that it may be used for malaria prophylaxis because not shown to be harmful at prophylactic doses (400 mg/week).
Hydroxyprogesterone	Category D. May cause ambiguous genitalia. In males, may cause less heterosexual experience and fewer masculine interests.
Hydroxyzine	Category C. Possible relation between fetal malformations and use during first trimester, but statistical significance not known.
Ibuprofen	Category B; category D in third trimester. No congenital anomalies reported. May cause closing of ductus arteriosus in utero, PPHN, and inhibition of labor.
Idoxuridine	Category C. No data available on use in human pregnancy.
Imipramine	Category D. May cause fetal malformations, withdrawal syndrome, and urine retention.
Immune globulin, intravenous	Category C. No adverse effects reported.
Indomethacin	Category B; category D if taken after 34 weeks' gestation or if used for longer than 48 h. May cause delayed labor, premature closure of ductus arteriosus, PPHN, renal failure, intestinal perforation, and death.
Insulin	Category B. Insulin rather than oral hypoglycemics should be used to control diabetes. Poorly controlled diabetes associated with increased risk of congenital defects.
Interferon alfa	Category C. Not a significant risk. Limited data. Because of the antiproliferative activity of these agents, use cautiously during gestation.
Intravenous fat emulsion	Category C. One case of placental fat deposits and fetal demise after 8 weeks of IV parenteral nutrition and lipid emulsion for hyperemesis gravidarum.
Iodine	Category D. Topical use may result in significant absorption of iodine, resulting in transient hypothyroidism in newborn. (See also Potassium iodide and Povidone iodine.)
Iron (ferrous sulfate)	Category B. No adverse effects reported.
Isocarboxazid	Category C. Increased risk of fetal malformations.
Isoetharine	Category C. Use in first trimester associated with possible increased risk of minor fetal malformations.
Isoniazid (INH)	Category C. Increased risk of fetal malformations found in 1 study but not confirmed by other studies. Use of INH for TB occurring during pregnancy is recommended because untreated TB represents far greater hazard to mother and fetus than does INH.
Isoproterenol	Category C. Use of sympathomimetics in first trimester associated with possible increased risk of minor fetal malformations. Inhibits contractions of pregnant uterus.

Drug or Substance	FDA Fetal Risk Category, Adverse Effects, and Clinical Comments
Isosorbide dinitrate	Category C. No data available.
Isotretinoin (Accutane, retinoic acid)	Category X. With first-trimester use, causes severe birth defects, including external ear, CNS, craniofacial, cardiac, and thymic anomalies. Prevent pregnancy during use. Use effective contraception 1 month before use, during therapy, and for 1 month after discontinuation.
Isoxsuprine	Category C. No congenital defects reported; however, fetal tachycardia and neonatal ileus may occur, and infants with cord levels exceeding 10 ng/mL may have RDS, hypotension, hypocalcemia, and death.
Itraconazole	Category C. Risk to fetus is probably low. However, avoid during first trimester if possible because fluconazole, a related antifungal, causes possible dose-related major malformations.
Kanamycin	Category D. May cause eighth cranial nerve damage.
Ketoconazole	Category C. No major birth defects reported.
Labetalol	Category C. May cause hypotension and bradycardia. Monitor infant for 48 h after birth.
Lactulose	Category B. No information available.
Laetrile	Category C. Theoretic risk of cyanide poisoning.
Lamotrigine	Category C. Probably not a major risk for congenital malformations or fetal loss in first trimester.
Levallorphan	Category D. May cause neonatal respiratory depression.
Levarterenol	Category D. No fetal malformations reported, but may cause reduction of uterine blood flow.
Levofloxacin	Category C. Avoid in pregnancy because of arthropathy in immature animals. Use safer alternative.
Levorphanol	Category B with therapeutic doses; category D if used at high doses for prolonged periods. May cause respiratory depression and withdrawal syndrome.
Levothyroxine	Category A. First-trimester use possibly associated with cardiovascular anomalies, Down syndrome, and polydactyly, but confirmation needed.
Lidocaine	Category B. No association with malformations found.
Lindane (Kwell)	Category B. May cause neurotoxicity and aplastic anemia. Use pyrethrins with piperonyl butoxide rather than lindane to treat lice during pregnancy.
Liothyronine	Category A. No adverse effects reported.
Liotrix	Category A. First-trimester use possibly associated with cardiovascular anomalies, Down syndrome, and polydactyly, but confirmation needed.
Lisinopril	Category D. Discontinue as soon as pregnancy detected. ACE inhibitors have caused malformations and fetal death.
Lithium	Category D. May cause cardiac congenital defects when used in first trimester and toxicity in newborn (cyanosis, hypotonia, bradycardia, nephrogenic diabetes insipidus, and other disorders) when used near term. Reduce risk by using lowest dose possible, monitoring serum concentrations, and avoiding sodium-restricted diets and sodium-wasting diuretics.
Loperamide	Category B. No adverse effects reported.
Loratadine	Category B. Data too limited to assess safety. Consider chlorpheniramine or tripelennamine instead.
Lorazepam	Category D. May cause neonatal respiratory depression and hypotonia. Other drugs in this class have been suspected of causing malformations.
Losartan	Category C first trimester (category D in second and third trimesters). Drugs that act on the renin-angiotensin system can cause fetal and neonatal morbidity and death when administered in pregnancy. Monitor newborn's BP and renal function closely. Avoid use during pregnancy.
Lovastatin	Category X. May cause malformations. Monitor renal function of newborn. Avoid using in pregnancy.
LSD	Category C. Available data indicate that pure LSD does not cause chromosomal abnormalities, spontaneous abortions, or congenital malformations.
Lynestrenol	Category D. Use of progestogens not recommended during pregnancy.
Lypressin	Category C. No adverse effects reported.
Magnesium salts	Category B. May cause neonatal respiratory depression and muscle weakness if used just before delivery and congenital rickets with prolonged infusion. Possible respiratory arrest when gentamicin given to newborns with high magnesium levels. Inhibits indomethacin effect for ductal closure.
Mannitol	Category C. No adverse effects reported.

Drug or Substance	FDA Fetal Risk Category, Adverse Effects, and Clinical Comments
Maprotiline	Category B. May cause oral cleft, but other factors may be involved. Very limited data.
Marijuana	Category C. May cause impaired fetal growth and acute nonlymphoblastic leukemia. Conflicting reports on safety.
Measles vaccine	Category C. Not for use during pregnancy because of risk of fetal malformations and abortion from this live virus vaccine.
Mechlorethamine	Category D. Possible fetal malformations with first-trimester use and low birth weight with use any time during pregnancy.
Meclizine	Category D. Possible fetal malformations reported; however, 3 studies involving large numbers of patients concluded that meclizine is not a human teratogen. Increased risk of retrolental fibroplasia in premature infant exposed to antihistamines during last 2 weeks of pregnancy.
Meclofenamate	Category D; category D if taken in third trimester near delivery. May cause delayed labor, premature closure of ductus arteriosus, and PPHN.
Medroxyprogesterone	Category X. Not recommended for use in pregnancy because of risk of fetal malformations associated with use of female sex hormones.
Melphalan	Category D. May cause low birth weight. Structurally similar to other alkylating agents that have produced defects.
Meperidine	Category B; category D with prolonged use of high doses. May cause respiratory depression and withdrawal syndrome. First-trimester use possibly associated with inguinal hernia, but confirmation needed.
Mephentermine	Category C. No adverse effects reported.
Mephenytoin	Category C. No adverse effects reported.
Mephobarbital	Category D. May cause withdrawal and hemorrhagic disease of newborn.
Mepindolol	Category C. May cause bradycardia and hypotension in infant exposed near term. Carefully monitor blood pressure and heart rate.
Meprobamate	Category D. May be associated with fetal malformations when used in first trimester. Avoid during pregnancy.
Mercaptopurine	Category D. May cause fetal malformations, pancytopenia, and low birth weight.
Meropenem	Category B. Most likely safe to use in perinatal period, 28 weeks' gestation or later.
Mesalamine	Category B. No teratogenic effects reported. Maternal benefits appear to outweigh potential risks to fetus.
Mesoridazine	Category C. No adverse effects reported.
Mestranol	Category X. May cause fetal malformations. Avoid estrogenic hormones during pregnancy.
Metaproterenol	Category C. Prevents premature labor. May cause fetal tachycardia and neonatal hypoglycemia.
Metaraminol	Category D. May reduce uterine blood flow.
Methadone	Category B; category D with prolonged use of high doses. May cause withdrawal syndrome, low birth weight, and death.
Methamphetamine	Category C. With amphetamine abuse, increased incidence of preterm labor, placental abruption, fetal distress, postpartum hemorrhage, IUGR, feeding difficulty, drowsiness, and lassitude that may last several months.
Methantheline	Category C. Possibly associated with minor fetal malformations.
Methaqualone	Category D. Not recommended during pregnancy.
Methenamine	Category C. Associated with fetal malformations, but confirmation needed.
Methicillin	Category B. No adverse effects reported.
Methimazole	Category D. May cause aplasia cutis (scalp defects) and other malformations. Use propylthiouracil rather than carbimazole or methimazole to treat hyperthyroidism during pregnancy.
Methotrexate	Category X. Associated with fetal malformations and low birth weight.
Methoxsalen	Category C. Probably not a significant human teratogen. Long-term effects of in-utero exposure need to be studied.
Methsuximide	Category C. No adverse effects reported.
Methyldopa	Category C. Probably not associated with fetal malformations. Monitor neonate for hypotension for 48 h after delivery.
Methylene blue	Category C; category D if injected intra-amniotically. Possibly associated with fetal malformations, but confirmation needed. May cause hemolytic anemia, hyperbilirubinemia, and methemoglobinemia with intra-amniotic injection of large doses.
Methylergonovine	Category C. Stimulates contractions of uterus. Indicated only for postpartum use and as an alternative to oxytocin for management of the third stage of labor.

Drug or Substance	FDA Fetal Risk Category, Adverse Effects, and Clinical Comments
Methylphenidate	Category C. No adverse effects reported.
Methysergide	Category X. Do not use in pregnancy because of oxytocic properties.
Metoclopramide	Category B. No adverse effects reported, but data limited.
Metolazone	Category D. Thiazide-related diuretics may cause increased risk of congenital defects if taken during first trimester. May also cause hypoglycemia, thrombocytopenia, hyponatremia, hypokalemia, and death and may inhibit labor. Use during pregnancy only if required for patients with heart disease. Carefully monitor infant's electrolytes, platelet count, and serum glucose after birth.
Metoprolol	Category D. Hypotension and bradycardia may occur. Monitor infant for 48 h after birth.
Metrizamide	Category D. Monitor infant's thyroid function at birth. A related drug, diatrizoate, has suppressed fetal thyroid gland when administered by intra-amniotic injection.
Metronidazole	Category B. Possible fetal malformations with first-trimester use. Contraindicated in first trimester in patients with trichomoniasis and bacterial vaginosis. Use in second and third trimesters for these indications is acceptable.
Miconazole	Category C. No adverse effects reported.
Mineral oil	Category C. No adverse effects reported but may inhibit maternal absorption of fat-soluble vitamins (A, D, E, and K).
Minocycline	Category D. Tetracyclines should be avoided during pregnancy because they may cause adverse effects, including yellow staining of teeth, inhibition of bone growth, maternal liver toxicity, and congenital defects.
Minoxidil	Category C. May cause hypertrichosis that gradually disappears over 2–3 months.
Misoprostol	Category X. Contraindicated in pregnancy because of risk of uterine bleeding and contractions, which may result in abortion. May cause malformations.
Mithramycin (Plicamycin)	Category X. May cause fetal harm. Avoid during pregnancy.
Molindone	Category C. No adverse effects reported.
Montelukast	Category B. Not a teratogen in animals, but human data are lacking.
Morphine	Category C; category D with prolonged use of high doses. May cause respiratory depression and withdrawal syndrome. First-trimester use possibly associated with inguinal hernia, but confirmation needed.
Mumps virus vaccine	Category X. Not for use in pregnancy because of risk of malformations. Live, attenuated vaccine.
Nadolol	Category D. May cause bradycardia and hypotension in infants exposed near term. Carefully monitor blood pressure and heart rate.
Nafcillin	Category B. No adverse effects reported.
Nalbuphine	Category B. May cause respiratory depression and withdrawal syndrome.
Nalidixic acid	Category C. No adverse effects reported.
Naloxone	Category B. No adverse effects reported.
Naltrexone	Category C. Embryocidal in rats and rabbits. Human data are lacking. Concern is warranted regarding potential long-term behavioral effects based on results of animal studies.
Naproxen	Category B; category D if given near term. May cause closure of ductus arteriosus, with resulting pulmonary hypertension of newborn. Avoid use near term.
Neomycin	Category C. No fetal malformations reported. May cause ototoxicity, which has been reported with use of other aminoglycosides.
Neostigmine	Category C. No fetal malformations reported.
Niacin/niacinamide	Category A for RDA doses; category C for doses above the RDA and for doses used to treat lipid disorders. No adverse effects reported.
Nicardipine	Category C. No adverse effects in treating hypertension during pregnancy, except a lower birth weight in the nicardipine group in 1 study.
Nicotine	Category X. May cause dose-related low birth weight, decreased placental blood flow, increased risk of stillborn or neonatal death, and SIDS.
Nifedipine	Category C. Experience limited. Severe adverse effects when combined with magnesium sulfate. Causes fetal hypoxemia and acidosis in pregnant rhesus monkeys. Try standard therapy first for severe hypertension.
Nitrofurantoin	Category B. No adverse effects reported. May theoretically cause hemolysis if given near term in patient with G6PD deficiency.
Nitroglycerin	Category C. No adverse effects reported. Data limited, especially with first-trimester use.
Nitroprusside	Category C. May cause fetal bradycardia. Avoid prolonged use.

Drug or Substance	FDA Fetal Risk Category, Adverse Effects, and Clinical Comments
Nonoxynol-9/ octoxynol-9	Category C. Vaginal spermicides do not pose a risk of congenital malformations.
Norethindrone	Category X. May cause masculinization of female infants.
Norethynodrel	Category X. May cause masculinization of female infants.
Norfloxacin	Category C. Not a risk of major malformations. Use caution in pregnancy, especially during first trimester. Best to avoid use in pregnancy and use a safer alternative.
Nortriptyline	Category D. May cause fetal malformations, but confirmation needed. May cause urinary retention in newborn.
Novobiocin	Category C. No adverse effects reported, but may cause hyperbilirubinemia if used near term.
Nystatin	Category C. No adverse effects reported.
Octreotide	Category B. Not a teratogen in animals. Normal outcome in 4 human pregnancies. Does cross the placenta. Data too limited to assess safety.
Oleandomycin	Category C. No adverse effects reported.
Omeprazole	Category C. No adverse effects reported in 20 infants of mothers given omeprazole the night before C-section. Teratogenic risk probably low. Dose-related gastric tumors occurred in rats given omeprazole. Avoid if possible, especially in first trimester.
Ondansetron	Category B. No adverse effects reported.
Oral contraceptives	See Contraceptives, oral.
Oxacillin	Category B. No adverse effects reported.
Oxazepam	Category C. No adverse effects reported.
Oxprenolol	Category D. May cause bradycardia and hypotension in infants exposed near term. Carefully monitor blood pressure and heart rate.
Oxtriphylline	Category C. No adverse effects reported.
Oxycodone	Category B for therapeutic doses; category D for prolonged use of high doses. May cause withdrawal syndrome and respiratory depression. No congenital malformations reported.
Oxymetazoline	Category C. Does not pose risk when administered at recommended frequency to healthy patient. High dose and frequency higher than recommended may cause persistent late fetal heart rate decelerations.
Oxymorphone	Category B for therapeutic doses; category D for prolonged use of high doses. May cause withdrawal syndrome and respiratory depression. No congenital malformations reported.
Oxytetracycline	Category D. Tetracyclines should be avoided during pregnancy because they may cause adverse effects, including yellow staining of teeth, inhibition of bone growth, maternal liver toxicity, and congenital defects.
Pancuronium	Category C. No data on use in early pregnancy. Has been administered to mother at C-section and to fetus during last half of pregnancy without harm to fetus.
Pantothenic acid	Category A for RDA doses; category C for excessive doses. No adverse effects reported.
Paraldehyde	Category C. Easily diffuses across placenta and may cause neonatal respiratory depression when used at term.
Paramethadione	Category D. Increased risk of spontaneous abortion and other abnormalities, including tetralogy of Fallot, mental retardation, and failure to thrive.
Paregoric	Category B for therapeutic doses; category D for prolonged use of high doses. May cause withdrawal syndrome and respiratory depression. No congenital malformations reported.
Parenteral nutrition	See Intravenous fat emulsion.
Paroxetine	Category C. May cause withdrawal. Also, see Fluoxetine.
Penicillamine	Category D. May cause connective tissue abnormalities (cutis laxa).
Penicillin G/ penicillin G benzathine/ penicillin V	Category B. Association with adverse effects very unlikely.
Penicillin G procaine	Category B. Association with congenital malformations unlikely.
Pentamidine	Category C. Aerosolized pentamidine 300 mg/month in 15 women in second and third trimesters had no adverse effects on fetus or newborn.
Pentazocine	Category B for therapeutic doses; category D for prolonged use of high doses. May cause withdrawal syndrome and respiratory depression. No congenital malformations reported.

Drug or Substance	FDA Fetal Risk Category, Adverse Effects, and Clinical Comments
Pentobarbital	Category D. May cause withdrawal syndrome and hemorrhage in newborn.
Pentoxifylline	Category C. Possibly associated with congenital defects, but other factors may be involved.
Permethrin	Category B. No adverse effects reported. Recommended by CDC as one treatment for pubic lice in pregnant women.
Perphenazine	Category C. No adverse effects reported.
Phenacetin	Category B. May cause fetal malformations (musculoskeletal malformations and kidney and adrenal anomalies), but confirmation needed.
Phenazopyridine	Category B. No adverse effects reported.
Phencyclidine (PCP)	Category X. May cause dysmorphic features, nystagmus, hypertonicity, respiratory distress, and withdrawal syndrome.
Phenelzine	Category C. May cause fetal malformations.
Pheniramine	Category C. First-trimester use possibly associated with fetal malformations; confirmation is needed. Increased risk of retrolental fibroplasia in premature infants exposed to antihistamines during last 2 weeks in utero.
Phenobarbital	Category D. May cause withdrawal syndrome, hemorrhagic disease in newborn, major and minor fetal malformations, and neurodevelopmental problems. Use at lowest possible level to control seizures.
Phenylephrine	Category C. Fetal malformations reported, but confirmation needed. May cause constriction of uterine vessels.
Phenylpropanolamine	Category C. May cause constriction of uterine vessels. May also cause malformations, but confirmation needed.
Phenytoin	Category D. May cause fetal hydantoin syndrome (craniofacial [broad nasal bridge, low-set hairline, short neck, and microcephaly]; limbs [hypoplasia of nails and distal phalanges]; impaired growth; and many other abnormalities). May also cause tumors and hemorrhage in newborn at delivery.
Phytonadione	Category C. No adverse effects reported.
Pindolol	Category D. May cause bradycardia and hypotension in infants exposed near term. Carefully monitor blood pressure and heart rate. May cause IUGR.
Piperacillin	Category B. No adverse effects reported.
Piperazine	Category B. Adverse effects unlikely.
Pneumococcal vaccine	Category C. No adverse effects reported; however, use during pregnancy for high-risk patients only.
Poliovirus vaccine	Category C. No adverse effects reported; however, use during pregnancy for patients with high risk of exposure only.
Polymyxin B	Category B. No adverse effects reported.
Potassium chloride/ citrate/acetate/ gluconate	Category A. No adverse effects reported.
Potassium iodide	Category D. May cause hypothyroidism and goiter with prolonged use; however, 10-day preparation for thyroid surgery is safe.
Povidone iodine	Category D. Topical use may result in significant absorption of iodine, resulting in transient hypothyroidism with goiter in newborn.
Pravastatin	Category X. Contraindicated in pregnancy.
Prazosin	Category C. No adverse effects reported.
Prednisone/ prednisolone	Category C (Category D in first trimester). May cause immunosuppression and cataracts; carries small risk of fetal malformations such as orofacial clefts.
Primaquine	Category C. No adverse effects reported. May theoretically cause hemolysis if given near term in patients with G6PD deficiency.
Primidone	Category D. Possible risk of fetal malformations similar to those associated with phenytoin and of tumors and hemorrhage of newborn at birth.
Probenecid	Category C. No adverse effects reported.
Procainamide	Category C. Not associated with congenital anomalies or adverse fetal effects.
Procarbazine	Category D. May cause fetal malformations and low birth weight.
Prochlorperazine	Category C. Fetal malformations reported rarely.
Promazine	Category C. Fetal malformations reported rarely.
Promethazine	Category C. May cause respiratory depression when given at term (*controversial*).
Propantheline	Category C. No adverse effects reported.
Propofol	Category B. When used during C-section, most studies show no difference in Apgar scores of infants exposed to propofol.
Propoxyphene	Category C. May cause fetal malformations and has caused neonatal withdrawal syndrome.

Drug or Substance	FDA Fetal Risk Category, Adverse Effects, and Clinical Comments
Propranolol	Category D. May cause low birth weight, fetal depression at birth, prolonged labor, neonatal hypoglycemia, hypotension, and bradycardia. Carefully monitor blood pressure, respirations, and heart rate for 24–48 h in infants exposed near term.
Propylthiouracil	Category D. Fetal malformations reported, but association with this drug unclear. May cause reversible hypothyroidism and goiter in infant. Drug of choice for treatment of hypothyroidism during pregnancy.
Protamine	Category C. No adverse effects reported.
Pseudoephedrine	Category C. May cause minor fetal malformations with first-trimester use.
Psyllium (Metamucil)	Category D. Psyllium or another bulk-producing laxative is preferred if laxative needed during pregnancy.
Pyrantel pamoate	Category C. No adverse effects reported.
Pyrethrins with piperonyl butoxide	Category C. No adverse effects reported.
Pyridostigmine	Category C. May cause premature labor when given near term.
Pyridoxine	Category A. Probably does not cause fetal malformations.
Pyrilamine	Category C. May cause fetal malformations and benign tumors. Increased risk of retrolental fibroplasia in premature infant exposed to antihistamines during last 2 weeks in utero.
Pyrimethamine	Category C. Probably does not cause birth defects. Administer with folinic acid or folic acid supplementation, especially during first trimester to avoid birth defects.
Pyrvinium pamoate	Category C. No adverse effects reported.
Quinacrine	Category C. May cause fetal malformations with first-trimester use.
Quinidine	Category C. Considered relatively safe for fetus. High doses have oxytocic properties and may cause abortion.
Quinine	Category X. Has caused malformations of limbs, CNS, heart, and GI tract as well as deafness and other abnormalities. Avoid during pregnancy.
Rabies immune globulin	Category B. No adverse effects reported.
Ranitidine	Category B. Not a major teratogen.
Reserpine	Category C. Nasal discharge, cyanosis, hypothermia, lethargy, and anorexia have occurred when used near term.
Ribavirin	Category X. Teratogenic in animals. No abnormalities seen, however, in 1 human exposure reported. Avoid in pregnancy.
Rifampin	Category C. Probably not a teratogen. May cause hemorrhagic disease of newborn; prevent with vitamin K administration.
Ritonavir	Category B. If indicated, do not withhold during pregnancy (with the possible exception of first trimester) because the benefit to HIV-positive mother probably outweighs the unknown risk to the fetus.
Rubella vaccine	Category X. This live virus vaccine should not be used during pregnancy because of risk of congenital rubella syndrome.
Scopolamine	Category C. May cause tachycardia, fever, and lethargy when given to mother during labor.
Secobarbital	Category D. May cause hemorrhagic disease of newborn; prevent with vitamin K administration. May cause withdrawal.
Selegiline	Category C. Limited data. No teratogenesis reported. Avoid, if possible, until more data available.
Selenium sulfide	Category C. No adverse effects reported.
Senna	Category C. No adverse effects reported.
Simethicone	Category C. No adverse effects reported.
Sodium iodide (^{131}I)	Category X. Has caused fetal malformations, damage to fetal thyroid gland, and hypothyroidism.
Sodium polystyrene sulfonate (Kayexalate)	Category C. No adverse effects reported.
Spectinomycin	Category B. No adverse effects reported.
Spironolactone	Category D. No adverse effects reported; however, potential risk of antiandrogenic effects.
Streptokinase	Category C. No adverse effects reported.
Streptomycin	Category D. May cause eighth cranial nerve damage.
Succinylcholine	Category C. Not teratogenic.
Sucralfate	Category B. No adverse effects reported.

Drug or Substance	FDA Fetal Risk Category, Adverse Effects, and Clinical Comments
Sufentanil	Category C (category D for prolonged use or high doses). Not a significant risk. Dose-related depression of fetus and newborn.
Sulfasalazine	Category B (category D when administered near term). May increase risk of kernicterus when given near term.
Sulfonamides	Category C (category D when administered near term). May increase risk of kernicterus when given near term.
Sulindac	Category B; category D if used during last trimester. No congenital anomalies reported. May cause closing of ductus arteriosus in utero, PPHN, and inhibition of labor.
Tacrolimus	Category C. May cause reversible hyperkalemia, renal toxicity, IUGR, and premature delivery.
Tamoxifen	Category D. Avoid during pregnancy because of toxicities reported in animals, increased incidence of abortions, and possible human teratogenicity. Ambiguous genitalia reported in 1 female infant.
Temazepam	Category X. Potential drug interaction between temazepam and diphenhydramine resulted in stillbirth. Avoid this combination.
Terbutaline	Category B. May cause fetal tachycardia and neonatal hypoglycemia.
Tetanus immune globulin	Category B. No adverse effects reported.
Tetanus toxoid	Category C. No adverse effects reported.
Tetracyclines	Category D. Tetracyclines should be avoided during pregnancy because they may cause adverse effects, including yellow staining of teeth, inhibition of bone growth, maternal liver toxicity, and congenital defects.
Thalidomide	Category X. Contraindicated. A potent teratogen involving limbs, skeleton, head, face, eyes, ears, tongue, teeth, CNS, and respiratory, cardiovascular, GU, and GI systems.
Theophylline	Category C. May cause transient tachycardia, irritability, and vomiting at birth, especially if mother's serum concentrations above therapeutic range. No congenital defects reported. Theophylline withdrawal with apneic spells responsive to theophylline therapy reported.
Thiabendazole	Category C. No adverse effects reported, but data limited.
Thiethylperazine	Category C. Do not use during pregnancy because of risk of fetal malformations.
Thioguanine	Category D. May cause fetal malformations and chromosomal abnormalities.
Thioridazine	Category C. Probably safe for use in pregnancy.
Thiotepa	Category D. No adverse effects reported, but data limited.
Thiothixene	Category C. No information available.
Thyroid extract	Category A. Probably safe for use in pregnancy.
Ticarcillin	Category B. No adverse effects reported.
Timolol	Category D. May cause bradycardia and hypotension in infants exposed near term. Carefully monitor blood pressure and heart rate.
Tobacco	Category X. Dose-related risk of low birth weight, decreased placental blood flow, decreased fetal breathing movements, stillbirth, neonatal death, and SIDS.
Tobramycin	Category D. No congenital defects reported. Potentiation of magnesium sulfate-induced neuromuscular weakness. Monitor infant for ototoxicity because this has occurred with other aminoglycosides (eg, kanamycin and streptomycin).
Tolazamide	Category C. May cause prolonged neonatal hypoglycemia when given near term.
Tolazoline	Category C. May cause fetal malformations.
Tolbutamide	Category C. May cause prolonged neonatal hypoglycemia when given near term.
Tolmetin	Category C; category D if given near term. No congenital anomalies reported. May cause closing of ductus arteriosus in utero, PPHN, and inhibition of labor.
Tranylcypromine	Category C. May cause fetal malformations.
Tretinoin	Category D. When used topically, teratogenic risk thought to be minimal.
Triamterene	Category D. No adverse effects reported.
Trifluoperazine	Category C. Probably safe for use in pregnancy.
Trihexyphenidyl	Category C. May cause congenital defects.
Trimeprazine	Category C. Has been associated with congenital defects, but confirmation needed.
Trimethadione	Category D. Causes adverse effects on fetus, including IUGR, mental and physical retardation, impaired hearing, cardiac defects, abnormally set ears, oral clefts, fetal demise, and GU, skeletal, and other abnormalities. Use other, safer anticonvulsants to treat petit mal.
Trimethaphan	Category C. No adverse effects reported.
Trimethobenzamide	Category C. May cause congenital defects and extrapyramidal dysfunction in neonate.

Drug or Substance	FDA Fetal Risk Category, Adverse Effects, and Clinical Comments
Trimethoprim	Category C. Folate antagonist, so there is risk of fetal malformations.
Tripelennamine	Category B. No adverse effects reported.
Urokinase	Category B. No adverse effects reported.
Ursodiol	Category B. No adverse effects reported.
Valproic acid	Category D. Increased risks of neural tube defects and defects of head, face, digits, GU tract, and mental and physical growth.
Vancomycin	Category B. No reports of congenital defects.
Vasopressin	Category B. No fetal malformations reported. May cause uterine contractions (infrequent).
Verapamil	Category C. May cause decreased uterine blood flow, hypotension, and fetal bradycardia.
Vidarabine	Category C. Insufficient data available.
Vincristine	Category D. Congenital defects may occur.
Vitamin A	Category A (category X with doses above RDA). Excessive doses are teratogenic as is marked maternal vitamin A deficiency.
Vitamin B_{12}	Category A. No adverse effects reported.
Vitamin C	Category A. No reports directly link this vitamin to congenital defects in humans. May cause scurvy in infant if used at high doses during pregnancy.
Vitamin D	Category A for RDA dose; category D for therapeutic and higher doses. High doses of vitamin D teratogenic in animals but not in humans. Because vitamin D raises calcium levels, may be associated with supravalvular aortic stenosis syndrome, which is often associated with hypercalcemia of infancy.
Vitamin E	Category A. No adverse effects reported.
Vitamin K	See Phytonadione.
Warfarin	Category X. Significant risk of congenital defects. May cause fetal warfarin syndrome (hypoplastic, flattened nasal bridge; stippled epiphyses; and other features, such as low birth weight, eye defects, development retardation, congenital heart disease, and death). May also cause hemorrhage. If anticoagulation is required during pregnancy, heparin given at lowest effective dose is probably safer choice.
Zidovudine	Category C. Neonatal anemia may occur. No pattern of birth defects found. If indicated, benefits of maternal AZT treatment to the infant outweigh the risks of AZT-induced toxicity.
Zinc sulfate	Category C. No information available. Manufacturer recommends that supplementation not be given during pregnancy.

ACE, angiotensin-converting enzyme; BP, blood pressure; CDC, Centers for Disease Control and Prevention; CMV, cytomegalovirus; CNS, central nervous system; C-section, cesarean section; GI, gastrointestinal; G6PD, glucose-6-phosphate dehydrogenase; GU, genitourinary. IUGR, intrauterine growth retardation; PPHN, persistent pulmonary hypertension of the newborn; RDA, recommended daily allowance; RDS, respiratory distress syndrome; SIDS, sudden infant death syndrome; t-PA, tissue-plasminogen activator.

REFERENCES

Briggs GG et al: *Drugs in Pregnancy and Lactation,* 6th ed. Lippincott Williams & Wilkins, 2002. Manufacturers' product information for medications listed.

Appendices

APPENDIX A. ABBREVIATIONS USED IN NEONATOLOGY

AFP	Alpha-fetoprotein
AGA	Appropriate for gestational age
ARC	AIDS-related complex
ASD	Atrial septal defect
ATN	Acute tubular necrosis
BG	Babygram (x-ray film that includes the chest and abdomen)
BPD	Biparietal diameter; bronchopulmonary dysplasia
BW	Birth weight; body weight
CBG	Capillary blood gases
CDH	Congenital diaphragmatic hernia
CHD	Congenital hip dislocation; congenital heart disease
CHF	Congestive heart failure
CID	Cytomegalovirus inclusion disease
CLD	Chronic lung disease
CPIP	Chronic pulmonary insufficiency of prematurity
CST	Contraction stress test
DDST	Denver Developmental Screening Test
ECMO	Extracorporeal membrane oxygenation
EDC	Estimated date of confinement
ET	Endotracheal tube/enterostomal therapist
FBS	Fasting blood sugar; fetal blood sample
FHR	Fetal heart rate
FHT	Fetal heart tone
GA	Gestational age; general anesthesia
GDM	Gestational diabetes mellitus
$G_xP_xAb_xLC_x$	Shorthand for gravida/para/abortion/living children (subscript variables represent numbers of each)
G_xP_x0000	First zero, full term; second zero, premature; third zero, abortion; fourth zero, living children
HC	Head circumference
HCM	Health care maintenance
HDON	Hemolytic disease of the newborn
HLHS	Hypoplastic left heart syndrome
HMD	Hyaline membrane disease
IDAM	Infant of drug-addicted mother
INF	Intravenous nutritional feedings
IODAM	Infant of drug-addicted mother
IODM	Infant of diabetic mother
ITB	Intrathecal
IUGR	Intrauterine growth retardation
IVH	Intraventricular hemorrhage
LBW	Low birth weight
LBWL	Low birth weight "lytes"
LGA	Large for gestational age
L-S ratio	Lecithin-sphingomyelin ratio
MAS	Meconium aspiration syndrome
MCA	Multiple congenital abnormalities
MCT	Medium-chain triglycerides
MSUD	Maple syrup urine disease
NEC	Necrotizing enterocolitis
NICU	Neonatal intensive care unit
NST	Nonstress test
OCT	Oxytocin challenge test
OFC	Occipital frontal circumference
P&PD	Percussion and postural drainage

PBLC	Premature birth, living child
PDA	Patent ductus arteriosus
PFC	Persistent fetal circulation
PIE	Pulmonary interstitial emphysema
PLAST	Percussion, lavage, suction, turn
PPH	Persistent pulmonary hypertension
PROM	Premature rupture of membranes
RDS	Respiratory distress syndrome
RLF	Retrolental fibroplasia
ROM	Range of motion; rupture of membranes
ROP	Retinopathy of prematurity
RT	Rubella titer
RVH	Right ventricular hypertrophy
Sao_2	Oxygen saturation of arterial blood
SC	Subcutaneous
SEH	Subependymal hemorrhage
SGA	Small for gestational age
SIDS	Sudden infant death syndrome
SVD	Spontaneous vaginal delivery
SVT	Supraventricular tachycardia
TAR	Thrombocytopenia–absent radii (syndrome)
TBLC	Term birth, living child
TD$_x$FLM	TD$_x$ fetal lung maturity
TEF	Tracheoesophageal fistula
THAM	Tris(hydroxymethyl)aminomethane (tromethamine)
THAN	Transient hyperammonemia of the newborn
TOF	Tetralogy of Fallot
TORCH	Toxoplasmosis, other, rubella, cytomegalovirus, herpes simplex
TORCHS	As above plus syphilis
TTN	Transient tachypnea of the newborn
UAC	Umbilical artery catheter
UVC	Umbilical vein catheter
VBG	Venous blood gas
VF	Ventricular fibrillation
VLBW	Very low birth weight
VT	Ventricular tachycardia

APPENDIX B. APGAR SCORING

Apgar scores are a numerical expression of the condition of a newborn infant on a scale of 0–10. The scores are usually recorded at 1 and 5 min after delivery and become a permanent part of the health record. They have clinical usefulness not only during the nursery stay but at later child health visits also, when clinical status at delivery may have a bearing on current diagnostic assessments. The system was originally described by Virginia Apgar, MD, an anesthesiologist, in 1953.

	Score		
Sign	**0**	**1**	**2**
Appearance (color)	Blue or pale	Pink body with blue extremities	Completely pink
Pulse (heart rate)	Absent	Slow (<100 beats/min)	>100 beats/min
Grimace (reflex irritability)	No response	Grimace	Cough or sneeze
Activity (muscle tone)	Limp	Some flexion	Active movement
Respirations	Absent	Slow, irregular	Good, crying

APPENDIX C. BLOOD PRESSURE DETERMINATIONS

Birth weight (g)	Mean pressure	Systolic (mm Hg)	Diastolic (mm Hg)
501–750	38–49	50–62	26–36
751–1000	35.5–47.5	48–59	23–36
1001–1250	37.5–48	49–61	26–35
1251–1500	34.5–44.5	46–56	23–33
1501–1750	34.5–45.5	46–58	23–33
1751–2000	36–48	48–61	24–35

Based on data from Hegyi T et al: Blood pressure ranges in premature infants: 1. The first hours of life. *J Pediatr* 1994;124:627.

APPENDIX D. CEREBROSPINAL FLUID NORMAL VALUES

Variable	Value
Opening pressure	
Newborn	80–110 mm H_2O
Infant	<200 mm H_2O
Glucose	
Premature	24–63 mg/dL (CSF-blood ratio 55–105%)
Term	44–128 mg/dL (CSF-blood ratio 44–128%)
Protein	
Premature	65–150 mg/dL
Term	20–170 mg/dL
White blood cell count	
Premature	0–25 mm^3 (57% PMNs)
Term	0–22/mm^3 (61% PMNs)

CSF, cerebrospinal fluid; PMNs, polymorphonuclear cells.

APPENDIX E. CHARTWORK
ADMISSION HISTORY

A. **Identification (ID).** State the name, age, sex, and weight of the infant. Include whether the patient or mother was transported from another facility or whether the infant was born at home or within the hospital.
  Infant James, a 3-h-old 1800-g white male, is an inborn patient from Baltimore, Maryland.
B. **Chief complaint (CC).** The major problems of the patient are usually listed in the order of severity of disease process or occurrence.
  1. *Respiratory distress syndrome.*
  2. *Suspected neonatal sepsis.*
  3. *Premature birth, living child (PBLC).*
C. **Referring physician.** Include the name, address, and telephone number of the referring physician.
  Dr. Nick Pavona, FSK Medical Center, Baltimore, Maryland (410) 852–8494.
D. **History of present illness (HPI).** The history of the present illness is more helpful if it is divided into four separate paragraphs.
  1. **Initial statement.** This part of the HPI includes the patient's name, gestational age, birth weight, sex, age of the mother, and the number of times she has been pregnant along with the number of living children she has.

2. **Prenatal history.** Discuss the maternal prenatal care and record the number of prenatal clinic visits. Include any medications the mother was taking, any pertinent prenatal tests done, and the results.
3. **Labor and delivery.** Include a detailed history of the labor and delivery: type of delivery, type of anesthesia, any medication used, and any fetal monitoring (including results).
4. **Infant history.** Discuss the initial condition of the infant and the need for resuscitation, and write a detailed description of what occurred. Include the Apgar scores and discuss when the infant became symptomatic or when problems were first noted.

> Infant James is a 1800-g white male delivered to a 19-year-old G_2 now P_2, LC_2 married white female.
> The mother had excellent prenatal care. She had her first prenatal visit at approximately 8 weeks' gestation and then saw her obstetrician routinely. She was on no medications nor has any history of ethanol or cigarette abuse.
> She had rupture of membranes (ROM) at 33 weeks with some mild contractions. At that time, she was seen by her obstetrician, who confirmed the premature rupture of the membranes. She was admitted to the hospital and started on IV ritodrine in an attempt to stop the labor. She was also closely observed for signs of infection. After 4 days of hospitalization, fever developed, with an increase in her white blood cell count. Because of suspicion of chorioamnionitis, ritodrine was stopped and Pitocin was begun to induce labor. Ampicillin and gentamicin were started after cervical cultures were obtained; results are pending. External fetal monitoring had been normal until 4 h after the Pitocin induction, at which time it showed late decelerations. At this point, an emergency cesarean section was performed. General anesthesia was used, and the infant was delivered within 6 min.
> The infant was delivered depressed at birth, with 1-min Apgar of 4. He required bag-mask ventilation with 100% oxygen. No medications were needed. The 5-min Apgar was 7. The infant appeared poorly perfused and had poor color without oxygen. He was stabilized and transported on 100% oxygen to the NICU.

E. **Family history (FH).** The family history should include any previous complicated births and their history, miscarriages, neonatal deaths, or premature births. Also include any major family medical problems (eg, hemophilia, sickle cell disease).

> Ms. James had 1 prior uncomplicated vaginal delivery that went to term. There is a history of myelodysplasia in infant James' maternal first cousin.

F. **Social history (SH).** In the social history, include a brief statement discussing the parent's age, marital status, siblings, occupation, and where they are from.

> The parents are separated and both live in Baltimore. Mother is a 19-year-old factory worker and cares for their 2-year-old daughter; the father is 24 and works as a custodial engineer.

G. **Laboratory data.** List the admission laboratory and radiology results.
H. **Assessment.** State your evaluation of the infant's problems. It can include a list of suspected and potential problems as well as a differential diagnosis.

> 1. Respiratory distress syndrome: Because the infant is premature, hyaline membrane disease must be considered. Pneumonia is also a likely cause because of the maternal history of suspected chorioamnionitis.
> 2. Suspected neonatal sepsis: Because of the high suspicion of chorioamnionitis and the premature onset of labor, there is an increased septic risk in this infant. Certain pathogens need to be ruled out. Group B streptococcus is the most common pathogen in this age group, but Listeria monocytogenes and gram-negative pathogens should be considered.

3. *Premature birth, living child: The infant is at 33 weeks' gestation by Ballard examination.*
I. **Plan.** Include the therapeutic and diagnostic plans for the infant. (See section on "Admission Orders," below.)

PROGRESS NOTES

The most commonly used format for daily progress notes is the *SOAP* method. *SOAP* is an acronym in which *S* = subjective, *O* = objective, *A* = assessment, and *P* = plan. Each problem should be discussed in this format. First, state the problems you are to discuss in the order of severity or occurrence and assign a number to them. Then discuss each problem in the *SOAP* format as outlined next.

A. **Subjective (S).** Include an overall subjective view of the patient by the physician.
B. **Objective (O).** Include data that can be objectively gathered, usually in three areas:
   1. **Vital signs (temperature, respiratory rate, pulse, blood pressure).**
   2. **Pertinent physical examination.**
   3. **Laboratory data and other test results.**
C. **Assessment (A).** Include evaluation of the above data.
D. **Plan (P).** Discuss the medication changes, laboratory orders, and any other new orders as well as the treatment plan.
E. **Example.** The following is an example of part of a progress note using the *SOAP* format.
   Problem 1. Respiratory distress syndrome
   Problem 2. Suspected neonatal sepsis
   Problem 3. Premature birth, living child (PBLC)

   Problem 1. Respiratory distress syndrome
   S: Infant James is now 4 days old and doing much better. He has been able to wean down to 30% oxygen with good arterial gases.
   O: Vital signs: temperature 98.7, respirations 52, pulse 140, blood pressure 55/35.
   Physical examination: The peripheral perfusion appears good with no obvious cyanosis. There is no grunting or nasal flaring, but the infant has mild substernal and intercostal retractions. The chest sounds slightly wet.
   Laboratory data and other test results: Arterial blood gases on 30% oxygen—pH 7.32, CO_2 48, O_2 67, 97% saturation. Chest x-ray shows mild haziness in both lung fields.
   A: Infant James has resolving mild hyaline membrane disease.
   P: The plan is to wean the oxygen as long as his arterial Pao_2 is greater than 55.

ADMISSION ORDERS

The following format is useful for writing admission orders. It involves the mnemonic *A.D.C. VAN DISSEL*. This stands for *A*dmit, *D*iagnosis, *C*ondition, *V*ital signs, *A*ctivity, *N*ursing procedures, *D*iet, *I*nput and Output, *S*pecific drugs, *S*ymptomatic drugs, *E*xtras, and *L*aboratory data.

A. **Admit.** Specify the location of the patient (neonatal intensive care unit, newborn nursery) and the attending physician in charge and the house officer along with their paging numbers.
B. **Diagnosis.** List the admitting diagnoses.
   1. *Respiratory distress syndrome.*
   2. *Suspected neonatal sepsis.*
   3. *Premature birth, living child.*

C. **Condition.** Note whether the patient is in stable or critical condition.

D. **Vital signs.** State the desired frequency of monitoring of vital signs. Specify rectal or axillary temperature. Rectal temperature is usually done initially to obtain a core temperature and also to rule out imperforate anus. Then, monitor axillary temperature. Other parameters include blood pressure, pulse, respiratory rate. Weight, length, and head circumference should also be obtained on admission.

E. **Activity.** All are at bed rest but one can specify "minimal stress or hands-off protocol" here. This notation is used for infants who react poorly to stress by dropping their oxygenation, as in patients with persistent pulmonary hypertension. At most centers, it means to handle the infant as little as possible and record all vital signs off the monitor.

F. **Nursing procedure.** Respiratory care (ventilator settings, chest percussion and postural drainage orders, endotracheal suctioning with frequency). Also require that a daily weight and head circumference be recorded. The frequency of Dextrostix (or Chemstrip-bG) testing is included in this section because it is a bedside procedure.

G. **Diet.** All infants admitted to the neonatal intensive care unit are usually made NPO (nothing by mouth) for at least 6–24 h until they are accessed and stabilized. When appropriate, write specific diet orders.

H. **Input and output (I and O).** Request that the nursing staff record accurate input and output of each infant. This record is especially important for infants on intravenous fluids and those just starting oral feedings. Specify how often you want the urine tested for specific gravity and glucose.

I. **Specific drugs.** State drugs to be administered, giving specific dosages and routes of administration. It is useful to also include the milligrams-per-kilogram-per-day dose of the drug to allow cross-checking and verification of the dose ordered. An example is as follows:

Ampicillin 150 mg IV q12h (300 mg/kg/d divided q12h).

For all infants, order the following medications at the time of admission.

1. Vitamin K (see Chapter 80) is given to prevent hemorrhagic disease of the newborn.
2. Erythromycin eyedrops (see Chapter 80) are given to prevent gonococcal ophthalmia.

J. **Symptomatic drugs.** These drugs are not routinely used in a neonatal intensive care unit and would include such items as pain and sleep medications.

K. **Extras.** Any other orders required but not included above, such as roentgenography, electrocardiography, and ultrasonography.

L. **Laboratory data.** Include laboratory data drawn on admission, plus routine laboratory orders with frequency (eg, arterial blood gases q2h, sodium and potassium bid).

DISCHARGE SUMMARY

The following information is written at the time of discharge and provides a summary of the infant's illness and hospital stay.

A. **Date of admission.**

B. **Date of discharge.**

C. **Admitting diagnosis.**

D. **Discharge diagnosis.** List in order of occurrence or severity.

E. **Attending physician and service caring for the patient.**

F. **Referring physician and address.**

G. **Procedures.** Include all invasive procedures.

H. **Brief history, physical examination, and laboratory data on admission.** Use the admission history, physical examination, and laboratory data as a guide.

I. **Hospital course.** The easiest way to approach this section of the discharge summary is to discuss each problem in paragraph form.

J. **Condition at discharge.** A complete physical examination is done at the time of discharge and is included in this section. It is important to include the discharge weight, head circumference, and length so that growth can be assessed at the time of the patient's initial checkup. Also include the type and amount of formula the patient is on and any pertinent discharge laboratory values.

K. **Discharge medications.** Include the name(s) of medication(s), the dosage(s), and length of treatment. If the patient is being sent home on an apnea monitor, it is helpful to include the monitor settings and the planned course of treatment.

L. **Disposition.** Note where the patient is being sent (outside hospital, home, foster home).

M. **Discharge instructions and follow-up.** Include instructions to the parents on medications and when the patient is to return to the clinic (and exact location). It is helpful to indicate tests that need to be done on follow-up and any results that need to be rechecked (eg, bilirubin, repeat phenylketonuria screen).

N. **Problem list.** Same list as the discharge diagnosis list.

APPENDIX F. GROWTH CHARTS

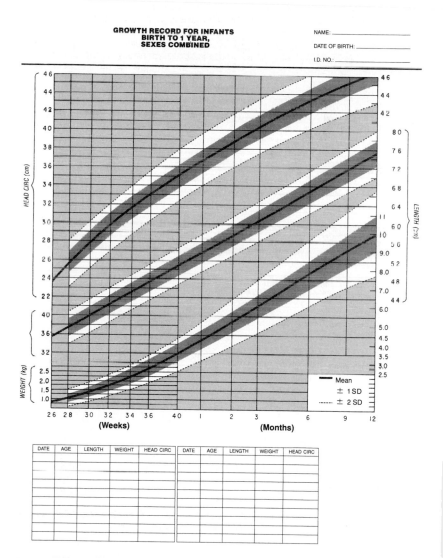

APPENDIX FIGURE F–1. Growth charts for infants. *(Adapted with permission: Babson SG, Benda GI: Growth graphs for the clinical assessment of infants of varying gestational age. J Pediatr 1976;89:814.)*

GIRLS: BIRTH TO 36 MONTHS
CDC US GROWTH CHARTS   Name _____ Record #_____

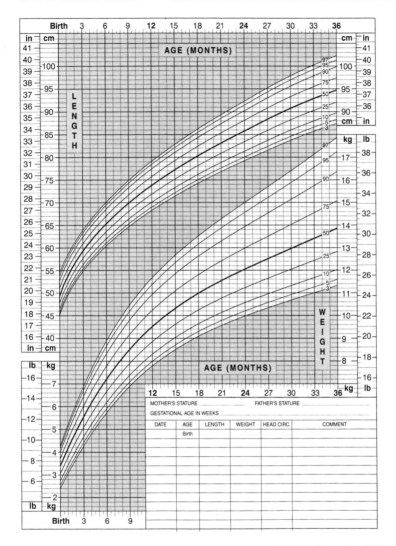

APPENDIX FIGURE F–2. Growth chart for girls: weight and length, birth to 36 months. NCHS, National Center for Health Statistics. *(Reprinted with the permission of Abbott Laboratories.)*

GIRLS: BIRTH TO 36 MONTHS
CDC US GROWTH CHARTS   Name _____ Record #_____

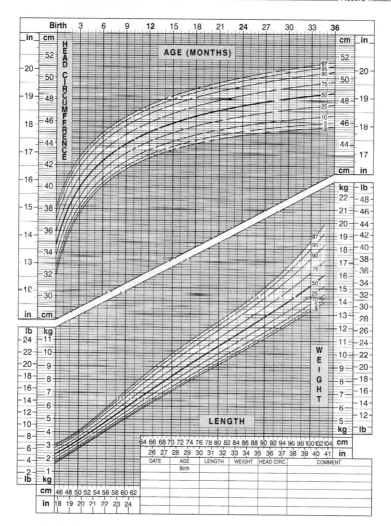

APPENDIX FIGURE F–3. Growth chart for girls: head circumference and weight, birth to 36 months. NCHS, National Center for Health Statistics. *(Reprinted with the permission of Abbott Laboratories.)*

BOYS: BIRTH TO 36 MONTHS
CDC US GROWTH CHARTS   Name _____ Record #_____

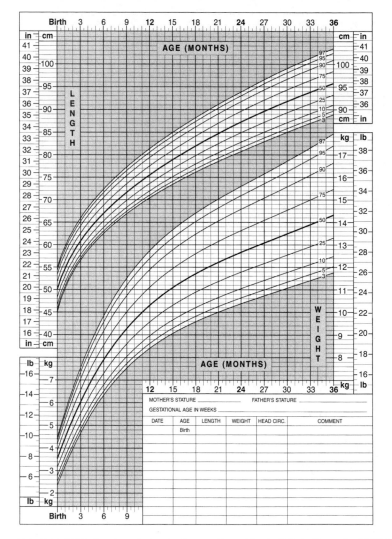

APPENDIX FIGURE F–4. Growth chart for boys: weight and length, birth to 36 months. NCHS, National Center for Health Statistics. *(Reprinted with the permission of Ross Laboratories.)*

BOYS: BIRTH TO 36 MONTHS
CDC US GROWTH CHARTS   Name _____ Record #_____

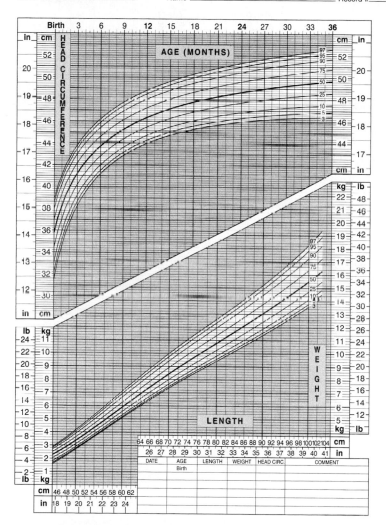

APPENDIX FIGURE F–5. Growth chart for boys: head circumference and weight, birth to 36 months. NCHS, National Center for Health Statistics. *(Reprinted with the permission of Ross Laboratories.)*

APPENDIX G. ISOLATION GUIDELINES[a]

Infection/disease	Maternal precautions	Neonatal precautions	Room-in	Mother may visit in nursery	Breast-feeding	Additional considerations
AIDS/HIV-positive		Bathe infant as soon as possible	Yes	Yes	No; HIV may be transmitted through breast milk	TB testing recommended for mothers. Report AIDS to Health Department.
Chickenpox (see varicella)						
Chlamydia trachomatis			Yes	Yes	Yes	Prophylactic use of topical erythromycin at birth prevents inclusion conjunctivitis.
Cytomegalovirus		Careful hand-washing after contact with urine or secretions	Yes	Yes	Yes	
Diarrhea			Yes	Yes	Yes	Report clusters of diarrhea to Health Department.
Gonococcal ophthalmia neonatorum			Yes, after 24 h of maternal treatment with antibiotics	Yes, after 24 h of maternal treatment with antibiotics	Yes, after 24 h of maternal treatment with antibiotics	
Hepatitis A, B, and C			Yes	Yes	Yes	Report hepatitis to Health Department. Vertical transmission from mother to newborn is rare; consider use of immune globulin.

Disease	Precautions					Comments
Herpes simplex virus Genital (mother with primary, recurrent active, or recurrent inactive herpes)			Yes	Yes	Yes	Avoid scalp monitors if possible for infants of women suspected of having genital herpes.[b]
Neonatal infection or positive culture in the absence of disease			No	No	Yes	Cultures from lesion or conjunctiva, oral pharynx, or skin 48 h or later after birth more likely to identify neonatal infection. A positive culture obtained >24 h after birth requires immediate antiviral treatment, even in absence of symptoms.[b]
Lice (see pediculosis)						
Measles (rubeola)	Labor, delivery, and postpartum recovery in private room. Wear mask if susceptible. Airborne precautions.	Private room. Wear mask in close contact	No	No	Not until mother judged to be noncontagious	Contagious during prodrome and up to 4 days of rash illness. Report rubeola to Health Department.
Mumps (infectious parotiditis)	Private room. Wear mask if susceptible. Droplet precautions.		No	No	Not until mother judged to be noncontagious	Contagious for 9 days after onset of swelling. Report mumps to Health Department.

(continued)

APPENDIX G. ISOLATION GUIDELINES[a] *(continued)*

Infection/disease	Maternal precautions	Neonatal precautions	Room-in	Mother may visit in nursery	Breast-feeding	Additional considerations
Pediculosis (lice)			Yes	Yes	Yes; instruct mother in cleaning breasts before feeding if medication applied in that area; stress good hand-washing.	Contacts should be examined and treated if infected.
Pertussis (whooping cough)	Private room. Wear mask within 3 ft. Droplet precautions.	Private room. Wear mask in close proximity.	No	No	Not until mother judged to be noncontagious	Contagious for 7 days after start of effective therapy. Report pertussis to Health Department.
Respiratory syncytial virus in infants		Transfer to ICU or pediatric ward. Droplet precautions.	Yes	Yes	Yes	
Rubella (German measles) Maternal	Private room. Wear mask if susceptible. Droplet precautions.	Wear mask.	Yes	No	No	Isolate for 7 days after onset of rash. Those who have had rubella do not need to wear mask. Susceptible persons stay out of room, if possible. Report rubella to Health Department.

Disease					Comments
Congenital		Yes	Yes	Yes	Continue universal body substance precautions until 1 year of age unless nasopharyngeal and urine cultures after 3 months of age are negative for rubella irus. Susceptible vpersons stay out of room if possible. Report rubella to Health Department.
				Yes	Treatment of household contact is recommended.
Scabies	Yes	Yes	Yes		Stress good handwashing. Instruct mother in cleaning breasts before feeding if medication applied in that area.
					Contact precautions for 24 h after treatment.
Staphylococcus aureus		No	Yes	Yes	Two or more concurrent S. aureus cases of impetigo related to a nursery or single case of breast abscess in a nursing mother or infant is presumptive evidence of an epidemic. Report immediately to attending physician and Infection Control Department.

(continued)

APPENDIX G. ISOLATION GUIDELINES[a] (continued)

Infection/disease	Maternal precautions	Neonatal precautions	Room-in	Mother may visit in nursery	Breast-feeding	Additional considerations
Streptococcus, group B			Yes	Yes	Yes	Refer to guidelines for preventing group B strep infection.[c]
Syphilis			Yes, after 24 h of treatment with antibiotics	Yes, after 24 h of treatment with antibiotics	Yes, after 24 h of treatment with antibiotics	Report syphilis to Health Department.
TB						Report TB to Health Department.
1. Mother with positive PPD and no evidence of current disease			Yes	Yes	Yes	Infant should be tested: at 4–6 weeks of age, 3–4 months, and 12 months of age.
2. Mother with untreated (newly diagnosed) minimal disease, or if treated for 2 or more weeks and is judged by pulmonary or ID to be noncontagious at delivery				Yes	Yes	Infant should have CXR and PPD at 4–6 weeks of age; if negative, retest at 3–4 and 6 months.
3. Mother with current pulmonary TB, suspected of being contagious at time of delivery	Labor and delivery and postpartum care in private room (negative-pressure, nonrecirculating air). Keep door closed. Mask required at all times. Airborne precautions.		No contact until mother judged to be noncontagious	No contact until mother judged to be noncontagious	No contact until mother judged to be noncontagious	Infant should be given INH until 6 months of age, then repeat PPD. If PPD is positive, continue INH for a total of 12 months.

4. Mother has extra-pulmonary spread of TB (eg, miliary, bone, or meningitis)		No contact until mother judged to be noncontagious	No contact until mother judged to be noncontagious	No contact until mother judged to be noncontagious	Infant should be given INH until 6 months of age, then repeat PPD. If PPD is positive, continue INH for 12 months.
Varicella (chickenpox) or herpes zoster in immunocompromised patient or if disseminated Maternal/neonatal	Labor and delivery postpartum care in private room with negative-pressure, non-recirculating air. Keep door closed. Gown, mask, and gloves required. Continue precautions until all lesions crusted. Airborne and contact precautions if susceptible.	Private room with negative-pressure nonrecirculating air. Gown, mask, and gloves required. If they must be hospitalized beyond 10 days of age, continue precautions until 21 days of age. If VZIG given, keep on precautions until 28 days after exposure.	Yes, after mother's lesions have crusted	Yes, after mother's lesions have crusted	May be contagious 1–2 days before the onset of rash. Persons who have had chickenpox do not need to wear mask. Hospitalized patients should be discharged before day 10 after exposure, if possible. Exposed susceptible patients should be placed on precautions beginning 10 days after exposure and continuing until 21 days after last exposure, or until 28 days if VZIG given.

CXR, chest x-ray film; ID, Infectious Diseases Department; INH, isoniazid; PPD, purified protein derivative; TB, tuberculosis; VZIG, varicella-zoster immune globulin.

[a]These are generally accepted guidelines. Individual institutions may have additional recommendations.

[b]See Brown ZA et al: Preventing vertical transmission of herpes simplex. *Contemp OB/GYN* 1995;40:27.

[c]See *Contemp OB/GYN* 1996;41; *Morb Mortal Wkly Rep* 1996;45(RR 7).

Modified from guidelines issued by Kaiser Permanente Hospital, Fontana, CA.

APPENDIX H. TEMPERATURE CONVERSION TABLE

Celsius	Fahrenheit	Celsius	Fahrenheit
34.0	93.2	37.6	99.6
34.2	93.6	37.8	100.0
34.4	93.9	38.0	100.4
34.6	94.3	38.2	100.7
34.8	94.6	38.4	101.1
35.0	95.0	38.6	101.4
35.2	95.4	38.8	101.8
35.4	95.7	39.0	102.2
35.6	96.1	39.2	102.5
35.8	96.4	39.4	102.9
36.0	96.8	39.6	103.2
36.2	97.1	39.8	103.6
36.4	97.5	40.0	104.0
36.6	97.8	40.2	104.3
36.8	98.2	40.4	104.7
37.0	98.6	40.6	105.1
37.2	98.9	40.8	105.4
37.4	99.3	41.0	105.8

Celsius = (Fahrenheit − 32) × 5/9.
Fahrenheit = (Celsius × 9/5) + 32.

APPENDIX I. WEIGHT CONVERSION TABLE[a]

Ounces	1 lb	2 lb	3 lb	4 lb	5 lb	6 lb	7 lb	8 lb
				Grams				
0	454	907	1361	1814	2268	2722	3175	3629
1	482	936	1389	1843	2296	2750	3204	3657
2	510	964	1418	1871	2325	2778	3232	3686
3	539	992	1446	1899	2353	2807	3260	3714
4	567	1021	1474	1928	2381	2835	3289	3742
5	595	1049	1503	1956	2410	2863	3317	3771
6	624	1077	1531	1985	2438	2892	3345	3799
7	652	1106	1559	2013	2466	2920	3374	3827
8	680	1134	1588	2041	2495	2948	3402	3856
9	709	1162	1616	2070	2523	2977	3430	3884
10	737	1191	1644	2098	2552	3005	3459	3912
11	765	1219	1673	2126	2580	3033	3487	3941
12	794	1247	1701	2155	2608	3062	3515	3969
13	822	1276	1729	2183	2637	3090	3544	3997
14	851	1304	1758	2211	2665	3119	3572	4026
15	879	1332	1786	2240	2693	3147	3600	4054

To convert from kilograms to pounds, multiply kilograms by 2.2.
To convert from pounds to grams, multiply pounds by 454.
[a]Values represent weight in grams.

Index

Note: Page numbers followed by *t* denote tabular material. Major discussions are in boldface type. When a drug trade name is listed, the reader is referred to the generic name.